CLINICAL APPLICATION
OF
MECHANICAL VENTILATION

David W. Chang

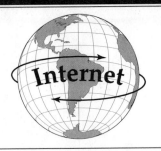

CLINICAL APPLICATION
OF
MECHANICAL VENTILATION

SECOND EDITION

David W. Chang, Ed.D., R.R.T.
Director of Clinical Education
Respiratory Therapy
Athens Technical College
Athens, Georgia

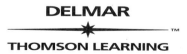

Africa • Australia • Canada • Denmark • Japan • Mexico • New Zealand • Philippines
Puerto Rico • Singapore • Spain • United Kingdom • United States

NOTICE TO THE READER

Delmar Staff:
Business Unit Director: William Brottmiller
Acquisitions Editor: Candice Janco
Development Editor: Deb Flis
Editorial Assistant: Elizabeth O'Keefe
Executive Marketing Manager: Cathy L. Esperti
Channel Manager: Tara Carter
Executive Production Manager: Karen Leet
Project Editor: Elizabeth B. Keller
Production Coordinator: Barbara a. Bullock
Art/Design Coordinator: Rich Killar
Cover Design: Bill Finnerty

Printed in the United States of America
1 2 3 4 5 6 7 8 9 10 XXX 05 04 03 02 01 00

For more information, contact Delmar, 3 Columbia Circle, PO Box 15015, Albany, NY 12212–0515; or find us on the World Wide Web at http://www.delmar.com

Asia
Thomson Learning
60 Albert Street, #15-01
Albert Complex
Singapore 189969
Tel: 65 336 6411
Fax: 65 336 7411

Japan
Thomson Learning
Palaceside Building 5F
1-1-1 Hitotsubashi, Chiyoda-ku
Tokyo 100 0003 Japan
Tel: 813 5218 6544
Fax: 813 5218 6551

Australia/New Zealand
Nelson/Thomson Learning
102 Dodds Street
South Melbourne, Victoria 3205
Australia
Tel: 61 39 685 4111
Fax: 61 39 685 4199

UK/Europe/Middle East
Thomson Learning
Berkshire House
168–173 High Holborn
London
WC1V7AA United Kingdom
Tel: 44 171 497 1422
Fax: 44 171 497 1426

Thomas Nelson & Sons LTD
Nelson House
Mayfield Road
Walton-on-Thames
KT 12 5PL United Kingdom
Tel: 44 1932 2522111
Fax: 44 1932 246574

Latin America
Thomson Learning
Seneca, 53
Colonia Polanco
11560 Mexico D.F. Mexico
Tel: 525-281-2906
Fax: 525-281-2656

South Africa
Thomson Learning
Zonnebloem Building
Constantia Square
526 Sixteenth Road
P.O. Box 2459
Halfway House, 1685
South Africa
Tel: 27 11 805 4819
Fax: 27 11 805 3648

Canada
Nelson/Thomson Learning
1120 Birchmount Road
Scarborough, Ontario
Canada M1K 5G4
Tel: 416-752-9100
Fax: 416-752-8102

Spain
Thomson Learning
Calle Magallanes, 25
28015-MADRID
ESPANA
Tel: 34 91 446 33 50
Fax: 34 91 445 62 18

International Headquarters
Thomson Learning
International Division
290 Harbor Drive, 2nd Floor
Stamford, CT 06902-7477
Tel: 203-969-8700
Fax: 203-969-8751

Library of Congress Cataloging-in-Publication Data

ISBN 0-7668-1375-4

Dedicated to

my wife, Bonnie

and our children, Michelle, Jennifer, and Michael

with love

CONTENTS

FOREWORD

Mechanical ventilation has been a cornerstone of intensive care medicine for over half a century. Indeed, the modern mechanical ventilator is capable of supplying a wide range of breath delivery patterns, airway pressures, patient interactive features, and breathing gas mixtures (e.g., supplemental oxygen, anesthetic gases, heliox and nitric oxide).

The goals of mechanical ventilation have changed in recent years. Initially, mechanical ventilation goals were simply to "normalize" the arterial blood gases by providing large tidal volumes and breathing frequencies in the physiologic range. Oxygen supplementation and positive expiratory pressure were later added to improve the ability of these devices to achieve these gas exchange goals. By the middle of the twentieth century, however, clinicians began to realize that mechanical ventilation could also injure the lungs. For instance, pneumothorax and other forms of extraalveolar air were noted to be linked to ventilator strategies that overdistended the lungs. Later came data showing that high oxygen concentrations also could injure patients. Finally, by the end of the twentieth century, it became apparent that even modest lung overdistention could produce lung injury and could also release cytokines into the systemic circulation to injure other organs. The term "biotrauma" was thus added to the term "barotrauma" to describe ventilator induced lung injury (VILI). Other complications of mechanical ventilation were also recognized and included impaired cardiac filling from high intrathoracic pressures, imposed breathing loads from insensitive/unresponsive assist systems, and infection risk associated with prolonged placement of an artificial airway.

The goals of mechanical ventilation now are to provide "lung protective" strategies that minimize distention, even if gas exchange is not "normalized." Such terms as "permissive" hypercapnia and hypoxemia have emerged to describe this shift in focus. In addition, more sensitive/responsive assist systems (to reduce sedation needs) and more aggressive "weaning" strategies have been developed in an effort to get patients off the ventilator as quickly as possible. Further, non-invasive systems have been developed in an effort to both avoid endotracheal intubation in impending respiratory failure as well as facilitate removal in recovering respiratory failure.

The first edition of Dr. Chang's book brought cohesiveness to the many clinical tradeoffs that must be made as clinicians try to balance the risks and benefits of mechanical ventilation. This second edition is an important update of these concepts. New design features for mechanical ventilators are reviewed. These are particularly important in these cost-conscious times. Mechanical ventilation strategies and the various tradeoffs required during total support, partial support (weaning), and long-term support (home and subacute) are reviewed. New case studies and self-assessment questions supplement the text appropriately. Because of all these features, this second edition is a welcome addition to the clinical literature and should help guide clinicians through the multiple tradeoffs that must be considered in delivering optimal mechanical ventilation.

Neil R. MacIntyre, M.D.

PREFACE

Since the beginning of mechanical ventilation, the design of ventilators and the techniques used to provide ventilation have undergone distinct and drastic changes. For example, it is now a common practice to ventilate patients in their homes using traditional ventilators with special designs as well as using simpler devices to provide noninvasive positive pressure ventilation. From these new innovations in equipment and clinical practice, we are capable of using different strategies of ventilation to meet different patient needs.

ORGANIZATION OF TEXT

Chapters 1 and 2 provide a review of the physiologic basis, rationale, and effects of positive pressure ventilation. Chapter 3 covers the common terminology in ventilator mechanics and the system used to classify mechanical ventilators. Chapter 4 describes the different operating modes of mechanical ventilation. Chapter 5 is a new chapter on temporary airways.

Chapter 6 provides a useful guide in the procedure of airway management—from intubation to extubation. Chapter 7 is a new chapter on noninvasive positive pressure ventilation.

Chapter 8 gives a step-by-step approach in the initiation of mechanical ventilation. The indications, contraindications, initial ventilator settings, and alarm settings relating to mechanical ventilation are also included. Chapter 9 outlines the essential methods of patient monitoring. Vital signs, chest auscultation, pulse oximetry, and capnography are also covered. Chapter 10 covers the basics of hemodynamic monitoring. Normal and abnormal hemodynamic values are also covered. Chapter 11 is a new chapter on basic ventilator waveform analysis.

Chapter 12 presents the common and basic strategies to improve ventilation and oxygenation. It describes the basic strategies to correct common ventilator alarms, and to recognize problems associated with fluid imbalance, electrolyte abnormalities, and nutritional concerns that may occur during mechanical ventilation. Chapter 13 summarizes the use of pharmacotherapy during mechanical ventilation. The drugs discussed in this chapter include bronchodilators, neuromuscular blocking agents, sedatives, narcotic analgesics, and barbiturates. Chapter 14 provides the weaning protocols. Weaning criteria, weaning indices, weaning failure, and terminal weaning are also included.

Chapter 15 covers neonatal mechanical ventilation. The unique characteristics of neonates make this chapter valuable to those respiratory care practitioners caring for "tiny patients." In a nontraditional setting, home mechanical ventilation is discussed in Chapter 16. This chapter provides a list of learning objectives that may be used as a working framework for those who use mechanical ventilator in this "primitive" and restrictive environment. Chapter 17 has a total of 15 case studies including four new cases.

The key terms are boldface within the text and appear in the margin along with definitions to provide a quick reference. Essential information is also highlighted in the margin and can be identified with the icon (☑).

CHANGES TO THE SECOND EDITION

This second edition provides updated coverage of the clinical application of mechanical ventilation. Three new chapters have been added: Chapter 5 Temporary Airways for Ventilation, Chapter 7 Noninvasive Positive Pressure Ventilation, and Chapter 11 Basic Ventilator Waveform Analysis. Four new case studies have also been added in Chapter 17 to enhance the clinical application of mechanical ventilation.

Chapter 5 Temporary Airways for Ventilation covers the design and application of temporary airways that may precede the use of endotracheal tubes. These temporary airways include esophageal obturator airway (EOA), esophageal gastric tube airway (EGTA), laryngeal mask airway (LMA) and pharyngealtracheal lumen airway (PTLA). Since they are used in many nontraditional settings (e.g., patient transport, emergency room, operating and recovery room), respiratory therapy students should find it helpful in becoming familiar with these temporary airways.

Chapter 7 Noninvasive Positive Pressure Ventilation provides coverage in the use of continuous positive airway pressure (CPAP) and bilevel positive airway pressure (bilevel PAP). In conjunction with these techniques of ventilation, the interfaces (e.g., nasal mask, facial mask, nasal pillows) are also covered in this chapter.

Chapter 11 Basic Ventilator Waveform Analysis provides the reader a practical look at the waveforms in mechanical ventilation. Many illustrations are used to show the normal and abnormal waveforms that are common in clinical practice.

Four new case studies (COPD, Guillain Barre Syndrome, Botulism, and Home Care and Case Management) have been added to Chapter 17 to enhance the understanding and use of mechanical ventilation under different clinical settings and patient conditions.

Like the first edition, the goal of this edition of Clinical Application of Mechanical Ventilation is to provide the reader with a textbook they will enjoy reading and using at school and at home. It is my hope that respiratory care practitioners and other health care professionals will also find this textbook a useful source of information for their clinical practice.

David W. Chang

ACKNOWLEDGMENTS

I am very grateful to my colleagues for writing the chapters and case studies in areas that are beyond my expertise. These include Frank Dennison (Chapter 11 Basic Ventilator Waveform Analysis), Wayne Lawson (Case Study 1: COPD), Paul Eberle (Case Study 11: Guillain Barre Syndrome and Case Study 12: Botulism), and Angela Roberts (Case Study 15: Home Care and Case Management). A comprehensive textbook in mechanical ventilation would not have been possible without their sincere commitment and tireless efforts.

My sincere thanks go to my colleagues who reviewed drafts and chapters of the manuscript. They pointed out areas in the first edition needing clarification and provided useful comments for this new edition. Their suggestions made this book more organized as a textbook and more complete as a reference source for clinical practice. A big thank you goes to my colleague Terry LeGrand for her effort in reviewing and making corrections to the manuscripts for the textbook, workbook, and Instructor's Manual.

Other reviewers include:

Ann Allen, RRT
Clinical Coordinator, Respiratory Care
Health Science Department
Piedmont Technical College
Greenwood, South Carolina

Allen W. Barbaro, MS, RRT
Program Director, Respiratory Care
Collin County Community College
McKinney, Texas

Sidney L. Coffin, MS, RRT
Respiratory Care Instructor
California Paramedical and Technical
   College
Riverside, California

Terry S. LeGrand, PhD, RRT
School of Allied Health Sciences
Department of Respiratory Care
The University of Texas Health
   Science Center at San Antonio
San Antonio, Texas

Carol J. Miller, EdD, RRT
Chair, Department of Cardiorespiratory
   Tech
Miami-Dade Community College
Miami, Florida

For clerical and copying assistance, I want to acknowledge our secretary Ms. Rita Snell for her help on this project. Like everything else that she does, her work has always been timely and accurate.

Publishing a textbook without editors and production team members is like producing a movie without directors, producers, and stage crew members. For their efforts in guiding this revision from beginning to end, my gratitude goes to Doris Smith, Deb Flis, Elizabeth Keller, Richard Killar, and Barb Bullock of Delmar Publishers and the staff of Publishers' Design and Production Services, Inc.

David W. Chang

CONTRIBUTORS

Valerie Thomas Aston, R.R.T.
Weber State University
Ogden, Utah

Walter C. Chop, M.S., R.R.T.
Southern Maine Technical College
South Portland, Maine

Frank Dennison, M.Ed., R.R.T., R.P.F.T.
Medical College of Georgia
Augusta, Georgia

Paul G. Eberle, Ph.D., R.R.T.
Weber State University
Ogden, Utah

Sandra Gaviola, R.R.T.
Greater Johnstown Career and
    Technology Center
Johnstown, Pennsylvania

Luis S. Gonzalez III, Pharm. D., B.C.P.S.
Conemaugh Memorial Hospital
Duquesne University
University of Pittsburg
Johnstown, Pennsylvania

Gary Hamelin, M.S., R.R.T.
Southern Maine Technical College
South Portland, Maine

James H. Hiers, M.Ed., R.R.T.
Columbus State University
Columbus, Georgia

Wayne Lawson, M.S., R.R.T.
University of Texas
Health Science Center at San Antonio
San Antonio, Texas

Terry S. LeGrand, Ph.D., R.R.T.
University of Texas
Health Science Center at San Antonio
San Antonio, Texas

Michell Oki, R.R.T., R.P.F.T.
Weber State University
Ogden, Utah

Angie Roberts, R.R.T.
Columbus State University
Columbus, Georgia

Randon K. Parker, B.S., R.R.T.
Weber State University
Ogden, Utah

Kent B. Whitaker, M.Ed., R.R.T.
formerly of Weber State University
Ogden, Utah

Gary C. White, M.Ed., R.R.T., C.P.F.T.
Spokane Community College
Spokane, Washington

CHAPTER ONE

PRINCIPLES OF MECHANICAL VENTILATION

David W. Chang

OUTLINE

KEY TERMS

- alveolar deadspace
- alveolar volume
- anatomic deadspace
- airway resistance
- deadspace ventilation
- diffusion defect
- hypoventilation
- hypoxic hypoxia
- intrapulmonary shunting
- lung compliance
- oxygenation failure
- peak airway pressure
- physiologic deadspace
- plateau pressure
- refractory hypoxemia
- V/Q mismatch
- ventilatory failure

INTRODUCTION

Mechanical ventilation is a useful modality for patients who are unable to sustain the level of ventilation necessary to maintain the gas exchange functions (oxygenation and carbon dioxide elimination). Indications for mechanical ventilation vary greatly among patients. Mechanical ventilation may be indicated in conditions due to physiologic changes (e.g., deterioration of lung parenchyma), disease states (e.g., chest trauma), medical/surgical procedures (e.g., postoperative recovery), as well as many other conditions leading to ventilatory failure or oxygenation failure.

Use of mechanical ventilation also varies greatly from short term to long term and from acute care in the hospital to extended care at home. One of the most frequent uses of mechanical ventilation is for the management of postoperative patients recovering from anesthesia and medications. In one study, postoperative procedures accounted for 35% of all patients who were placed on mechanical ventilation for more than 24 hours. Other major uses of mechanical ventilation include respiratory failure with multisystem failure, preexisting lung disease, trauma, uncomplicated acute lung injuries, and other severe medical problems (Gillespie et al., 1986).

Regardless of the diagnosis or disease state, patients who require mechanical ventilation generally have developed ventilatory failure, oxygenation failure, or both. Specifically, when a patient fails to ventilate or oxygenate adequately, the problem may be caused by one of six pathophysiological factors: (1) increased airway resistance, (2) changes in lung compliance, (3) hypoventilation, (4) V/Q mismatch, (5) intrapulmonary shunting, and (6) diffusion defect.

AIRWAY RESISTANCE

Airway resistance is defined as air flow obstruction in the airways. In mechanical ventilation, the degree of airway resistance is primarily affected by the length, size, and patency of the airway, endotracheal tube, and ventilator circuit.

FACTORS AFFECTING AIRWAY RESISTANCE

Airway resistance causes obstruction of air flow in the airways. It is increased when the patency or diameter of the airways is reduced. Obstruction of air flow may be caused by changes: (1) inside the airway (e.g., retained secretions), (2) in the wall of the airway (e.g., neoplasm of the bronchial muscle structure), or (3) outside the airway (e.g., tumors surrounding and compressing the airway) (West, 1998). When one of these conditions occurs, the radius of the airway decreases and airway resistance increases. According to the simplified form of Poiseuille's Law, the driving pressure ($\triangle P$) to maintain the same air flow ($\dot{V}$) must increase by a factor of 16-fold when the radius (r) of the airway is reduced by only half of its original size.

☑ Based on Poiseuille's Law, the work of breathing increases by a factor of 16-fold when the radius (r) of the airway is reduced by half its original size.

$$\text{Simplified form of Poiseuille's Law: } \triangle P = \frac{\dot{V}}{r^4}$$

One of the most common causes of increased airway resistance is chronic obstructive pulmonary disease (COPD). This type of lung disease includes emphysema, chronic bronchitis, chronic asthma, and bronchiectasis. Mechanical conditions that may increase airway resistance include postintubation obstruction and foreign body aspiration. Infectious processes include laryngotracheobronchitis (croup), epiglottitis, and bronchiolitis (Cherniack et al., 1983). Table 1-1 lists three categories of clinical conditions that increase airway resistance.

Normal airway resistance is between 0.6 and 2.4 cm H_2O/L/sec. at a flow rate of 30 L/min. (0.5 L/sec.) (Burton et al., 1997). It is higher in intubated patients, depending on the size of the endotracheal (ET) tube. Airway resistance varies directly with the length and inversely with the diameter of the ET tube. In the clinical setting, the ET tube is sometimes cut shorter for ease of airway management, reduction of mechanical deadspace, and reduction of airway resistance. However, the major contributor to increased airway resistance is the internal diameter of the ET tube. Therefore, during intubation, the largest appropriate size ET tube must be used so that the airway resistance contributed by the ET tube may be minimized. Once the ET tube is in place, its patency must be maintained as secretions retained on the inside wall of the ET tube greatly increase airway resistance.

☑ Airway resistance varies directly with the length and inversely with the diameter of the ET tube.

Besides the ET tube, the ventilator circuit may also impose mechanical resistance to air flow and contribute to total airway resistance. This

TABLE 1-1 Clinical Conditions That Increase Airway Resistance

TYPE	CLINICAL CONDITIONS
COPD	Emphysema Chronic bronchitis Asthma Bronchiectasis
Mechanical obstruction	Postintubation obstruction Foreign body aspiration Endotracheal tube Condensation in ventilator circuit
Infection	Laryngotracheobronchitis (croup) Epiglottitis Bronchiolitis

is particularly important when there is a significant amount of water in the ventilator circuit due to condensation.

AIRWAY RESISTANCE AND THE WORK OF BREATHING ($\triangle$P)

Airway resistance is calculated by $\dfrac{\text{Pressure Change } (\triangle P)}{\text{Flow}}$

$$\text{Raw} = \frac{\triangle P}{\dot{V}}$$

Raw : Airway resistance
  $\triangle$P : Pressure change (Peak airway pressure – plateau pressure)
  $\dot{V}$: Flow

☑ An increase in airway resistance means an increase in the work of breathing.

The pressure change ($\triangle$P) in the equation can be treated as the amount of work of breathing imposed on the patient. Since airway resistance is directly related to pressure change (the work of breathing), an increase in airway resistance means an increase in the work of breathing. In a clinical setting, airway obstruction is one of the most frequent causes of increased work of breathing (Beachey et al., 1990).

If pressure change (work of breathing) in the equation above is held constant, an increase in airway resistance will cause a decrease in flow and subsequently a decrease in minute ventilation. This is because airway resistance and flow in the equation are inversely related. In a clinical setting, **hypoventilation** may result if the patient is unable to overcome the airway resistance by increasing the work of breathing.

As a result of chronic air trapping, patients with chronic airway obstruction may develop highly compliant lung parenchyma and use

hypoventilation: Inadequate alveolar ventilation leading to CO_2 retention.

ventilatory failure:
Failure of the lungs to eliminate carbon dioxide. Without supplemental oxygen, it leads to hypoxemia.

oxygenation failure:
Failure of the heart and lungs to provide adequate oxygen for metabolic needs.

a breathing pattern that is deeper but slower. Patients with restrictive lung disease breathe more shallowly but faster, since air flow resistance is not the primary disturbance in these patients.

EFFECTS ON VENTILATION AND OXYGENATION

The work of breathing imposed on a patient is increased when airway resistance is high. This creates a detrimental effect on the patient's ventilatory and oxygenation status. If an abnormally high airway resistance is sustained over a long time, fatigue of the respiratory muscles may occur, leading to ventilatory and oxygenation failure (Rochester, 1993). **Ventilatory failure** occurs when the patient's minute ventilation cannot keep up with CO_2 production. **Oxygenation failure** usually follows when the pulmonary system cannot provide adequate oxygen needed for metabolism.

LUNG COMPLIANCE

lung compliance:
The degree of lung expansion per unit pressure change.

Lung compliance is volume change (lung expansion) per unit pressure change (work of breathing) and it is calculated by $C = \triangle V / \triangle P$ where C = Compliance, $\triangle V$ = Volume change, and $\triangle P$ = Pressure change. A method to measure compliance is outlined in Table 1-2.

COMPLIANCE MEASUREMENT

Abnormally low or high lung compliance impairs the patient's ability to maintain efficient gas exchange. Low compliance typically makes lung expansion difficult and high compliance induces incomplete exhalation and CO_2 elimination. These abnormalities are often contributing factors to the need for mechanical ventilation.

plateau pressure:
The pressure needed to maintain lung inflation in the absence of air flow.

peak airway pressure: *The pressure used to deliver the tidal volume by overcoming non-elastic (airways) and elastic (lung parenchyma) resistance.*

TABLE 1-2 Method to Measure Static and Dynamic Compliance

(1) Obtain corrected expired tidal volume.

(2) Obtain **plateau pressure** by applying inspiratory hold or occluding the exhalation port at end-inspiration.

(3) Obtain **peak airway pressure**.

(4) Obtain **positive end-expiratory pressure** (PEEP) level, if any.

$$\text{Static compliance} = \frac{\text{Corrected tidal volume}}{\text{(plateau pressure–PEEP)}}$$

$$\text{Dynamic compliance} = \frac{\text{Corrected tidal volume}}{\text{(peak airway pressure–PEEP)}}$$

TABLE 1-3   **Clinical Conditions That Decrease the Compliance**

TYPE OF COMPLIANCE	CLINICAL CONDITIONS
Static compliance	Atelectasis ARDS Tension pneumothorax Obesity Retained secretions
Dynamic compliance	Bronchospasm Kinking of ET tube Airway obstruction

✓ ↓ Lung compliance = ↑ Work of breathing

refractory hypoxemia: Low oxygen tension in blood that responds very poorly to oxygen therapy.

✓ In extreme high compliance situations, exhalation is often incomplete due to lack of elastic recoil by the lungs.

✓ Static compliance reflects the elastic properties (elastic resistance) of the lung and chest wall.

Low Compliance.   Low compliance (high elastance) means that the volume change is small per unit pressure change. Under this condition, the lungs are "stiff" or noncompliant. The work of breathing is high when compliance is low. In many clinical situations (e.g., atelectasis), low lung compliance is responsible for **refractory hypoxemia.**

Low compliance measurements are usually related to conditions that reduce the patient's functional residual capacity. Patients with noncompliant lungs often have a restrictive lung defect, low lung volumes, and low minute ventilation. This condition may be compensated for by an increased respiratory rate. Table 1-3 shows some examples that lead to a decreased compliance measurement.

High Compliance.   High compliance means that the volume change is large per unit pressure change. In extreme high compliance situations, exhalation is often incomplete due to lack of elastic recoil by the lungs. Emphysema is an example of high compliance where the gas exchange process is impaired. This condition is due to chronic air trapping, destruction of lung tissues, and enlargement of terminal and respiratory bronchioles.

High compliance measuremenst are usually related to conditions that increase the patient's functional residual capacity. Patients with extremely compliant lungs often have an obstructive lung defect, air flow obstruction, incomplete exhalation, and poor gas exchange.

STATIC AND DYNAMIC COMPLIANCE

Assessment of compliance can be divided into static compliance and dynamic compliance measurements. The relationship and clinical significance of these measurements are discussed in the following sections.

Static Compliance.   Static compliance is measured when there is no air flow (using the plateau pressure – PEEP). When air flow is absent,

☑ Dynamic compli-
ance reflects the
airway resistance
(nonelastic resis-
tance) and the elastic
properties of the
lung and chest wall
(elastic resistance).

☑ In general,
conditions caus-
ing changes in static
compliance invoke
similar changes
in dynamic
compliance.

☑ In conditions
where airway
resistance is the
only abnormality,
dynamic compliance
can change inde-
pendently without
a corresponding
change in static
compliance.

airway resistance is not a determining factor. Thus, static compliance reflects the elastic resistance of the lung and chest wall.

Dynamic Compliance. Dynamic compliance is measured when air flow is present (using the peak airway pressure–PEEP). Since air flow is present, airway resistance becomes a critical factor in the measurement of compliance. Dynamic compliance therefore reflects the condition of airway resistance (nonelastic resistance) as well as the elastic properties of the lung and chest wall (elastic resistance).

Changes of Static and Dynamic Compliance. In general, conditions causing changes in static compliance invoke similar changes in dynamic compliance. For example, in atelectasis both static and dynamic compliance measurements are decreased simultaneously. When atelectasis is resolved, both compliance measurements are increased and returned to normal concurrently (Figure 1-1).

In conditions where airway resistance is the only abnormality, dynamic compliance can change independently without a corresponding change in static compliance. For example, bronchospasm can decrease dynamic compliance while leaving static compliance unaffected. When bronchospasm is resolved, dynamic compliance is increased and returns to normal (Figure 1-2).

Compliance measurements should be made so that a trend can be established. Interpretation is of little value with a single compliance

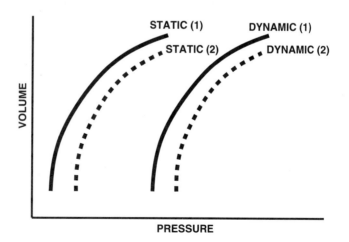

Figure 1-1 Shifting of the dynamic and static compliance curves. Both curves shift to the right with a decrease in static compliance (increase in elastic or lung parenchymal resistance). Note that the static compliance curve and the dynamic compliance curve are both shifted to the right (static [2] and dynamic [2]). Improvement in elastic or lung parenchymal resistance to its normal state will cause both compliance curves to return to their original positions (static [1] and dynamic [1]).

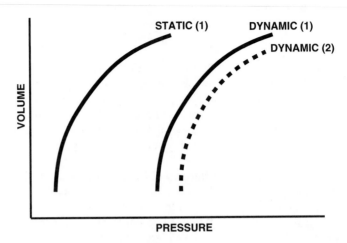

Figure 1-2 Shifting of the dynamic compliance curve. The dynamic compliance curve shifts to the right with a decrease in dynamic compliance (increase in nonelastic or airway resistance). Note that shifting of the dynamic compliance curve occurs independently (dynamic [2]) and that the position of the static compliance curve is unchanged. Improvement in nonelastic or airway resistance to its normal state will cause the dynamic compliance curve to return to its original position (dynamic [1]).

measurement. It is also essential not to compare static compliance with dynamic compliance measurements as this can cause erroneous interpretations.

Normal Ranges. Normal dynamic compliance is between 30 and 40 mL/cm H_2O and normal static compliance is between 40 and 60 mL/cm H_2O. It is lower in intubated patients, depending on the internal diameter of the ET tube. See Table 1-2 for the method to measure compliance. The equations for static compliance (C_{ST}) and dynamic compliance (C_{DYN}) are:

☑ See Appendix 1 for example.

$$C_{ST} = \frac{\text{Corrected tidal volume}}{(\text{Plateau pressure} - \text{PEEP})}$$

☑ See Appendix 1 for example.

$$C_{DYN} = \frac{\text{Corrected tidal volume}}{(\text{Peak airway pressure} - \text{PEEP})}$$

COMPLIANCE AND THE WORK OF BREATHING

Since compliance is inversely related to pressure change (work of breathing), a decrease in compliance means an increase in the work of breathing. In a clinical setting, atelectasis is one of the frequent causes of increased work of breathing.

If the plateau pressure and peak airway pressure (work of breathing) in the previous equations are held unchanged, a decrease in compliance will cause a decrease in volume. This is because compliance and volume change in the equation are directly related. In a clinical setting, hypoventilation usually results when a patient is unable to compensate for the decrease in compliance by increasing and maintaining a higher level of work of breathing. In low compliance situations such as ARDS, fibrosis, and kyphoscoliosis, the decrease in minute ventilation is characterized by small tidal volumes and fast respiratory rates—a sign of volume restriction (Cherniack et al., 1983).

EFFECTS ON VENTILATION AND OXYGENATION

Abnormal compliance impairs the gas exchange mechanism. When an abnormally low or high compliance is uncorrected and prolonged, muscle fatigue may occur and lead to the development of ventilatory and oxygenation failure (Rochester, 1993). Ventilatory failure develops when the patient's minute ventilation cannot keep up with the CO_2 production. Oxygenation failure usually follows when the pulmonary system cannot supply the oxygen needed for metabolism.

DEADSPACE VENTILATION

deadspace ventilation: Ventilation in excess of perfusion; wasted ventilation.

Deadspace ventilation is defined as wasted ventilation or a condition in which ventilation is in excess of perfusion. There are three types of deadspace: anatomic, alveolar, and physiologic.

ANATOMIC DEADSPACE

anatomic deadspace: The volume occupying the conducting airways that does not take part in gas exchange (estimated to be about 1 milliliter per pound ideal body weight).

Normally, the conducting airways contribute to about 30% of deadspace ventilation. For a tidal volume of 500 mL, about 150 mL of this volume is wasted since it does not take part in gas exchange. This volume in the conducting airways is called **anatomic deadspace** and it can be estimated to be about 1 mL per pound of ideal body weight (Shapiro et al., 1991).

☑ Decrease in tidal volume causes a higher anatomic deadspace to tidal volume percent.

Decrease in tidal volume causes a higher anatomic deadspace to tidal volume percent. Using the above example, the deadspace to tidal volume percent would increase from 30% (150/500) to 50% (150/300) if the tidal volume was decreased from 500 mL to 300 mL. See equations below for comparison:

$$\frac{150}{500} = 0.3 \text{ or } 30\%$$

$$\frac{150}{300} = 0.5 \text{ or } 50\%$$

ALVEOLAR DEADSPACE

In addition to anatomic deadspace, **alveolar deadspace** may occur in some clinical conditions. Alveolar deadspace contributes to wasted

alveolar deadspace:
The normal lung volume that has become unable to take part in gas exchange because of reduction or lack of pulmonary perfusion (e.g., pulmonary embolism).

ventilation, and it occurs when the ventilated alveoli are not adequately perfused by pulmonary circulation. Pulmonary perfusion may be absent or low because of decreased cardiac output (e.g., congestive heart failure, blood loss), or due to obstruction of the pulmonary blood vessels (e.g., pulmonary vasoconstriction, pulmonary embolism) (Shapiro et al., 1991). Figure 1-3 shows the relationship between ventilation and perfusion during alveolar deadspace ventilation.

PHYSIOLOGIC DEADSPACE

Physiologic deadspace is the sum of anatomic and alveolar deadspace volumes. Under normal conditions, the physiologic deadspace approximates the anatomic deadspace. In diseased conditions where anatomic or alveolar deadspace ventilation is increased, physiologic deadspace is always higher than anatomic deadspace. Table 1-4 shows some clinical conditions that increase physiologic (anatomic and alveolar) deadspace.

physiologic deadspace: *Sum of anatomic and alveolar deadspace. Under normal conditions, it is about the same as anatomic deadspace.*

Physiologic deadspace to tidal volume ratio (V_D/V_T) can be calculated as follows:

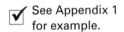 See Appendix 1 for example.

$$V_D/V_T = \frac{(PaCO_2 - P\bar{E}CO_2)}{PaCO_2}$$

$PaCO_2$ is arterial CO_2 and $P\bar{E}CO_2$ is PCO_2 of a mixed expired gas sample. They are collected simultaneously. In patients on mechanical ventilation, V_D/V_T of less than 60% predicts normal ventilatory function upon weaning from mechanical ventilation (Shapiro et al., 1991).

Severe and prolonged deadspace ventilation causes inefficient ventilation, muscle fatigue, ventilatory and oxygenation failure.

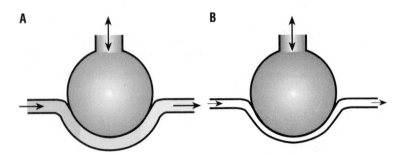

Figure 1-3 (A) Normal ventilation/perfusion relationship; (B) Alveolar deadspace ventilation occurs when the ventilated alveoli are not adequately perfused by pulmonary circulation (i.e., ventilation in excess of perfusion). Examples of deadspace ventilation include decrease in cardiac output and obstruction of pulmonary blood vessels.

TABLE 1-4 Clinical Conditions That Increase Physiologic Deadspace

TYPE OF CHANGE	CLINICAL CONDITIONS
↓ Tidal volume	Relative increase in V_D/V_T ratio (drug overdose, neuromuscular disease)
↑ Alveolar deadspace	Decreased cardiac output (congestive heart failure, blood loss) Obstruction of pulmonary blood vessels (pulmonary vasoconstriction, pulmonary embolism)

V/Q mismatch: An abnormal distribution of ventilation and pulmonary blood flow. High V/Q is related to deadspace ventilation, whereas low V/Q is associated with intrapulmonary shunting.

intrapulmonary shunting: Pulmonary blood flow in excess of ventilation; wasted perfusion (e.g., atelectasis).

diffusion defect: Pathologic condition leading to impaired gas exchange through the alveolar-capillary membrane (e.g., interstitial or pulmonary edema).

VENTILATORY FAILURE

Ventilatory failure is the inability of the pulmonary system to maintain proper removal of carbon dioxide. Hypercapnia (increase in $PaCO_2$) is the key feature of ventilatory failure. When carbon dioxide production exceeds its removal, respiratory acidosis results. Hypoxemia can be the secondary complication of ventilatory failure but this type of hypoxemia usually responds well to oxygen therapy. Without supplemental oxygen, the degree of hypoxemia corresponds to the severity of ventilatory failure.

Table 1-5 lists five mechanisms leading to the development of ventilatory failure. They are: (1) hypoventilation, (2) persistent ventilation-perfusion (**V/Q) mismatch**, (3) persistent **intrapulmonary shunting**, (4) persistent **diffusion defect**, and (5) persistent reduction of inspired oxygen tension (PIO_2) (Greene et al., 1994).

TABLE 1-5 Development of Ventilatory Failure

MECHANISM	CLINICAL FINDING
Hypoventilation	$PaCO_2$ greater than 45 mm Hg (>50 mm Hg for COPD patients)
Persistent V/Q mismatch	Hypoxemia that responds well to oxygen therapy
Persistent intrapulmonary shunt	Q_S/Q_T greater than 20% (>30% in critical shunt)
Persistent diffusion defect	Gas diffusion rate less than 75% of predicted normal
Persistent reduction of P_IO_2	Low barometric pressure as in high altitude

HYPOVENTILATION

Hypoventilation can be caused by depression of the central nervous system, neuromuscular diseases, airway obstruction, and other conditions. In a clinical setting, hypoventilation is characterized by a reduction of alveolar ventilation (V_A) and an increase of arterial carbon dioxide tension ($PaCO_2$).

alveolar volume: The portion of tidal volume that takes part in gas exchange.

Alveolar Volume. Alveolar volume (V_A) is the difference between tidal volume (V_T) and deadspace volume (V_D), as shown below:

$$V_A = V_T - V_D$$

The equation shows that alveolar volume can be increased by raising the tidal volume or by reducing the deadspace volume. In mechanical ventilation, a decrease in alveolar volume occurs when the tidal volume delivered to the patient is decreased or the deadspace volume is increased.

Hypoventilation caused by a reduction in tidal volume can be corrected by increasing the tidal volume on the ventilator. Unlike tidal volume, deadspace volume is difficult to change because anatomic deadspace stays rather constant and physiologic deadspace is caused by a lack of perfusion, thus requiring a different strategy to improve blood flow.

☑ $\dot{V}_A = (V_T - V_D)$ $\times$ RR (See Appendix 1 for example).

Minute Alveolar Ventilation ($\dot{V}_A$). When the measurements are made over one minute, minute alveolar ventilation ($\dot{V}_A$) becomes a function of the respiratory rate. Hypoventilation can result when the respiratory rate is too slow or absent (apnea). Hypoventilation due to a reduction in respiratory rate can be corrected by increasing the respiratory rate on the ventilator.

A patient's ventilatory status can best be monitored by the $PaCO_2$ measurement. The equation below shows the inverse relationship between $\dot{V}_A$ and $PaCO_2$. When the minute alveolar ventilation is low (hypoventilation), an elevated $PaCO_2$ is the typical finding in blood gas analysis.

☑ Hypoventilation is characterized by an increase of $PaCO_2$.

$$\dot{V}_A = \frac{\dot{V}CO_2}{PaCO_2}$$

VENTILATION/PERFUSION (V/Q) MISMATCH

Ventilation/perfusion (V/Q) ratio reflects the amount of ventilation in relation to the amount of pulmonary blood flow (perfusion). Since blood flow is gravity dependent, the V/Q ratio ranges from about 0.4 in the lower lung zone to 3.0 in the upper lung zone (West, 1999).

Pulmonary embolism is an example that decreases pulmonary perfusion and leads to a high V/Q. Airway obstruction and interstitial lung disease are two examples that can cause a decrease in ventilation and lead to a low V/Q.

V/Q mismatch is responsible for the development of hypoxemia. With sufficient pulmonary reserve, a patient can usually compensate for the hypoxemic condition by hyperventilation. Hypoxemia caused by uncomplicated V/Q mismatch is readily reversible by oxygen therapy.

In mechanical ventilation, hypoxemia caused by V/Q mismatch can be compensated by increasing the rate, tidal volume, or F_IO_2 on the ventilator (Shapiro et al., 1991).

INTRAPULMONARY SHUNTING

✓ Shunted pulmonary blood flow is not useful in gas exchange.

In contrast with deadspace ventilation (ventilation in excess of perfusion), shunting refers to perfusion in excess of ventilation ("wasted" perfusion) (Figure 1-4). Shunted pulmonary blood flow is not useful in gas exchange because it does not come in contact with ventilated and oxygenated alveoli. Intrapulmonary shunting causes refractory hypoxemia—low oxygen levels in the blood that respond very poorly to oxygen therapy alone.

✓ Intrapulmonary shunting causes refractory hypoxemia.

In healthy individuals, the physiologic shunt approximates the anatomic shunt and it is less than 5%. For non-critically ill patients, the normal physiological shunt is less than 10%. In other disease states, the physiologic shunt may be greater than 30% (Shapiro et al., 1994). See Table 1-6 for interpretation of shunt percent in hospitalized patients.

The shunt percent can be calculated or estimated by many methods, ranging from simple (less accurate) to complex (more accurate). The clinical use of two common calculations are discussed here: an estimated shunt equation and a classic shunt equation.

✓ The estimated physiologic shunt equation requires only an arterial blood sample.

Estimated Physiologic Shunt Equation. The estimated physiologic shunt equation requires only an arterial blood sample. It does not require a mixed venous blood sample from the pulmonary artery and

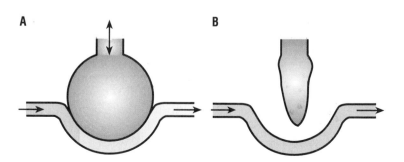

Figure 1-4 (A) Normal ventilation/perfusion relationship; (B) Intrapulmonary shunting occurs when the perfused alveoli are not adequately ventilated (i.e., perfusion in excess of ventilation). Atelectasis is an example that leads to intrapulmonary shunting.

TABLE 1-6   Interpretation of Shunt Percent

PHYSIOLOGIC SHUNT	INTERPRETATION
< 10%	Normal
10% to 20%	Mild shunt
20% to 30%	Significant shunt
> 30%	Critical and severe shunt

therefore it is noninvasive and rather simple to compute. This estimated method is more meaningful when serial measurements are used to establish a trend. Two forms of this equation are possible: one for noncritical patients (e.g., spontaneously breathing, moderate level of F_IO_2, moderate level of continuous positive airway pressure) and one for critically ill patients (e.g., mechanical ventilation, high F_IO_2, high level of positive end-expiratory pressure).

For noncritical patient:

$$\text{Estimated } Q_S/Q_T = \frac{(CcO_2 - CaO_2)}{[5 + (CcO_2 - CaO_2)]}$$

☑ See Appendix 1 for example.

For critical patient:

$$\text{Estimated } Q_S/Q_T = \frac{(CcO_2 - CaO_2)}{[3.5 + (CcO_2 - CaO_2)]}$$

☑ The classic physiologic shunt equation requires arterial and mixed venous blood samples.

Classic Physiologic Shunt Equation.   The classic physiologic shunt equation requires an arterial blood sample and a mixed venous blood sample from the pulmonary artery. It is the most accurate among all shunt equations.

$$\text{Classic } Q_S/Q_T = \frac{(CcO_2 - CaO_2)}{(CcO_2 - C\dot{v}O_2)}$$

☑ See Appendix 1 for example.

When the shunt percent is too high, oxygenation becomes an extremely difficult task for the cardiopulmonary system to support. Over time, the respiratory muscles will fatigue resulting in ventilatory failure. This is usually followed by oxygenation failure if ventilatory interventions are unsuccessful (Rochester, 1993).

DIFFUSION DEFECT

Diffusion of oxygen and carbon dioxide across the alveolar-capillary (A-C) membrane is due to the gas pressure gradients. Oxygen diffuses from the lungs (PAO_2 = 109 mm Hg) to the pulmonary arteries ($P\dot{v}O_2$ = 40 mm Hg) with a pressure gradient of 69 mm Hg. Carbon dioxide diffuses from the pulmonary arteries ($P\dot{v}CO_2$ = 46 mm Hg) to the

TABLE 1-7   **Causes of Decreased Diffusion Rate**

TYPE OF DIFFUSION PROBLEM	CLINICAL CONDITIONS
Decrease in pressure gradient	High altitude Fire combustion
Thickening of A-C membrane	Pulmonary edema Retained secretions
Decreased surface area of A-C membrane	Emphysema Pulmonary fibrosis
Insufficient time for diffusion	Tachycardia

hypoxic hypoxia:
Lack of oxygen
in the organs and
tissues due to a
reduction in inspired
oxygen tension.

lungs ($PACO_2 = 40$ mm Hg) with a net pressure gradient of only 6 mm Hg. This is possible because the gas diffusion coefficient for carbon dioxide is 19 times greater than that for oxygen.

Diffusion of oxygen is greatly impaired when the inspired oxygen tension (PIO_2) is reduced. The inspired oxygen tension is directly related to the barometric pressure. At high altitude where the barometric pressure is low, the inspired oxygen tension is also low. This leads to a condition known as **hypoxic hypoxia**.

The PIO_2 is also reduced in a burning enclosure as combustion consumes oxygen in the air. Patients who suffer from smoke inhalation are at risk for developing hypoxic hypoxia. In addition to the reduced oxygen concentration and tension, the lung functions are impaired by the presence of carbon monoxide, toxic gases, and inert particles found in a fire (Wilkins et al., 1998).

In addition to the pressure gradient and diffusion coefficient, the gas diffusion rate is also affected by the thickness of the A-C membrane, the surface area of the A-C membrane, and the time available for diffusion to take place. Factors that can decrease the diffusion rate are shown in Table 1-7.

Conditions in Table 1-7 induce poor or inappropriate gas diffusion and can severely hinder the oxygenation process. Hypoxemia and hypoxia are usually the end results. Severe hypoxemia and hypoxia may lead to hypoxic pulmonary vasoconstriction, pulmonary hypertension, and cor pulmonale.

OXYGENATION FAILURE

Oxygenation failure is defined as severe hypoxemia ($PaO_2 < 40$ mm Hg) that does not respond to moderate to high levels (50 to 100%) of supplemental oxygen. It may be caused by hypoventilation, ventilation/perfusion mismatch, or intrapulmonary shunting. Regardless of the etiology of oxygenation failure, mechanical ventilation may be needed to minimize the work of breathing and provide oxygenation support.

HYPOXEMIA AND HYPOXIA

Hypoxemia is present when the oxygen level (e.g., PO_2, SaO_2) is decreased in arterial blood. The presence of hypoxia ($\downarrow PO_2$ in organs and tissues) may not be always apparent. Hypoxemia reflects the likelihood of hypoxia, but it is important to remember that hypoxia can occur in the absence of hypoxemia. For example, anemic hypoxia (e.g., $\downarrow$ hemoglobin, carbon monoxide poisoning), histotoxic hypoxia (e.g., cyanide poisoning), and circulatory hypoxia (e.g., $\downarrow$ cardiac output) may show normal PaO_2 measurements (Shapiro et al., 1991).

Hypoxemia.   Hypoxemia is reduced oxygen in the blood. The PaO_2 is most often used to evaluate a patient's oxygenation status. Since PaO_2 reflects only the oxygen that is dissolved in the plasma, it does not represent all oxygen carried by the blood (hemoglobin and plasma). For precise assessment, oxygen content should be used as it includes the oxygen combined with hemoglobins as well as oxygen dissolved in the plasma.

When PaO_2 is used for oxygenation assessment, Table 1-8 may be used for interpretation of an adult's oxygenation status.

Hypoxia.   Hypoxia is reduced oxygen in the body organs and tissues. While hypoxemia and hypoxia are two terms sometimes used interchangably, it is important to understand that hypoxia can occur with a normal PaO_2. For example, cyanide poisoning causes histotoxic hypoxia in which the tissues cannot carry out aerobic metabolism. In anemic hypoxia, the low hemoglobin level causes a low oxygen content while the PaO_2 may be normal. Since PaO_2 measures the oxygen tension of the plasma only, it cannot be used for assessment of anemic or histotoxic hypoxia. Arterial oxygen content (CaO_2) should be measured and used to assess the oxygenation status of a patient. In addition to the PaO_2 and CaO_2 measurements, hypoxia

☑ Hypoxia can occur with a normal PaO_2.

TABLE 1-8   **Interpretation of Oxygenation Status Using PaO_2**

HYPOXEMIA STATUS	PaO_2 (P_B = 760 mm Hg)	PaO_2 (P_B = 630 mm Hg)
Normal	80 to 100 mm Hg	60 to 79 mm Hg
Mild	60 to 79 mm Hg	50 to 59 mm Hg
Moderate	40 to 59 mm Hg	40 to 49 mm Hg
Severe	Less than 40 mm Hg	Less than 40 mm Hg

✓ Oxygenation failure may develop when severe hypoxemia (PaO$_2$ < 40 mm Hg) does not respond to a moderate to high level (50 to 100%) of supplemental oxygen.

✓ The important clinical signs of oxygenation failure and hypoxia include hypoxemia, dyspnea, tachypnea, tachycardia, and cyanosis.

produces some clinical signs that may be used as a secondary assessment tool.

Signs of Hypoxia. In most clinical situations, hypoxemia is readily corrected by a moderate amount of supplemental oxygen. Oxygenation failure may develop when severe hypoxemia (PaO$_2$ < 40 mm Hg) does not respond to moderate to high levels (50 to 100%) of supplemental oxygen.

The important clinical signs of oxygenation failure and hypoxia include hypoxemia, dyspnea, tachypnea, tachycardia, and cyanosis (Rochester, 1993). In addition, patients often appear to have shortness of breath and may become disoriented. These signs are usually readily available in the medical records or at the bedside. They should be used in conjunction with laboratory results during "routine" ventilator rounds to assess the patient so that appropriate action may be taken.

CLINICAL CONDITIONS LEADING TO MECHANCIAL VENTILATION

✓ Mechanical ventilation is often used to support ventilatory or oxygenation failure.

Mechanical ventilation is often used to support ventilatory or oxygenation failure. Failure to ventilate or oxygenate adequately may be caused by pulmonary or nonpulmonary conditions. For example, adult respiratory distress syndrome is a pulmonary condition commonly associated with mechanical ventilation and mortality. Many nonpulmonary conditions (e.g., hypovolemic shock, head trauma) also contribute to the need for mechanical ventilation (Gillespie et al., 1986; Kelly et al., 1993).

These pulmonary and nonpulmonary conditions often lead to a combination of deadspace ventilation, V/Q mismatch, shunt, diffusion defect, ventilatory failure, and oxygenation failure. For logical discussion and ease of patient management, they are separated into three distinct groups: (1) depressed respiratory drive (e.g., drug overdose), (2) excessive ventilatory workload (e.g., air flow obstruction), and (3) failure of ventilatory pump (e.g., chest trauma).

DEPRESSED RESPIRATORY DRIVE

✓ Depressed or insufficient respiratory drive may lead to ventilatory and oxygenation failure.

Depressed or insufficient respiratory drive may lead to a decrease in tidal volume, respiratory rate, or both. These patients may have normal pulmonary function but the respiratory muscles do not have adequate neuromuscular impulses to function properly. Mechanical ventilation is used to support these patients until the cause of insufficient respiratory drive has been reversed.

Table 1-9 lists the clinical conditions that may lead to a depressed respiratory drive. They are drug overdose (Parsons, 1994), acute spinal cord injury (Bach, 1991), head trauma (Hemmer, 1985), neurologic

TABLE 1-9   Causes of Depressed Respiratory Drive

TYPE OF RESPIRATORY DRIVE DEPRESSION	CLINICAL CONDITIONS
Drug overdose	Central hypoventilation (narcotics, alcohol, sedatives). Acute respiratory insufficiency (cocaine, heroin, methadone, propoxyphene, phenothiazines, alcohol, barbiturates). Severe pulmonary complications (poisons and toxins such as paraquat, petroleum distillates, organophosphates, mushrooms of *Amanita* genus, hemlock, botulism.
Acute spinal cord injury	Respiratory paralysis (Quadriplegic with injury at C1-C3 level).
Head trauma	Abnormal respiratory patterns (apnea, tachypnea, Cheyne-Stokes respiration, apneustic breathing, ataxic breathing) Neurogenic pulmonary edema (increase in intracranial pressure) Delayed pulmonary dysfunction (Intrapulmonary shunt, increased pulmonary vascular resistance, V/Q mismatch)
Neurologic dysfunction	Coma Cerebral vascular accident (stroke) Altered mental status (Hypoxic brain)
Sleep disorders	Sleep apnea (Central, obstructive, mixed) Sleep deprivation
Metabolic alkalosis	Hypoventilation to compensate for elevated pH in metabolic alkalosis

dysfunction (Kelly et al., 1993), sleep disorders, and compensation for metabolic alkalosis (Greene et al., 1994).

EXCESSIVE VENTILATORY WORKLOAD

✔️ Excessive ventilatory workload may lead to muscle fatigue, ventilatory and oxygenation failure.

Ventilatory workload is influenced by many clinical conditions (Table 1-10). When it exceeds the patient's ability to carry out the workload, ventilatory and oxygenation failure ensues and mechanical ventilation becomes necessary. The ventilatory workload is increased in the presence of acute air flow obstruction (Beachey et al., 1990), increased deadspace ventilation (Greene et al., 1994), acute lung injury (Kraus et al., 1993), congenital heart disease (DiCarlo et al., 1994), cardiovas-

TABLE 1-10   Causes of Excessive Ventilatory Workload

TYPE	CLINICAL CONDITIONS
Acute airflow obstruction	Status asthmaticus Epiglotittis COPD
Deadspace ventilation	Pulmonary embolism Decrease in cardiac output Emphysema
Acute lung injury	ARDS IRDS
Congenital heart disease	Hypoplastic left heart syndrome Tetralogy of Fallot Persistent pulmonary hypertension
Cardiovascular decompensation	Decreased cardiac output V/Q mismatch Deadspace ventilation
Shock	Blood loss Peripheral vasodilation Congestive heart failure
Increased metabolic rate	Fever Increased work of breathing
Drugs	Acute pulmonary edema (narcotics, salicylates, nonsteroidal anti-inflamma-tory agents, naloxone, thiazide diuretics, contrast media, insulin) Bronchospasm (salicylates, nonsteroidal anti-inflammatory agents, hydrocortisone, beta-blockers, neuromuscular blocking agents, contrast media)
Decreased compliance	Atelectasis Tension pneumothorax Post-thoracic surgery Obesity Diaphragmatic hernia

☑ Failure of the ventilatory pump may lead to an increased work of breathing, eventual ventilatory and oxygenation failure.

cular decompensation, shock (Hinson et al., 1992), increased metabolic rate, and decreased lung and chest wall compliance (Greene et al., 1994).

FAILURE OF VENTILATORY PUMP

Failure of the ventilatory pump is the structural dysfunction of the respiratory system to include the lung parenchyma and respiratory muscles.

TABLE 1-11 Causes of Ventilatory Pump Failure

TYPE	CLINICAL CONDITIONS
Chest trauma	Flail chest
	Tension pneumothorax
Premature birth	Idiopathic respiratory distress syndrome
Electrolyte imbalance	Hyperkalemia
Geriatric patients	Fatigue of respiratory muscles

If uncorrected, this condition may lead to increased work of breathing and eventual ventilatory and oxygenation failure.

Table 1-11 lists some clinical examples of conditions that may lead to ventilatory pump failure. They include chest trauma, prematurity (Watchko et al., 1994), electrolyte imbalance (Freeman et al., 1993), and problems in geriatric patients (Krieger, 1994).

SUMMARY

Mechanical ventilation is used for many different clinical conditions. Essentially all uses of mechanical ventilation are targeted toward patients who fail to ventilate or oxygenate adequately. Ventilatory and oxygenation failure may be due to the adverse changes in a patient's physiologic functions (i.e., depressed respiratory drive, excessive ventilatory workload, and failure of ventilatory pump). These abnormal physiologic functions should be identified early on so that the indications for mechanical ventilation are clearly delineated.

While mechanical ventilation does not treat any ventilation or oxygenation abnormalities per se, it is a useful adjunct to support the gas exchange function until effective spontaneous breathing is restored.

Self-Assessment Questions

1. Airway resistance may be increased in all of the following clinical conditions *except:*

   A. airway obstruction.
   B. endotracheal tube with small internal diameter.

   C. condensation in ventilator circuit.
   D. tachycardia.

2. Static compliance is primarily affected by a patient's:

   A. elastic properties of the lungs.
   B. airway resistance.

   C. spontaneous tidal volume.
   D. A and B only.

3. Dynamic compliance is primarily affected by a patient's:

A. elastic properties of the lungs.
B. airway resistance.

C. spontaneous tidal volume.
D. A and B only.

4. Low compliance limits the patient's ability to provide _____, whereas high compliance hinders the patient's ability to support _____.

A. deadspace ventilation, intrapul-
    monary shunting.
B. intrapulmonary shunting, deadspace
    ventilation.

C. gas exchange, lung expansion.

D. lung expansion, efficient gas
    exchange.

5. The most recent blood gas report shows that a patient is hypoventilating ($PaCO_2$ = 65 mm Hg). The physician asks you to improve the patient's alveolar ventilation by making changes to the ventilator. You would proceed to:

A. decrease the tidal volume.
B. increase the mechanical deadspace
    on the ventilator circuit.

C. increase the rate.
D. decrease the tidal volume and rate.

6. Hypoventilation is characterized by a(n):

A. increased PaO_2.
B. increased pH.

C. increased $PaCO_2$.
D. decreased pH and $PaCO_2$.

7. Ventilation/perfusion (V/Q) mismatch is common in lung diseases. For example, a low V/Q ratio may be seen in _____ and a high ratio in _____.

A. atelectasis, pulmonary embolism.
B. pulmonary embolism, atelectasis.

C. atelectasis, airway obstruction.
D. airway obstruction, atelectasis.

8. Which of the following causes of hypoxemia is *least* likely to be treated by oxygen therapy alone?

A. hypoventilation
B. V/Q mismatch

C. intrapulmonary shunting
D. low PIO_2

9. In managing a critically ill patient who has been on the ventilator for six days, the physician asks you to calculate the estimated shunt percent using only one arterial blood gas sample. You would use:

A. Estimated $Q_S/Q_T = (CcO_2 - CaO_2) /$
    $[5 + (CcO_2 - CaO_2)]$.
B. Estimated $Q_S/Q_T = (CcO_2 - CaO_2) /$
    $[3.5 + (CcO_2 - CaO_2)]$.

C. Classic $Q_S/Q_T = (CcO_2 - CaO_2) /$
    $(CcO_2 - C\dot{v}O_2)$.
D. B or C only.

10 to 13. Match the types of gas diffusion problem with the clinical conditions affecting the diffusion rate.

Type of Diffusion Problem	Clinical Condition
10. Decreased pressure gradient	A. Emphysema
11. Thickening of A-C membrane	B. High altitude
12. Decreased surface area of A-C membrane	C. Tachycardia
13. Insufficient time for diffusion	D. Pulmonary edema

14. The ABG report for an abdominal postoperative patient shows respiratory acidosis with severe hypoxemia. In order to determine whether *hypoxia* is present, you would evaluate all of the following *except:*

A. $PaCO_2$.
B. heart rate.
C. color of skin.
D. spontaneous respiratory rate.

15 to 20. Ventilatory and oxygenation failure may occur when the respiratory drive is diminished. Match the types of respiratory depression with the respective clinical conditions.

Type of Depression	Clinical Conditions
15. Drug overdose	A. Altered mental status (Hypoxic brain)
16. Acute spinal cord injury	B. Neurogenic pulmonary edema (Increase of intracranial pressure)
17. Head trauma	C. Sleep apnea (Central, obstructive, mixed)
18. Neurologic dysfunction	D. Hypoventilation to compensate for elevated pH
19. Sleep disorders	E. Respiratory paralysis (Quadriplegic with injury at C1-C3 level)
20. Metabolic alkalosis	F. Narcotic and sedative use

21. Excessive and prolonged increase in the patient's respiratory workload may lead to fatigue of the _____ muscles. If uncorrected, _____ failure is the likely end result.

A. heart, ventilatory and oxygenation

B. heart, congestive heart

C. respiratory, ventilatory and oxygenation

D. respiratory, congestive heart

References

Bach, J. R. (1991). Alternative methods of ventilatory support for the patient with ventilatory failure due to spinal cord injury. *Journal of the American Paraplegia Society, 14*(4), 158–174.

Beachey, W. D. et al. (1990). Quantifying ventilatory reserve to predict respiratory failure in exacerbations of COPD. *Chest, 97*, 1086–1091.

Burton, G. G. et al. (1997). *Respiratory care: A guide to clinical practice* (4th ed.). Philadelphia: Lippincott-Raven Publishers.

Cherniack, R. M. et al. (1983). *Respiration in health and disease* (3rd ed.). Philadelphia: W.B. Saunders Co.

DiCarlo, J. V. et al. (1994). Respiratory failure in congenital heart disease. *Pediatric Clinics of North America, 41*(3), 525–542.

Freeman, S. J. et al. (1993). Muscular paralysis and ventilatory failure caused by hyperkalemia. *British Journal of Anaesthesia, 70,* 226–227.

Gillespie, D. J. et al. (1986). Clinical outcome of respiratory failure in patients requiring prolonged (>24 hours) mechanical ventilation. *Chest, 90*(3), 364–369.

Greene, K. E. et al. (1994). Pathophysiology of acute respiratory failure. *Clinics in Chest Medicine, 15*(1), 1–12.

Hemmer, M. (1985). Ventilatory support for pulmonary failure of the head trauma patient. *Bull Eur Physiopathol Respir, 21,* 287–293.

Hinson, J. R. et al. (1992). Principles of mechanical ventilator use in respiratory failure. *Annu Rev Med, 43,* 341–361.

Kelly, B. J. et al. (1993). Prevalence and severity of neurologic dysfunction in critically ill patients—Influence on need for continued mechanical ventilation. *Chest, 104,* 1818–1824.

Kraus, P. A. et al. (1993). Acute lung injury at Baragwanath ICU, an eight-month audit and call for consensus for other organ failure in the adult respiratory distress syndrome. *Chest, 103,* 1832–1836.

Krieger, B. P. (1994). Respiratory failure in the elderly. *Clinics in Geriatric Medicine, 10*(1), 103–119.

Parsons, P. E. (1994). Respiratory failure as a result of drugs, overdoses, and poisonings. *Clinics in Chest Medicine, 15*(1), 93–102.

Rochester, D. F. (1993). Respiratory muscles and ventilatory failure. *The American Journal of the Medical Sciences, 305*(6), 394–402.

Schuster, D. P. (1990). A physiologic approach to initiating, maintaining, and withdrawing mechanical ventilatory support during acute respiratory failure. *The American Journal of Medicine, 88,* 268–278.

Shapiro, B. A. et al. (1991). *Clinical application of respiratory care* (4th ed.). St. Louis: Mosby-Year Book.

Shapiro, B. A. et al. (1994). *Clinical application of blood gases* (5th ed.). St. Louis: Mosby-Year Book.

Watchko, J. F. et al. (1994). Ventilatory pump failure in premature newborns. *Pediatric Pulmonology, 17,* 231–233.

West, J. B. (1998). *Pulmonary pathophysiology—The essentials* (5th ed.). Baltimore: Williams & Wilkins.

West, J. B. (1999). *Respiratory physiology—the essentials* (6th ed.). Philadelphia: Lippincott-Raven Publishers.

Wilkins, R. L., et al. (1998). *Respiratory disease—Principles of patient care* (2nd ed.). Philadelphia: F.A. Davis Co.

Suggested Reading

Chang, D. W. (1999). *Respiratory care calculations* (2nd ed.). Albany, NY: Delmar Publishers, Inc.

Misasi, R. S. et al. (1994). The pathophysiology of hypoxia. *Critical Care Nurse, 14*(4), 55–64.

CHAPTER TWO

EFFECTS OF POSITIVE PRESSURE VENTILATION

David W. Chang
Terry S. LeGrand

OUTLINE

KEY TERMS

- **central venous pressure (CVP)**
- **continuous positive airway pressure (CPAP)**
- **hepatic perfusion**
- **intra-abdominal pressure (IAP)**
- **mean airway pressure (MAWP)**
- **oxygen delivery**
- **peak airway pressure (PAP)**
- **positive end-expiratory pressure (PEEP)**

- **positive pressure ventilation**
- **pressure-limited**
- **pulmonary artery pressure**
- **pulmonary capillary wedge pressure**
- **renal perfusion**
- **stroke volume**
- **thoracic pump mechanism**
- **total parenteral nutrition (TPN)**
- **volume-limited**

INTRODUCTION

Positive pressure ventilation is an essential life support measure in the intensive care and extended care environments. The physiological effects of positive pressure ventilation have complex interactions with the lungs and other organ systems. Some of these physiological effects are beneficial while others may cause complications. This chapter discusses the side effects of positive pressure ventilation on the major organ systems of the body.

PULMONARY CONSIDERATIONS

This section compares the physiologic differences between spontaneous breathing and positive pressure ventilation. Two of the major effects are the changes in airway pressure and compliance.

SPONTANEOUS BREATHING

☑ During negative pressure ventilation, pressures in the airways, alveoli, and pleura are *decreased* during inspiration.

During spontaneous ventilation, the diaphragm and other respiratory muscles create gas flow by lowering the pleural, alveolar, and airway pressures. When alveolar and airway pressures drop below atmospheric pressure, air flows into the lungs (Pinsky, 1990). Negative pressure ventilation uses this principle by creating a negative pressure on the chest wall. When negative pressure is used for ventilation, the pressures in the airways, alveoli, and pleura are *decreased* during inspiration. Table 2-1 shows the relationship of barometric pressure (P_B) and alveolar pressure (P_A) during spontaneous breathing.

Pressures shown in Table 2-1 are for illustration purposes only. The barometric pressure is assigned 0 cm H_2O for easy comparison of pressure changes during spontaneous breathing. (Scanlan et al., 1999).

TABLE 2-1   Relationship of Barometric Pressure (P$_B$) and Alveolar Pressure (P$_A$) During Spontaneous Breathing

SPONTANEOUS BREATHING	P$_B$ (cm H$_2$O)	P$_A$ (cm H$_2$O)	$\triangle$P	FLOW
Inspiration	0	−5	−5	Into lungs
End-inspiration	0	0	0	None
Expiration	0	+5	+5	Out of lungs
End-expiration	0	0	0	None

positive pressure ventilation:
Mechanical ventilation in which the volume is delivered by a positive pressure gradient (i.e., airway pressures higher than alveolar pressure).

pressure-limited:
Termination of the inspiratory cycle when the preset pressure is reached.

volume-limited:
Termination of the inspiratory cycle when the preset volume is reached.

POSITIVE PRESSURE VENTILATION

During **positive pressure ventilation**, gas flow is delivered to the lungs under a positive pressure gradient (i.e., airway pressure is greater than alveolar pressure). Therefore, the tidal volume delivered to the lungs is directly related to the positive pressure when a **pressure-limited** ventilator is used. In **volume-limited** ventilators, the level of positive pressure is dependent on the mechanical tidal volume, as well as the patient's compliance and airway resistance.

When positive pressure is used for ventilation, the pressures in the airways, alveoli, and pleura are *increased* during inspiration (Pinsky, 1990). Table 2-2 shows the relationship of inspiratory pressure (P$_I$) and alveolar pressure (P$_A$) during positive pressure ventilation. Pressures in Table 2-2 are for illustration purposes only. The barometric pressure is assigned 0 cm H$_2$O for easy comparison of pressure changes during positive pressure ventilation.

Since the pressure gradient and tidal volume are directly related, a higher peak airway pressure observed during mechanical ventilation is usually related to a larger volume delivered. However, there are some exceptions to this relationship and some examples are presented in Table 2-3.

TABLE 2-2   Relationship of Inspiratory Pressure (P$_I$) and Alveolar Pressure (P$_A$) During Positive Pressure Ventilation

POSITIVE PRESSURE VENTILATION	P$_I$ (cm H$_2$O)	P$_A$ (cm H$_2$O)	$\triangle$P	FLOW
Inspiration	20	0	+20	Into lungs
End-inspiration	20	20	0	No flow
Expiration	0	20	−20	Out of lungs
End-expiration	0	0	0	No flow

TABLE 2-3   Conditions That Limit the Volume Delivered by Positive Pressure Ventilation

CONDITIONS	EXAMPLES
Peak airway pressure reached too soon	Airway obstruction Kinking of ET tube Bronchospasm Low lung compliance Pressure limit set too low
Unable to reach peak airway pressure	ET tube cuff leak Ventilator circuit leak

peak airway pressure (PAP): Maximum pressure measured during one respiratory cycle, usually at the end of inspiration.

AIRWAY PRESSURES

With a pressure-limited ventilator, the **peak airway pressure (PAP)** is preset according to the estimated tidal volume requirement of a patient. The inspiratory phase terminates once the preset pressure is reached. For this reason, the patient may receive a smaller volume when the preset pressure is reached prematurely as would happen under conditions of low compliance or high airway resistance.

With a volume-limited ventilator, the volume is preset and the pressure used by the ventilator to deliver this preset volume is variable. The PAP observed at the end of the inspiratory phase is higher under conditions of low compliance or high airway resistance. On the other hand, the PAP is lower under conditions of high compliance or low airway resistance.

mean airway pressure (MAWP): Average pressure within the airway during one complete respiratory cycle. It is directly related to the inspiratory time, respiratory rate, peak inspiratory pressure, and positive end-expiratory pressure (PEEP).

When using a volume ventilator, all airway pressures (including PAP and **mean airway pressure [MAWP]**) are directly related to tidal volume, airway resistance, and peak inspiratory flow rate; and inversely related to compliance.

These airway pressures (and lung volumes) have a direct impact on the intrathoracic pressure, blood flow, and blood pressure. Indirectly, they can affect the functions of different organ systems.

COMPLIANCE

In lungs with normal compliance, about 50% of the airway pressure is transmitted to the thoracic cavity. In noncompliant or "stiff" lungs (atelectasis, ARDS), the pressure transmitted to the thoracic cavity is much less due to the dampening effect of the nonelastic lung tissues. For this reason, high levels of PAP or positive end-expiratory pressure (PEEP) may be required to ventilate and oxygenate patients with low compliance. The decrease in cardiac output due to excessive PAP or PEEP is less severe, however, than if the same pressures are applied to lungs with normal or high compliance (Perkins et al., 1989).

CARDIOVASCULAR CONSIDERATIONS

positive end-expiratory pressure (PEEP): PEEP is an airway pressure strategy in ventilation that increases the end-expiratory or baseline airway pressure to a value greater than atmospheric pressure. It is used to treat refractory hypoxemia caused by intrapulmonary shunting.

Mechanical ventilation creates air flow by generating a pressure gradient. In turn, the pressures in the airways, thoracic cage, and pulmonary blood vessels are altered. In a clinical setting, the cardiovascular functions should be evaluated and monitored to prevent the adverse effects of mechanical ventilation on the heart and its vessels.

MEAN AIRWAY PRESSURE AND CARDIAC OUTPUT

Positive pressure ventilation increases MAWP and decreases cardiac output. Regardless of the mode of ventilation selected on the ventilator, a higher MAWP usually results in a lower cardiac output (Perkins et al., 1989). Since MAWP is a function of inspiratory time, respiratory rate, peak inspiratory pressure, and **positive end-expiratory pressure (PEEP)**, these four parameters should be kept to a minimum in order to maintain the MAWP at the lowest level possible.

continuous positive airway pressure (CPAP): The end-expiratory pressure applied to the airway of a spontaneously breathing patient.

In comparing **continuous positive airway pressure (CPAP)** and PEEP, PEEP reduces the cardiac output more severely as it causes a higher MAWP. This is because PEEP is used in addition to positive pressure ventilation, whereas CPAP is used in spontaneously breathing patients (Figure 2-1).

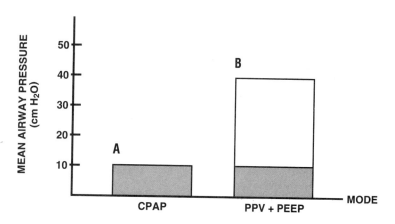

Figure 2-1 Comparison of mean airway pressure between (A) CPAP and (B) PEEP. The mean airway pressure is higher in (B) because PEEP (10 cm H_2O) is used in addition to positive pressure ventilation.

DECREASE IN CARDIAC OUTPUT AND O_2 DELIVERY

stroke volume:
Blood volume output delivered by one ventricular contraction.

Use of positive pressure ventilation can reduce the amount of oxygen available to the body. An increase in positive airway pressure generally causes a higher intrathoracic pressure. In turn, this pressure is transmitted to the airways and alveoli, as well as to the mediastinum, great vessels that return blood to the heart (Martini et al., 1989). This change in pressure leads to a reduction in **stroke volume** and cardiac output.

oxygen delivery:
Total amount of oxygen carried by blood. It is the product of O_2 content and cardiac output.

Since O_2 delivery is the product of O_2 content and cardiac output, reduction in stroke volume and cardiac output results in a decrease in **oxygen delivery.** As shown in the equation below and Figure 2-2, decreased cardiac output reduces O_2 delivery.

$$O_2 \text{ Content} \times \downarrow \text{Cardiac Output} = \downarrow O_2 \text{ Delivery}$$

BLOOD PRESSURE CHANGES

✓ For patients with cardiopulmonary disease or compromised cardiovascular reserve, positive pressure ventilation may cause blood pressure measurements to decrease.

During spontaneous inspiration, there is a transient decrease of arterial blood pressure readings. In certain disease states, such as acute asthma exacerbation, this physiologic decrease becomes exaggerated and is referred to as pulsus paradoxus (Wright et al., 1996). During positive pressure ventilation, reverse pulsus paradoxus is observed in which the arterial blood pressure is slightly higher than that measured during spontaneous breathing. During positive pressure ventilation, pressures measured in the aorta, left atrium, pulmonary artery, and right atrium are also slightly higher than those measured during spontaneous ventilation Because left ventricular end systolic volume has been shown to be reduced during a positive pressure inspiration while there is no change in left ventricular end diastolic volume, the mechanism of reverse pulsus paradoxus appears to be a reduction in left ventricular afterload (Abel, 1987). For patients with cardiopulmonary disease or compromised cardiovascular reserve, however, positive pressure ventilation may cause these pressure measurements to decrease. These measurements may also decrease when PAP or PEEP is at a level that compromises the cardiovascular function.

thoracic pump mechanism:
Alternations in pulmonary blood flow caused by changes in intrathoracic pressure during positive pressure ventilation. In hypotensive conditions, positive pressure ventilation decreases the blood flow to the left heart. In hypertensive conditions, this mechanism enhances the outflow of blood from the right ventricle and into the left heart.

PULMONARY BLOOD FLOW AND THORACIC PUMP MECHANISM

During positive pressure ventilation, intrathoracic pressure changes according to the pressure transmitted across the lung parenchyma. In turn, changes in intrathoracic pressure can affect the pulmonary blood flow entering and leaving the ventricles.

Left ventricle. In the left ventricle, the effect of an increase in lung volume on pulmonary venous blood flow is dependent on the relative state of filling of the pulmonary circulation. In patients who are hypotensive, an increase in tidal volume causes a decrease in pulmonary venous return to the left ventricle (Figure 2-3) (Pinsky, 1990).

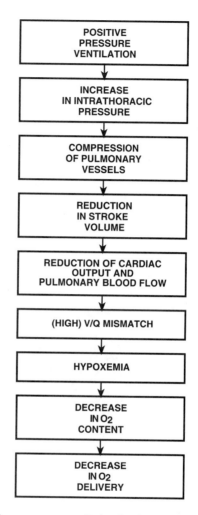

Figure 2-2 Positive pressure ventilation leads to a decrease in O_2 delivery.

In hypertensive patients, use of large tidal volumes increases venous return to the left ventricle (Figure 2-4) (Pinsky, 1990). This is because compression of pulmonary blood vessels is minimal in hypertensive conditions. It is also due in part to the **thoracic pump mechanism** where the blood flow from right to left ventricle is enhanced during the expiratory phase of positive pressure ventilation (DiCarlo et al., 1994).

Right ventricle. In the right ventricle, high airway pressures and large tidal volumes used in positive pressure ventilation stretch and compress the pulmonary blood vessels and limit their capacity to hold blood volume. During expiration the pulmonary vessels, no longer

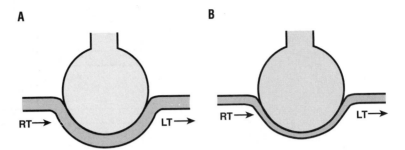

Figure 2-3 In hypotensive conditions, positive pressure ventilation decreases the blood flow to left heart. (A) spontaneous breathing; (B) positive pressure ventilation causes compression of the pulmonary blood vessels in hypotensive conditions.

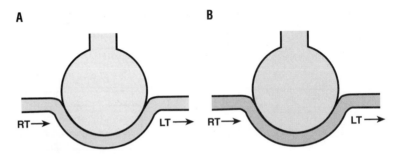

Figure 2-4 In hypertensive conditions, positive pressure ventilation increases the blood flow to left heart in part due to the thoracic pump mechanism (see text). (A) spontaneous breathing; (B) positive pressure ventilation does not cause significant compression of the pulmonary blood vessels in hypertensive conditions.

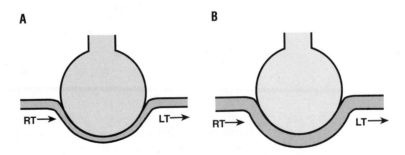

Figure 2-5 Thoracic pump mechanism. (A) During the inspiratory phase of positive pressure ventilation, the pulmonary blood vessels are compressed and the blood flow from right to left ventricle is decreased. (B) During the expiratory phase, the pulmonary blood vessels are no longer under alveolar compression and the blood flow from right to left ventricle is increased.

central venous pressure (CVP): Pressure measured in the vena cava or right atrium. It reflects the status of blood volume in the systemic circulation. Right ventricular preload.

pulmonary artery pressure: Pressure measured in the pulmonary artery. It reflects the volume status of the pulmonary artery and the functions of the ventricles. Right ventricular afterload.

pulmonary capillary wedge pressure: Pressure measured in the pulmonary artery with a balloon inflated to stop pulmonary blood flow. It reflects the volume status and functions of the left heart. Left ventricular preload.

under high pressure and large tidal volumes, are free to fill to their holding capacity with the blood leaving the right ventricle. This thoracic pump mechanism facilitates the outflow of blood from the right ventricle (Figure 2-5) (DiCarlo et al., 1994).

In children with right ventricular dysfunction, high positive pressure (up to 40 cm H_2O) and large tidal volumes (20 to 30 mL/kg) may reduce the work load of the right heart by the action of the thoracic pump mechanism (DiCarlo et al., 1994).

HEMODYNAMIC CONSIDERATIONS

One of the major adverse effects of mechanical ventilation is the changes in a patient's hemodynamic status. The major hemodynamic measurements affected by positive pressure ventilation include **central venous pressure (CVP),** and **pulmonary artery pressure.** The **pulmonary capillary wedge pressure** is not affected to a great extent because of the capability of the systemic venous circulation to compensate for changes in blood pressure and volume.

POSITIVE PRESSURE VENTILATION
Positive pressure ventilation causes an increase in intrathoracic pressure and compression of the pulmonary blood vessels. Partial recovery is observed during the expiratory phase. It is estimated that 15 to 20% of pulmonary blood volume is shifted to the systemic circulation at a tidal volume of 1 liter. An increase in intrathoracic pressure and compression of the pulmonary blood vessels causes an overall decrease in ventricular output, stroke volume, and pressure readings (Versprille, 1990).

Table 2-4 shows the general effects of positive pressure ventilation on hemodynamic measurements. It is essential to remember that the severity of these hemodynamic changes is dependent on the level of airway pressures, lung volume, and compliance characteristics of the patient.

POSITIVE END-EXPIRATORY PRESSURE
Positive end-expiratory pressure (PEEP) is a modality used in conjunction with positive pressure ventilation and it significantly increases the PAP and MAWP. In one study, when PEEP was initiated and increased to 15 cm H_2O over 90 seconds, the central venous pressure and pulmonary artery pressure showed a drastic increase while the aortic pressure and cardiac output showed a significant decrease (Versprille, 1990). PEEP must be used with extreme care in a clinical setting because PEEP, in addition to positive pressure ventilation, can potentiate the reduction in cardiac output.

Table 2-5 outlines the general effects of PEEP on hemodynamic measurements. It is important to remember that PEEP is used in conjunction

☑ PEEP increases peak airway and mean airway pressures.

☑ PEEP increases CVP and PAP but decreases aortic pressure and cardiac output.

TABLE 2-4   Effects of Positive Pressure Ventilation on Hemodynamic Measurements

PRESSURE OR VOLUME CHANGES	NOTES
Increase in intrathoracic pressure	Positive pressure applied to the lungs causes compression of the lung parenchyma against the chest wall.
Decrease in pulmonary blood volume and *Increase* in systemic blood volume	During the inspiratory phase of positive pressure ventilation, a fraction of the pulmonary blood volume is shifted to the systemic circulation. This does not increase the central venous pressure (CVP) because the systemic venous circulation can readily absorb this extra volume.
Decrease in venous return (CVP)	Higher intrathoracic pressure impedes systemic blood return to right ventricle.
Decrease in right ventricular stroke volume*	Decreased venous return to right ventricle leads to lower right ventricular output.
Decrease in pulmonary arterial pressure (PAP)	Decreased right ventricular stroke volume leads to lower blood volume (pressure) in the pulmonary arteries.
Decrease in filling pressures	Lower blood volume entering and leaving the ventricles.
Decrease in left ventricular stroke volume*	Decreased right ventricular stroke volume and pulmonary artery pressure lead to lower left ventricular input and output.

NOTE: In the absence of compensation by increasing the heart rate, decrease in right and left ventricular stroke volumes generally leads to a decreased cardiac output.

with positive pressure ventilation. For this reason, the hemodynamic changes may be different from those caused by positive pressure ventilation alone. The severity of these hemodynamic changes is also dependent on the lung volume and compliance.

The decrease in cardiac output due to positive pressure ventilation and PEEP can be managed by using intravascular volume expansion and positive inotropic support. A patient with adequate intravascular volume or one who receives a positive inotrope may have a smaller decline in cardiac output during positive pressure ventilation and PEEP (Perkins et al., 1989).

RENAL CONSIDERATIONS

Kidneys play an important role in eliminating wastes, clearance of certain drugs, and regulating fluid, electrolyte, and acid-base balance. The kidneys are highly vascular and at any one time receive about 25% of the body's circulating blood volume (Brundage, 1992). Because of these characteristics, they are highly vulnerable to decreases in blood flow as it would occur during positive pressure ventilation.

TABLE 2-5 **Effects of Positive End-Expiratory Pressure on Hemodynamic Measurements**

PRESSURE OR CARDIAC OUTPUT CHANGE	NOTES
Increase in pulmonary artery pressure (PAP)	PEEP and positive pressure applied to the lungs cause significant compression of pulmonary blood vessels.
Increase in central venous pressure (CVP)	Incease in PAP causes a higher right ventricular pressure and hinders blood return from systemic circulation to right heart. This causes backup of blood flow and increase in pressure in the systemic venous circulation.
Decrease in aortic pressure	This is due to the significant increase in intra-thoracic pressure and significant *decrease* in left and right ventricular stroke volumes.
Decrease in cardiac output	This is due to the significant increase in intra-thoracic pressure and significant *decrease* in left and right ventricular stroke volumes.

renal perfusion:
Blood flow to the kidneys. It is decreased when blood volume or cardiac output is low.

RENAL PERFUSION

When **renal perfusion** or perfusion of the glomeruli of the kidneys is decreased, filtration becomes less effective (Baer et al., 1992). Subsequently, the urine output is decreased as the kidneys try to correct the hypovolemic condition by retaining fluid. If hypoperfusion of the kidneys persists or worsens, renal failure may result.

INDICATORS OF RENAL FAILURE

For adequate removal of body wastes, urine output must be above 400 ml in a 24-hour period. Decreased urine output is an early sign of renal failure. This condition is called oliguria and is defined as urine output less than 400 ml in 24 hours (or less than 160 ml in 8 hours) (Kraus et al., 1993). Other early signs of renal failure include elevation of serum BUN (blood urea nitrogen) and creatinine, products of nitrogen metabolism (King, 1994). The kidney is responsible for eliminating these nitrogenous wastes to prevent toxic accumulation in the body; thus an increase in serum levels of BUN and creatinine indicates compromised renal function. See Table 2-6 for other major serum indicators of renal failure.

☑ Oliguria is defined as urine output < 400 ml in 24 hours (or < 160 ml in 8 hours).

EFFECTS OF RENAL FAILURE ON DRUG CLEARANCE

Whenever the kidneys are not functioning properly, their performance is hindered. Renal dysfunction from any cause can affect all normal kidney functions, including fluid and electrolyte regulation and drug clearance.

TABLE 2-6 **Serum Indicators of Renal Failure**

SERUM MEASUREMENTS	NORMAL	RENAL FAILURE
Blood urea nitrogen (BUN)	10 to 20 mg/dl	Increased
Creatinine	0.7 to 1.5 mg/dl	Increased
BUN to creatinine ratio	10:1	Normal or increased
Potassium	3 to 5 mEq/L	Usually increased
Sodium	138 to 142 mEq/L	Usually decreased

✓ Hypoperfusion of the kidneys may affect the rate of drug clearance and lead to a higher drug concentration in the circulation.

Hypoperfusion. Hypoperfusion of the kidneys may affect the rate of drug clearance. For example, the duration of neuromuscular blockade after short-term use of pancuronium or vecuronium may be prolonged in renal failure. The duration of muscle paralysis may be as long as 7 days after receiving vecuronium for more than 2 days (Hansen-Flaschen et al., 1993). It is therefore essential to note the effects of renal failure and the possibility of prolonged neuromuscular blockade when measuring a patient's lung mechanics or attempting to wean a patient from mechanical ventilation.

Glomerular Filtration Rate (GFR). Decreased renal function caused by positive pressure ventilation may also affect other drugs whose clearance is mainly dependent on the glomerular filtration rate (GFR) of the kidneys. Glomerular filtration results from high pressure within the glomerulus or renal capillary. This is caused by differences in the tone of the afferent and efferent arterioles, the vessels that lead into and out of the glomerulus. The afferent arteriole is maintained in a somewhat dilated state relative to the efferent arteriole, which is always somewhat constricted. When blood flow to the kidney is normal, a hydrostatic pressure head causes the high rate of renal perfusion seen in the normovolemic state. When coupled with back pressure from the partially constricted efferent arteriole, pressures within the glomerulus are maintained at an elevated state and are responsible for its ultrafiltration function. When renal perfusion drops, the pressure causing glomerular filtration decreases, leading to a decrease in filtration.

Examples of drugs that are eliminated by this mechanism include digoxin, vancomycin, beta-lactam antibiotics, and the aminoglycosides (Perkins et al., 1989). A decrease in GFR causes a relatively higher concentration of these drugs in the circulation.

Tubular Secretion. Another group of drugs whose elimination could be reduced by a lower renal blood flow are drugs undergoing tubular secretion. Tubular secretion is the mechanism whereby substances are secreted from the blood via the peritubular capillaries into the renal tubule to become a part of the urine. Examples of drugs that are eliminated by this mechanism include digoxin, furosemide, procainamide, and some penicillins (Perkins et al., 1989). Decrease of renal tubular secretion causes a relatively higher concentration of these drugs in the circulation.

Reabsorption. The third group of drugs whose elimination could be decreased are those being reabsorbed at a higher rate. Reabsorption in the renal tubules is the mechanism whereby required substances that are filtered by the glomerulus are reclaimed by the cells lining the renal tubule and are ultimately reabsorbed into the blood. Some of these substances are reabsorbed down their concentration gradient; thus an enhanced concentration gradient could lead to increased reabsorption.

As cardiac output is reduced by mechanical ventilation, renal blood flow and, thus, urine volume are also reduced. As the urine becomes more concentrated, the drugs in the glomerular filtrate also become more concentrated. This causes an increase in the reabsorption gradient of the drugs in the filtrate. Some of the drugs used in critically ill patients include aminoglycosides, theophylline, and phenobarbital (Perkins et al., 1989). Decreased renal perfusion causes a higher reabsorption rate of these drugs back into the circulation.

HEPATIC CONSIDERATIONS

hepatic perfusion: Blood flow to the liver. It is decreased when the blood volume or cardiac output is low.

Hepatic perfusion accounts for about 15% of total cardiac output. Positive pressure ventilation alone does not alter the blood flow to the liver to any significant degree. But when PEEP is added to mechanical ventilation, the blood flow to the liver is noticeably reduced (Bonnet et al., 1982).

PEEP AND HEPATIC PERFUSION

The decrease in hepatic blood flow is inversely related to the level of PEEP. In one study, the hepatic blood flow decreased 3, 12, and 32% at PEEP of 10, 15, and 20 cm H_2O, respectively (Bonnet et al., 1982). The decrease in hepatic blood flow is solely caused by a reduction in cardiac output as a result of PEEP. This inference is made because the ratio of hepatic blood flow to cardiac output remains unchanged at 15% during mechanical ventilation without PEEP (Perkins et al., 1989).

INDICATORS OF LIVER DYSFUNCTION

☑ Impairment of liver function is likely when prothrombin time is > 4 seconds, bilirubin level is ≥ 50 mg/L, or albumin level is ≤ 20 g/L.

Liver dysfunction may be monitored by measuring the prothrombin time and bilirubin and albumin levels (Kraus et al., 1993). Impairment of liver function is likely when coagulation time is increased (prothrombin time > 4 seconds over control, bilirubin level is increased (≥ 50 mg/L), or albumin level is decreased (≤ 20 g/L).

EFFECTS OF DECREASED HEPATIC PERFUSION ON DRUG CLEARANCE

☑ Hypoperfusion of the liver may affect the rate of drug clearance and lead to a higher drug concentration in the circulation.

A decrease in hepatic blood flow may diminish the drug clearance mechanism of the liver. Drugs most likely to be affected by changes in hepatic blood flow are agents whose clearance relies on the liver and its perfusion. Examples of such drugs commonly used in the intensive care unit include lidocaine, meperidine, propranolol, and verapamil (Perkins et al., 1989). When hepatic perfusion is inadequate, use of these drugs may lead to a relatively higher serum concentration due to diminished drug clearance.

ABDOMINAL CONSIDERATIONS

intra-abdominal pressure (IAP): Pressure measured by a transducer via a transurethral bladder catheter.

Increases in **intra-abdominal pressure (IAP)** are related to clinical conditions such as bowel edema or obstruction and ascites. IAP may also be increased in procedures such as use of pneumatic antishock garments and surgical repair of abdominal wall hernias. When these patients are placed on mechanical ventilation, conditions that are conducive to an increase in IAP should be monitored to avert potential complications.

EFFECTS OF PEEP AND INCREASED INTRA-ABDOMINAL PRESSURE

☑ Elevated intra-abdominal pressure transmits excessive pressure across the diaphragm to the heart and great vessels. In turn, this excess pressure leads to decreased cardiac output and decreased renal perfusion.

An elevated IAP transmits excessive pressure across the diaphragm to the heart and great vessels. In turn, this excessive pressure leads to decreased cardiac output (Cullen et al., 1989) and decreased renal perfusion (Harman et al., 1982). Excessive IAP also compresses the lungs and reduces the functional residual capacity (Burchard et al., 1985). It has been shown that use of PEEP on patients with elevated IAP may lead to cardiovascular, renal, and pulmonary dysfunction (Burchard et al., 1985; Cullen et al., 1989; Harman et al., 1982). These types of dysfunction are summarized in Table 2-7.

Use of high levels of PEEP (>15 cm H_2O) in the presence of high IAP (>20 mm Hg) requires caution because of potentiation of the pressures exerted on the heart and great vessels (Sussman et al., 1991). However, the pressures transmitted to the heart and great vessels are not as severe in patients with low pulmonary compliance due to the dampening effects of the noncompliant lungs and chest wall.

NUTRITIONAL CONSIDERATIONS

Malnutrition in critically ill patients can create muscle fatigue, ventilatory insufficiency, and ventilatory failure. This sequence of events can lead to a need for mechanical ventilation. It can also make weaning from mechanical ventilation difficult or unsuccessful. Adequate

TABLE 2-7 **Effects of PEEP and Increased Intra-abdominal Pressure**

SYSTEM	EFFECTS
Cardiovascular	Increased peripheral vascular resistance Decreased compliance of ventricles Decreased cardiac output
Renal	Decreased renal perfusion Decreased glomerular filtration rate
Pulmonary	Decreased functional residual capacity Increased atelectasis Impaired gas exchange Increased V/Q mismatch and venous admixture

nutritional support is therefore essential in the management of critically ill patients. However, excessive nutritional support is undesirable since it may cause excessive carbon dioxide production, as well as increased work of breathing from the need to eliminate excessive CO_2 (van den Berg and Stam, 1988).

MUSCLE FATIGUE

✓ COPD patients have higher caloric needs because of the increased work of breathing associated with chronic air flow obstruction.

The work of breathing can be affected by mechanical aberrations such as changes in airway resistance and lung or chest wall compliance. In clinical conditions where there is a persistent increase in airway resistance (e.g., COPD) or reduction in compliance (e.g., atelectasis), the respiratory muscles must work strenuously to overcome the abnormal resistance and compliance. For instance, COPD patients use 430 to 720 kcal per day to carry out the work of breathing. This caloric cost of breathing for COPD patients is about 10 times that of normal individuals (normal = 38 to 72 kcal/d) (Brown et al., 1983) because of the increased work of breathing necessary to overcome the high airway resistance and V/Q abnormalities.

Over time, these abnormalities may cause fatigue of the respiratory muscles, and ventilatory failure with concurrent CO_2 retention and hypoxemia (Brown et al., 1994).

Other than the mechanical aberrations that can lead to increased work of breathing and eventual muscle fatigue, there are nonmechanical factors as well. Malnutrition is an example of a nonmechanical cause of muscle fatigue that may lead to ventilatory failure (Fiaccadori et al., 1991).

Table 2-8 shows the major mechanical and nonmechanical factors that may lead to reduced respiratory muscle efficiency and muscle fatigue.

TABLE 2-8 **Factors Leading to Respiratory Muscle Fatigue**

MECHANICAL FACTORS	NONMECHANICAL FACTORS
High airway resistance	Malnutrition
Low lung compliance	Endocrine diseases (high metabolic rate)
Low chest wall compliance	Electrolyte disorders
	Drugs
	Persistent hypoxemia

(Data from Fiaccadori et al., 1991; Grassino et al., 1984; Rochester, 1986.)

NUTRITIONAL SUPPORT

Adequate nutrition is a therapeutic necessity in order to provide and preserve inspiratory muscle strength and prevent ventilatory failure. Patients who have respiratory disorders are likely to lose weight due to increased work of breathing, decreased nutritional intake, and infectious states causing increased metabolic rate (Mlynarek and Zarowitz, 1987).

Undernutrition in patients with or without COPD is found to deplete their stores of glycogen and protein in the diaphragm. In addition, COPD patients who suffer from decreased protein synthesis in the diaphragm may lose diaphragm muscle mass (Mlynarek and Zarowitz, 1987). Since the diaphragm is the major respiratory muscle, loss of muscle mass in the diaphragm may reduce the efficiency of ventilation.

It has been demonstrated that patients who receive 2,000 to 3,000 kcal per day exhibit better inspiratory strengths and endurance than those receiving only 400 kcal per day (Bassili et al., 1981). Energy requirements for critically ill patients are normally computed using the Harris-Benedict equation. This equation estimates the resting energy expenditure (REE) based on weight, height, age, and sex (Roza et al., 1984). In ventilator patients who are hypermetabolic or hypercatabolic (i.e., infection, trauma, burns), a correction factor is included to allow for additional metabolic needs. It ranges from 1.0 to 1.2 times the REE for maintenance of lean body mass and 1.4 to 1.6 times the REE for restoration of lean body mass (Mlynarek and Zarowitz, 1987).

NUTRITION AND THE WORK OF BREATHING

Total parenteral nutrition (TPN) or hyperalimentation is a complete nutritional program provided to patients by any method (usually intravenous) other than the intestinal route. It is often used to support and supplement a patient's nutritional needs with a hypertonic solution consisting of amino acids, glucose, vitamins, electrolytes, and fat

total parenteral nutrition (TPN): *Complete nutritional support provided to the patient by any method (usually intravenous) other than the intestinal route.*

emulsion. When TPN is used, it is essential to keep the amount of dextrose (a form of glucose) to a minimum as it can cause lipogenesis and increase O_2 consumption and CO_2 production. Contribution to the total caloric needs by glucose should be in the range of 40 to 60% (Brown et al., 1984).

Since hydrous dextrose generates 3.4 kcal per gram and fat emulsion provides 9.1 kcal per gram, fat is the ideal source of energy for patients who have restricted fluid intake. Fat also reduces CO_2 production, a by-product of glucose metabolism, thus reducing the work of breathing (Brown et al., 1983). A fat-based TPN should be considered for patients with significant or persistent CO_2 retention as fat emulsion may provide maximum caloric intake with minimum CO_2 production.

> ✔ Since fat emulsion provides 9.1 kcal per gram, it provides maximum caloric intake with minimum CO_2 production.

It is important to note that the work of breathing is significantly increased in patients receiving high caloric intake by means of TPN. The increase in work of breathing is primarily due to increases in oxygen consumption and carbon dioxide production during TPN (van den Berg and Stam, 1988). Mechanical ventilation and weaning strategies must take this fact into account in order to provide adequate support for a patient's ventilatory needs.

The increase in $\dot{V}CO_2$ causes a rise in $PaCO_2$, resulting in respiratory acidosis. Ventilatory failure can occur if the patient is unable to increase ventilation in proportion to the increase of CO_2 production. This is particularly important in patients with impaired ventilatory reserves such as those with obstructive or restrictive lung diseases.

NEUROLOGICAL CONSIDERATIONS

Among many other monitoring systems that influence the respiratory drive, the central and peripheral chemoreceptors respond rapidly to the levels of CO_2, H+, and O_2 in the blood. For this reason, the degree of ventilation (CO_2, H+) and oxygenation (O_2) can affect the normal functions of the brain.

HYPERVENTILATION

Carbon dioxide acts as a vasodilator in cerebral blood vessels. During mechanical ventilation, intentional hyperventilation is sometimes used to constrict these blood vessels, and thus minimize intracranial pressure in patients with head injury. Sustained hyperventilation of less than 24 hours causes respiratory alkalosis, reducing cerebral blood flow and intracranial pressure. After 24 hours, the buffer systems of the body return the pH toward normal, negating the vasoconstrictor effect of controlled hyperventilation.

> ✔ Sustained hyperventilation of less than 24 hours causes respiratory alkalosis and reduces cerebral blood flow and intracranial pressure.

If hyperventilation is prolonged, cerebral tissue hypoxia may result due to the leftward shift of the oxyhemoglobin curve. A left shift

TABLE 2-9 Neurological Changes in Hyperventilation

CONDITION	PATHOPHYSIOLOGIC CHANGES
Respiratory alkalosis (<24 hours)	Decreased cerebral blood flow Reduced intracranial pressure
Respiratory alkalosis (Prolonged >24 hours)	Leftward shift of oxyhemoglobin curve Increased O_2 affinity for hemoglobin Reduced O_2 release to tissues Cerebral tissue hypoxia Neurologic dysfunction Hypophosphatemia

causes higher oxygen affinity for hemoglobin but reduced oxygen release to tissues. Sustained hyperventilation also produces significant hypophosphatemia because of movement of phosphate into the cells. Hypophosphatemia interferes with cerebral tissue metabolism by reducing ATP stores and 2,3-DPG levels, which further increases the leftward shift of the oxyhemoglobin curve (Jozefowicz, 1989). Table 2-9 summarizes the neurological changes in short-term (< 24 hours) and sustained (> 24 hours) hyperventilation.

VENTILATORY AND OXYGENATION FAILURE

Ventilatory and oxygenation failure has serious and detrimental effects on the central nervous system (CNS). Such failure may occur in patients on mechanical ventilation because of preexisting clinical conditions, making ventilation and oxygenation extremely difficult to accomplish in spite of high F_IO_2 and PEEP.

Abnormalities in ventilation and gas exchange can cause hypercapnia (increase in $PaCO_2$), respiratory acidosis (decrease in pH as a result of the increased $PaCO_2$), hypoxemia (decrease in PaO_2), secondary polycythemia (increase in red blood cell concentration and thus hemoglobin level), and electrolyte disturbances. These changes may lead to neurological impairment.

INDICATORS OF NEUROLOGICAL IMPAIRMENT

☑ Headache, mental status changes, motor disturbances, and ocular abnormalities may be signs of neurological impairment.

When neurological functions are impaired due to ventilatory and oxygenation failure, the patient may experience headache, mental status changes, motor disturbances, and ocular abnormalities (Jozefowicz, 1989).

The patient usually describes the headache as "pressure in the head" having a higher intensity during night and early morning hours. The headache is the result of cerebral vasodilation in response to hypoventilation and CO_2 retention during sleep.

Hypoxia, hypercapnia, and acidosis are responsible for the changes in a patient's mental status. Early mental disturbances include

TABLE 2-10   Neurological Changes in Hypercapnia and Hypoxemia

CONDITION	PHYSIOLOGIC CHANGES
Hypercapnia (with normal pH)	Increased cerebral blood flow Increased intracranial pressure
Hypercapnia (with low pH)	Impaired cerebral metabolism
Hypoxemia	Decreased mental and motor functions

drowsiness, forgetfulness, and irritability. In severe or chronic cases of hypoxia and hypercapnia, stupor and coma may occur.

Hypercapnia may also cause muscle tremor and ocular abnormalities. Muscle tremor is the result of excessive stimulation of the sympathetic nervous system and catecholamine release from the adrenal medulla. Ocular abnormalities such as papilledema, swelling of the area where the optic nerve exits the back of the eye, is the result of cerebral vasodilation and elevated intracranial pressure. Table 2-10 illustrates some neurological changes in hypercapnia and hypoxemia.

SUMMARY

Positive pressure ventilation is beneficial to support a patient's ventilatory and oxygenation needs. However, it has many inherent physiological side effects on other organ systems. When caring for critically ill patients with positive pressure ventilation, it is vital to observe and monitor the patients carefully for occurrence of side effects. If side effects and their causes are identified, appropriate strategies should be used to resolve them.

Self-Assessment Questions

1. During the inspiratory phase of positive pressure ventilation, gas flows into the lung because the pressure in the:

    A. airway is higher than the pressure in the lungs.

    B. airway is lower than the pressure in the lungs.

    C. lungs is higher than the barometric pressure.

    D. lungs and airway are the same.

2. A neonate is being ventilated by a pressure-limited ventilator. The physician asks you to adjust the ventilator to increase the patient's mechanical tidal volume. You would:

    A. increase the tidal volume setting.

    B. increase the pressure setting.

    C. decrease the flow rate.

    D. decrease the inspiratory time.

3. A postoperative patient is recovering in the intensive care unit on a volume-limited ventilator. For a volume-limited ventilator, the _____ is preset with a variable _____ depending on the compliance and airway resistance characteristics.

   A. peak airway pressure, tidal volume   C. tidal volume, peak airway pressure
   B. peak airway pressure, peak flow   D. tidal volume, peak flow

4. Positive pressure ventilation decreases the oxygen delivery to a patient with normal hemodynamic status because it causes all of the following changes *except:*

   A. increase in intrathoracic pressure.   C. increase in pulmonary blood flow.
   B. reduction in stroke volume.   D. decrease in cardiac output.

5. In children with right ventricular dysfunction, the thoracic pump mechanism _____ the outflow of blood from the _____ ventricle.

   A. increases, left   C. increases, right
   B. decreases, left   D. decreases, right

6 to 11. For *positive pressure ventilation,* match the volume and pressure changes with the respective reasons.

Pressure or Volume Change	Reasons
6. *Increase* in intrathoracic pressure	A. Decreased venous return to right ventricle leads to lower right ventricular output.
7. *Decrease* in venous return or central venous pressure	B. Decreased right ventricular stroke volume and pulmonary artery pressure lead to lower left ventricular input and output.
8. *Decrease* in right ventricular stroke volume	C. Higher intrathoracic pressure impedes systemic blood return to right ventricle.
9. *Decrease* in pulmonary arterial pressure	D. Positive pressure applied to the lungs causes compression against the chest wall.
10. *Decrease* in filling pressures	E. Decreased right ventricular stroke volume leads to lower blood volume (pressure) in the pulmonary arteries.
11. *Decrease* in left ventricular stroke volume	F. Lower blood volume entering and leaving the ventricles.

12 to 15. For *positive end-expiratory pressure,* match the pressure and cardiac output changes with the respective reasons. You may use any answer *more than once.*

Pressure or Cardiac Output Change	Reasons
12. *Increase* in pulmonary artery pressure	A. Increase in pulmonary artery pressure causes a higher right ventricular pressure and hinders the blood return from systemic circulation to right heart. This causes backup of blood flow and increase in pressure in the systemic venous circulation.
13. *Increase* in central venous pressure (CVP)	B. This is due to the significant increase in intrathoracic pressure and significant *decrease* in left and right ventricular stroke volumes.
14. *Decrease* in aortic pressure	C. PEEP and positive pressure applied to the lungs cause significant compression of pulmonary blood vessels.
15. *Decrease* in cardiac output	

16. A patient in the renal dialysis unit has recently been placed on a ventilator because of ventilatory and oxygenation failure. In caring for this patient, which of the following laboratory results would indicate that the patient's renal functions are failing?

A. blood urea nitrogen of 30 mg/dl
B. creatinine of 1.0 mg/dl
C. potassium of 3 mEq/L
D. sodium of 140 mEq/L

17. For patients with renal _____ or failure, the drug concentration in the circulation is usually _____ than normal when clearance of those drugs is dependent on proper renal perfusion.

A. hyperperfusion, higher
B. hyperperfusion, lower
C. hypoperfusion, higher
D. hypoperfusion, lower

18. Perfusion to the liver is usually affected by a high level of _____ and hepatic failure may be present when the _____.

A. positive pressure ventilation, bilirubin level is less than 50 mg/L.
B. positive pressure ventilation, albumin level is less than 20 mg/L.
C. positive end-expiratory pressure, bilirubin level is greater than 50 mg/L.
D. positive end-expiratory pressure, albumin level is greater than 20 mg/L.

19. Cardiovascular, renal, and pulmonary dysfunction may occur in patients with an intra-abdominal pressure _____ when positive end-expiratory pressure _____ is used during mechanical ventilation.

    A. greater than 15 mm Hg, greater than 15 cm H_2O

    B. greater than 20 mm Hg, greater than 15 cm H_2O

    C. less than 15 mm Hg, greater than 15 cm H_2O

    D. greater than 20 mm Hg, less than 15 cm H_2O

20. For patients with increased work of breathing and CO_2 retention, the caloric intake should be _____ than normal and the source of nutrition should be _____-based so as to provide maximum calorie intake and minimum CO_2 production.

    A. higher, fat

    B. higher, dextrose

    C. lower, fat

    D. lower, dextrose

21. Hyperventilation is sometimes provided for patients with increased intracranial pressure. This is done because respiratory _____ can reduce the intracranial pressure by _____ the cerebral blood vessels.

    A. acidosis, dilating

    B. acidosis, constricting

    C. alkalosis, dilating

    D. alkalosis, constricting

22. Headache, drowsiness, and irritability are some signs of altered _____ status resulting from hypoxemia and hypercapnia.

    A. renal

    B. hepatic

    C. nutritional

    D. neurological

References

Abel, J. G. et al. (1987). Cardiovascular effects of positive pressure ventilation in humans. *Ann Thorac Surg, 43,* 198–206.

Baer, C. L. et al. (1992). Acute renal failure. *Critical Care Nursing Quarterly, 14*(4), 1.

Bassili, H. R. et al. (1981). Effect of nutritional support on weaning patients off mechanical ventilators. *J Parenter Enter Nutr, 5,* 161–163.

Bonnet, F. et al. (1982). Changes in hepatic flow induced by continuous positive-pressure ventilation in critically ill patients. *Crit Care Med, 10,* 703–705.

Brown, B. R. (1994). Understanding mechanical ventilation: Indications for and initiation of therapy. *J Okla State Med Assoc, 87,* 353–357.

Brown, R. O. et al. (1984). Nutrition and respiratory disease. *Clin Pharm, 3,* 152–160.

Brown, S. E. et al. (1983). What is now known about protein-energy depletion: When COPD patients are malnourished. *J Respir Dis, 4*(5), 36–50.

Brundage, D. J. (1992). *Renal disorders.* St. Louis: Mosby-Year Book.

Burchard, K. W. et al. (1985). Positive end-expiratory pressure with increased intra-abdominal pressure. *Surg Gynecol Obstet, 161,* 313–318.

Cullen, D. J. et al. (1989). Cardiovascular, pulmonary and renal effect of massively increased intra-abdominal pressure in critically ill patients. *Crit Care Med, 17,* 118–121.

DiCarlo, J. V. et al. (1994). Respiratory failure in congenital heart disease. *Pediatric Clinics of North America, 41*(3), 525–542.

Fiaccadori, E. et al. (1991). Pathophysiology of respiratory muscles in course of under-nutrition. *Ann Ital Med Int, 6,* 402–407.

Grassino, A. et al. (1984). Respiratory muscle fatigue and ventilatory failure. *Am Rev Respir Dis, 35,* 625–647.

Hansen-Flaschen, J. et al. (1993). Neuromuscular blockade in the intensive care unit—More than we bargained for. *Am Rev Respir Dis, 147,* 234–236.

Harman, P. K. et al. (1982). Elevated intra-abdominal pressure and renal function. *Ann Surg, 196,* 594–597.

Jozefowicz, R. F. (1989). Neurologic manifestations of pulmonary disease. *Neurologic Clinics, 7*(3), 605–616.

King, B. A. (1994, March). Detecting acute renal failure. *RN,* 34–40.

Kraus, P. A. et al. (1993). Acute lung injury at Baragwanath ICU—An eight-month audit and call for consensus for other organ failure in the adult respiratory distress syndrome. *Chest, 103*(6), 1832–1836.

Marini, J. J., & Wheeler, A. P. (1989). *Critical care medicine: The essentials.* Baltimore: Williams & Wllkins.

Mlynarek, M., & Zarowitz, B. J. (1987). Individualizing nutrition in patients with acute respiratory failure requiring mechanical ventilation. *Drug Intell Clin Pharm (EBU), 21*(11), 865–870.

Perkins, M. W. et al. (1989). Physiologic implications of mechanical ventilation on pharmacokinetics. *DICP, The Annals of Pharmacotherapy, 23,* 316–323.

Pinsky, M. R. (1990). The effects of mechanical ventilation on the cardiovascular system. *Critical Care Clinics, 6*(3), 663–678.

Rochester, D. F. (1986). Respiratory effects of respiratory muscle weakness and atrophy. *Am Rev Respir Dis, 134,* 1083–1086.

Roza, A. M. et al. (1984). The Harris-Benedict equation reevaluated: Resting energy requirements and the body cell mass. *Am J Clin Nutr, 40,* 168–182.

Scanlan, C. L. et al. (1999). *Egan's fundamentals of respiratory care* (7th ed.). St. Louis: Mosby-Year Book.

Sussman, A. M. et al. (1991). Effect of positive end-expiratory pressure on intra-abdominal pressure. *Southern Med J, 84*(6), 697–700.

van den Berg, B., & Stam, H. (1988). Metabolic and respiratory effects of enteral nutrition in patients during mechanical ventilation. *Intensive Care Med, 14,* 206–211.

Versprille, V. (1990). The pulmonary circulation during mechanical ventilation. *Acta Anaesthesiol Scand, 34, Supplementum, 94,* 51–62.

Wright, R. O. et al. (1996) Continuous, noninvasive measurement of pulsus paradoxus in patients with acute asthma. *Archives of Pediatric and Adolescent medicine, 150*(9): 914–918.

CHAPTER THREE

CLASSIFICATION OF MECHANICAL VENTILATORS

Gary C. White

OUTLINE

KEY TERMS

- compressor
- controller
- cycle
- flow triggered
- microprocessor
- pneumatic drive mechanism

- pressure triggered
- reducing valve
- servo
- sine wave
- solenoid valve
- time triggered

INTRODUCTION

The role of patient management in many situations is dependent upon the respiratory care practitioner's understanding of mechanical ventilators and their characteristics. This applies to the acute care setting for all ages: adults, pediatrics, and neonatal patients. The same is also true in the transport and long-term care environments. Therefore, it is important for the respiratory care practitioner to understand classification of mechanical ventilators and the design characteristics employed by a ventilator to achieve the task of supporting a patient's ventilation.

In this chapter, you learn how ventilators are classified according to Chatburn's classification system and how the common ventilators employed in various patient care settings are classified.

VENTILATOR CLASSIFICATION

Ventilator technology has evolved since the introduction of mechanical ventilators over thirty years ago. Since that time, a multitude of manufacturers have produced and marketed ventilators of all sizes, descriptions, and capabilities. Many manufacturers have coined new terms to describe their ventilators and to accentuate how their product is different from the others. Several different ventilator classification systems may be employed to describe mechanical ventilators. The majority of these systems focus on the differences between ventilators rather than the similarities.

Robert Chatburn (1992) has proposed a new way to classify mechanical ventilators based on related features, physics, and engineering. Chatburn's ventilator classification system has been featured in several articles and textbooks. It allows flexibility as ventilator technology evolves in contrast to other systems that employ more narrowly defined design principles or rely to a greater extent on manufacturer's terms.

As ventilator technology evolves over the next decade or more, the flexibility of Chatburn's classification system will be validated. Unfortunately today, not all practitioners or educators have adopted this newer classification system. This author believes this system is important enough to include in this text and others that describe ventilator operational characteristics. Students and practitioners learning about this classification system should refer to the bibliography at the conclusion of this chapter and read Chatburn's original contributions.

VENTILATORY WORK

Pulmonary physiologists have described the work ventilatory muscles perform during inspiration, and how muscles can actively assist during exhalation. During inspiration, the primary ventilatory muscles cause the size (volume) of the thoracic cage to increase, overcoming the elastic forces of the lungs and thorax and the resistance of the airways. As the volume of the thoracic cage increases, intrapleural pressure becomes more negative, resulting in lung expansion as the visceral pleura expands with the parietal pleura. Gas flows from the atmosphere into the lungs as a result of the transairway pressure gradient. During expiration, the muscles of inspiration relax. The elastic forces of the lung and thorax cause the chest to decrease in volume. Exhalation occurs as a result of the greater pressure at the alveolus when compared to atmospheric pressure. All of this muscle activity to overcome the elastic and resistance properties of the lungs and thorax requires energy and work.

The work that the muscles and/or the ventilator must perform is proportional to the pressure required for inspiration times the tidal volume. The pressure required to deliver the tidal volume is referred to as the "load" either the muscles or the ventilator must work against. There is an elastic load (proportional to volume and inversely proportional to compliance) and a resistance load (proportional to airway resistance and inspiratory flow). These variables are related by the equation of motion for the respiratory system:

$$\text{Muscle Pressure} + \text{Ventilator Pressure} = \frac{\text{Volume}}{\text{Compliance}} + (\text{Resistance} \times \text{Flow})$$

Compliance is defined as a change in volume divided by a change in pressure, which is a measure of the elastic forces of the lungs and thorax. Flow as defined earlier, is a unit of volume divided by a unit of time. Resistance is the force that must be overcome to move gas through the conducting airways, which is best described by Poiseulle's Law.

A mechanical ventilator is simply a machine or device that can fully or partially substitute for the ventilatory work accomplished by the patient's muscles. If the patient's ventilatory muscles contribute no work (sedation, paralysis, etc.), the mechanical ventilator provides full ventilatory support. If the patient's muscles are able to sustain all of the patient's ventilatory requirements, no support is provided by the machine and ventilatory support is zero. Between the two extremes, partial support can be provided by the mechanical ventilator in assisting the ventilatory muscles.

INPUT POWER

Mechanical ventilators may be first classified as to the power source that is used to provide the energy required to support the patient's ventilation. As described earlier, ventilation requires work and therefore, energy.

Pneumatically powered ventilators use compressed gas as an energy source for their operation. Medical gases are anhydrous, and oil-free at a pressure of 50 psi. Examples of ventilators that utilize pneumatic power include the Bennett PR-2, Bird Mark 7, Percussionaire IPV, Monaghan 225/SIMV and the Percussionaire VDR.

Ventilators may also be electrically powered, utilizing 120 V 60 Hz alternating current (AC) or 12 V direct current (DC) for a power source. The electrical power can be used to run electric motors to drive pistons, **compressors** or other mechanical devices that generate gas flow. Examples of electrically powered ventilators include the Emerson 3-MV, Aequitron Medical LP-10, BEAR Medical Systems BEAR 33, and the Puritan-Bennett 2801 Companion.

Some ventilators are powered by a combination of both pneumatic and electric power sources. Many third-generation ventilators require both an electrical (for **microprocessor** control systems) and pneumatic power source. These ventilators include the BEAR 1000, Hamilton Veolar, Puritan-Bennett 7200ae, and others.

DRIVE MECHANISM

The drive mechanism is the system used by the ventilator to transmit or convert the input power to useful ventilatory work. The type of drive mechanism determines the characteristic flow and pressure patterns each ventilator produces. The use of microprocessors and proportional **solenoid valves** allows these newer ventilators to produce a variety of user-selected inspiratory flow or pressure patterns. An understanding of the different drive mechanisms will allow you to apply a ventilator more effectively in the clinical environment. Drive mechanisms include pistons, bellows, **reducing valves** and pneumatic circuits.

compressor: A device capable of building up pressure by compressing the volume of air.

microprocessor: Minute computer that is designed to perform specific functions.

solenoid valve: A valve controlled by an electronic switching device that is used to regulate the specific functions of a ventilator.

reducing valve: A device that decreases the delivery pressure of a gas.

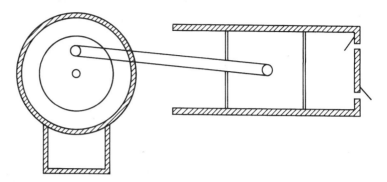

Figure 3-1 A schematic diagram of a rotary-driven piston drive mechanism for a mechanical ventilator.

PISTON DRIVE MECHANISM

An electrically driven piston with an inspiratory one-way valve can be used to generate a pressure gradient to drive a ventilator (Figure 3-1). During the backstroke of the piston, gas enters the cylinder through the one-way valve. When the piston travels in the opposite direction, a second one-way valve opens, delivering the compressed gas to the patient.

Pistons are usually electrically powered. However, they may be rotary or linear driven. Figure 3-2 compares a linear-driven and rotary-

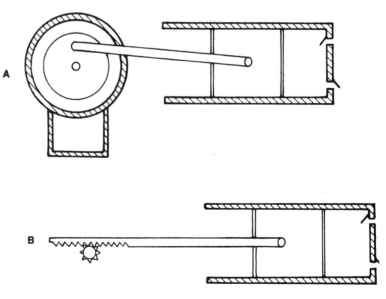

Figure 3-2 A comparison between (A) a rotary-driven piston and (B) a linear-driven piston drive mechanism for a mechanical ventilator.

driven piston. Output waveforms, which are discussed later in this chapter, vary depending on how the piston is driven.

BELLOWS DRIVE MECHANISM

Ventilators may also use a bellows to compress the gas for delivery to the patient (Figure 3-3). A bellows may be compressed by a spring, a weight, or by gas pressure if it is in a sealed chamber. A one-way valve admits gas to the bellows expanding the bellows. When it is compressed, the one-way valve closes, causing gas delivery to the patient.

REDUCING VALVE DRIVE MECHANISM

A reducing valve may be used to drive a ventilator and to provide enough of a pressure gradient to cause ventilation. The Bennett PR-2 is one example of a ventilator that uses a reducing valve.

MICROPROCESSOR-CONTROLLED PNEUMATIC DRIVE MECHANISM

Although technically both pistons and bellows are pneumatic systems, a separate classification is required for the newer ventilators that use proportional solenoid valves and microprocessor controls. Current

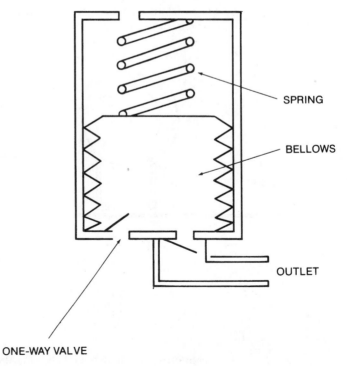

Figure 3-3 A bellows drive mechanism for a mechanical ventilator.

generation ventilators use programmed algorithms in the microprocessors to open and close the solenoid valves to mimic virtually any flow or pressure wave pattern.

pneumatic drive mechanism: *Operation of a ventilator with pressurized gas as a power source.*

This is called a microprocessor-controlled **pneumatic drive mechanism**. Furthermore, with advances in clinical medicine, the microprocessors can be reprogrammed to deliver new patterns that may not yet be described in the literature. Ventilator manufacturers, using microprocessors and the associated proportional solenoid valves, have greater flexibility in designing and updating ventilator technology.

CONTROL CIRCUIT

The control circuit is the system that governs or controls the ventilator drive mechanism or output control valve. The control circuit is the system that is responsible for the characteristic output waveforms that will be discussed later in this chapter. Control circuits may be classified as open or closed loop control circuits, mechanical, pneumatic, fluidic, electric, and electronic.

An open loop control circuit is one where the desired output is selected and the ventilator achieves the desired output without any further input from the clinician or the ventilator itself.

A closed loop control circuit is one where the desired output is selected and then the ventilator measures a specific parameter or variable (flow, pressure, or volume) continuously, and the input is constantly adjusted to match the desired output. This type of control circuit may also be referred to as **servo** controlled.

servo: *A feedback system that typically consists of a sensing element, an amplifier, and a servomotor, used in the automatic control of the mechanical device of a ventilator.*

MECHANICAL
Mechanical control circuits employ simple machines such as levers, pulleys, or cams to control the drive mechanism. Early mechanical ventilators used these systems to control their outputs. Being mechanical, some of these control systems were very durable but lacked flexibility by being an open loop type control system.

PNEUMATIC
Pneumatic devices can be used as control circuits. These devices include valves, nozzles, ducted ejectors, and diaphragms. The IPPB ventilators and the Percussionaire IPV and VDR ventilators all use pneumatic control circuits.

FLUIDIC
Fluidics is the application of gas flow and pressure to control the direction other gas flows and to perform logic functions. The logic functions of fluidics have their origin in digital electronics. Fluidic elements, just

as do digital electronic gates, control their outputs according to the inputs received. By combining fluidic elements in specific ways, a ventilator can be designed to function in a similar way to other ventilators that are electronically controlled.

Fluidic elements operate using the Coanda effect. If a jet of gas exits at high velocity adjacent to a wall (Figure 3-4), the gas flow will attach to the adjacent wall. An area of reduced pressure forms a separation bubble, which attaches the flow to the adjacent surface. Fluidic elements use a flow splitter located beside adjacent walls to control the direction of flow and to perform logic functions (Figure 3-5).

ELECTRIC

Electric control circuits use simple switches to control the drive mechanism. Some home care ventilators control tidal volume delivery using electric switches to control the travel limit of the piston that

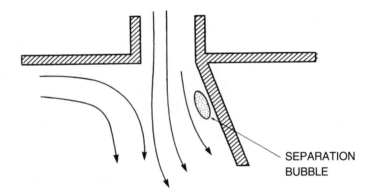

Figure 3-4   A schematic illustrating the Coanda effect.

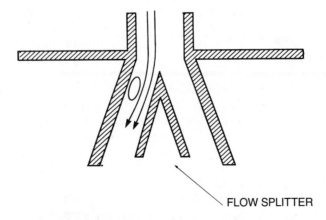

Figure 3-5   A schematic illustrating a fluidic flow splitter.

drives the ventilator. The Emerson 3-MV ventilator uses two micro-switches to control the inspiratory and expiratory time.

ELECTRONIC

Electronic devices such as resistors, diodes, transistors, integrated circuits, and microprocessors can be used to provide sophisticated levels of control over the drive mechanisms of contemporary ventilators. Electronic control systems provide greater flexibility but often at the expense of complexity.

CONTROL VARIABLES

When providing ventilatory support, the mechanical ventilator can control four primary variables during inspiration. These four variables are pressure, volume, flow, and time. Figure 3-6 illustrates an algorithm that can be applied to determine which variable the ventilator is controlling.

PRESSURE CONTROLLER

controller: The mechanism that provides a mode of ventilation within a specific parameter (pressure, time, volume, or flow).

A ventilator is classified as a pressure **controller** if the ventilator controls the transrespiratory system pressure (airway pressure minus body surface pressure). Further classification of a ventilator as a positive or negative pressure ventilator depends on whether the airway pressure rises above baseline (positive) or body surface pressure is lowered below baseline (negative).

A positive pressure ventilator applies pressure inside the chest to expand it. This type of ventilator requires the use of a tight-fitting

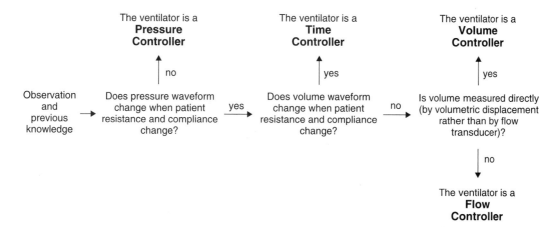

Figure 3-6 Criteria for determining the control variable during a ventilator-assisted inspiration. (From R. L. Chatburn [1991]. *Respir Care, 36*[10]. Used with permission.)

mask, or more commonly, an artificial airway. A pressure greater than atmospheric pressure is applied to the lungs, causing them to expand (Figure 3-7). Once positive pressure is no longer applied, the patient is allowed to exhale passively to ambient pressure. Exhalation occurs because of the pressure differential between the lungs and the atmosphere and through the elastic recoil of the lungs and thorax. This is the type of ventilator most commonly used today.

Negative pressure ventilators apply subatmospheric pressure outside of the chest to inflate the lungs. The negative pressure causes the chest wall to expand, and the pressure difference between the lungs and the atmosphere causes air to flow into the lungs (Figure 3-8). Once negative pressure is no longer applied, the patient is allowed to exhale passively to ambient pressure. Positive pressure may also be applied to further assist the patient during exhalation.

Regardless of whether a ventilator is classified as positive or negative pressure, the lungs expand as a result of the positive transrespiratory system pressures generated. It is the transrespiratory pressure gradient that largely determines the depth or volume of inspiration. A typical pressure controller is unaffected by changes in the patient's compliance or resistance. That is, the pressure level that is delivered to the patient will not vary in spite of changes in patient compliance or resistance.

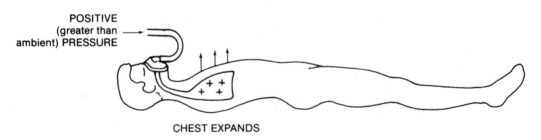

Figure 3-7   A schematic illustrating positive pressure ventilation.

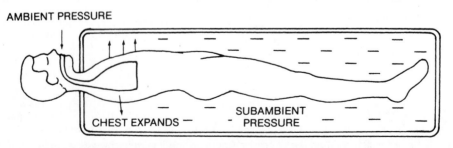

Figure 3-8   A schematic illustrating negative pressure ventilation.

VOLUME CONTROLLER

To be classified as a volume controller, volume must be measured and used as a feedback signal to control the output (volume) delivered. A volume controller allows pressure to vary with changes in resistance and compliance while volume delivery remains constant.

Volume controllers can measure volume by the displacement of the piston or bellows that serves as the ventilator's drive mechanism. If the displacement of the bellows or piston is controlled, volume therefore is also controlled. Examples of this type of ventilator include the Bennett MA-1 and MA-2+2 and the Emerson 3-MV. The Bennett ventilators control bellows displacement whereas the Emerson 3-MV controls piston displacement. Another way to control volume is to measure flow and turn it into a volume signal electronically.

FLOW CONTROLLER

Flow controllers allow pressure to vary with changes in the patient's compliance and resistance while directly measuring and controlling flow. Flow may be measured by vortex sensors, heated wire grids, venturi pneumotachometers, strain gauge flow sensors, and other devices. What is important is that the ventilator directly measures flow, and uses the flow signal as a feedback signal to control its output.

Many ventilators are incorrectly classified as "volume ventilators." Even though a tidal volume is set or displayed, many ventilators measure flow and then derive volume from the flow measurement [Volume (L) = Flow (L/sec) × Inspiratory Time (sec)]. However, if a ventilator is operated in pressure support or pressure control mode, the ventilator then becomes a pressure controller, since pressure is the variable that is measured and controlled.

TIME CONTROLLER

Time controllers are ventilators that measure and control inspiratory and expiratory time. These ventilators allow pressure and volume to vary with changes in pulmonary compliance and resistance. Since neither pressure or volume is directly measured or used as a control signal, time (inspiratory, expiratory, or both) remains the only variable that may be controlled.

PHASE VARIABLES

A ventilator-supported breath may be divided into four distinct phases: 1) the change from expiration to inspiration, 2) inspiration, 3) the change from inspiration to expiration, and 4) expiration. More detail can be learned by studying what occurs to the four variables (pressure, volume, flow, and time) during these phases. When the variable is examined during a particular phase, it is termed a phase variable.

TRIGGER VARIABLE

The trigger variable is the variable that determines the start of inspiration. Pressure, volume, flow, or time may be measured by the ventilator and used as a variable to initiate inspiration. Most ventilators use time or pressure as trigger variables.

Control: Time Triggered. A **time-triggered** breath is initiated and delivered by the ventilator when a preset time interval has elapsed. The respiratory rate control on the ventilator is a time-triggering mechanism.

For example, if the ventilator respiratory rate is preset at 12 breaths per minute (60 seconds), the time triggering interval for each complete breath is 5 seconds. At this time trigger interval, the ventilator automatically delivers one mechanical breath every 5 seconds without regard to the patient's breathing effort or requirement.

60 sec / 12 breaths = 5 sec / breath

time triggered: Initiation of a mechanical breath based on the set time interval for one complete respiratory cycle (inspiratory time and expiratory time).

pressure triggered: Initiation of a mechanical breath based on the drop in airway pressure that occurs at the beginning of a spontaneous inspiratory effort.

Pressure Triggered. A **pressure-triggered** breath is initiated and delivered by the ventilator when it senses the patient's spontaneous (negative pressure) inspiratory effort. The patient may trigger the ventilator by generating a pressure gradient or a flow gradient.

Pressure triggering uses the drop in airway pressure that occurs at the beginning of a spontaneous inspiratory effort to signal the ventilator to begin inspiration (Figure 3-9). The amount of negative pressure below the patient's baseline airway pressure (or end-expiratory pressure) a patient must generate to trigger the ventilator into inspiration is the sensitivity level. The range of acceptable sensitivity levels for pressure triggering varies from –1 to –5 cm H_2O below the patient's baseline pressure.

☑ Comparing to a sensitivity setting of –3 cm H_2O, –5 cm H_2O requires *more* patient effort to trigger the ventilator to inspiration.

For example, if the sensitivity for pressure triggering is set at –3 cm H_2O, then the patient must generate a pressure of –3 cm H_2O at the airway opening to trigger the ventilator into inspiration. If the sensitivity for pressure triggering is changed from –3 to –5 cm H_2O, the ventilator becomes *less* sensitive to the patient's inspiratory effort as more effort is needed to trigger the ventilator into inspiration. Changing the sensitivity from –3 to –5 cm H_2O is *decreasing* the sensitivity setting on the ventilator.

flow triggered: Flow- triggering strategy uses a combination of continuous flow and demand flow. Before inspiration, the delivered flow equals the return flow. As the patient initiates a breath, the return flow to the ventilator is decreased and this flow differential triggers a mechanical breath.

Flow Triggered. Some third-generation ventilators measure flow. When the patient's inspiratory flow reaches a specific value, a ventilator-supported breath is delivered. Flow triggering has been shown to be more sensitive and responsive to a patient's efforts than pressure triggering. A **flow-triggered** breath uses a strategy that combines the continuous flow and demand flow mechanisms, and it is used to reduce the inspiratory effort imposed on the patient during mechanical ventilation. It is considered to be more sensitive to the

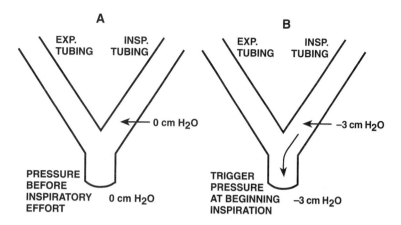

Figure 3-9 Pressure-trigger mechanism. (A) Before an inspiratory effort, the pressure in the airway and ventilator tubing equals 0 cm H_2O. A mechanical breath is not initiated because there is no pressure drop to trigger the ventilator sensitivity settings. (B) At beginning inspiration, the pressure in the airway and ventilator tubing is –3 cm H_2O. A mechanical breath is initiated because the pressure drop is sufficient to trigger the ventilator sensitivity setting (assuming it is set as –3 cm H_2O or less).

patient's inspiratory effort and therefore usually requires less inspiratory work than pressure triggering.

In flow triggering, a continuous flow passes through the ventilator circuit and returns to the ventilator (i.e., delivered flow = returned flow). As the patient initiates a breath, part of the delivered flow goes to the patient and the return flow to the ventilator is therefore reduced (i.e., delivered flow > return flow). The ventilator senses this flow differential and instantly supplies enough flow to satisfy the mechanical or spontaneous tidal volume. CMV, SIMV, and PSV can all be flow triggered (Figure 3-10).

One infant ventilator (Sechrist IV-200) uses inductive plethysmography to initiate a ventilator-supported breath. When the infant's chest expands, a small electrical signal is generated between two chest leads, which is commonly used to monitor the infant's respiratory rate. The ventilator is interfaced to the respiratory rate monitor, and inspiratory triggering occurs when the signal is detected by the ventilator. This type of triggering is much faster and responsive than pressure or flow triggering, since it is directly measuring the infant's inspiratory efforts or exertions.

How hard the patient must work to initiate or trigger a breath is termed the ventilator sensitivity. If the ventilator is made more sensitive to the patient's efforts (pressure, flow, or volume), it is easier for the patient to trigger a breath. The converse is also true.

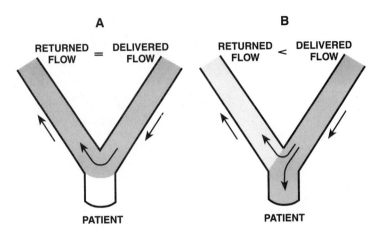

A

RETURNED $=$ DELIVERED
FLOW   FLOW

B

RETURNED $<$ DELIVERED
FLOW   FLOW

PATIENT   PATIENT

Figure 3-10 Flow-trigger mechanism. (A) Before an inspiratory effort, the delivered flow equals the returned flow. Flow trigger is not activated because there is no drop in returned flow. (B) At beginning inspiration, some of the delivered flow goes to the patient and this leads to a lower returned flow. Flow trigger is activated when the ventilator senses an inspiratory effort (the returned flow is lower than the delivered flow).

LIMIT VARIABLE

During a ventilator-supported breath, volume pressure and flow all rise above their respective baseline values. Inspiratory time is defined as the time interval between the start of inspiratory flow and the beginning of expiratory flow. If one or more variables (pressure, flow, or volume), is not allowed to rise above a preset value during the inspiratory time, it is termed a limit variable. Note that in this definition, inspiration does not end when the variable reaches its preset value. The breath delivery continues, but the variable is held at the fixed, preset value. Figure 3-11 provides a useful algorithm for determining the limit variable (pressure-limited, volume-limited, or flow-limited) during the inspiratory phase.

CYCLE VARIABLE

cycle: The length of one complete breathing cycle.

Inspiration ends when a specific **cycle** variable (pressure cycled, volume cycled, flow cycled, or time cycled) is reached (Figure 3-11). This variable must be measured by the ventilator and used as a feedback signal to end inspiratory flow delivery, which then allows exhalation to begin.

Again it is easy to make false assumptions regarding many ventilators by classifying them as volume cycled. Most newer ventilators

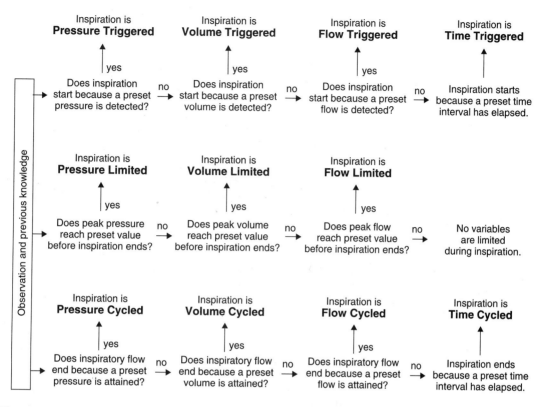

Figure 3-11 Criteria for determining the phase variables during a ventilator-assisted breath. (From R. L. Chatburn [1991]. *Respir Care, 36*[10]. Used with permission.)

measure flow and are flow controllers. Since flow is measured and used as a feedback signal for gas delivery, volume becomes a function of flow and time [Volume (L) = Flow (L/sec) × Inspiratory Time (sec)]. Therefore, these ventilators are really time cycled, rather than "volume cycled." Inspiration ends because a preset time interval has passed, and volume has not been directly measured.

BASELINE VARIABLE

Expiratory time is defined as the interval between the start of expiratory flow and the beginning of inspiratory flow. This is also termed the expiratory phase. The variable that is controlled during the expiratory phase or expiratory time is termed the baseline variable. Most commonly, pressure is controlled during the expiratory phase.

Application of positive end-expiratory pressure (PEEP) and continuous positive airway pressure (CPAP) are used to increase the functional residual capacity (FRC), to improve gas distribution, and oxygenation. These pressures when applied above baseline (ambient pressure) during exhalation, maintain the lungs in a partially inflated state. This helps to prevent alveolar collapse, recruit previously collapsed alveoli, and distend those alveoli that are already patent. PEEP and CPAP pressures must be titrated carefully to monitor hemodynamic functions, blood gases or oximetry, and compliance to achieve the greatest benefit with the least amount of detrimental side effects.

CONDITIONAL VARIABLE

Conditional variables are defined as patterns of variables that are controlled by the ventilator during the ventilatory cycle. Early ventilators, such as the Puritan Bennett MA-1, used relatively simple conditional variables (volume cycled, pressure limited, pressure triggered, and PEEP). Newer third-generation microprocessor-controlled ventilators, such as the Puritan-Bennett 7200ae, are capable of delivering complex ventilatory patterns. Figure 3-12 summarizes the ventilator classification system.

OUTPUT WAVEFORMS

Output waveforms are graphical representations of the control or phase variables in relation to time. Output waveforms are typically presented in the order of pressure, volume, and flow. The ventilator determines the shape of the control variable, whereas the other two depend on the patient's compliance and resistance. Convention dictates that flow values above the horizontal axis are inspiratory, whereas flow below the horizontal axis is expiratory. This corresponds to pressure and flow values rising above the horizontal axis for inspiration and falling back to the baseline during expiration. The ideal waveforms are represented in Figure 3-13.

Careful observation and assessment of waveforms during mechanical ventilation can provide useful information for the clinician. Waveforms can assist the clinician in the detection of inadvertent PEEP, the patient's ventilatory work, resistance and compliance changes as well as many other events or changes. Some ventilators are able to present pressure versus volume waveforms to assist in minimizing the patient's work of breathing. Still other ventilators can present flow versus volume waveforms, to aid in the assessment of bronchodilator therapy during mechanical ventilation and the assessment of airway obstruction. As waveforms become widely used, their usefulness will approach that of the ECG tracing in the assessment of the heart.

Mode	Mandatory Breath				Spontaneous Breath				Control Logic		
	Control	Trigger	Limit	Cycle	Control	Trigger	Limit	Cycle	Supported	Conditional Variable	Action
CMV*	Pressure, volume, or flow	Time	Pressure, volume, or flow	Time, pressure, volume, or flow	—	—	—	—	—	—	—
A/C	Pressure, volume, or flow	Time, pressure, volume, or flow	Pressure, volume, or flow	Time, pressure, volume, or flow	—	—	—	—	—	Time or patient effort	Machine-to-patient triggered
AMV	Pressure, volume, or flow	Pressure, volume, or flow	Pressure, volume, or flow	Time, pressure, volume, or flow	—	—	—	—	—	—	—
IMV	Pressure, volume, or flow	Time	Pressure, volume, or flow	Time, pressure, volume, or flow	Pressure	Pressure, volume, or flow	Pressure	Pressure	No	—	—
SIMV	Pressure, volume, or flow	Time, pressure, volume, or flow	Pressure, volume, or flow	Time, pressure, volume, or flow	Pressure	Pressure, volume, or flow	Pressure	Pressure	No	Time or patient effort	Machine-to-patient triggered
CPAP	—	—	—	—	Pressure	Pressure, volume, or flow	Pressure	Pressure	No	—	—
PCV	Pressure	Time	Pressure	Time	—	—	—	Pressure	—	—	—
PC-IMV	Pressure	Time	Pressure	Time	Pressure	Pressure, volume,	Pressure	Pressure	No	—	—

(continued)

Figure 3-12 Summary of the ventilator classification system as described by Robert L. Chatburn. (From R. L. Chatburn [1992]. "Technical description and classification of modes of ventilator operation." *Respir Care, 37*[9]. Used with permission.)

| | Mandatory Breath | | | | Spontaneous Breath | | | | Control Logic | | |
Mode	Control	Trigger	Limit	Cycle	Control	Trigger	Limit	Cycle	Supported	Conditional Variable	Action
PC-SIMV	Pressure	Time, pressure, volume, or flow	Pressure	Time	Pressure	Pressure, volume, or flow	Pressure	Pressure	No	Time or patient effort	Machine-to-patient triggered
PCIRV	Pressure	Time	Pressure	Time	Pressure						
APRV	Pressure	Time or pressure	Pressure	Time	Pressure	Pressure, volume, or flow	Pressure	Pressure	No	Time or patient effort	Machine-to-patient triggered
PSV	—	—	—	—	Pressure	Pressure, volume, or flow	Pressure	Volume	Yes		
MMV	Volume or flow	Time	Volume or flow	Time, volume, or flow	Pressure	Pressure, volume, or flow	Pressure	Pressure or volume	Yes*	Minute ventilation, time	Spontaneous to-mandatory breath
VAPS	Flow	Time or pressure	Flow	Time or volume	Pressure	Pressure or flow	Pressure	Flow	Yes*	Tidal volume	Pressure-to-volume control
BiPAP	Pressure	Time	Pressure	Time	Pressure	Pressure	Pressure	Pressure	No	—	—

*CMV = continuous mandatory ventilation; NA = not applicable; A/C = assist/control; AMV = assisted mechanical ventilation; IMV = intermittent mandatory ventilation; SIMV = synchronized mandatory ventilation; CPAP = continuous positive airway pressure; PCV = pressure-controlled ventilation; PC-IMV = pressure-controlled IMV; PCIRV = PC inverse-ratio ventilation; APRV = airway pressure release ventilation; PSV = pressure support ventilation; MMV = mandatory minute ventilation; VAPS = volume-assisted pressure support; BiPAP = bilevel positive airway pressure.

From "Technical description and classification of modes of ventilator operation" by R. D. Branson and R. L. Chatburn, Respiratory Care, September 1992, 37, (9) p. 1029. Copyright 1992 Daedalus Enterprises, Inc.. Adapted with permission.

Figure 3-12 (continued)

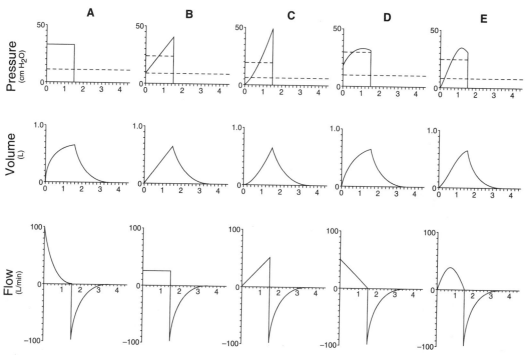

Figure 3-13 Theoretical output waveforms for (A) pressure-controlled inspiration with rectangular pressure waveform, identical to flow-controlled inspiration with an exponential-decay flow waveform; (B) flow-controlled inspiration with rectangular flow waveform, identical to volume-controlled inspiration with an ascending-ramp flow waveform; (C) flow-controlled inspiration with an ascending-ramp flow waveform; (D) flow-controlled inspiration with a descending-ramp flow waveform; and (E) flow-controlled inspiration with a sinusoidal flow waveform. The short dashed lines represent mean inspiration pressure, whereas the longer dashed lines denote mean airway pressure (assuming zero end-expiratory pressure). For the rectangular pressure waveform in A, the mean inspiratory pressure is the same as the peak inspiratory pressure. These output waveforms were created by (1) defining the control waveform (e.g., an ascending-ramp flow waveform is specified as flow = constant × time) and specifying that tidal volume equals 644 mL (about 9 mL/kg for a normal adult); (2) specifying the desired values for resistance and compliance (for these waveforms, compliance = 20 mL/cm H_2O and resistance = 20 cm H_2O/L/sec, according to ANSI recommendations); (3) substituting the above information into the equation of motion; and (4) using a computer to solve the equation for pressure, volume, and flow and plotting the results against time. (From R. L. Chatburn [1991]. *Respir Care, 36*[10]. Used with permission.)

PRESSURE WAVEFORMS

Pressure waveforms include rectangular, exponential, sinusoidal and oscillating (Figure 3-14). Each of these waveforms would have these characteristic shapes, providing that pressure is the control variable. The descriptors used to describe each waveform are based upon their respective shapes.

The rectangular waveform is characterized by a near instantaneous rise to a peak pressure value that is held to the start of exhalation. During expiration, the pressure rapidly drops to baseline.

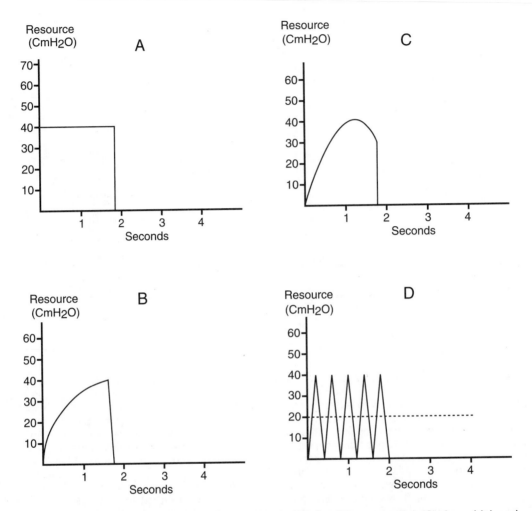

Figure 3-14 Four types of pressure waveforms: (A) rectangular, (B) exponential, (C) sinusoidal, and (D) oscillating.

The exponential waveform is depicted by a more gradual increase in pressure when compared with the rectangular waveform. This type of waveform is common in some infant ventilators and has become an option on some adult ventilators. Ventilator settings such as flow and inspiratory time regulate how steep the waveform rises toward peak inspiratory pressure.

The sinusoidal waveform resembles the positive half of a **sine wave.** Sinusoidal waveforms are characteristically produced by ventilators having a rotary-driven piston drive mechanism (Figure 3-15). Ventilators using this drive mechanism include the Emerson 3-MV, Lifecare PLV-100, BEAR 33, Puritan-Bennett 2801 Companion, and the Aequitron Medical LP-10.

sine wave: A graphic presentation of flow and time that has a horizontal "S" appearance.

VOLUME WAVEFORMS

Volume waveforms can be classified into two types, ascending ramp and sinusoidal (Figure 3-16). The ascending ramp waveform is produced by a constant (i.e., rectangular) inspiratory flow pattern. The shape is characterized by a linear rise to the peak inspiratory pressure value. Sinusoidal volume waveforms are produced by ventilators that have a rotary-driven piston drive mechanism. Ventilators using this drive mechanism include the Emerson 3-MV, Lifecare PLV-100, BEAR 33, Puritan-Bennett 2801 Companion, and the Aequitron Medical LP-10.

FLOW WAVEFORMS

The four types of flow waveforms are shown in Figure 3-17. The waveforms include rectangular, ascending ramp, descending ramp, and sinusoidal.

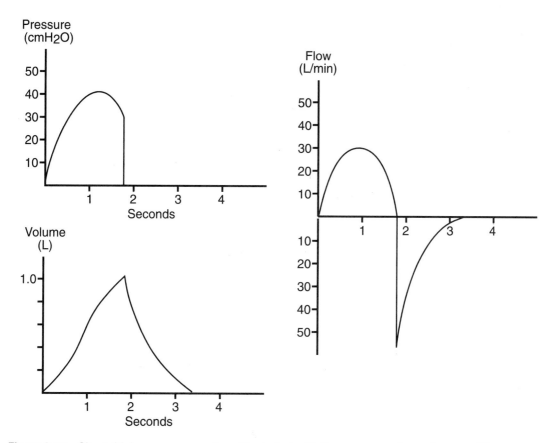

Figure 3-15   Sinusoidal pressure waveform illustrated with the corresponding volume and flow waveforms. This type of pattern is typical of a rotary-driven piston drive mechanism.

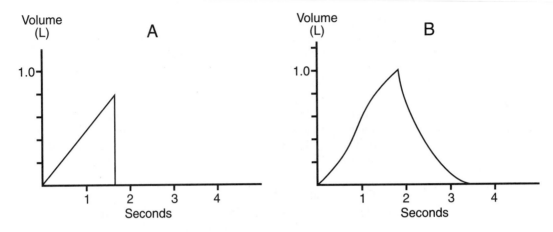

Figure 3-16 Two types of volume waveforms: (A) ascending ramp, and (B) sinusoidal.

The rectangular waveform is produced when volume is the control variable and the output is an ascending ramp. The flow waveform (a derivative of the volume waveform with respect to time), assumes the characteristic rectangular shape.

The ramp waveform can be ascending or descending. If flow rises as the breath is delivered, it is termed ascending. If flow falls during the ventilator-supported breath, it is called a descending ramp.

The sinusoidal waveform resembles the positive portion of a sine wave. It is generated by a rotary-driven piston drive mechanism.

ALARM SYSTEMS

Alarm systems are designed to alert the clinician to undesirable technical or patient events. Triggering of an alarm that requires clinician awareness or action. As the complexity of mechanical ventilators has increased, so have the number and complexity of the alarm systems. Technical events are those events limited to the performance of the ventilator, while patient events are those relating to the patient's condition. Alarms can be visual, audible, or both depending on the seriousness of the event.

INPUT POWER ALARMS
Input power alarms can be further classified as to loss of electrical or pneumatic power.

Loss of electrical power usually results in the ventilator activating a backup alarm that is battery powered. Most battery backup alarms are powered by rechargeable nickel cadmium batteries, which are

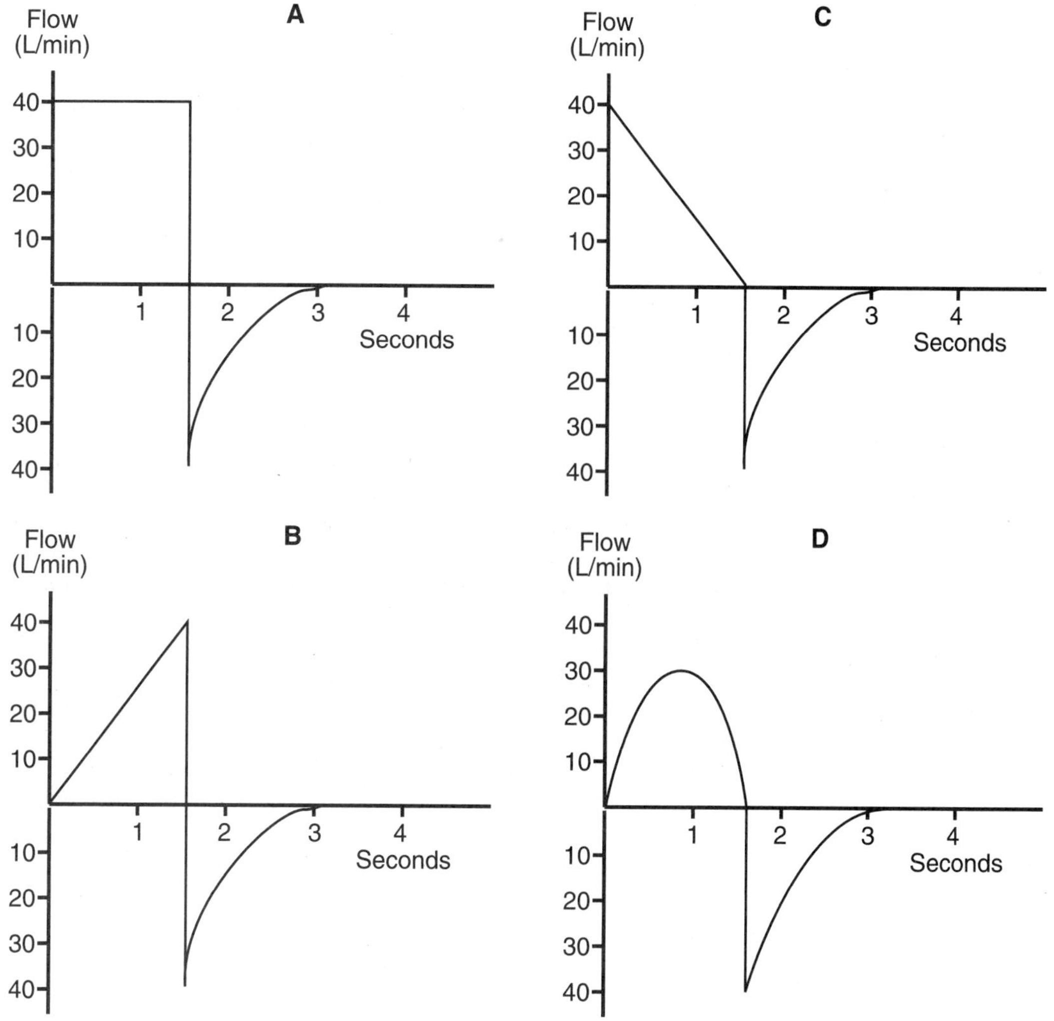

Figure 3-17 Four types of flow waveforms: (A) rectangular, (B) ascending ramp, (C) descending ramp, and (D) sinusoidal.

recharged when alternating current (AC) power is available. When AC power is lost, the backup batteries activate audible and visual alarms.

Loss of either air or oxygen pneumatic sources will result in a technical event alarm. If either input pressure falls below a specified value from 50 psi, the alarm will result. Some alarms are electronic (BEAR 1000, BEAR I, II and III, Puritan-Bennett 7200ae), whereas others are pneumatic reed alarms such as those employed in oxygen blenders.

CONTROL CIRCUIT ALARMS

Control circuit alarms alert the clinician to settings or parameters that are not within acceptable ranges or specifications, or they warn the clinician that the ventilator has failed some part of a self-diagnostic test. In the event of an incompatible setting or parameter, the clinician is allowed the opportunity to change the input to one that is compatible. Failure of the self-diagnostic test may render the ventilator inoperative, and the clinician is alerted by a message display that test failure has occurred.

OUTPUT ALARMS

Output alarms can be further subdivided into pressure, volume, flow, time, inspiratory, and expiratory gas.

Pressure alarms include high/low peak and mean and baseline airway pressures. High and low values may be set for each of these output parameters to alert the clinician of changes in the patient's physiological status. Additionally, an alarm may be provided to detect failure of the airway pressure to return to the baseline valve. This could be caused by airway obstructions, circuit obstructions, or ventilator malfunctions.

Volume alarms include high/low exhaled tidal volumes for both ventilator-supported breaths and spontaneous breaths. Low volumes may result from sedation (spontaneous volumes), disconnection, or apnea (spontaneous volumes).

Flow alarms are limited to exhaled minute volume. High and low values may be set on some ventilators to alert the clinician to changes in the patient's minute ventilation.

Time alarms include high/low frequency or rate, excessive or inadequate inspiratory time, and excessive or inadequate expiratory time. High/low ventilatory rate alarms alert the clinician to changes in the patient's ventilatory rate. Inspiratory and expiratory time alarms may alert the practitioner to circuit obstructions or malfunctions, changes in gas distribution, or inappropriate ventilator settings.

Inspired gas alarms alert the clinician to changes in oxygen concentration or gas temperature. Some ventilators incorporate an oxygen analyzer to detect changes in F_IO_2. High/low alarms alert the clinician to these changes. Inspired gas temperature may be controlled by a servo-controlled humidifier or monitored by an independent ventilator temperature alarm. High/low temperature alarms can alert the clinician to changes in the inspiratory gas temperature.

Exhaled oxygen tension or end tidal carbon dioxide tension can be monitored and high/low alarms can be sent to the exhaled gas monitoring system. These monitors can assist the clinician in determining the V_D/V_T, gas exchange and determining the respiratory exchange ratio (R).

──── SUMMARY ────

As computer and medical technologies are getting more advanced, future mechanical ventilators are likely to have more new features than the current ventilators. No one knows for certain whether more new features will make the ventilators more complex and less user-friendly. But no matter what the future ventilators become, the practitioners who use mechanical ventilators must learn and maintain the theory, skills, and practice in the use of mechanical ventilation.

The ability to use mechanical ventilation will be enhanced if the practitioners are able to classify the ventilator properly and apply the unique characteristics of each ventilator in patient care situations.

Self-Assessment Questions

1. The primary forces that the ventilatory muscles must overcome include:

    I. Resistive forces
    II. Compliance forces
    III. Elastic forces
    IV. Inductive forces

    A. I and II.   C. II and III.
    B. I and III.   D. II and IV.

2. When the ventilator assumes all of the ventilatory work, this is termed:

    A. partial ventilatory support.   C. incomplete ventilatory support.
    B. full ventilatory support.   D. no ventilatory support.

3. A type of control circuit that relies on cams, pulleys, and levers is termed a/an:

    A. electronic control circuit.   C. electric control circuit.
    B. fluidic control circuit.   D. mechanical control circuit.

4. A ventilator that measures flow and uses that measurement to control the output of the ventilator is termed a:

    A. pressure controller.   C. volume controller.
    B. flow controller.   D. time controller.

5. If pressure rises to a preset level and is maintained at that level until inspiration ends, this is termed a:

    A. time limit.   C. pressure limit.
    B. volume limit.   D. flow limit.

6. An alarm that results from the loss of 50 psi gas pressure is termed a/an:

        A. input power alarm.   C. output alarm.
        B. control circuit alarm.   D. gas pressure alarm.

Suggested Reading

Barnes, Thomas A. et al. (1994). *Core textbook of respiratory care practice* (2nd ed.). St. Louis: Mosby-Year Book.

Branson, R. D. (1992). Intrahospital transport of critically ill, mechanically ventilated patients. *Respir Care, 37*(7), 775–795.

Branson, R. D. et al. (1992). Technical description and classification of modes of ventilator operation. *Respir Care, 37*(9), 1026–1044.

Chatburn, R. L. (1991). A new system for understanding mechanical ventilators. *Respir Care, 36*(10), 1123–1155.

Chatburn, R. L. (1992). Classification of mechanical ventilators. *Respir Care, 37*(9), 1009–1025.

Dupis, Y. (1992). *Ventilators: Theory and clinical application* (2nd ed.). St. Louis, MO: Mosby-Year Book.

Gietzen, J. W. et. al. (1991). Effect of PEEP-Valve placement on function of a home-care ventilator. *Respir Care, 36*(10), 1093–1098.

White, G. C. (1999). *Equipment theory for respiratory care* (3rd ed.). Albany, NY: Delmar Publishers.

CHAPTER FOUR

OPERATING MODES OF MECHANICAL VENTILATION

David W. Chang
James H. Hiers

OUTLINE

KEY TERMS

- **airway pressure release ventilation (APRV)**
- **assist/control (AC)**
- **Bi-level positive airway pressure (BiPAP)**
- **continuous positive airway pressure (CPAP)**
- **control mode**

- **eucapnic ventilation**
- **intermittent mandatory ventilation (IMV)**
- **mandatory minute ventilation (MMV)**
- **positive end-expiratory pressure (PEEP)**
- **pressure control ventilation (PCV)**
- **synchronized intermittent mandatory ventilation (SIMV)**

INTRODUCTION

This chapter provides an introduction to different operating modes available on most mechanical ventilators. Since the information associated with mechanical ventilation is immense, the reader should learn the operating modes and study them in the order presented in this chapter. The definition and unique characteristics of each operating mode are described here. The initiation and application of these operating controls may be found in subsequent chapters.

NEGATIVE AND POSITIVE PRESSURE VENTILATION

☑ Mechanical ven-
tilators generate
gas flow and volume
by creating either a
negative or positive
pressure gradient.

Every ventilator must generate an inspiratory flow in order to deliver a tidal volume. Since gas flow requires a pressure gradient, a mechanical ventilator must produce a pressure gradient (i.e., pressure difference) between the airway opening and the alveoli in order to produce inspiratory flow and volume delivery. The pressure gradient that must be generated between the airway opening and the alveoli is known as the transairway pressure (Des Jardins, 1998).

Transairway pressure is the difference between the airway opening pressure (Pao) and alveolar pressure (P_A):

Transairway Pressure = Pressure @ airway opening (Pao) – alveolar pressure (P_A)

At end-exhalation and prior to the beginning of inspiration, the pressures at the airway opening and the alveoli are both equal to atmospheric pressure. Since these two pressures are equal at this point, there is no pressure gradient and therefore no flow.

Since a pressure gradient is needed to generate gas flow and volume, mechanical ventilators achieve this condition by creating either a negative or positive pressure gradient.

NEGATIVE PRESSURE VENTILATION

Negative pressure ventilation creates a transairway pressure gradient by decreasing the alveolar pressures to a level below the airway opening pressure, usually below the atmospheric pressure. Unless airway obstruction is present, negative pressure ventilation does not require an artificial airway. Two classical devices that provide negative pressure ventilation are the "iron lung" and the chest cuirass or chest shell.

☑ The tidal vol-
ume delivered
by a negative pres-
sure ventilator is
directly related to
the negative pres-
sure gradient.

Iron Lungs.   An "iron lung" ventilator encloses the patient's body except for the head and neck in a tank and the air in it is evacuated to produce a negative pressure around the chest cage. This negative pressure surrounding the chest and underlying alveoli results in chest wall and alveolar expansion. The tidal volume delivered to the patient is directly related to the negative pressure gradient. For example, a more negative pressure applied to the chest wall will yield a larger tidal volume. Since negative pressure ventilation does not require tracheal intubation, this noninvasive method of ventilation has been used extensively and successfully to support chronic ventilatory failure (Corrado et al., 1994; Frederick, 1994).

Disadvantages and complications associated with the iron lung type of negative pressure ventilator are (1) poor patient access, and (2) potential for a decreased cardiac output known as "tank shock" (Frederick, 1994).

Since the iron lung encloses the patient, it restricts access to the patient for routine health care. Tank shock may result from a decreased venous blood return to the right atrium. Normally, the heart and vena cava are surrounded by negative pleural pressure while the remainder of the vascular system outside the thorax is subjected to atmospheric pressure. This creates a vascular pressure gradient between the vena cava and the venous drainage that enhances venous blood return to the right atrium. However, if a patient is placed in an iron lung, this vascular pressure gradient is lost because the peripheral vasculature is subjected to negative pressures that closely approximate the pleural pressure. This results in a potential decrease in venous return that could lead to a decreased cardiac output.

Chest Cuirass. The chest cuirass or chest shell is a form of negative pressure ventilation that was intended to alleviate the problems of patient access and tank shock associated with iron lungs. This shell device covers only the patient's chest and leaves the arms and lower body exposed. Although the chest shell improves patient access and decreases the potential for tank shock, ventilation with this device may be limited by the difficulties in maintaining an airtight seal between the shell and the patient's chest wall (Newman et al., 1988).

To overcome the problem of air leakage, individually designed cuirass "respirators" minimize air leaks, and they have been used successfully to ventilate patients with chest wall diseases such as scoliosis (Kinnear, Hockley, Harvey et al., 1988; Kinnear, Petch, Taylor et al., 1988). Because of the availability of positive pressure ventilators, chest cuirass ventilators are seldom used in an acute care facility. However, they are rather useful in selected home care settings because of the ease to maintain and the capability to ventilate without an artificial airway. All subsequent discussions on mechanical ventilation in this text refer to positive pressure ventilation unless negative pressure ventilation is specifically mentioned.

POSITIVE PRESSURE VENTILATION

Positive pressure ventilation is achieved by applying positive pressure (a pressure greater than atmospheric pressure) at the airway opening. Increasing the pressure at the airway opening produces a transairway pressure gradient that generates an inspiratory flow. This flow in turn results in the delivery of a tidal volume. Therefore, tidal volume is directly related to the transairway pressure gradient. All other factors being held constant, increasing the positive pressure being applied to the lungs will result in a larger tidal volume being delivered.

☑ The tidal volume delivered by a positive pressure ventilator is directly related to the positive pressure gradient.

OPERATING MODES OF MECHANICAL VENTILATION

A ventilator mode can be defined as a set of operating characteristics that control how the ventilator functions. An operating mode can be described by the way a ventilator is triggered into inspiration and cycled into exhalation, what variables are limited during inspiration, and whether or not the mode allows only mandatory breaths, spontaneous breaths, or both.

Many different functions are commonly available on modern ventilators regardless of the mode. These functions include control of the F_IO_2, control of the inspiratory flow rate, and control of various alarms.

There are 13 essential ventilator modes available in different ventilators. Two or more of these modes are often used together to achieve certain desired effects. For example, spontaneous plus PEEP is the same as CPAP, and it is used to oxygenate a patient who has adequate ventilation. SIMV may be used with PSV to provide ventilation and reduce the work of breathing.

1. Spontaneous
2. Positive End-Expiratory Pressure (PEEP)
3. Continuous Positive Airway Pressure (CPAP)
4. Bi-level Positive Airway Pressure (BiPAP)
5. Controlled Mandatory Ventilation (CMV)
6. Assist Control (AC)
7. Intermittent Mandatory Ventilation (IMV)
8. Synchronized Intermittent Mandatory Ventilation (SIMV)
9. Mandatory Minute Ventilation (MMV)
10. Pressure Support Ventilation (PSV)
11. Pressure Control Ventilation (PCV)
12. Airway Pressure Release Ventilation (APRV)
13. Inverse Ratio Ventilation (IRV)

SPONTANEOUS

Spontaneous mode is not an actual mode on the ventilator since the rate and tidal volume during spontaneous breathing are determined by the patient. Even though the spontaneous mode is not a direct ventilator function, the role of the ventilator during the spontaneous mode is to provide the (1) inspiratory flow to the patient in a timely manner, (2) flow adequate to fulfill a patient's inspiratory demand (i.e., tidal volume or inspiratory flow), and (3) provide adjunctive modes such as PEEP to complement a patient's spontaneous breathing effort. The graphical tracing of spontaneous breaths is shown in Figure 4-1.

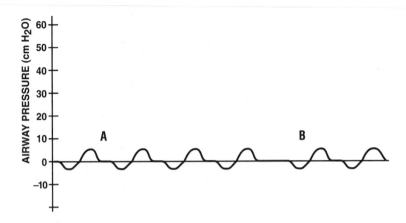

Figure 4-1 Spontaneous breathing pressure tracing. (A) The spontaneous rate is at a normal pattern. (B) The spontaneous breath is delayed by the patient.

positive end expiratory pressure (PEEP): PEEP is an airway pressure strategy in ventilation that increases the end-expiratory or baseline airway pressure to a value greater than atmospheric. It is used to treat refractory hypoxemia caused by intrapulmonary shunting.

continuous positive airway pressure (CPAP): CPAP is PEEP applied to the airway of a patient who is breathing spontaneously. It is used to treat refractory hypoxemia in patients who are able to maintain adequate spontaneous ventilation.

assist/control (AC): In the assist/control (AC) mode, the patient may increase the respiratory rate (assist) in addition to the preset mechanical respiratory rate (control). Each assist breath provides the preset mechanical tidal volume, not the spontaneous tidal volume.

APNEA VENTILATION

Apnea ventilation is a safety feature incorporated with the spontaneous breathing mode. In the event of apnea or an extremely slow respiratory rate, back up ventilation is invoked by the apnea ventilation feature and it delivers a predetermined tidal volume, respiratory rate, F_IO_2, and other essential options to the patient.

POSITIVE END-EXPIRATORY PRESSURE (PEEP)

Positive end-expiratory pressure (PEEP) increases the end-expiratory or baseline airway pressure to a value greater than atmospheric (0 cm H_2O on the ventilator manometer). It is often used to improve the patient's oxygenation status, especially in hypoxemia that is refractory to increasing F_IO_2.

PEEP is not commonly regarded as a "stand alone" mode, rather it is applied in conjunction with other ventilator modes. For example, when PEEP is applied to spontaneous breathing patients, the airway pressure is called **continuous positive airway pressure** (CPAP). Figure 4-2 shows an **assist/control** pressure tracing with 10 cm H_2O of PEEP.

INDICATIONS FOR PEEP

Two major indications for PEEP are (1) intrapulmonary shunt and refractory hypoxemia, and (2) decreased functional residual capacity (FRC) and lung compliance.

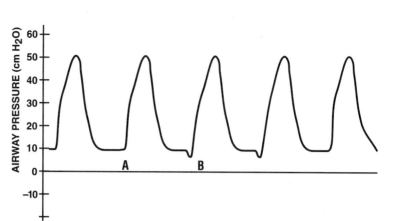

Figure 4-2 Positive end-expiratory pressure (PEEP). An assist/control pressure tracing with 10 cm H_2O of PEEP. (A) A controlled breath with PEEP. (B) An assisted breath with PEEP; note the negative deflection at the beginning of inspiration.

☑ PEEP is effective in refractory hypoxemia caused by intrapulmonary shunting.

☑ Refractory hypoxemia is present when the PaO_2 is ≤ 60 mm Hg at an F_IO_2 of ≥ 50%.

Intrapulmonary Shunt and Refractory Hypoxemia. The primary indication for PEEP is refractory hypoxemia induced by intrapulmonary shunting. This condition may be caused by a reduction of the functional residual capacity (FRC), atelectasis, or low V/Q mismatch (Tyler, 1983). Refractory hypoxemia is defined as hypoxemia that responds poorly to moderate to high levels of oxygen. A helpful clinical guideline for refractory hypoxemia is when the patient's PaO_2 is 60 mm Hg or less at an F_IO_2 of 50% or more.

Decreased FRC and Lung Compliance. A severely diminished FRC and reduced lung compliance greatly increase the alveolar opening pressure. If the patient is breathing spontaneously, a decreased lung compliance always increases the work of breathing and if severe enough can lead to fatigue of the respiratory muscles and ventilatory failure. Since PEEP increases the FRC, this pulmonary impairment may be prevented or improved by early application of PEEP therapy.

PHYSIOLOGY OF PEEP THERAPY

PEEP reinflates collapsed alveoli and maintains alveolar inflation during exhalation. Once "recruitment" of these alveoli has occurred, PEEP lowers the alveolar distending pressure and facilitates gas diffusion and oxygenation (Tyler, 1983).

Normally, the alveolar end-expiratory pressure equilibrates with atmospheric pressure (i.e., zero pressure) and the average pleural pressure is approximately –5 cm H_2O. Under these conditions, the alveolar distending pressure is 5 cm H_2O (alveolar-pleural). This distending pressure is sufficient to maintain a normal end-expiratory alveolar volume to overcome the elastic recoil of the alveolar wall.

However, if the force of elastic recoil is increased due to a decrease in compliance, the alveolar volume will decrease. If the lung compliance continues to deteriorate, the elastic recoil forces can become great enough to completely overcome the normal alveolar distending pressure, thus resulting in alveolar collapse and the creation of intrapulmonary shunting. PEEP increases the alveolar end-expiratory pressure which increases the alveolar distending pressure, and therefore reexpands or "recruits" these collapsed alveoli.

PEEP
↓
Increases alveolar distending pressure
↓
Increases FRC by alveolar recruitment
↓
Improves ventilation
↓
(1) Increases V/Q,
(2) Improves oxygenation,
(3) Decreases work of breathing

COMPLICATIONS ASSOCIATED WITH PEEP

Complications and hazards associated with PEEP include: (1) decreased venous return and cardiac output; (2) barotrauma; (3) increased intracranial pressure; and (4) alterations of renal functions and water metabolism.

Decreased Venous Return.   Assuming a normal intravascular volume, venous return to the right atrium is influenced by the difference in the central venous pressure and the negative pleural pressure that surrounds the heart. During PEEP, the pleural pressure becomes less negative and the pressure gradient between the central venous drainage and the right atrium will decrease resulting in a decreased venous return. This in turn results in a decreased cardiac output and hypotension (Qvist et al., 1975).

Experience has shown that significant increases in the mean airway pressure are more likely to increase pleural pressures sufficiently to decrease venous return. Since PEEP increases both peak inspiratory pressures and mean airway pressures, it has the potential to decrease venous return and cardiac output. It is vital to closely monitor the patient receiving PEEP therapy for any drop in blood pressure, especially when PEEP is either first applied or increased to high levels. If PEEP decreases the blood pressure, first be sure that the patient is not hypovolemic (Shapiro et al., 1991). If the blood volume is adequate, then the PEEP should be decreased until an adequate blood pressure is reestablished.

A given amount of PEEP does not impede venous return to the same degree in different patients. If a patient has an extremely low

☑ Since PEEP increases both peak inspiratory pressures and mean airway pressures, it has the potential to decrease venous return and cardiac output.

☑ The detrimental effects of PEEP are dependent on the compliance characteristics of the patient.

lung compliance, the airway pressure is less readily transmitted into the pleural space. In effect, the low lung compliance shields the pleural space from the full effects of the increased alveolar pressure. Patients with adult respiratory distress syndrome (ARDS) usually have a very low lung compliance and often require very high PEEP levels. However, despite high PEEP levels, hemodynamic instability is seldom a problem unless the patient has preexisting cardiovascular disease (Shapiro et al., 1991).

In contrast, if a patient has a normal or elevated lung compliance, the increased alveolar pressure due to the PEEP will more readily be transmitted into the pleural space. In other words, PEEP therapy in patients with normal or high lung compliance will more likely produce an elevated pleural pressure and therefore a decreased venous return (Shapiro et al., 1991).

Barotrauma.   Barotrauma is lung injury that results from the hyperinflation of alveoli past the rupture point. Although each patient is different, a PEEP greater than 10 cm H_2O (or mean airway pressure > 30 cm H_2O, or a peak inspiratory pressure > 50 cm H_2O) are associated with an increased incidence of alveolar rupture or barotrauma (Bezzant et al., 1994; Slutsky, 1994). Alveolar rupture can produce pneumothorax, tension pneumothorax, pneumomediastinum, pneumopericardium and pneumoperitoneum. Subcutaneous emphysema or crepitus of unknown cause should always be interpreted as a sign that barotrauma has occurred.

☑ PEEP greater than 10 cm H_2O (or mean airway pressure > 30 cm H_2O, peak inspiratory pressure > 50 cm H_2O) are associated with an increased incidence of barotrauma.

Since PEEP increases alveolar pressures and alveolar volumes, it has the potential to produce barotrauma (Petersen et al., 1983), especially when combined with volume-cycled ventilation. Therefore plateau pressures should be closely monitored in these patients as well as being vigilant for any signs of barotrauma.

☑ In patients with normal lung compliance, PEEP may increase the intracranial pressure due to impedance of venous return from the head.

Increased Intracranial Pressure.   In patients with normal lung compliance, PEEP may increase the intracranial pressure (ICP) due to an impedance of venous return from the head. However, in patients with ARDS or noncompliant lungs, transmission of the excessive pressure generated by PEEP is minimal and it does not cause as much adverse effect on a patient's ICP.

☑ Positive pressure ventilation can reduce the blood flow to the kidneys and affect its normal functions.

Alterations of Renal Functions and Water Metabolism.   Kidneys play an important role in eliminating wastes, clearance of certain drugs, and regulating fluid, electrolyte, and acid-base balance. They are highly vascular and at any one time receive about 25% of the body's circulating blood volume (Brundage, 1992). Because of these characteristics, the kidneys are highly vulnerable to a decrease in blood flow as would occur during positive pressure ventilation.

When perfusion to the glomeruli of the kidneys is decreased, filtration becomes less effective (Baer et al., 1992). Subsequently, the urine

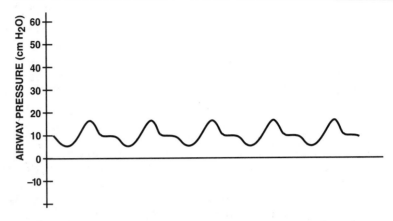

Figure 4-3 Continuous positive airway pressure (CPAP) of 10 cm H₂O.

output is decreased as the kidneys try to correct the hypovolemic condition by retaining fluid. If hypoperfusion of the kidneys persists or worsens, renal failure may result.

CONTINUOUS POSITIVE AIRWAY PRESSURE (CPAP)

Continuous positive airway pressure (CPAP) is PEEP applied to the airway of a patient who is breathing spontaneously (Figure 4-3). The indications for CPAP are essentially the same as for PEEP with the addition requirement that the patient must have adequate lung functions that can sustain **eucapnic ventilation** documented by the $PaCO_2$. In adults, CPAP may be given via a face mask, nasal mask, or endotracheal tube. In neonates, nasal CPAP is the method of choice.

eucapnic ventilation:
The amount of ventilation needed to bring the patient's $PaCO_2$ to normal.

BI-LEVEL POSITIVE AIRWAY PRESSURE (BIPAP)

Bi-level positive airway pressure (BiPAP): An airway pressure strategy that applies independent positive airway pressures (PAP) to both inspiration and expiration.

Bi-level positive airway pressure (BiPAP)® allows the clinician to apply independent positive airway pressures to both inspiration and expiration. IPAP (inspiratory) and EPAP (expiratory) are used to define when the positive airway pressure is present. IPAP provides positive pressure breaths and it improves hypoxemia and/or hypercapnia. EPAP is in essence CPAP and it improves oxygenation by increasing the functional residual capacity and enhancing alveolar recruitment.

INDICATIONS FOR BIPAP

☑ BiPAP appears to be of value in preventing intubation of the end-stage COPD patient and in supporting patients with chronic ventilatory failure.

BiPAP appears to be of value in preventing intubation of the end-stage COPD patient (Ambrosino et al., 1992; Confalonieri et al., 1994; Renston et al., 1994) and in supporting patients with chronic ventilatory failure (Strumpf, 1990). Other indications of BiPAP include patients with restrictive chest wall disease (Hill, 1992), neuromuscular disease (Ellis et al., 1987), and nocturnal hypoventilation (Carroll et al., 1988; Waldhorn, 1992).

INITIAL SETTINGS

☑ The initial settings of IPAP and EPAP are 8 cm H_2O and 4 cm H_2O, respectively.

Since the BiPAP system may be used in one of three modes: spontaneous, spontaneous/time, and timed, mode selection depends on a patient's needs and ability to breath spontaneously. In general, if the patient is breathing spontaneously, the IPAP and EPAP may be set at 8 cm H_2O and 4 cm H_2O, respectively. The spontaneous/timed mode is used as a backup mechanism and the breaths per minute (BPM) is set two to five breaths below the patient's spontaneous rate. In the timed mode, set IPAP and EPAP as above and the BPM slightly higher than the patient's spontaneous rate. The %IPAP may be set at 33% or 50% for an I:E ratio of 1:2 or 1:1, respectively.

☑ A BiPAP device can be used as a CPAP device by setting the IPAP and EPAP at the same level.

ADJUSTMENTS OF IPAP AND EPAP

IPAP levels are generally determined by monitoring the patient's clinical and physiologic response to gradual changes of IPAP, rather than by directly measuring the volume delivered.

☑ IPAP may be increased in increments of 2 cm H_2O to enhance the "pressure boost" to improve alveolar ventilation, normalize $PaCO_2$, and reduce the work of breathing.

When the cardiopulmonary responses are positive, the IPAP may be increased in increments of 2 cm H_2O to enhance the "pressure boost" to improve alveolar ventilation, normalize $PaCO_2$, and reduce the work of breathing. Since IPAP does not provide volume-cycled ventilation, the volume delivered by IPAP is directly related to the IPAP and EPAP pressure difference and the compliance characteristics of the lung/thorax system. The volume delivered is inversely related to the air flow resistance. In other words, a larger delivered volume may be obtained by (1) increasing the IPAP level, (2) decreasing the EPAP level, (3) increasing the compliance, and (4) reducing the air flow resistance.

☑ The EPAP should be increased by 2 cm H_2O increments to increase functional residual capacity and oxygenation in patients with intrapulmonary shunting.

The EPAP should be increased by 2 cm H_2O increments to increase functional residual capacity and oxygenation in patients with intrapulmonary shunting. When the EPAP is the same as the IPAP, CPAP results. It is not possible to increase the EPAP higher than the IPAP. Since IPAP and EPAP are methods to manipulate the airway pressures, all adverse effects of positive pressure ventilation and PEEP should be monitored. The patient should be advised to report any unusual chest discomfort, shortness of breath, or severe headache when using the BiPAP system.

CONTROLLED MANDATORY VENTILATION (CMV)

control mode: In control mode, the ventilator delivers the preset tidal volume at a set time interval (time-triggered respiratory rate).

With controlled mandatory ventilation or **control mode,** the ventilator delivers the preset tidal volume at a time-triggered respiratory rate (Figure 4-4). Since the ventilator controls both the patient's tidal volume and respiratory rate, the ventilator "controls" the patient's minute volume. In the control mode, a patient cannot change the ventilator respiratory rate or breath spontaneously. For example, if the tidal volume and respiratory rate of a ventilator are set at 800 ml and 10 BPM, respectively, the minute volume will be 8,000 ml.

The control mode should only be used when the patient is properly medicated with a combination of sedatives, respiratory depressants, and neuromuscular blockers. The control mode ventilation should not be instituted by decreasing the ventilator's triggering sensitivity to the point that no amount of patient effort can trigger the ventilator into inspiration. The problem with this approach should be obvious since any spontaneous inspiratory effort would be like attempting to inspire through a completely obstructed airway. Regardless of how vigorous the patient's inspiratory effort is, no gas flow would be delivered to the patient until the ventilator automatically becomes time triggered. If the control mode is improperly established in this way, it may not be physically harmful to the patient. However, it would most likely be psychologically devastating for the patient to realize that he or she has no control over his or her breathing requirements.

✓ The RCP must recognize any spontaneous breathing efforts during control mode ventilation.

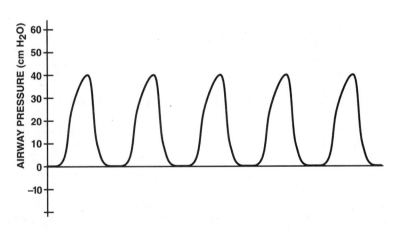

Figure 4-4 Control mode pressure tracing. The time intervals between mechanical breaths are equal when a control mode is used.

INDICATIONS FOR THE CONTROL MODE

The control mode is most often indicated if the patient "fights" the ventilator in the initial stages of mechanical ventilatory support. "Fighting" or "bucking" the ventilator often means that the patient is severely distressed and vigorously struggling to breathe. Their rapid spontaneous inspiratory efforts become asynchronous with the ventilator's ability to provide an adequate inspiratory flow. The typical result is that the patient will be attempting to actively exhale while the ventilator is delivering a breath. This results in high pressure limit cycling, which decreases the ventilator delivered tidal volume.

Other indications for control mode ventilation include (1) tetanus or other seizure activities that interrupt the delivery of mechanical ventilation (Linton et al., 1992), (2) complete rest for the patient typically for a period of 24 hours (Perel et al., 1991), and (3) patients with a crushed chest injury in which spontaneous inspiratory efforts produce significant paradoxical chest wall movement (Burton et al., 1991).

COMPLICATIONS ASSOCIATED WITH THE CONTROL MODE

✓ In a sedated or apneic patient, the primary hazard of the control mode is the potential for apnea and hypoxia if the patient should become disconnected from the ventilator or the ventilator should fail to operate.

Since the patient's spontaneous respiratory drive will have been blunted with sedation in the control mode, the patient is totally dependent on the ventilator for ventilation and oxygenation. As a result, the primary hazard associated with the control mode is the potential for apnea and hypoxia if the patient should become accidentally disconnected from the ventilator or the ventilator should fail to operate.

Because of the patient's dependence on the ventilator, the most important alarms in the control mode become those that alert the caregiver of any interruption in the patient's ventilation. The important ventilator alarms include the low exhaled volume alarm and the low inspiratory pressure alarm.

OVERVIEW

Table 4-1 summarizes the major characteristics of the control mode.

TABLE 4-1   **Characteristics of the Control Mode**

CHARACTERISTIC	DESCRIPTION
Type of breath	Each breath delivers a mechanical tidal volume.
Triggering mechanism	Every breath in the control mode is time triggered.
Cycling mechanism	Inspiration is terminated by the delivery of a preset tidal volume (volume cycled).

ASSIST CONTROL (AC)

With the assist/control (AC) mode, the patient may increase the ventilator respiratory rate (assist) in addition to the preset mechanical respiratory rate (control). Each control breath provides the patient with a pre-set, ventilator delivered tidal volume. Each assist breath also results in a preset, ventilator delivered tidal volume. The assist-control mode does not allow the patient to take spontaneous breaths (Figure 4-5).

ASSIST CONTROL TRIGGERING MECHANISM

The mandatory mechanical breaths may be either patient triggered by the patient's spontaneous inspiratory efforts (assist) or time triggered by a preset respiratory rate (control). If a breath is patient triggered, it is referred to as an assisted breath; if a breath is time triggered, the breath is referred to as a control breath.

For example, if the patient has a stable assist rate of 12 breaths per minute, then the patient is triggering breaths every 5 seconds. If the control rate is preset at 10 breaths per minute, the ventilator would deliver time-triggered breaths every 6 seconds. However, since the interval between the assisted breaths is shorter than 6 seconds, no time-triggered breaths will be delivered. If however, the patient's spontaneous breaths were to decrease less than the preset control rate, then the ventilator would begin delivering time-triggered breaths.

ASSIST CONTROL CYCLING MECHANISM

Inspiration in the AC mode is terminated by volume cycling. When the preset tidal volume is delivered, the ventilator is cycled to expiration.

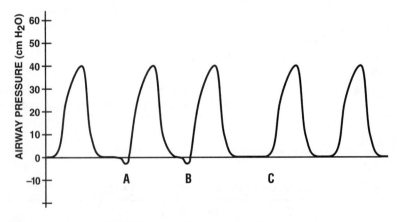

Figure 4-5   Assist/control mode pressure tracing. Each assisted or controlled breath triggers a mechanical tidal volume. (A) An assisted breath; note the negative deflection at the beginning of inspiration. (B) Another assisted breath that is initiated by the patient sooner than (A). (C) A controlled breath; note the absence of a negative deflection at the beginning of inspiration.

INDICATIONS FOR THE AC MODE

The AC mode is most often used to provide full ventilatory support for patients when they are first placed on mechanical ventilation. Full ventilatory support is defined as any ventilator mode that provides all of the work of breathing.

The AC mode is typically used for patients who have a stable respiratory drive (a stable rate of spontaneous inspiratory efforts of at least 10 to 12 per minute) and can therefore trigger the ventilator into inspiration. Essentially, the time-triggering control rate is generally considered as a safety net to provide adequate ventilation in the event that the patient stops triggering the ventilator at an acceptable respiratory rate (Sassoon et al., 1990). The generally accepted minimum control respiratory rate in the AC mode is 2 to 4 breaths per minute less than the patient's assist rate, or a minimum control rate of from 8 to 10 breaths per minute.

ADVANTAGES OF THE AC MODE

☑ The AC mode allows the patient to control the respiratory rate and therefore the minute volume required to normalize the patient's $PaCO_2$.

There are two primary advantages with the AC mode. First, the patient's work of breathing requirement in the AC is very small when the triggering sensitivity (pressure or flow) is set appropriately and the ventilator supplies an inspiratory flow that meets or exceeds the patient's inspiratory flow demand. The second advantage of AC is that if the patient has an appropriate ventilatory drive, this mode allows the patient to control the respiratory rate and therefore the minute volume required to normalize the patient's $PaCO_2$ (Kirby, 1988).

COMPLICATIONS ASSOCIATED WITH THE AC MODE

intermittent mandatory ventilation (IMV): IMV is a mode in which the ventilator delivers control (mandatory) breaths and allows the patient to breathe spontaneously to any tidal volume the patient is capable of between the mandatory breaths.

The potential hazard associated with AC is alveolar hyperventilation (respiratory alkalosis). In two separate studies, the pH was found to be higher and the $PaCO_2$ was lower in the AC mode than the results obtained in the **intermittent mandatory ventilation (IMV)** mode (Culpepper et al., 1985; Hopper et al., 1985). If the patient's respiratory center is either injured or diseased, the patient may have an inappropriately high respiratory drive leading to an excessive assist rate despite a low $PaCO_2$. If the patient is assisting at a high respiratory rate (i.e., > 20 to 25 breaths/minute) and the tidal volume is preset at 10 to 15 ml/kg, this will usually result in hypocapnia and respiratory alkalosis.

Mechanical deadspace may be used in this situation, but it is generally considered safer to switch the patient to another mode of ventilation (e.g., SIMV) that limits the patient's ability to generate excessive minute volumes.

OVERVIEW

Table 4-2 summarizes the major characteristics of the assist control mode.

TABLE 4-2 Characteristics of the Assist Control Mode

CHARACTERISTIC	DESCRIPTION
Type of breath	Each breath, assist or control, delivers a preset mechanical tidal volume.
Triggering mechanism	Mechanical breaths may be either patient triggered (assist) or time triggered (control).
Cycling mechanism	Inspiration is terminated either by the delivery of a preset tidal volume (volume cycled) or by the high pressure limit (pressure cycled).

INTERMITTENT MANDATORY VENTILATION (IMV)

☑ Since IMV breaths are delivered at a rate independent of the patient's spontaneous respiratory rate, breath stacking may occur.

Intermittent mandatory ventilation (IMV) is a mode in which the ventilator delivers control (mandatory) breaths and allows the patient to breathe spontaneously at any tidal volume the patient is capable of in between the mandatory breaths (Figure 4-6).

Historically, IMV was a separate circuit adapted to ventilators that were designed to provide either assist/control or control mode ventilation. As such, it was the first widely used mode that allowed partial

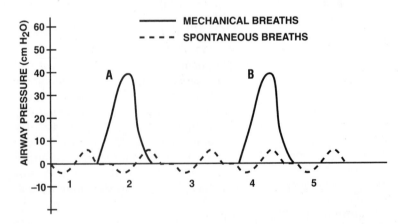

Figure 4-6 Intermittent mandatory ventilation (IMV) pressure tracing with two mandatory breaths and five anticipated spontaneous breaths (only three active). IMV mode may cause breath stacking since the mandatory breaths are delivered at a set time interval with no regard to the patient's breathing frequency. Mandatory breath (A) begins before the patient is ready for the anticipated spontaneous breath #2. Mandatory breath (B) begins shortly after the initiation of the anticipated spontaneous breath #4. The anticipated spontaneous breaths #2 and #4 did not occur as they turned into mechanical breaths during the mandatory cycle.

ventilatory support (i.e., a mode that allowed the patient to breathe spontaneously in addition to receiving ventilator delivered breaths) (Heenan et al., 1980).

The primary complication associated with IMV was the random chance for breath stacking. This occurs when the patient is taking a spontaneous breath and the ventilator delivers a time-triggered mandatory breath at the same time. If this occurs, the patient's lung volume and airway pressure could increase significantly. Setting appropriate high pressure limits will reduce the risk of barotrauma in the event of breath stacking. As long as the breath stacking only occurs occasionally, the IMV mode is an acceptable mode of ventilation with few complications.

The sophistication of ventilator technology has progressed to the point that no new adult ventilators offer the IMV mode. Rather, all ventilators currently available have been designed to provide synchronized IMV (SIMV) (Shapiro et al., 1976).

SYNCHRONIZED INTERMITTENT MANDATORY VENTILATION (SIMV)

synchronized intermittent mandatory ventilation (SIMV): SIMV is a mode in which the ventilator delivers control (mandatory) breaths to the patient at or near the time of a spontaneous breath. The mandatory breaths are synchronized with the patient's spontaneous breathing efforts so as to avoid breath stacking.

Synchronized intermittent mandatory ventilation (SIMV) is a mode in which the ventilator delivers either assisted breaths to the patient at the beginning of a spontaneous breath or time-triggered mandatory breaths. The mandatory breaths are synchronized with the patient's spontaneous breathing efforts so as to avoid breath stacking (Figure 4-7).

SIMV MANDATORY BREATH-TRIGGERING MECHANISM

The SIMV mandatory breaths may be either time triggered or patient triggered. The triggering mechanism is determined by whether or not the patient makes a spontaneous inspiratory effort just prior to the delivery of a time-triggered breath. For example, if the SIMV mandatory respiratory rate is set at 10 breaths per minute, then the ventilator would time trigger a breath every 6 seconds if the patient is not attempting to inspire spontaneously. However, if the patient is breathing spontaneously between the mandatory breaths, and if by random chance, the patient begins to inspire just prior to the point at which the ventilator would be expected to time trigger, then the ventilator senses this spontaneous effort and delivers the mandatory breath as an assisted patient-triggered breath. The mandatory breath whether time or patient-triggered is controlled by all applicable mechanical tidal volume settings.

Synchronization Window. The time interval just prior to time triggering in which the ventilator is responsive to the patient's spontaneous

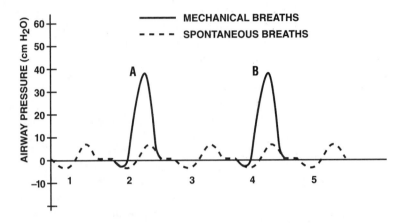

Figure 4-7 Synchronized intermittent mandatory ventilation (SIMV) pressure tracing with two synchronized mandatory breaths and five anticipated spontaneous breaths (only three active). SIMV mode does not cause breath stacking since the mandatory breaths are delivered slightly sooner or later than the preset time interval but within a time window. Mandatory breaths (A) and (B) occur during a spontaneous inspiratory effort. The anticipated spontaneous breaths #2 and #4 did not occur as they turned into mechanical breaths during the mandatory cycle.

inspiratory effort is commonly referred to as the "synchronization window" (Sassoon, 1991). Although the exact time interval of the synchronization window is slightly different from manufacturer to manufacturer, 0.5 second is representative. For example, given an SIMV mandatory rate of 10 breaths per minute, the ventilator would be expected to time trigger every 6 seconds. If the synchronization window is 0.5 second, then at 5.5 seconds from the beginning of the previous mandatory breath, the ventilator automatically becomes sensitive to any spontaneous inspiratory effort; i.e., the synchronization window becomes active. If the patient makes a spontaneous inspiratory effort when the synchronization window is active, the ventilator is patient triggered to deliver an assisted mandatory breath. Patient triggering may be based either on pressure or flow. If however, no spontaneous inspiratory effort exists while the synchronization window is active, the ventilator will time trigger when the full time triggering interval elapses.

SIMV SPONTANEOUS BREATH-TRIGGERING MECHANISM

☑ Spontaneous rate and tidal volume taken by the patient in the SIMV mode are totally dependent on the patient's breathing effort.

In between the mandatory breaths, SIMV permits the patient to breathe spontaneously to any tidal volume the patient desires. The gas source for spontaneous breathing in the SIMV mode is typically supplied by a demand valve. The demand valve is always patient triggered, either by pressure or flow depending on the ventilator.

It is important to understand that the spontaneous breaths taken by the patient in the SIMV mode are truly spontaneous. The ventilator provides the humidified gas at the selected F_1O_2, but the spontaneous rate and spontaneous tidal volume are totally dependent on the patient's breathing effort.

INDICATIONS FOR THE SIMV MODE

✓ The primary indication for SIMV is to provide partial ventilatory support to the patient.

The primary indication for SIMV is to provide partial ventilatory support; i.e., a desire to have the patient actively involved in providing part of the minute volume. In a practical sense, when a patient is first placed on ventilatory support, full ventilatory support is appropriate to provide a period of rest, typically for the first 24 hours. After this initial period of full ventilatory support, it is typical practice to place the patient on a trial run of partial ventilatory support with SIMV. It is customary to ease the patient from full support to partial support by gradually decreasing the mandatory rate as tolerated by the patient. This depends on, of course, reversal of the clinical conditions that committed the patient to the ventilator in the first place.

ADVANTAGES OF THE SIMV MODE

Since SIMV promotes spontaneous breathing and use of respiratory muscles, SIMV (1) maintains respiratory muscle strength/avoids muscle atrophy, (2) reduces ventilation to perfusion mismatch, (3) decreases mean airway pressure, and (4) facilitates weaning.

Maintains Respiratory Muscle Strength/Avoids Muscle Atrophy. SIMV helps to maintain respiratory muscle activity and strength. Patients maintained in full ventilatory support for extended periods tend to experience partial loss of ventilatory muscle strength. This can be minimized by using the respiratory muscles during spontaneous breathing (Zelt et al., 1972).

Reduces Ventilation to Perfusion Mismatch. Deadspace ventilation (i.e., high ventilation to low perfusion) is typical in the upper zone of the lungs because pulmonary perfusion is gravity dependent and favors the lower lung zone. This problem is intensified during positive pressure ventilation as the lung units in the upper zone are hyperinflated. Spontaneous breathing during SIMV tends to distribute the spontaneous tidal volume more evenly thus reducing alveolar deadspace ventilation (Weisman et al., 1983).

Decreases Mean Airway Pressure. The mean airway pressure is directly related to the peak inspiratory pressure and inspiratory time (Note: Two other factors are respiratory rate and positive end-expiratory pressure). Since spontaneous breaths during SIMV have a lower peak inspiratory pressure and inspiratory time, SIMV tends to have a lower mean airway pressure.

The mean airway pressure is an important consideration because the greater the mean airway pressure, the greater the potential for a

TABLE 4-3 Characteristics of the Synchronized IMV Mode

CHARACTERISTIC	DESCRIPTION
Type of breath	The ventilator delivers mechanical tidal volume at a preset respiratory rate. The patient may breathe spontaneously between mandatory breaths.
Triggering mechanism	Mandatory breaths may be either time triggered or patient triggered. Spontaneous breaths are patient triggered (i.e., the demand flow valve opens in response to the patient's spontaneous inspiratory effort).
Cycling mechanism	The mandatory breaths are volume cycled. The patient controls spontaneous rate and volume.

reduced venous return, cardiac output, and arterial perfusion pressure. Reduction of the mean airway pressure during SIMV indirectly enhances the patient's cardiovascular functions (Scanlan et al., 1999).

Facilitates Weaning. SIMV facilitates weaning due to its ability to decrease the mandatory rate in small increments. This may offer some advantage to those "hard-to-wean" patients who cannot tolerate an abrupt decrease of the mechanical respiratory rate (Downs et al., 1973).

COMPLICATIONS ASSOCIATED WITH THE SIMV MODE

The ideal approach of SIMV weaning is to provide a spontaneous breathing workload that gradually increases a patient's muscle strength and endurance. The primary disadvantage associated with SIMV is the desire to wean the patient too rapidly, leading first to a high work of spontaneous breathing and ultimately to muscle fatigue and weaning failure. The best way to avoid this is to decrease the SIMV mandatory respiratory rate slowly and monitor the patient closely for signs of fatigue (Scanlan et al., 1999).

OVERVIEW

Table 4-3 summarizes the major characteristics of the synchronized IMV mode.

MANDATORY MINUTE VENTILATION (MMV)

mandatory minute ventilation (MMV): MMV is a feature of some ventilators that causes an increase of the mandatory rate (Note: In Hamilton Veolar, the pressure support level), when the patient's spontaneous breathing level becomes inadequate. This compensation by the ventilator ensures a safe minimal minute ventilation.

Mandatory minute ventilation (MMV), also called minimum minute ventilation, is a feature of some ventilators that provides a predetermined minute ventilation when the patient's spontaneous breathing effort becomes inadequate. For example, an apnea episode (lack of spontaneous breathing) may cause the actual minute ventilation to drop below the preset level. When this occurs, the mandatory rate is increased automatically to compensate for the decrease in minute ventilation caused by the apnea. This compensation by the ventilator ensures a desired minute ventilation.

MMV is an additional function of the SIMV mode and is intended to prevent hypercapnia by "automatically" insuring that the patient receives a minimum preset minute volume. It is especially useful in preventing hypoventilation and respiratory acidosis in the final stages of weaning with SIMV when the patient's spontaneous breathing is assuming a significant portion of the total minute volume.

For example, a patient may have been weaned down to a mandatory SIMV rate of 4/min with a mandatory tidal volume of 800 ml; the patient's ventilator delivered minute volume would then be 3.2 liters/minute ($\dot{V}_E = RR \times V_T$). If this patient's spontaneous minute volume is 6 liters/minute, then the total minute volume is the sum of the ventilator-delivered minute volume and the spontaneous breathing minute volume 9.2 liters/minute in this example. If the patient's spontaneous minute volume suddenly decreases by a significant amount or if the patient becomes apneic, then without MMV the reduced minute volume would cause hypercapnia and respiratory acidosis. However, on MMV-equipped ventilators, a decrease in the patient's spontaneous minute volume would trigger an automatic increase in the ventilator's mandatory respiratory rate.

The way that MMV functions on the majority of ventilators is that a desired minimum minute volume is preset on the ventilator; usually only slightly less than the minute volume required to "normalize" the $PaCO_2$. The ventilator then measures the total minute volume and compares it with the preset minimum minute volume. As long as the patient's total minute volume equals or exceeds the preset minimum minute volume, the MMV function is not activated. However, if the patient's spontaneous minute volume decreases to the point that the total minute volume becomes less than the preset mandatory minute volume, then the ventilator will automatically increase the SIMV mandatory respiratory rate until it reaches the preset mandatory minute volume.

In the MMV mode, it is important to monitor not only the patient's spontaneous minute volume, but also the patient's estimated spontaneous alveolar minute volume. The reason for this is that if the patient becomes distressed, the tendency is to increase the spontaneous respiratory rate at the expense of a decreased tidal volume (i.e., the patient will typically adopt the spontaneous breathing pattern that minimizes the work of breathing). A minute volume supported by a rapid respiratory rate and low tidal volume may avert the MMV function but at the same time provides a significant amount of deadspace ventilation. This results in a decreased alveolar minute volume.

☑ A minute volume supported by rapid respiratory rate and low tidal volume (e.g., distressed patient) may avert the MMV function but at the same time provides a significant amount of deadspace ventilation. This results in a decreased alveolar minute volume.

TABLE 4-4   Characteristics of the Mandatory Minute Ventilation Mode

CHARACTERISTIC	DESCRIPTION
Type of breath	The ventilator increases the mandatory respiratory rate (Note: Hamilton Veolar increases the pressure support level).
Triggering mechanism	Increase of the mandatory respiratory rate (or the pressure support level in the Hamilton Veolar) is triggered when the actual minute volume is less than the preset minimal minute volume.
Cycling mechanism	All mandatory breaths are volume cycled. Patients control their own spontaneous rates and volumes.

Perhaps the most efficient method of insuring that this condition does not occur is to set the high respiratory rate alarm at approximately ten breaths/minute greater than the patient's "baseline" spontaneous respiratory rate.

Although MMV operates in the manner previously described on most ventilators, one exception is seen in the Hamilton Veolar ventilator. Selecting the MMV mode on this ventilator automatically places the patient in a "pure" pressure support mode (i.e., every breath is a spontaneous pressure-supported breath and no mandatory breaths are given). A minimum desired mandatory minute volume is selected and the ventilator automatically compares the patient's total minute volume with the preset minimum minute volume. On the Veolar, if the patient's total minute volume is less than the preset minimum minute volume, the ventilator automatically increases the pressure support level until the minimum minute volume is obtained (Scanlan et al., 1999).

OVERVIEW

Table 4-4 summarizes the major characteristics of the mandatory minute ventilation mode.

PRESSURE SUPPORT VENTILATION (PSV)

☑ PSV lowers the work of spontaneous breathing and augments the spontaneous tidal volume.

Pressure support ventilation (PSV) is used to lower the work of spontaneous breathing and augment a patient's spontaneous tidal volume. When PSV is used with SIMV, it significantly lowers the oxygen consumption requirement presumably due to the reduced work of breathing (Kanak et al., 1985).

PSV applies a preset pressure plateau to the patient's airway for the duration of a spontaneous breath (Figure 4-8). Pressure-supported breaths are considered spontaneous because (1) they are patient triggered, (2) the tidal volume varies with the patient's inspiratory flow

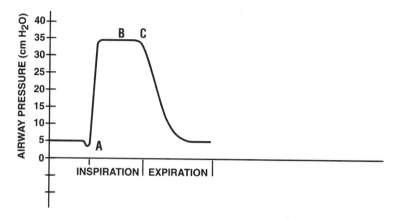

Figure 4-8 Pressure support ventilation (PSV) with PEEP of 5 cm H_2O. (A) Inspiratory effort; (B) Pressure support plateau of 30 cm H_2O (Peak airway pressure of 35 cm H_2O, PEEP of 5 cm H_2O); (C) Beginning expiratory phase when the inspiratory flow drops to 25% (or other predetermined %) of its peak flow.

demand, (3) inspiration lasts only for as long as the patient actively inspires, and (4) inspiration is terminated when the patient's inspiratory flow demand decreases to a preset minimal value. PSV can be used in conjunction with spontaneous breathing in any ventilator mode.

A pressure-supported breath is therefore patient triggered, pressure limited, and flow cycled. It is pressure limited because the maximum airway pressure cannot exceed the preset pressure support level. It is flow cycled because a pressure-supported breath cycles to expiration when the flow reaches a minimal level.

It is important to understand how the pressure plateau is created and maintained. Essentially, when the pressure-supported breath is patient triggered (either by pressure or flow), the ventilator demand valve generates a flow high enough to rapidly increase the airway pressure to the preset pressure limit and then maintain the pressure plateau (via servo control and demand valve) for the duration of the patient's spontaneous inspiratory effort. Typically, the flow pattern associated with pressure support is a steeply descending tapered flow pattern. As previously described, the demand valve flow terminates when it decreases to a preset lower flow limit. The point at which flow cycling occurs varies with different ventilators but 5L/min is representative.

INDICATIONS FOR THE PSV MODE

Pressure support is commonly applied in the SIMV mode when the patient takes spontaneous breaths. Pressure support is not active during the mandatory breaths. Pressure support has been advocated as a stand-alone mode by some clinicians, however this requires close monitoring because as a stand-alone mode, every breath is patient triggered.

☑ **Pressure support (1)** ↑ spontaneous tidal volume, **(2)** ↓ spontaneous respiratory rate, and **(3)** ↓ work of breathing.

☑ **The level of pressure support is titrated until (1)** spontaneous tidal volume = 10 to 15 ml/kg or **(2)** spontaneous respiratory rate < 25/min.

Pressure support is typically used in the SIMV mode to facilitate weaning in a difficult to wean patient. In this application, pressure support (1) increases the patient's spontaneous tidal volume, (2) decreases the patient's spontaneous respiratory rate, and (3) decreases the work of breathing.

These three effects have been used to titrate the proper level of pressure support. For example, one physician may increase the pressure support level until a desired spontaneous tidal volume is achieved (e.g., 10 to 15 ml/kg). Another physician may increase the pressure support level until the patient's spontaneous respiratory rate decreases to a target value (usually 25 breaths/min or less) (MacIntyre, 1987).

The third endpoint for the pressure support level is to decrease the work of breathing (MacIntyre, 1986). This approach is probably less commonly used for the patient in immediate respiratory distress, but is more often used as a "routine" method to decrease the work of breathing. Since an endotracheal tube provides an increased airway resistance and increased the work of breathing, pressure support has been used successfully to overcome this gas flow resistance. The airway resistance on most modern ventilators may be obtained easily but in ventilators not equipped with this function, the following equation may be used to estimate the airway resistance:

☑ **See Appendix 1 for example.**

$$\text{Airway Resistance} = \frac{(\text{Peak airway pressure} - \text{Plateau pressure})}{\text{Mean Flow}}$$

OVERVIEW

Table 4-5 summarizes the major characteristics of the pressure support ventilation mode.

TABLE 4-5   Characteristics of the Pressure Support Ventilation Mode

CHARACTERISTIC	DESCRIPTION
Type of breath	Pressure-supported breaths are considered spontaneous. (Note: Pressure support may be applied in any mode that permits spontaneous breathing such as SIMV).
Triggering mechanism	Pressure-supported breaths are always patient triggered.
Cycling mechanism	Pressure-supported breaths are technically flow cycled by a minimum spontaneous inspiratory flow threshold. This minimum inspiratory flow is controlled entirely by the patient's spontaneous inspiratory flow demand.

NOTES: *The tidal volume delivered by a pressure-supported breath is influenced both by the pressure support level (cm H$_2$O) and the patient's spontaneous inspiratory flow demand. The inspiratory time of the pressure-supported breath is also completely controlled by the patient's spontaneous inspiratory flow demand.*

PRESSURE CONTROL VENTILATION (PCV)

pressure control ventilation (PCV): Once inspiration begins, a pressure plateau is created and maintained for a preset inspiratory time.

In **pressure control ventilation (PCV)**, the pressure-controlled breaths are time triggered by a preset respiratory rate. Once inspiration begins, a pressure plateau is created and maintained for a preset inspiratory time. Pressure-controlled breaths are therefore time triggered, pressure limited, and time cycled.

Pressure control is a newer mode of controlled ventilation that has some functional similarities to pressure support ventilation, but they have very different indications. Pressure-controlled breaths are time triggered by a preset respiratory rate and as in the control mode, the patient should be sedated. Once a pressure-controlled breath has been time triggered, a pressure plateau is created and maintained by servo-controlled inspiratory flow in a manner similar to pressure support. Recall that the pressure plateau in pressure support is maintained for as long as the patient maintains a spontaneous inspiratory flow. In pressure control however, the pressure plateau is maintained for a preset inspiratory time (Figure 4-9).

☑ Pressure control can minimize the peak inspiratory pressure while still maintaining adequate oxygenation and ventilation.

Pressure control is usually indicated for patients with severe ARDS who require extremely high peak inspiratory pressures during mechanical ventilation in a volume-cycled mode. As a result of these high airway pressures, they have a higher incidence of barotrauma (Gurevitch et al., 1986).

The advantage of switching these patients from conventional volume-cycled ventilation to pressure control is that by doing so, the peak inspiratory pressure can be reduced while still maintaining

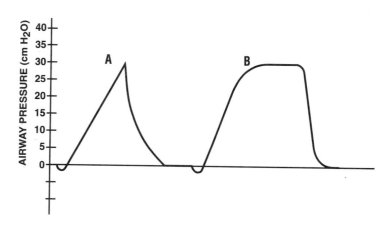

Figure 4-9 (A) Pressure tracing of a volume-controlled mechanical breath; (B) Pressure tracing of a pressure-controlled mechanical breath; note the prolonged inspiratory pressure plateau with pressure control ventilation.

TABLE 4-6   Characteristics of the Pressure Control Ventilation Mode

CHARACTERISTIC	DESCRIPTION
Type of breath	Only mandatory breaths are available to the patient in the pressure control mode.
Triggering nechanism	The mandatory breaths in the pressure control mode are all time triggered by a preset respiratory rate.
Cycling mechanism	The mandatory breaths are time cycled by a preset inspiratory time.

NOTES: The peak inspiratory pressure is controlled by the preset pressure limit. As with any pressure limited ventilator, the tidal volume will vary directly with lung compliance and inversely with airway resistance. It may be necessary to "invert" the I:E ratio beyond 1:2 to maintain oxygenation. I:E ratios as high as 4:1 have been reported with successful outcome.

adequate oxygenation (PaO_2) and ventilation ($PaCO_2$) (Lain et al., 1989). Being able to decrease the PIP significantly reduces the risk of barotrauma for these patients.

OVERVIEW

Table 4-6 summarizes the major characteristics of the pressure control ventilation mode.

PROPORTIONAL ASSIST VENTILATION

☑ PAV may be flow assist or volume assist and it is active in assist breaths only.

☑ With PAV, the pressure supplied by the ventilator is variable and it is proportional to the patient's breathing effort.

Proportional Assist Ventilation (PAV) is a mode of assisted ventilation where pressure is applied by the ventilator in proportion to the patient-generated flow and volume. Flow assist (FA) is a term used to describe a strategy of PAV where the applied pressure is used to satisfy the patient's inspiratory flow demand. FA reduces the inspiratory effort needed to overcome airflow resistance (i.e., obstructive defects). Volume assist (VA) occurs when PAV provides the applied pressure to meet the patient's volume demand. VA reduces the inspiratory effort needed to overcome systemic elastance (i.e., restrictive defects) (Navalesi, Hernandez, Wongsa et al., 1996). With PAV, there is no target flow, volume, or pressure during mechanical ventilation. The pressure supplied by the ventilator is variable and it is in proportion to the patient's breathing effort (Appendini, Purro, Gudjonsdottir et al., 1999).

PAV is achieved by a positive feedback control that amplifies airway pressure in proportion to instantaneous inspiratory flow and volume. Unlike traditional modes of mechanical ventilation that deliver a preset tidal volume or inspiratory pressure, with PAV the level of applied pressure is designed to change with the patient's effort. The advantage of PAV is its ability to track changes of ventilatory effort that may occur over time. By varying the applied pressure to augment flow and volume, a more uniform breathing pattern becomes possible (Bigatello, Nishimura, Imanaka et al., 1997). PAV has been reported to provide mechanical support while promoting patient-ventilator synchrony (Younes, 1992).

In terms of physiologic response, PAV improves ventilation and reduces both P0.1 (neuromuscular drive) and work of breathing in ventilator-dependent patients with COPD. When PAV is used with CPAP, the reduction of inspiratory muscle work reaches values close to those found in normal subjects. Exercise tolerance may be improved with this strategy of combining PAV with CPAP (Appendini, Purro, Gudjonsdottir et al., 1999; Dolmage & Goldstein, 1997).

OVERVIEW

Table 4-7 summarizes the major characteristics of the proportional assist ventilation mode.

AIRWAY PRESSURE RELEASE VENTILATION (APRV)

airway pressure release ventilation (APRV): A mode of ventilation in which the spontaneous breaths are at an elevated baseline (i.e., CPAP). This elevated baseline is periodically "released" to facilitate expiration.

Airway pressure release ventilation (APRV) is similar to CPAP in that the patient is allowed to breathe spontaneously without restriction. During spontaneous exhalation, the PEEP is dropped (released) to a lower level and this action simulates an effective exhalation maneuver. The length of pressure release time is usually between one to two seconds. When the pressure release time is shorter than the spontaneous effort, it resembles pressure-controlled (from high to low baseline pressure) with an inverse inspiratory-expiratory (I:E) ratio.

To provide APRV, the ventilator must have a high flow CPAP circuit that has been modified with the addition of a release valve. When the release valve opens, the CPAP pressure is vented and the circuit

TABLE 4-7   Characteristics of Proportional Assist Ventilation

CHARACTERISTIC	DESCRIPTION
Type of breath	PAV occurs during assisted breaths only.
Triggering mechanism	Pressure or flow triggered by the patient.
Cycling mechanism	PAV terminates once the flow or volume satisfies patient's demand

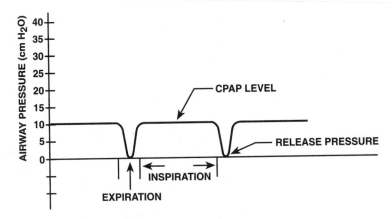

Figure 4-10 Airway pressure release ventilation (APRV) at a CPAP level of 10 cm H_2O and pressure release to 0 cm H_2O with a net release pressure gradient of 10 (10–0) cm H_2O. During APRV, the expiratory phase occurs when the airway pressure is released from 10 to 0 cm H_2O. On inspiration, the CPAP level is maintained at 10 cm H_2O. Since the pressure release time period is rather short, an inversed I:E ratio is usually observed when the mechanical rate is less than 20 breaths per minute (or more than 3 seconds per breath). The tidal volume during APRV is determined by the pressure gradient between CPAP and final pressure after pressure release.

pressure decreases to zero or a lower CPAP level. Figure 4-10 shows the airway pressure release during CPAP mode.

A mandatory inspiration begins with time-triggered closing of the release valve. The airway pressure rapidly increases to the baseline CPAP pressure and is maintained for the duration of inspiration (for as long as the release valve remains closed). The mandatory inspiration ends with time-triggered opening of the release valve, which allows the circuit pressure to decrease as the patient exhales. What is unique about this mode is that the patient is allowed to inspire spontaneously at any point during a mandatory breath. Since APRV mandatory breaths are pressure limited, for a given pressure gradient (difference between the CPAP circuit pressure and the release pressure), the patient's tidal volume will vary directly with changes in lung compliance and inversely with changes in airway resistance. For this reason, the patient's exhaled tidal volume should be closely monitored.

INDICATIONS FOR THE APRV MODE

This is a relatively new mode of ventilation that has yet to gain wide acceptance. At present, the primary indication for this mode is similar to that of pressure control, namely, as an alternative to conventional volume-cycled ventilation for patients with significantly decreased lung compliance such as patients with ARDS. Conventional volume-

☑ With APRV, the patient's tidal volume will vary directly with changes in lung compliance and inversely with changes in airway resistance.

☑ APRV can provide effective partial ventilatory support with lower peak airway pressure than that provided by the PSV and SIMV modes.

TABLE 4-8   Characteristics of the Airway Pressure Release Ventilation Mode

CHARACTERISTIC	DESCRIPTION
Type of breath	Time-triggered mandatory breaths will continue in this mode and the patient is allowed to breathe spontaneously between mandatory breaths.
Triggering mechanism	The mandatory breaths are time triggered, and the patient assumes all spontaneous breaths.
Cycling mechanism	The mandatory breaths are time cycled by a preset inspiratory time.

cycled ventilation in these patients is associated with excessive peak airway pressures and barotrauma. APRV can provide effective partial ventilatory support with lower peak airway pressure than that provided by the PSV and SIMV modes (Chiang et al., 1994). However, APRV may be less comfortable than the PSV and SIMV mode, and synchronization with mechanical breaths may also be a problem.

OVERVIEW
Table 4-8 summarizes the major characteristics of the airway pressure release ventilation mode.

INVERSE RATIO VENTILATION (IRV)

The ratio of inspiratory time (I time) to expiratory time (E time) is known as the I:E ratio. In conventional mechanical ventilation, the I time is traditionally lower than the E time so that the I:E ratio ranges from about 1:1.5 to 1:3. This resembles the normal I:E ratio during spontaneous breathing, and it is considered physiologically beneficial to normal cardiopulmonary function.

Since the mid-1980s, investigators have been extending the inspiratory time during mechanical ventilation to promote oxygenation in patients with ARDS (Gurevitch et al., 1986; Marcy et al., 1991). The inverse I:E ratio in use is between 2:1 to 4:1 and often it is used in conjunction with pressure control ventilation (Lain et al., 1989; Tharratt et al., 1988).

☑ Inverse ratio ventilation (IRV) improves oxygenation by (1) ↓ intrapulmonary shunting, (2) ↑ V/Q matching, and (3) ↓ deadspace ventilation.

PHYSIOLOGY OF IRV
Inverse ratio ventilation (IRV) improves oxygenation by (1) reduction of intrapulmonary shunting, (2) improvement of V/Q matching, and (3) decrease of deadspace ventilation. From the review of available literature, Shanholtz et al. (1994) concluded that these mechanisms were also achievable by use of conventional ventilation with PEEP. However, two notable changes are observed during IRV. They are

(1) increase of mean airway pressure, and (2) presence of auto-PEEP. These two changes are likely the reason for the improvement of shunting and hypoxemia in ARDS patients.

✓ The increase in MAWP during IRV helps to reduce shunting and improve oxygenation in ARDS patients.

Increase of Mean Airway Pressure.   To achieve the same degree of ventilation and oxygenation, IRV requires a lower peak airway pressure and PEEP, but a higher mean airway pressure (MAWP) than conventional mechanical ventilation. The increase in MAWP during IRV helps to reduce shunting and improve oxygenation in ARDS patients (Shanholtz et al., 1994).

✓ The presence of auto-PEEP during IRV may help to reduce shunting and improve oxygenation in ARDS patients.

Addition of Auto-PEEP.   Since IRV provides a longer I time and shorter E time, breath stacking with an increase of end-expiratory pressure is likely when there is not enough time for complete expiration (Duncan et al., 1987; Kacmarek et al., 1990). The presence of auto-PEEP during IRV may help to reduce shunting and improve oxygenation in ARDS patients (Shanholtz et al., 1994).

ADVERSE EFFECTS OF IRV

During IRV, the increase in MAWP and the presence of auto-PEEP both contribute to the increase of mean alveolar pressure and volume, the incidence of barotrauma may be as high as that obtained by conventional ventilation with high levels of PEEP (Tharratt et al., 1988).

Another potential hazard of IRV is a higher rate of transvascular fluid flow or flooding induced by an increased alveolar pressure (Permutt et al., 1979). This condition may induce or worsen preexisting pulmonary edema.

Patients receiving IRV are often agitated. They may require sedation and neuromuscular blocking agents to facilitate ventilation. The associated complications with these drugs can be serious and they should be monitored carefully when used in conjunction with IRV (Hansen-Flaschen et al., 1993).

PRESSURE CONTROL-IRV (PC-IRV)

✓ When PC is used with IRV, the peak airway pressure may be kept at a safe level.

Since IRV may increase the MAWP, create auto-PEEP, and increase the incidence of barotrauma, it is sometimes used in conjunction with pressure control due to its pressure-limiting capability. By using pressure control, the peak airway pressure may be kept at a safe level. This strategy helps to minimize pressure-induced lung injuries. When an inverse I:E ratio is used with pressure control ventilation, it is called pressure control inverse ratio ventilation (PC-IRV).

Several studies compare the outcomes of ARDS patients before and after the implementation of PC-IRV. The changes that may occur when positive pressure ventilation with PEEP (PPV + PEEP) is switched over to the PC-IRV mode of ventilation are summarized in Table 4-9.

TABLE 4-9 Observed Changes after Switching from PPV + PEEP to PC-IRV

INCREASE	DECREASE	NO CHANGE
Mean airway pressure	PEEP requirement	F_IO_2 requirement
Central venous pressure	Peak airway pressure	Intrinsic PEEP
Pulmonary artery pressure	Cardiac output	Blood pressure
PaO_2 (Lain et al., 1989)		$PaCO_2$
		PaO_2 (East et al., 1992)

(Data from East et al., 1992; Lain et al., 1989 and 1990.)

SUMMARY

There are many different ventilator operating modes and the number is expected to increase in coming years. As each mode is designed to accomplish a set of specific functions, it is essential to understand its capabilities, as well as its limitations and complications. When two or more operating modes are used in tandem, care and caution must be used because the combined outcomes are often complex and difficult to predict or manipulate.

An excellent source of obtaining detailed technical information is to consult the operation manual or contact the technical professionals of each ventilator manufacturer. Quality patient care is possible when the appropriate operating modes are selected and applied. A willingness to participate in continuing education is highly desirable and sometimes mandatory in this ever-changing field of mechanical ventilation.

Self-Assessment Questions

1. Volume cycled ventilators deliver a predetermined _____ to the patient using variable _____ according to the changing compliance and resistance.

   A. tidal volume, peak inspiratory pressure

   B. tidal volume, PEEP

   C. peak airway pressure, tidal volume

   D. PEEP, pressure support

2. Positive end-expiratory pressure (PEEP) is most commonly used to correct:

   A. hypercapnia.

   B. mild hypoxemia.

   C. refractory hypoxemia.

   D. respiratory acidosis.

3. In the assist/control (AC) mode of a volume-limited ventilator, the tidal volume initiated by the assist breath should be _____ the tidal volume initiated by the control breath.

   A. greater than
   B. less than

   C. about 150 ml less than
   D. equal to

4. When PEEP is applied to the airway of a patient who is breathing spontaneously, it is called:

   A. airway pressure release ventilation.
   B. continuous positive airway pressure.

   C. pressure support ventilation.
   D. pressure control ventilation.

5. _____ is a mode in which the ventilator delivers control (mandatory) breaths and allows the patient to breathe spontaneously to any tidal volume the patient is capable of in between the mandatory breaths.

   A. Intermittent mandatory ventilation
   B. Continuous positive airway pressure

   C. Mandatory minute ventilation
   D. Airway pressure release ventilation

6. _____ delivers control (mandatory) breaths to the patient at or near the beginning of a spontaneous breath, thus avoiding breath stacking.

   A. Continuous positive airway pressure
   B. Airway pressure release ventilation

   C. Intermittent mandatory ventilation
   D. Synchronized intermittent mandatory ventilation

7. _____ is primarily used to reduce the work of breathing imposed by the endotracheal tube and ventilator circuit.

   A. Pressure support ventilation
   B. Pressure control ventilation

   C. Airway pressure release ventilation
   D. Continuous positive airway pressure

8. _____ is a feature of some ventilators that leads to an increase of the mandatory rate when the patient's spontaneous breathing level becomes inadequate.

   A. Pressure control ventilation
   B. Pressure support ventilation

   C. Mandatory minute ventilation
   D. Inverse I:E ratio ventilation

9. Pressure control ventilation delivers _____ triggered breaths and a _____ is created and maintained for a preset inspiratory time.

   A. pressure, PEEP
   B. time, pressure plateau

   C. flow, pressure plateau
   D. patient, PEEP

10. One distinctive characteristic of airway pressure release ventilation is that during exhalation, the _____ level is lowered (released) to the baseline or a lower level.

    A. peak airway pressure
    B. plateau pressure

    C. continuous positive airway pressure
    D. positive end expiratory pressure

11. Inverse ratio ventilation has been used successfully to reduce intrapulmonary shunting and improve oxygenation. These effects are likely the result of _____ and _____.

    A. deadspace ventilation, increase of peak airway pressure.
    B. deadspace ventilation, auto-PEEP.

    C. increase of mean airway pressure, auto-PEEP.
    D. increase of peak airway pressure, auto-PEEP.

References

Ambrosino, N. et al. (1992). Physiologic evaluation of pressure support ventilation by nasal mask in patients with stable COPD. *Chest, 101,* 385–391.

Appendini, L., Purro, A., & Gudjonsdottir, M. et al. (1999). Physiologic response of ventilator-dependent patients with chronic obstructive pulmonary disease to proportional assist ventilation and continuous positive airway pressure. *Am J Respir Crit Care Med, 159*(5 Pt 1):1510–1517.

Baer, C. L. et al. (1992). Acute renal failure. *Critical Care Nursing Quarterly, 14*(4), 1.

Bezzant, T. B. et al. (1994). Risk and hazards of mechanical ventilation: A collective review of published literature. *Dis Mon, 40*(11), 583–638.

Bigatello, I. M., Nishimura, M., & Imanaka, H. et al. (1997). Unloading of the work of breathing by proportional assist ventilation in a lung model. *Crit Care Med, 25*(2): 267–272.

Brundage, D. J. (1992). *Renal disorders.* St. Louis: Mosby-Year Book.

Burton, G. B. et al. (1991). *Respiratory care: A guide to clinical practice* (3rd ed.). Philadelphia: J.B. Lippincott.

Carroll, N. et al. (1988). Control of nocturnal hypoventilation by nasal intermittent positive pressure ventilation. *Thorax, 43,* 349–353.

Chiang, A. A. et al. (1994). Demand-flow airway pressure release ventilation as a partial ventilatory support mode: Comparison with synchronized intermittent mandatory ventilation and pressure support ventilation. *Crit Care Med, 22*(9), 1431–1437.

Confalonieri, M. et al. (1994). Severe exacerbations of chronic obstructive pulmonary disease treated with BiPAP by nasal mask. *Respiration, 61*(6), 310–316.

Corrado, A. et al. (1994). Iron lung treatment of acute or chronic respiratory failure: 16 years of experience. *Monaldi Arch Chest Dis, 49*(6), 552–555.

Culpepper, J. A. et al. (1985). Effect of mechanical ventilator mode on tendency towards respiratory alkalosis. *Am Rev Respir Dis, 132*(5), 1075–1077.

Des Jardins, T. R. (1998). *Cardiopulmonary anatomy and physiology: Essentials for respiratory care* (3rd ed.). Albany, NY: Delmar Publishers, Inc.

Dolmage, T. E., & Goldstein, R. S. (1997). Proportional assist ventilation and exercise tolerance in subjects with COPD. *Chest, 111*(4): 948–954.

Downs, J. B. et al. (1973). Intermittent mandatory ventilation: A new approach to weaning patients from mechanical ventilators. *Chest, 64,* 331–335.

Duncan, S. R. et, al. (1987). Inverse ratio ventilation. PEEP in disguise? *Chest, 92,* 390–391.

East, T. D. et al. (1992). A successful computerized protocol for clinical management of pressure control inverse ratio ventilation in ARDS patients. *Chest, 101*(3), 697–710.

Ellis, E. R. et al. (1987). Treatment of respiratory failure during sleep in patients with neuro-muscular disease. *Am Rev Respir Dis, 135,* 148–152.

Frederick, C. (1994). Noninvasive mechanical ventilation with the iron lung. *Crit Care Nurs Clin North Am, 6*(4), 831–840.

Gurevitch M. J. et al. (1986). Improved oxygenation and lower peak airway pressure in severe adult respiratory distress syndrome: Treatment with inverse ratio ventilation. *Chest, 89,* 211–213.

Hansen-Flaschen, J. et al. (1993). Neuromuscular blockade in the intensive care unit: More than we bargain for. *Am Rev Respir Dis, 147,* 234–236.

Heenan, T. J. et al. (1980). Intermittent mandatory ventilation. *Chest, 77,* 598–602.

Hill, N. S. (1992). Efficacy of nocturnal nasal ventilation in patients with restrictive thoracic disease. *Am Rev Respir Dis, 145,* 365–371.

Hopper, R. G. et al. (1985). Acid-base changes and ventilator mode during maintenance ventilation. *Crit Care Med, 13*(1), 44–45.

Kacmarek, R. M. et al. (1990). Pressure-controlled inverse-ratio ventilation: Panacea or auto-PEEP? *Respir Care, 35,* 945–948.

Kanak, R. et al. (1985). Oxygen cost of breathing: Changes dependent upon mode of mechanical ventilation. *Chest, 87*(1), 126–127.

Kinnear, W., Hockley, S., & Harvey, J. et al. (1988). The effects of one year of nocturnal cuirass-assisted ventilation in chest wall disease. *Eur Respir J, 1*(3), 204–208.

Kinnear, W., Petch, M., & Taylor, G. et al. (1988). Assisted ventilation using cuirass respirators. *Eur Respir J, 1*(3), 198–203.

Kirby, R. R. (1988). Modes of mechanical ventilation. In R. M. Kacmarek et al. (Eds.), *Current respiratory care.* Philadelphia: B. C. Becker, Inc.

Lain, D. et al. (1990). Reduction of peak inflation and positive end-expiratory pressures using pressure control with inverse-ratio ventilation: A case report. *Heart Lung, 19*(4), 358–361.

Lain, D. C. et al. (1989). Pressure control inverse ratio ventilation as a method to reduce peak inspiratory pressure and provide adequate ventilation and oxygenation. *Chest, 95*(5), 1081–1088.

Linton, D. M. et al. (1992). Metabolic requirements in tetanus. *Crit Care Med, 20*(7), 950–952.

MacIntyre, N. R. (1986). Respiratory function during pressure support ventilation. *Chest, 89*(5), 677–683.

MacIntyre, N. R. (1987). Pressure support ventilation: Effects on ventilatory reflexes and ventilatory muscle workload. *Resp Care, 32,* 447–457.

Marcy, T. W. et al. (1991). Inverse ratio ventilation in ARDS: Rationale and implementation. *Chest, 100,* 494–504.

Navalesi, P., Hernandez, P., & Wongsa, A. et al. (1996). Proportional assist ventilation in acute respiratory failure: Effects on breathing pattern and inspiratory effort. *Am J Respir Crit Care Med, 154*(5): 1330–8.

Newman, J. H. et al. (1988). Fabrication of a customized cuirass for patients with severe thoracic asymmetry. *Am Rev Respir Dis, 137*(1), 202–203.

Perel, A. et al. (1991). *Handbook of mechanical ventilatory support.* Baltimore: Williams and Wilkins.

Permutt, S. et al. (1979). Mechanical influences on water accumulation in the lungs. In A. E. Fishman, *Pulmonary edema* (pp. 175–193). Bethesda, MD: American Physiological Society.

Petersen, G. W. et al. (1983). Incidence of pulmonary barotrauma in a medical ICU. *Crit Care Med, 11,* 67–69.

Qvist, J. et al. (1975). Hemodynamic responses to mechanical ventilation with PEEP. *Anesthesiology, 42,* 45–55.

Renston, J. P. et al. (1994). Respiratory muscle rest using nasal BiPAP ventilation in patients with stable severe COPD. *Chest, 105*(4), 1053–1060.

Sassoon, C. S. H. et al. (1990). Ventilator modes: Old and new. *Crit Care Clin, 6*(3), 605–634.

Sassoon, C. S. H. (1991). Positive pressure ventilation: Alternate modes. *Chest, 100,* 1421–1429.

Scanlan, C. L. et al. (1999). *Egan's fundamentals of respiratory care* (7th ed.) St. Louis: Mosby-Year Book.

Shanholtz, C. et al. (1994). Should inverse ratio ventilation be used in adult respiratory distress syndrome? *Am J Respir Crit Care Med, 149,* 1354–1358.

Shapiro, B. A. et al. (1976). Intermittent demand ventilation (IDV): A new technique for support ventilation in critically ill patients. *Respir Care, 21,* 521–525

Shapiro, B. A. et al. (1991). *Clinical application of respiratory care.* St. Louis: Mosby-Year Book.

Slutsky, A. S. (1994). Consensus conference on mechanical ventilation—January 28–30, 1993 at Northbrook, IL, USA, Part I. *Int Care Med, 20,* 64–79.

Strumpf, D. A. (1990). An evaluation of the Respironics BiPAP bi-level CPAP device for delivery of assisted ventilation. *Respir Care, 35,* 415–422.

Tharratt, R. S. et al. (1988). Pressure controlled inverse ratio ventilation in severe adult respiratory failure. *Chest, 94,* 755–762.

Tyler, D. C. (1983). Positive end expiratory pressure: A review. *Crit Care Med, 11*(4), 300–308.

Waldhorn, R. E. (1992). Nocturnal nasal intermittent positive pressure ventilation with bi-level positive airway pressure (BiPAP) in respiratory failure. *Chest, 101,* 516–521.

Weisman, L. M. et al. (1983). Intermittent mandatory ventilation. *Am Rev Respir Dis, 127,* 641–647.

Younes, M. (1992) Proportional assist ventilation, a new approach to ventilatory support: Theory. *Am Rev Respir Dis, 145*:114–120.

Zelt, B. A. et al. (1972). Prolonged nasotracheal intubation and mechanical ventilation in the management of asphyxiating thoracic dystrophy: A case report. *Anesth Analg, 51,* 342–348.

Suggested Reading

PEEP/Pressure Support

MacIntyre, N. R., Cheng, K. C., & McConnell, R. (1997). Applied PEEP during pressure support reduces the inspiratory threshold load of intrinsic PEEP. *Chest, 111*(1):188–193.

Proportional Assist Ventilation

Ambrosino, N., Vitacca, M., & Polese, G. et al. (1997). Short-term effects of nasal *proportional* assist ventilation in patients with chronic hypercapnic respiratory insufficiency. *Eur Respir J, 10*(12):2829–2834.

Bianchi, L., Foglio, K., & Pagani, M. et al. (1998). Effects of *proportional* assist ventilation on exercise tolerance in COPD patients with chronic hypercapnia. *Eur Respir J, 11*(2):422–427.

Marantz, S., Patrick, W., & Webster, K. et al. (1996). Response of ventilator-dependent patients to different levels of proportional assist. *J Appl Physiol, 80*(2):397–403.

Ranieri, V. M., Giuliani, R., & Mascia, L. et al. (1996). Patient-ventilator interaction during acute hypercapnia: Pressure-support vs. proportional-assist ventilation. *J Appl Physiol, 81*(1):426–436.

Ranieri, V. M., Grasso, S., & Mascia, L. et al. (1997). Effects of proportional assist ventilation on inspiratory muscle effort in patients with chronic obstructive pulmonary disease and acute respiratory failure. *Anesthesiology, 86*(1):79–91.

Tejeda, M., Boix, J. H., & Alvarez, F. et al. (1997). Comparison of pressure support ventilation and assist-control ventilation in the treatment of respiratory failure. *Chest, 111*(5):1322–1325.

CHAPTER FIVE

TEMPORARY AIRWAYS FOR VENTILATION

David W. Chang

OUTLINE

KEY TERMS

- autoclave
- blind distal end
- blind intubation
- esophageal gastric tube airway (EGTA)

- esophageal obturator airway (EOA)
- laryngeal mask airway (LMA)
- pharyngealtracheal lumen airway (PTLA)

INTRODUCTION

In situations involving respiratory arrest, bag and mask ventilation is typically used and may be followed by endotracheal intubation. Occasionally, endotracheal intubation may not be successful due to unusual anatomy or difficult intubation. In these cases, a temporary airway such as the esophageal obturator airway, the esophageal gastric tube airway, the laryngeal mask airway, and the pharyngealtracheal lumen airway may serve as a stopgap measure for providing ventilation when bag and mask ventilation is deemed inadequate.

ESOPHAGEAL OBTURATOR AIRWAY (EOA)

esophageal obdurator airway (EOA): An EOA has a closed (blind) distal end and it is inserted into the esophagus.

blind distal end: The far end of a tube without an opening.

Unlike an endotracheal tube, an **esophageal obturator airway (EOA)** is inserted into the esophagus. It is used as an alternative to bag and mask ventilation. The EOA is a disposable tube; its structure consists of an opening at the proximal (top) end, many small holes near the upper end, and a **blind distal end.** Near the distal end is a large cuff that is inflated during use. The inflated cuff prevents air from entering the stomach and subsequent regurgitation and aspiration. A mask fits over the tube to prevent leaks around the patient's face during ventilation (Burton, Hodgkin & Ward, 1997; White 1999). Figure 5-1 shows an esophageal obturator airway.

The opening at the proximal end of the tube attaches to a ventilation bag. The small holes at the hypopharyngeal level allow ventilation to the lungs. The closed distal end of the EOA prevents aspiration or removal of air or gastric contents from the stomach. Since an EOA is inserted into the esophagus, the cuff at the distal end must be inflated during use to prevent air from entering the stomach (Scanlan, Wilkins & Stoller, 1999; White, 1999).

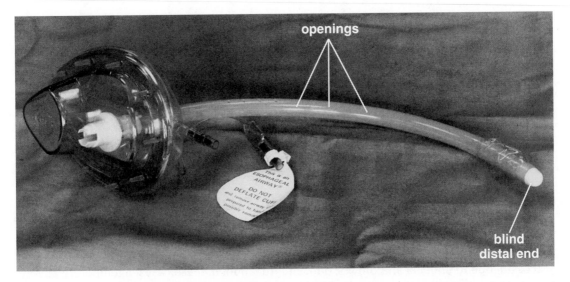

Figure 5-1 An Esophageal Obturator Airway (EOA).

INSERTION OF AN EOA

☑ Since an EOA is inserted into the esophagus, the cuff at the distal end must be inflated during use to prevent air from entering the stomach.

The cuff of an EOA is first inflated with 20 to 30 cc of air to check for cuff integrity and leaks. The cuff is then deflated, and the proximal end of the EOA is inserted through the opening of a mask. The distal end of the tube is lubricated with a water-soluable lubricant and then inserted into the patient's esophagus until the mask rests on the patient's face. Due to the large volume of air used to inflate the cuff, it is extremely important to check for proper tube placement before cuff inflation and ventilation. Asphyxia and tracheal damage are severe complications if the cuff is inflated while the tube is misplaced in the trachea (Scanlan, Wilkins & Stoller, 1999; White, 1999). Table 5-1 lists other precautions during use of the EOA.

TABLE 5-1 **Precautions in the Use of an Esophageal Obturator Airway**

An EOA should not be used in awake or semiconscious patients.

An EOA should not be used in children under 16 years of age or under 5 feet tall.

An EOA should not be used in patients with known esophageal disease.

Do not remove the EOA until patient has regained consciousness.

> ☑ The EOA is not designed to be used as an artificial airway for positive pressure ventilation.

The EOA is not designed to be used as an artificial airway for positive pressure ventilation. Since it is used as a temporary airway, it should be replaced with an endotracheal intubation as soon as feasible. With the EOA in place, endotracheal intubation is done using the standard procedure. After endotracheal intubation, bilateral breath sounds should be verified as the endotracheal tube may follow the EOA and enter the esophagus. After ascertaining proper placement, the endotracheal tube is secured prior to removal of the EOA. Suction setup should be ready in case of vomiting during removal of the EOA.

ESOPHAGEAL GASTRIC TUBE AIRWAY (EGTA)

esophageal gastric tube airway: A tube used in esophageal intubation. It has a patent distal end to relieve gastric distention.

The **esophageal gastric tube airway (EGTA)** is similar in design to the EOA. Whereas the EOA has a closed distal end, the EGTA has an opening at the distal end (Figure 5-2). The opening allows removal or aspiration of air and gastric contents from the stomach via a gastric tube. The advantage of this design is the relief of gastric distention that may occur during bag to mask ventilation (Scanlan, Wilkins & Stoller, 1999; White, 1999).

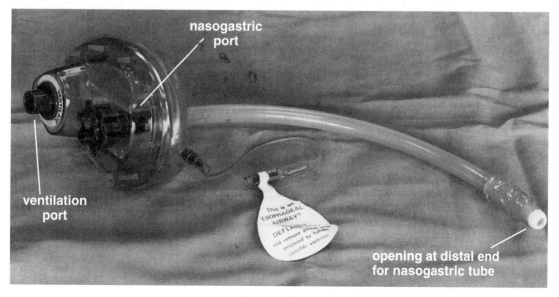

nasogastric port

ventilation port

opening at distal end for nasogastric tube

Figure 5-2 An Esophageal Gastric Tube Airway (EGTA).

TABLE 5-2   **Distinct Features of the EOA and the EGTA**

ESOPHAGEAL OBTURATOR AIRWAY	ESOPHAGEAL GASTRIC TUBE AIRWAY
Esophageal intubation	Esophageal intubation
Ventilation holes along tube	No ventilation holes along tube
Blind distal end	Patent distal end
One port on mask for ventilation	Two ports on mask (ventilation/gastric tube)

☑ There are two ports on the EGTA mask. The resuscitation bag must be attached to the ventilation port.

With an EGTA, the ventilation holes along the proximal end of the tube are absent. Ventilation is provided through the mask by a traditional manual resuscitation bag. Since there are two ports on the mask, the resuscitation bag must be attached to the ventilation port. Table 5-2 outlines the distinct features of the EOA and the EGTA.

LARYNGEAL MASK AIRWAY (LMA)

laryngeal mask airway: A tube with a small cushioned mask on the distal end that provides a seal over the laryngeal opening.

The **laryngeal mask airway (LMA)** resembles a short endotracheal tube with a small cushioned, oblong-shaped mask on the distal end (Figure 5-3) (Brain, Verghese & Addy et al., 1997; Brimacombe, Keller & Morris et al., 1998; Verghese, Berlet & Kapila et al. 1998). It was invented in England in 1981 by anesthesiologist Archie Brain and was available commercially in 1988. In 1991, this airway device was

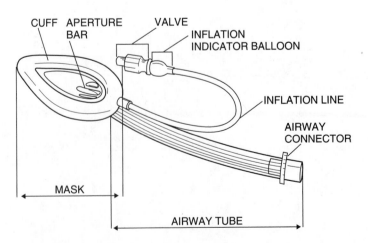

Figure 5-3   The components of the Laryngeal Mask Airway (LMA). (Courtesy of LMA North America, Inc.)

☑️ With proper care and sterilization, LMA can be reused up to 40 times.

approved by the Food and Drug Administration for clinical use in the United States (Ferson, Nesbitt & Nesbitt et al., 1997). The original LMA (LMA-Classic) is a reusable device, made primarily of medical-grade silicone rubber and is latex-free. With proper care and sterilization, it can be reused up to 40 times.

USE AND APPLICATION OF THE LMA

☑️ The cushioned mask of the LMA provides a seal over the laryngeal opening. It is not necessary for the LMA to enter the larynx or trachea.

The LMA fills a niche as an airway management tool between a face mask and an endotracheal tube (Brimacombe & Berry, 1996; Fetzer, 1998). When the cushioned mask of the LMA is inflated, it provides a seal over the laryngeal opening. It is not necessary therefore for the LMA to enter the larynx or trachea. Figure 5-4 shows the dorsal view of the position of the LMA in relation to the pharyngeal anatomy. After proper placement, spontaneous ventilation or low-level (up to 20 cm H_2O) positive pressure ventilation is possible without an endotracheal tube (LMA North America, Inc., 1999).

The LMA is also indicated as a method of establishing a patent airway during resuscitation in the profoundly unconscious patient with absent glossopharyngeal and laryngeal reflexes who may need

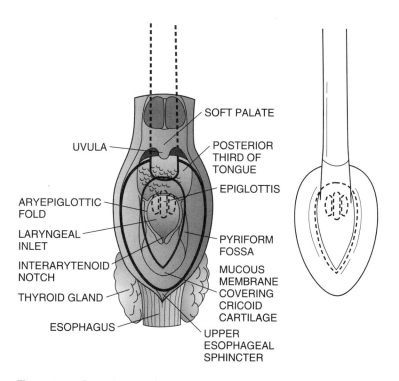

Figure 5-4 Dorsal view of the LMA showing position in relation to pharyngeal anatomy. (Courtesy of LMA North America, Inc.)

☑ LMA should be considered when tracheal intubation is precluded by lack of expertise or equipment or when attempts at endotracheal intubation have failed.

☑ The LMA does not protect an airway from the effects of regurgitation and aspiration.

☑ The LMA may not withhold airway pressures greater than 20 cm H_2O.

☑ For most adults, size 4 should be used for females and size 5 for males.

assisted ventilation. The LMA should be considered when tracheal intubation is precluded by lack of expertise or equipment or when attempts at endotracheal intubation have failed (LMA North America, Inc., 1999). Other uses and application of the LMA are outlined in Table 5-3.

CONTRAINDICATIONS FOR THE LMA

The design of the LMA does not protect an airway from the effects of regurgitation and aspiration. For this reason, the LMA should not be used in patients who have not fasted or those with hiatal hernia. Since the seal provided by the LMA may not withhold pressures over 20 cm H_2O, a leak may occur during high airway pressure situations. Patients with low lung compliance should use a traditional endotracheal tube instead of an LMA. In addition, the LMA should not be used in patients who are not profoundly unconscious and in those with severe oropharyngeal trauma.

SELECTION OF THE LMA

LMA is either reusable (silicone-based) or disposable (polyvinyl chloride). The disposable LMA-Unique performs similarly to the reusable LMA in clinical situations (Verghese, Berlet & Kapila et al., 1998). For most adult females, size 4 should be used and size 5 should be used for most adult males (Asai, Howell & Koga et al.,

TABLE 5-3 Uses and Application of a Laryngeal Mask Airway

Establishes airway in proven difficult intubations

Provides spontaneous and controlled ventilation in infants and children

Serves as a bridge to more secured airways

Provides complete survey of the larynx and trachea prior to thoracotomy

Provides lower work of breathing than endotracheal tube

Provides less hemodynamic response during surgical procedures

Provides less airway reaction

Offers benefit of shorter stay in hospital due to avoidance of endotracheal intubation

(Data from Ferson, Nesbitt & Nesbitt et al., 1997; Fukutome, Amaha & Nakazawa, 1998; Joo & Rose, 1998; Joshi, Morrison & White, 1998; Kim & Bishop, 1999; Lopez-Gil, Brimacombe & Alvarez, 1996; Marietta, Lunn & Ruby et al., 1998; Parmet, Colonna-Romano & Horrow et al., 1998; Stanwood, 1997; Webster, Morley-Forster & Janzen et al., 1999; Zerafa, Baulch & Elliott et al., 1999.)

1998). The standard cuff pressure is 60 cm H_2O (Berry, Brimacombe & McManus et al., 1998), but the air in the cuff should be adjusted to the minimal effective volume so as to decrease intracuff pressure, pressure on the pharynx (Asai, Howell & Koga et al., 1998), and incidence of sore throat (Nott, Noble & Parmar, 1998). Table 5-4 provides the suggested LMA size for patients ranging from neonates to large adults and the maximal cuff inflation volume (LMA North America, Inc., 1999).

INSERTION OF THE LMA

Prior to insertion of the LMA, the patient is in a supine position, and the head is advanced slightly. The chin is depressed to open the mouth. With the cuff completely deflated or partially inflated (Dingley & Asai, 1996), the LMA is inserted blindly without a laryngoscope through the mouth and advanced along the hard palate. It is then further advanced to the posterior pharynx and turned toward the trachea and larynx. At this point, the LMA may be guided with fingers to ascertain that it makes the proper turn (Watson, Hokanson & Maltby et al., 1999). Figure 5-5 A–G show the standard insertion technique of LMA.

REMOVAL OF THE LMA

☑ The LMA may be removed safely when the patient is anesthetized or awake.

The LMA may be discontinued when an upper airway is no longer needed for ventilation and oxygenation. Removal can be done safely when the patient is anesthetized or awake. During removal of the LMA, the patient must be monitored carefully for complications such as regurgitation, laryngeal spasm, bronchospasm, coughing, retching, excessive salivation, and oxygen desaturation (Nunez, Hughes & Wareham et al., 1998; Samarkandi, 1998).

TABLE 5-4   Selection of Laryngeal Mask Airway and Maximum Cuff Inflation Volume

SIZE	PATIENT GROUP	MAXIMUM CUFF VOLUME
1	Neonates and infants up to 5 kg	up to 4 mL
1.5	Infants between 5–10 kg	up to 7 mL
2	Infants and children between 10–20 kg	up to 10 mL
2.5	Children between 20–30 kg	up to 14 mL
3	Children over 30 kg and small adults	up to 20 mL
4	Normal and large adults	up to 30 mL
5	Larger adults	up to 40 mL

(Data from LMA North America, Inc., 1999.)

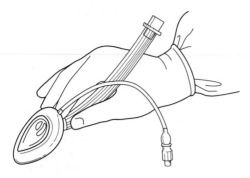

Figure 5-5A Method for holding the LMA for insertion. (Courtesy of LMA North America, Inc.)

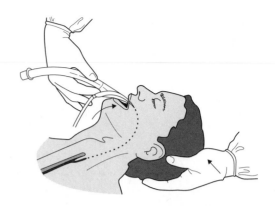

Figure 5-5B With the head extended and the neck flexed, carefully flatten the LMA tip against the hard palate. (Courtesy of LMA North America, Inc.)

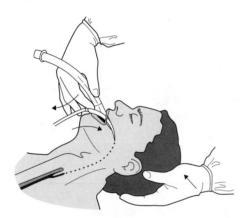

Figure 5-5C To facilitate LMA introduction into the oral cavity, gently press the middle finger down on the jaw. (Courtesy of LMA North America, Inc.)

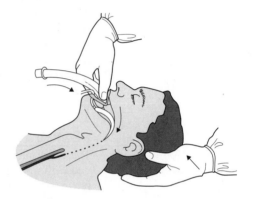

Figure 5-5D The index finger pushes the LMA in a cranial direction following the contours of the hard and soft palates. (Courtesy of LMA North America, Inc.)

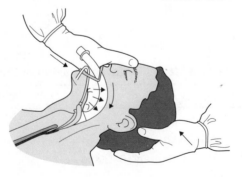

Figure 5-5E Maintaining pressure with the finger on the tube in the cranial direction, advance the mask until definite resistance is felt at the base of the hypopharynx. Note the flexion of the wrist. (Courtesy of LMA North America, Inc.)

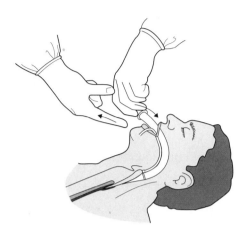

Figure 5-5F Gently maintain cranial pressure with the nondominant hand while removing the index finger. (Courtesy of LMA North America, Inc.)

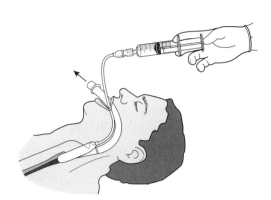

Figure 5-5G Inflation without holding the tube allows the mask to seat itself optimally. (Courtesy of LMA North America, Inc.)

LIMITATIONS OF THE LMA

Due to the unique position of its mask, rotation or turning of the LMA may cause misplacement of the mask and result in gastric insufflation and air leakage from the mask seal (Latorre, Eberle & Weiler et al., 1998). For this reason, the patient's head position and alignment of the LMA should be checked frequently to ensure adequate ventilation. Positive pressure ventilation may be provided via the LMA at peak airway pressures of up to 20 cm H_2O. For patients with low compliance or high air flow resistance, the LMA may not be able to withstand the pressure and air leaks may develop. When high peak inspiratory pressure is anticipated, the LMA should be replaced with an endotracheal tube (LMA North America, Inc., 1999).

The LMA is not a secured airway and it does not protect the lower airway from aspiration. The esophagus, which lies posterior to the LMA, has complete access to the larynx, and thus regurgitation or aspiration is a potential complication (Norton, Germonpré & Semple, 1998).

The reusable version of the LMA is handmade, thus the cost is rather significant. With proper sterilization by steam **autoclave** and careful handling, it can be reused up to 40 times as long as the mask is not damaged during use, handling, and steam autoclaving. Table 5-5 outlines the limitations of LMA.

☑ The LMA is sterilized by steam autoclave.

autoclave: A method of sterilization using steam pressure, usually at 250°F (121°C) for a specific length of time.

TABLE 5-5   Limitations of the Laryngeal Mask Airway

Rotation of the LMA may cause misplacement of mask, gastric inflation, and air leaks

Cuff does not provide seal at pressures greater than 20 cm H_2O

The LMA does not protect the lower airway from aspiration

Reusable version is costly but it can be reused after cleaning and sterilization

Steam autoclaving is the only recommended method of sterilization

PHARYNGEALTRACHEAL LUMEN AIRWAY (PTLA)

pharyngealtracheal lumen airway:
A tube that may be inserted into the trachea or esophagus.

☑ The PTLA is inserted blindly either into the trachea or esophagus.

☑ Both lumens on the PTLA can be used to provide ventilation. Lumen A is used when the tube enters the esophagus and lumen B is used when it is in the trachea.

The **pharyngealtracheal lumen airway (PTLA),** also called esophageal-tracheal airway, is a combination of esophageal and endotracheal tube in one unit (e.g., Combitube, by Kendall, Mansfield, Mass.). Due to its design, ventilation is possible when the PTLA is inserted blindly either into the trachea or esophagus (Liao & Shalit, 1996). The PTLA can be inserted easily by unskilled personnel (Yardy, Hancox & Strang, 1999), and it has been used successfully as an alternate artificial airway in patients outside the hospital (Blostein, Koestner & Hoak, 1998; Hoak & Koestner, 1997; Rumball & MacDonald, 1997). Ventilation is provided via a 15-mm airway connector at the proximal end of the PTLA.

There are two cuffs on the PTLA, a proximal latex pharyngeal cuff (100 cc) and a PVC cuff (15 cc) near the distal end of the tube (Figure 5-6). Both lumens on the PTLA can be used to provide ventilation. Lumen A is used when the tube enters the esophagus and the distal cuff seals off the esophagus. Lumen B is used when it is in the trachea and the proximal cuff seals off the trachea. Figure 5-7 shows the relative positions of the PTLA when it enters the esophagus or trachea.

INSERTION AND USE OF THE PTLA

The PTLA can be inserted with or without a laryngoscope. The tube is properly inserted once the black rings lie opposite the front teeth. After insertion, both cuffs are inflated immediately. Since the PTLA is designed to provide ventilation when the tube is in the trachea or esophagus, it does not matter whether the tube enters the esophagus or trachea.

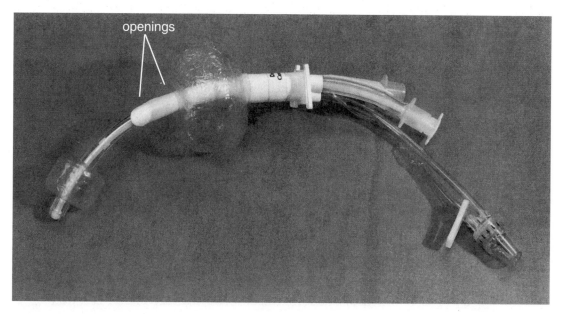

Figure 5-6   A Pharyngealtracheal Lumen Airway (PTLA).

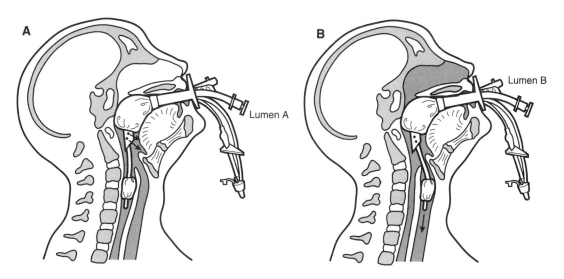

Figure 5-7   After placement of the Pharyngealtracheal Lumen Airway (PTLA), both cuffs are inflated. (A) When the tube is in the esophagus, lumen A is used to provide ventilation through the openings below the proximal cuff and air enters the trachea. (B) When the tube enters the trachea, lumen B is used to provide ventilation directly into the trachea.

blind intubation: Insertion of an artificial airway without use of visual aid.

☑ Following blind intubation with a pharyngealtracheal lumen airway (PTLA), ventilation should be attempted initially through lumen A of the PTLA.

During **blind intubation,** the PTLA is more likely to go into the esophagus. Therefore, ventilation through the PTLA should be done via lumen A first. When the distal end of the PTLA is in the esophagus, air goes through the side ports, becomes trapped between the cuff, and is forced into the trachea. If ventilation via lumen A is poor, lumen B should be used to provide ventilation as the distal end of the PTLA may be in the trachea.

If ventilation is poor with lumens A and B, a cuff leak may be present. This problem may be corrected by inflating the proximal cuff with more air. Try lumen A again and check for adequacy of ventilation. If ventilation is still poor, the entire procedure described earlier can be repeated after denitrogenating the patient with oxygen.

COMPLICATIONS WITH USE OF THE PTLA

Cases of complications associated with the use of the PTLA have been reported. These complications are related to either hemodynamic stress or air leaks. In one report, the hemodynamic and catecholamine stress response after insertion of the PTLA were significantly higher compared to laryngeal mask airway or endotracheal intubation. This observation might be attributed to the pressure of the pharyngeal cuff of the PTLA (Oczenski, Krenn & Dahaba et al., 1999). In another report, different types of air leak (subcutaneous emphysema, pneumomediastinum, and pneumoperitoneum) were observed as a result of using the PTLA. Esophageal laceration appears to be the cause of these air leaks (Richards, 1998; Vézina, Lessard & Bussières et al., 1998).

SUMMARY

The four types of temporary airways discussed in this chapter are useful in situations where bag and mask ventilation is inadequate and endotracheal intubation is not readily achievable. Since these temporary airways are not suitable for positive pressure ventilation, an endotracheal airway must be established as soon as feasible when mechanical ventilation is imminent. The purpose of using a temporary airway is to provide ventilation to the patient with minimal delay and to allow endotracheal intubation to be done under a controlled environment.

Self-Assessment Questions

1. An esophageal obturator airway (EOA) has a(n) _____ distal end and it is inserted into the _____.

   A. open, trachea
   B. open, esophagus

   C. closed, trachea
   D. closed, esophagus

2. Since an EOA is inserted into the _____, the cuff at the distal end must be _____ before ventilation is initiated.

   A. tracheal, deflated
   B. trachea, inflated

   C. esophagus, deflated
   D. esophagus, inflated

3. Since there are two ports on the mask of the _____, the resuscitation bag must be attached to the ventilation port.

   A. esophageal obturator airway
   B. laryngeal mask airway

   C. esophageal gastric tube airway
   D. pharyngealtracheal lumen airway

4. The silicone-based laryngeal mask airway may be reused up to _____ times with proper handling and _____.

   A. 40, chemical sterilization
   B. 40, steam autoclaving

   C. 100, chemical sterilization
   D. 100, steam autoclaving

5. Since the cushioned mask of a laryngeal mask airway (LMA) provides a seal over the _____, it is not necessary for the LMA to enter the larynx or trachea.

   A. tracheal opening
   B. laryngeal opening

   C. esophageal opening
   D. vocal cords

6. Which of the following is *not* true concerning the laryngeal mask airway (LMA)?

   A. LMA does not protect an airway from regurgitation and aspiration.
   B. LMA is sterilized by steam autoclave.

   C. Size 4 and size 5 LMAs are suitable for most adults.
   D. LMA may withhold airway pressures up to 40 cm H_2O.

7. A pharyngealtracheal lumen airway (PTLA) is inserted into the:

   A. trachea
   B. esophagus

   C. trachea or esophagus
   D. esophagus or larynx

8. Both lumens on the PTLA can be used to provide ventilation. Lumen A is used when the tube enters the _____ and lumen B is used when it is in the _____.

    A. trachea, esophagus

    B. esophagus, trachea

    C. trachea, larynx

    D. esophagus, larynx

9. Following blind intubation with a pharyngealtracheal lumen airway (PTLA), ventilation should be attempted initially through lumen A of the PTLA because:

    A. an airway usually goes into the trachea during blind intubation.

    B. an airway usually goes into the esophagus during blind intubation.

    C. lumen A has a closed distal end.

    D. lumen B has a closed distal end.

References

Asai, T., Howell, T. K., & Koga, K. et al. (1998). Appropriate size and inflation of the laryngeal mask airway. *Br J Anaesth, 80*(4):470–474.

Berry, A. M., Brimacombe, J. R., & McManus, K. F. et al. (1998). An evaluation of the factors influencing selection of the optimal size of laryngeal mask airway in normal adults. *Anaesthesia, 53*(6):565–570.

Blostein, P. A., Koestner, A. J., & Hoak, S. (1998). Failed rapid sequence intubation in trauma patients: Esophageal tracheal combitube is a useful adjunct. *J Trauma, 44*(3):534–537.

Brain, A. I., Verghese, C., & Addy, E. V. et al. (1997). The intubating laryngeal mask. I: Development of a new device for intubation of the trachea. *Br J Anaesth, 79*(6):699–703.

Brimacombe, J., & Berry, A. (1996). The laryngeal mask airway—anatomical and physiological implications. *Acta Anaesthesiol Scand, 40*(2):201–209.

Brimacombe, J., Keller, C., & Morris, R. et al. (1998). A comparison of the disposable versus the reusable laryngeal mask airway in paralyzed adult patients. *Anesth Analg, 87*(4):921–924.

Burton, G. G., Hodgkin, J. E., & Ward, J. J. (1997). *Respiratory care: A guide to clinical practice* (4th ed.). Philadelphia: J. B. Lippincott Company.

Dingley, J., & Asai, T. (1996). Insertion methods of the laryngeal mask airway. A survey of current practice in Wales. *Anaesthesia, 51*(6):596–599.

Ferson, D. Z., Nesbitt, J. C., & Nesbitt, K. et al. (1997). The laryngeal mask airway: A new standard for airway evaluation in thoracic surgery. *Ann Thorac Surg, 63*(3):768–772.

Fetzer, S. J. (1998). Laryngeal mask airway: Indications and management for critical care. *Crit Care Nurse, 18*(1):83–87.

Fukutome, T., Amaha, K., & Nakazawa, K. et al. (1998). Tracheal intubation through the intubating laryngeal mask airway (LMA-Fastrach) in patients with difficult airways. *Anaesth Intensive Care, 26*(4):387–391.

Hoak, S., & Koestner, A. (1997). Esophageal tracheal Combitube in the emergency department. *J Emerg Nurs, 23*(4):347–350.

Joo, H., & Rose, K. (1998). Fastrach—a new intubating laryngeal mask airway. Successful use in patients with difficult airways. *Can J Anaesth, 45*(3):253–256.

Joshi, G. P., Morrison, S. G., & White, P. F. et al. (1998). Work of breathing in anesthetized patients: Laryngeal mask airway versus tracheal tube. *J Clin Anesth, 10*(4):268–271.

Kim, E. S., & Bishop, M. J. (1999). Endotracheal intubation, but not laryngeal mask airway insertion, produces reversible bronchoconstriction. *Anesthesiology, 90*(2):391–394.

Latorre, F., Eberle, B., & Weiler, N. et al. (1998). Laryngeal mask airway position and the risk of gastric insufflation. *Anesth Analg, 86*(4):867–871.

Liao, D., & Shalit, M. (1996). Successful intubation with the Combitube in acute asthmatic respiratory distress by a Paramedic. *J Emerg Med, 14*(5):561–563.

LMA North America, Inc. (1999). *Instruction Manual LMA-Classic/LMA-Flexible.* San Diego, Calif.

Lopez-Gil, M., Brimacombe, J., & Alvarez, M. (1996). Safety and efficacy of the laryngeal mask airway. A prospective survey of 1400 children. *Anaesthesia, 51*(10):969–972.

Marietta, D. R., Lunn, J. K., & Ruby, E. I. et al. (1998). Cardiovascular stability during carotid endarterectomy: Endotracheal intubation versus laryngeal mask airway. *J Clin Anesth, 10*(1):54–57.

Norton, A., Germonpré, J., & Semple, T. (1998). Pulmonary aspiration of blood following traumatic laryngeal mask airway insertion. *Anaesth Intensive Care, 26*(2):213–215.

Nott, M. R., Noble, P. D., & Parmar, M. (1998). Reducing the incidence of sore throat with the laryngeal mask airway. *Eur J Anaesthesiol, 15*(2):153–157.

Nunez, J., Hughes, J., & Wareham, K. et al. (1998). Timing of removal of the laryngeal mask airway. *Anaesthesia, 53*(2):126–130.

Oczenski, W., Krenn, H., & Dahaba, A. A. et al. (1999). Hemodynamic and catecholamine stress responses to insertion of the Combitube, laryngeal mask airway or tracheal intubation. *Anesth Analg, 88*(6):1389–1394.

Parmet, J. L., Colonna-Romano, P., & Horrow, J. C. et al. (1998). The laryngeal mask airway reliably provides rescue ventilation in cases of unanticipated difficult tracheal intubation along with difficult mask ventilation. *Anesth Analg, 87*(3):661–665.

Richards, C. F. (1998). Piriform sinus perforation during Esophageal-Tracheal Combitube placement. *J Emerg Med, 16*(1):37–39.

Rumball, C. J., & MacDonald, D. (1997). The PTL, Combitube, laryngeal mask, and oral airway: A randomized prehospital comparative study of ventilatory. *Prehosp Emerg Care, 1*(1):1–10.

Samarkandi, A. H. (1998). Awake removal of the laryngeal mask airway is safe in paediatric patients. *Can J Anaesth, 45*(2): 150–152.

Scanlan, C. L., Wilkins, R. L., & Stoller, J. K. (1999). *Egan's fundamentals of respiratory care* (7th ed.). St. Louis: Mosby-Year Book.

Stanwood, P. L. (1997). The laryngeal mask airway and the emergency airway. *AANA J, 65*(4):364–370.

Verghese, C., Berlet, J., & Kapila, A. et al. (1998). Clinical assessment of the single use laryngeal mask airway—the LMA-unique. *Br J Anaesth, 80*(5):677–679.

Vézina, D., Lessard, M. R., & Bussières, J. et al. (1998). Complications associated with the use of the Esophageal-Tracheal Combitube. *Can J Anaesth, 45*(1):76–80.

Watson, N. C., Hokanson, M., & Maltby, J. R. et al. (1999). The intubating laryngeal mask airway in failed fibreoptic intubation. *Can J Anaesth, 46*(4):376–378.

Webster, A. C., Morley-Forster, P. K., & Janzen, V. et al. (1999). Anesthesia for intranasal surgery: A comparison between tracheal intubation and the flexible reinforced laryngeal mask airway. *Anesth Analg, 88*(2):421–425.

White, G. C. (1999). *Equipment theory for respiratory care* (3rd ed.) Albany, NY: Delmar Publishers.

Yardy, N., Hancox, D., & Strang, T. (1999). A comparison of two airway aids for emergency use by unskilled personnel. The Combitube and laryngeal mask. *Anaesthesia, 54*(2):181–183.

Zerafa, M., Baulch, S., & Elliott, M. J. et al. (1999). Use of the laryngeal mask airway during repair of atrial septal defect in children. *Paediatr Anaesth, 9*(3):257–259.

CHAPTER SIX

AIRWAY MANAGEMENT IN MECHANICAL VENTILATION

David W. Chang

OUTLINE

Introduction

Intubation
Indications

Common Artificial Airways in Mechanical Ventilation
Oral Endotracheal Tube
Nasal Endotracheal Tube
Tracheostomy Tube

Intubation Procedure
Supplies
Selection of Endotracheal Tube
Ventilation and Oxygenation
Oral Intubation
Nasal Intubation
Common Errors
Signs of Endotracheal Intubation
Signs of Esophageal Intubation

Management of Endotracheal and Tracheostomy Tubes
Securing Endotracheal and Tracheostomy Tubes

Cuff Pressure
Minimal Occlusion Volume and Minimal Leak Technique
Irrigation and Suction

Extubation
Predictors of Successful Extubation
Procedure
Unplanned Extubation

Complications of Endotracheal Intubation
During Intubation
While Intubated
Immediately after Extubation
Following Extubation

Summary

Self-Assessment Questions

References

Suggested Reading

KEY TERMS

- carina
- endotracheal tube
- laryngoscope
- Magill forceps
- pilot balloon
- radiopaque
- sniffing position

- stylet
- tracheostomy tube
- unplanned extubation
- vagus nerve
- vallecula
- vocal cords

INTRODUCTION

In mechanical ventilation, artificial airways provide a vital link between the ventilator and the patient. Two common artificial airways used in conjunction with mechanical ventilators are the endotracheal (ET) and tracheostomy tubes. For these airways to work properly and efficiently, they must be used and maintained correctly. This chapter provides a practical presentation on oral and nasal intubation, suctioning, and extubation. Supplies commonly used for intubation and suctioning are also included.

INTUBATION

✓ The surgical procedure that creates an opening at the trachea is called *tracheotomy.*

tracheostomy tube: An artificial airway inside the trachea that is inserted through a surgical opening at the trachea.

Endotracheal (ET) intubation is the placement of an ET tube inside the trachea through the mouth or nostril. It is estimated that 15 million patients undergo ET intubation annually (Coppolo et al., 1990).

ET intubation is a simpler procedure than tracheotomy—a surgical procedure that creates an airway opening by cutting into the trachea. Compared to an ET tube (Figure 6-1), a **tracheostomy tube** (Figure 6-2) is much shorter and it provides closer access to the lower airways. It has a lower mechanical deadspace volume than an ET tube. It also ventilates the patient more efficiently and enhances secretion removal. In spite of many advantages of a tracheostomy tube, ET intubation is preferred as the initial means of establishing an artificial airway.

Oral and nasal intubations are commonly done by respiratory care practitioners. When these two routes are not accessible or when the need for a long-term artificial airway is expected, a tracheotomy is done by a physician who is proficient in this surgical procedure.

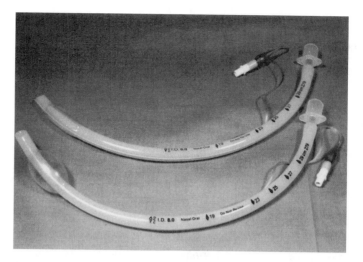

Figure 6-1 Two adult endotracheal tubes (8.0 mm ID). Note that one's cuff is inflated and the other's is not. Also note the markings visible on the tubes.

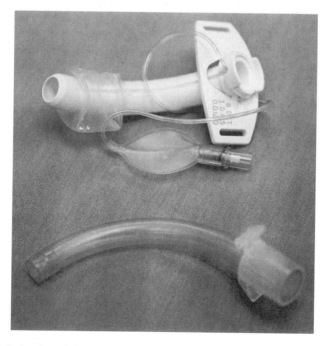

Figure 6-2 An adult tracheostomy tube with a disposable inner cannula that may be replaced as required to maintain patency.

TABLE 6-1   **Indications for Using Artificial Airway**

INDICATION	EXAMPLES
Relief of airway obstruction	Epiglottitis Facial burns and smoke inhalation Vocal cord edema
Protection of the airway	Prevention of aspiration Absence of coordinated swallow
Facilitation of suctioning	Excessive secretions Inadequate cough
Support of ventilation	Ventilatory failure / Respiratory arrest Chest trauma Postanesthesia recovery Hyperventilation to ↓ intracranial pressure

(Data from Shapiro et al., 1991; White, 1998; Whitten, 1997.)

INDICATIONS

The decision to perform ET intubation versus tracheotomy is based on the expected duration of need. In general, if the patient requires an artificial airway for a brief period (e.g., 10 days or less) and full recovery is expected, an ET tube is used. On the other hand, if the patient's condition is critical and recovery is not expected any time soon (e.g., more than 21 days), a tracheostomy tube is preferred (Shapiro et al., 1991).

Choosing when to intubate is also a difficult clinical decision because delayed intubation may lead to hypoventilation, hypoxemia, and hypoxia. The timing of intubation can be based on four indications: (1) Relief of airway obstruction, (2) Protection of the airway, (3) Facilitation of suctioning, and (4) Support of ventilation (Shapiro et al., 1991). Some examples for each of these indications are listed in Table 6-1.

COMMON ARTIFICIAL AIRWAYS IN MECHANICAL VENTILATION

An ET tube may be inserted orally (oral intubation) or nasally (nasal intubation) through the larynx and into the trachea. Oral intubation is easy to perform and it is often done in emergency situations. Nasal intubation is more time-consuming and it is more suitable in elective intubations.

ORAL ENDOTRACHEAL TUBE

Intubation through the mouth is the preferred method of establishing an artificial airway (Figure 6-3). An oral route allows the passage of a

☑ Oral intubation is easy to perform and is often done in emergency situations.

☑ An oral route of intubation allows the passage of a larger ET tube than nasal intubation.

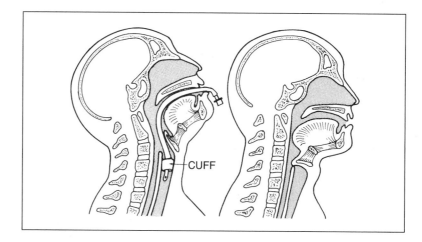

Figure 6-3 This illustration shows how an inflated cuff seals the trachea.

A larger ET tube lowers the peak, plateau, and mean airway pressures.

larger ET tube than nasal intubation. A larger tube has less air flow resistance, and it lowers the airway pressure requirements. However, oral intubation is less comfortable to the patient and may cause gagging and excessive secretion production. Agitated patients may bite down on the tube and cause air flow obstruction.

NASAL ENDOTRACHEAL TUBE

Disadvantages of nasal intubation include difficulty to insert, use of a smaller ET tube, and potential development of sinusitis.

Intubation through the nostril is better tolerated by the patient. It provides an ideal access to the lower airway in conditions where oral access is limited (e.g., oral trauma). The disadvantages of nasal intubation include difficulty to insert, use of a smaller ET tube, and potential development of sinusitis.

TRACHEOSTOMY TUBE

The decision to change from an ET tube to a tracheostomy tube is based on the patient's condition and prognosis.

A tracheostomy tube is inserted through a surgical opening into the trachea. In long-term mechanical ventilation, it is used to replace the ET tube that has been in place for 21 days or longer (Shapiro et al., 1991).

The tracheostomy tube bypasses the upper airway and the glottis and therefore avoids any potential injury in these areas and offers lower air flow resistance. It is also easier to maintain, stabilize, and suction. In addition, the patient can eat and drink with the tracheostomy cuff properly inflated (Shapiro et al., 1991).

Sterile technique must be followed during tracheostomy tube care and suctioning.

Tracheostomy tubes are not without drawbacks. Since a tracheostomy tube is inserted through a surgical opening, infection and trauma to the surgical site are always a threat. To reduce the potential complications of tracheostomy, sterile and aseptic techniques must be followed during tracheostomy care and suctioning (White, 1998).

laryngoscope: An instrument that is used to displace the tongue and soft tissues, and visualize the larynx and vocal cords during endotracheal intubation.

stylet: A flexible but semirigid wire placed inside an endotracheal tube to provide it with a desired curvature.

Magill forceps: Special forceps used to perform nasal intubation under direct vision.

☑ The laryngoscope handle is held by the left hand.

☑ Common laryngoscope blades range from size 0 (neonates) to 4 (adults).

INTUBATION PROCEDURE

Intubation is a fairly simple procedure. In order to become proficient in this procedure one may need to exercise good organization and frequent practice. The procedure described below provides the basics and it may vary somewhat depending on the preference of an individual and existing protocol of the respiratory therapy department.

SUPPLIES

The minimum supplies needed for ET intubation include (1) **laryngoscope** handle, (2) blade, (3) ET tube, (4) 10 cc syringe, (5) water-soluble lubricant, (6) tape, (7) stethoscope. Optional supplies for ET intubation include (8) **stylet**, (9) topical anesthetic, and (10) **Magill forceps**.

In addition to the intubation supplies, proper airway management also requires oral airway, nasal airway, oxygen supply, and resuscitation bag/mask system.

Laryngoscope Handle. The laryngoscope handle contains batteries and it allows attachment of the blade and manipulation of the blade during intubation. Figure 6-4 shows a laryngoscope handle with a Miller blade.

The laryngoscope handle is held in the left hand since all standard blades attached to the handle are designed for right-hand intubations.

Blade. The laryngoscope blade attaches its flange onto the post of the handle (Figure 6-5). Once snapped into position, the built-in light

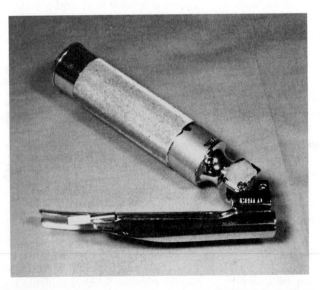

Figure 6-4 A conventional laryngoscope with a Miller blade attached.

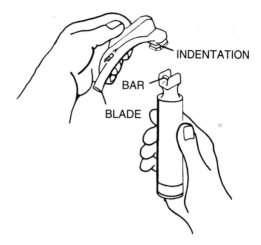

Figure 6-5   Attaching the laryngoscope blade to the handle. The blade locks into place when it is properly engaged. (Reproduced with permission. *Textbook of Advanced Cardiac Life Support*, 1994.

✓ A straight blade lifts the tongue *and* epiglottis upward to expose the vocal cord and related structures.

✓ A curved blade lifts the tongue only.

vallecula: An area between the base of the tongue and epiglottis; an anatomical landmark for the placement of the curved blade.

✓ A straight blade works better in patients with short necks, high or rigid larynxes, or obesity.

vocal cords: Two thin, almost parallel folds of tissue within the larynx that vibrate as air passes between them; an important landmark as the entry point to the trachea during intubation.

source at the distal end of the blade comes on. A laryngoscope blade is either straight or curved and ranges from size 0 (neonates) to 4 (adults). Size 3 and size 4 blades are intended for small and large adults, respectively. The straight (Miller) blade is used to pick up the epiglottis during intubation. The curved (MacIntosh) blade is placed in an area called **vallecula**, and indirectly moves the epiglottis out of the way.

The basic technique of intubation is the same no matter which type of blade is used. The primary difference between these two blades is that a straight blade lifts the tongue *and* epiglottis upward to expose the vocal cords and related structures (Figure 6-6). The epiglottis is not visible when a straight blade is placed properly. The tip of a curved blade rests at the vallecula (between base of tongue and epiglottis) and lifts the tongue only (Figure 6-7). The epiglottis may be seen through the mouth when a curved blade is used properly.

Patients with short necks, high larynxes, or who are obese often need straight blades to displace the tongue and attached soft tissues upward. A straight blade also works better in patients with rigid larynxes due to scar formation or trauma (Whitten, 1997).

A curved blade is easy to learn to use as it can be easily positioned by advancing to the base of the tongue. Once the tongue is lifted upward, the epiglottis moves upward with the attached soft tissues thus exposing the **vocal cords**.

Despite one's training and preference, it is essential to gain experience and proficiency in using both types of laryngoscope blades, since in some emergency situations, the preferred type of blade may not be readily available.

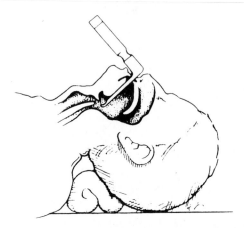

Figure 6-6 Laryngoscopic technique with a straight blade; the epiglottis is elevated anteriorly to expose the glottic opening. (Reproduced with permission. *Textbook of Advanced Cardiac Life Support*, 1994. Copyright American Heart Association.)

CURVED BLADE

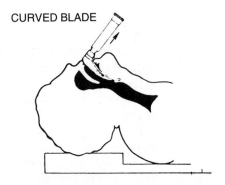

Figure 6-7 When a curved blade is used, the epiglottis is displaced anteriorly by upward traction, with the tip of the blade in the vallecula. (Reproduced with permission. *Textbook of Advanced Cardiac Life Support*, 1994. Copyright American Heart Association.)

endotracheal tube:
An artificial airway inside the trachea that is inserted through the mouth or nostril.

radiopaque: *Impenetrable to X-rays or other forms of radiation. It appears as a light area on the radiograph.*

Endotracheal Tube. **Endotracheal tubes** come in sizes ranging from 2 to 10. The size refers to the internal diameter (I.D.) of the tube in millimeters (mm) and it comes in 0.5 mm increments. To reduce air flow resistance, the largest size appropriate to a patient should be used.

The proximal end of an ET tube has a 15-mm adapter that fits all standard ventilator circuits and aerosol therapy adapters. Along the body of the tube, a **radiopaque** line runs lengthwise for the verification of tube location by chest radiograph. Markings in millimeters (mm) are also shown along the body for easy determination of the depth of intubation. The volume of air in the cuff at the distal end of *pilot balloon: The small balloon on the proximal end of an endotracheal or tracheostomy tube. It is used to regulate the volume of air in the cuff and to serve as an indicator of air volume in the cuff.*

☑ For adult ET tubes, the syringe used to inflate the cuff should have a capacity of 10 cc or larger.

☑ Use only a water-soluble lubricant on the distal end of an ET tube.

☑ Petroleum or oil-based lubricants must not be used as they can cause adverse reactions to the lungs.

☑ If the ET tube is not secured properly, inadvertent extubation or main-stem intubation may result.

☑ A stylet is not required for successful oral intubation and it is not used in nasal intubation.

the ET tube is controlled by using a large (10 cc or larger) syringe via the **pilot balloon.**

The ET tube is normally held in the right hand with the curvature facing forward. When intubating a spontaneously breathing patient, the tube is advanced into the trachea during spontaneous inspiratory efforts (when the vocal cords are opened wide). During expiration, the ET tube may bounce off the closed vocal cords and enter the esophagus.

10 cc Syringe.   A syringe with a capacity of 10 cc or larger is used to test the pilot balloon and ET tube cuff before intubation and to inflate the cuff after intubation. After testing the integrity of the pilot balloon and cuff, air is withdrawn from the cuff to the syringe. The air-filled syringe may be left attached to the pilot balloon for rapid inflation of the cuff immediately after intubation.

Water-Soluble Lubricant.   A water-soluble lubricant is used to lubricate the distal end of the ET tube for easy insertion into the trachea. Petroleum or oil-based lubricants must *not* be used in ET intubation. Once entering the lungs, they can cause adverse reactions to the airways and lung parenchyma.

Tape.   Tape is used to secure the ET tube so that the tube will not move too high causing inadvertent extubation, or too low leading to main-stem intubation. Benzoin or other commercially available solutions may be effective in making the tape more adhesive to the damp skin. Zinc oxide base tape (by Hy Tape Corporation, New York) also sticks well to the skin when it is exposed to moisture.

Stethoscope.   A stethoscope is needed to auscultate bilateral breath sounds immediately after intubation.

Stylet.   A flexible stylet wire guide is placed inside the ET tube to form a desired curvature and to make it more rigid for ease of intubation. Use of a stylet is not required for successful oral intubation. A stylet is not used in nasal intubation.

When a stylet is used, make certain that its end does not extend below the tip of the ET tube because the stylet can traumatize the tracheal wall. As a standard practice, the portion of stylet extending from the proximal end of the ET tube (outside the patient's mouth) is bent before intubation to prevent it from slipping deep inside the ET tube.

Topical Anesthetic.   A mild, topical anesthetic may be used to numb the mucosal membrane that may come in contact with the blade or ET tube. Use of a topical anesthetic is not feasible in emergency intubation or necessary in unconscious patients. It is useful to reduce the incidence of bronchospasm and vomiting when elective intubation is done in conscious and alert patients.

Magill Forceps. Magill forceps are used to perform nasal intubation. After the ET tube has been inserted through the nostril and becomes visible through the mouth, the laryngoscope blade and Magill forceps are used together to guide the ET tube into the trachea under direct vision.

SELECTION OF ENDOTRACHEAL TUBE

☑ Select the *largest* tube that is appropriate to the patient.

The size of an ET tube should be the largest one appropriate to a patient. Comparing to a smaller ET tube, a larger one offers lower airway resistance, and lower (peak, plateau, mean) airway pressures. A larger ET tube also improves dynamic compliance and facilitates secretion removal.

Table 6-2 shows the estimated size of the ET tube based on body size. In addition to the body weight or body size, final selection of an ET tube should be based on the clinical condition and tolerance of the patient.

VENTILATION AND OXYGENATION

☑ Mentally count from 1 to 30 when you begin the intubation attempt.

☑ Intubation attempts lasting longer than 30 seconds may cause hypoxia and arrhythmias.

Before each intubation attempt, the patient must be adequately ventilated and oxygenated. If the patient is not breathing spontaneously, a resuscitation bag/mask system is used to provide ventilation and oxygenation (Figure 6-8).

If an intubation attempt is not successful after 30 seconds, the ET tube and laryngoscope blade should be removed immediately and the patient ventilated with a bag/mask system and 100% oxygen. Ventilation and oxygenation should continue for at least 30 seconds or until the pulse oximetry (SpO_2) reading returns to the baseline level or in the 90s.

ORAL INTUBATION

The sequence outlined in Table 6-3 provides a general procedure for oral intubation. It should be modified to suit individual situations and to comply with existing protocols.

TABLE 6-2 **Estimation of ET Tube Size**

PATIENT		ESTIMATED SIZE
Neonate	<1000 gm	2.5 mm I.D.
Neonate	1000 to 2000 gm	3.0 mm I.D.
Neonate	2000 to 3000 gm	3.5 mm I.D.
Neonate	>3000 gm	4.0 mm I.D.
Child	1 to 2 years	4.5 mm I.D.
Child	2 to 12 years	4.5 + (age / 4) mm I.D.
Average adult female		7.5 to 8.5 mm I.D.
Average adult male		8.0 to 9.0 mm I.D.

☑ For an 8-year-old, the calculated ET tube size would be 4.5 + (8/4) = 4.5 + 2 = 6.5 mm I.D.

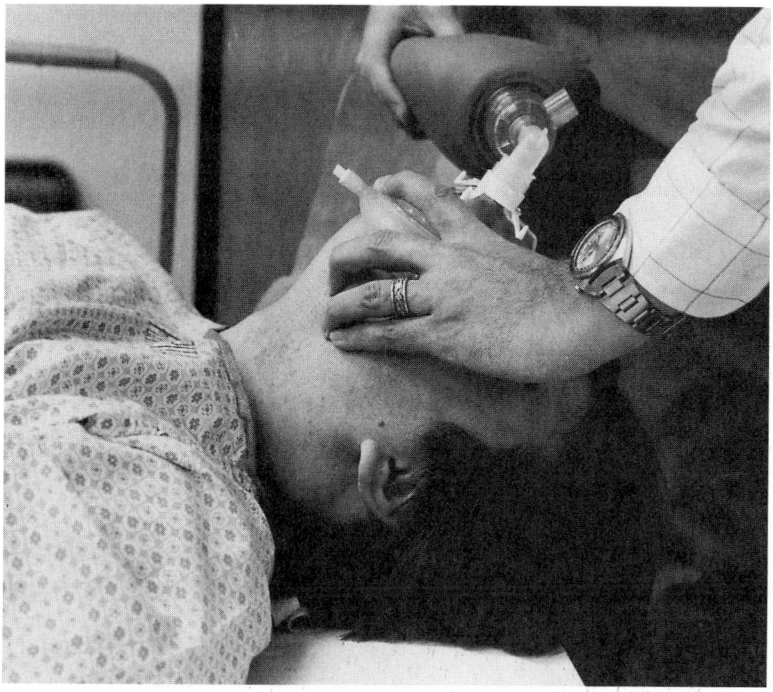

Figure 6-8   Correct use of a mask to manually ventilate a patient.

NASAL INTUBATION

The procedure for nasal intubation is similar to that for oral intubation. In nasal intubation, the ET tube is inserted through the nostril and then guided by the Magill forceps into the trachea (Table 6-4, page 142).

☑ "Blind" nasal intubation is done by advancing the ET tube slowly during spontaneous inspiratory efforts by listening for air movement through the ET tube.

Blind Intubation.   In alert and cooperative patients who are breathing spontaneously, "blind" nasal intubation may be done by inserting the ET tube into a nostril and advancing it slowly during inspiratory efforts. When the distal end of the ET tube approaches the trachea, air movement can be heard through the ET tube. The general depth of nasal intubation is guided by the distance marking (e.g., 23 cm) on the ET tube. Breath sounds and a chest radiograph are then assessed to confirm proper placement of the ET tube.

COMMON ERRORS

Errors can occur when intubation is done in a hurried fashion. They are also more likely to occur when it is done by someone who is not proficient or experienced with the intubation procedure. By staying

---

TABLE 6-3 Procedure for Oral Intubation

---

1. Assemble and test supplies (e.g., check light source, lubricate ET tube cuff).

2. Lubricate the deflated cuff with a water-soluble lubricant.

3. Explain procedure to patient.

4. Ventilate and preoxygenate patient with 100% oxygen.

5. Tilt the head back and place in the **sniffing position** (Figure 6-9).

6. Hold laryngoscope handle with left hand.

7. Open mouth and insert blade into the right side of mouth.

8. Slide blade to the base of tongue and sweep blade to the left.

9. Maneuver the tip of straight blade underneath the epiglottis or the tip of curved blade at the vallecula.

10. Lift handle and blade up anteriorly to displace the tongue and attached soft tissues (Figure 6-10).

11. Locate the (epiglottis [curve blade only]), larynx, and vocal cords (Figure 6-11).

12. Insert ET tube through the vocal cords under direct vision.

13. Inflate cuff and check for bilateral breath sounds.

14. Confirm proper ET tube placement with chest radiograph.

---

sniffing position: *An ideal head position for endotracheal intubation. It is done by tilting the forehead back slightly and moving the chin anteriorly to the patient.*

calm during an intubation attempt and updating the intubation skills in a controlled setting (e.g., in operating room), errors can be minimized or avoided.

Table 6-5 (page 143) outlines some problems that may be encountered during an intubation attempt. The potential cause and solution to each problem are provided.

SIGNS OF ENDOTRACHEAL INTUBATION

After intubation and inflation of the cuff, correct placement of the ET tube in the trachea must be checked immediately. If the patient is breathing spontaneously, bilateral breath sounds should be heard. Speech will not be possible since the vocal cords are bypassed by the ET tube and no longer receive air flow for making sound. In addition, air flow may be felt over the ET tube opening. Moisture or condensa-

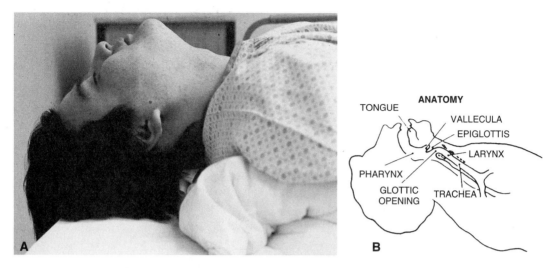

Figure 6-9   (A) A patient in the "sniffing" position. (B) Essential anatomical landmarks in direct laryngoscopy. (Reproduced with permission. *Textbook of Advanced Cardiac Life Support*, 1994. Copyright American Heart Association.)

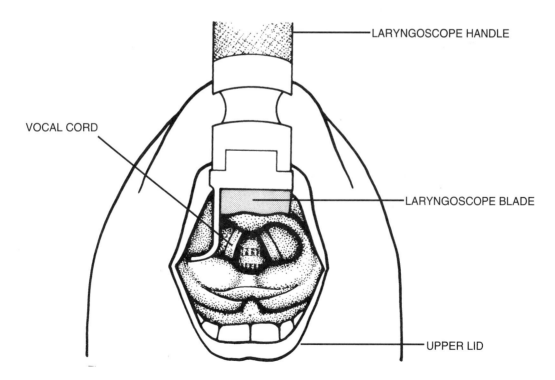

Figure 6-10   Anatomy of the upper airway as viewed with a laryngoscope in place.

ANATOMY

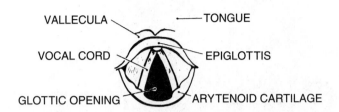

Figure 6-11 Anatomical structures seen during direct laryngoscopy. (Reproduced with permission. *Textbook of Advanced Cardiac Life Support*, 1994. Copyright American Heart Association.)

TABLE 6-4 **Procedure for Nasal Intubation**

1. Assemble and test supplies (e.g., check light source, lubricate ET tube cuff).

2. Lubricate the deflated cuff with a water-soluble lubricant.

3. Explain procedure to patient.

4. Ventilate and preoxygenate patient with 100% oxygen.

5. Tilt the head back and place in the sniffing position.

6. Insert ET tube into a nostril and advance slowly until the distal end is near the tongue.

7. Open mouth and insert blade into the right side of mouth.

8. Slide blade to the base of tongue and sweep blade to the left.

9. Lift handle and blade up anteriorly to displace the tongue and attached soft tissues.

10. Locate the epiglottis, larynx, and vocal cords.

11. Use right hand to insert Magill forceps into mouth and guide ET tube through the vocal cord under direct vision.

12. Inflate cuff and check for bilateral breath sounds.

13. Confirm proper ET tube placement with chest radiograph.

TABLE 6-5   **Common Problems During Intubation**

PROBLEM (POTENTIAL CAUSE)	SOLUTION
Difficult to put blade or tube in mouth (Improper head position)	Use "sniffing" position by (1) tilting head back slightly and (2) moving chin anteriorly.
Trauma to teeth and soft tissues (Improper use of handle and blade)	Open mouth wider. Do not pivot on teeth to lift blade and tongue.
Unable to see epiglottis, larynx, or vocal cords (Blade is inside esophagus)	Withdraw *curved* blade until it reaches the vallecula (between base of tongue and epiglottis). Withdraw *straight* blade until it reaches the epiglottis.
Unable to advance ET tube when straight blade is used (ET tube is blocked by the light bulb on the right side of straight blade)	Rotate blade slightly counterclockwise (top of handle to left) to move light bulb out of the way.
Esophageal intubation, vomiting, and aspiration (Inserting the ET tube into *any* "opening" hoping it is the tracheal opening)	Find vocal cords and insert ET tube through the cords under direct vision.
Arrhythmias (Hypoxia caused by prolonged intubation attempt)	Stop intubation. Ventilate and oxygenate.

✓ Presence of bilateral breath sounds, air flow, condensations on ET tube, and CO_2 are signs of successful ET intubation.

carina: The point at the lower end of the trachea separating openings of the main-stem bronchi.

✓ For adult patients, the tip of an ET tube should be about 1.5" above the carina.

tion will form inside the ET tube on exhalation. A carbon dioxide (CO_2) indicator or end-tidal CO_2 monitor may be attached to the end of the ET tube to detect CO_2 in the expired gas sample.

The CO_2 detection device contains a chemical that changes color in the presence of carbon dioxide (Figure 6-12). After intubation, the detection device is attached to the endotracheal tube and the color on the device is observed. If the color turns from purple to yellow, it is an indication of successful endotracheal intubation since expired air from the lungs contains approximately 5% carbon dioxide.

If the patient is not breathing spontaneously, bilateral breath sounds should be checked by manual ventilation with a resuscitation bag. The placement of the stethoscope diaphragm should be along the midaxillary line. When the ET tube is properly placed (about 1.5 inches above the **carina**), the chest should expand and the abdomen should not have a gurgling sound during manual ventilation. Breath sounds heard on one side of the chest may suggest main-stem intubation. In the absence of obvious lung pathology (e.g., atelectasis), borderline main-stem intubation produces uneven bilateral breath sounds.

Finally, the definitive confirmation of correct placement of the ET tube is done by a chest radiograph. For adult patients, the depth of

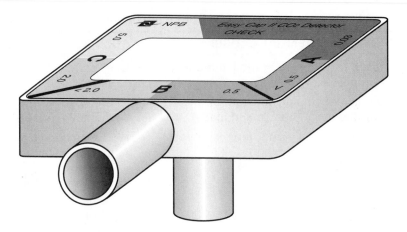

Figure 6-12 A carbon dioxide detection device that is attached to the end of an endotracheal tube immediately after intubation.

intubation may be adjusted accordingly so that the distal end of the ET tube is about 1.5 inches above the carina (Tasota et al., 1987). This distance from the carina is considered ideal as the ET tube may move *down* by an average of about one inch (1.9 cm) with neck flexion (Conrady et al., 1976).

SIGNS OF ESOPHAGEAL INTUBATION

Placing an ET tube into the esophagus is a grave error. Hypoventilation, tissue and cerebral hypoxia are certain and immediate following esophageal intubation of an apneic patient. Furthermore, manual ventilation via an ET tube that has been placed in the esophagus may lead to aspiration of stomach contents and make subsequent intubations extremely difficult.

In almost all instances, esophageal intubation can be avoided by confirming that the ET tube passes through the vocal cords under *direct vision*. If the vocal cords are not seen or cannot be identified, the ET tube *must not* be inserted. Another experienced physician or practitioner should attempt to reintubate. Valuable time must not be wasted when a difficult intubation is encountered.

Esophageal Detection Device. The Esophageal Detection Device (EDD) is a sensitive and specific tool to detect esophageal intubation in the emergency setting (Kasper & Deem, 1998). This device provides a negative-pressure test using a compressible and self-inflating bulb with two openings. The upper end contains a one-way valve to allow air to escape from the bulb. The lower end has an adaptor that connects to the endotracheal tube. After intubation, the bulb is attached to the endotracheal tube and then compressed. With tracheal placement,

☑ Do not check breath sounds at anterior chest locations close to the trachea since air flow in the *esophagus* can give false "breath sounds" in neonates and thin adults.

☑ In the absence of obvious lung pathology, uneven bilateral breath sounds may suggest main-stem intubation.

☑ Esophageal intubation can be avoided by inserting the ET tube through the vocal cords under *direct vision*.

the bulb draws air from the trachea and should reinflate to its original shape within 10 seconds. With esophageal placement, the bulb receives little or no air from the constricted esophagus and it remains deflated (Scanlan, Wilkins & Stoller, 1999). Since false positive and false negative results have been reported, the EDD test results should be used in conjunction with other clinical signs following an intubation attempt.

MANAGEMENT OF ENDOTRACHEAL AND TRACHEOSTOMY TUBES

Once the patient is successfully intubated with an artificial airway, it must be managed properly to prevent complications. Failure to secure the airway may lead to inadvertent or self-extubation. Excessive cuff pressures may lead to tracheal mucosal tissue injuries. Finally, failure to humidify the secretions makes removal of secretions from the artificial airway difficult and this condition may lead to pneumonia and atelectasis.

SECURING ENDOTRACHEAL AND TRACHEOSTOMY TUBES

The ET tube can be secured by using adhesive tape or commercially made harness. As shown in Figure 6-13A (oral intubation) and 6-13B (nasal intubation) they are used around the base of the head or neck for maximal security. Caution must be exercised as this technique may cause facial swelling and injuries to the lips when applied around the neck too tightly.

Since moisture often gathers between the tape and skin, tapes that can withstand moisture are more desirable. Zinc oxide base tape (by Hy Tape Corporation, New York) is one that sticks well to the skin when exposed to moisture.

Tracheostomy tubes are secured by tying a string to the two openings on the collar. The string goes around the neck for good fit and security.

CUFF PRESSURE

The estimated capillary perfusion pressure in the trachea is about 30 cm H_2O. If the cuff pressure is greater than the capillary perfusion pressure, ischemic injury and tissue necrosis may occur.

☑ The ET tube cuff pressure should be 25 cm H_2O or less to minimize pressure-induced injuries to the trachea.

The ET tube cuff pressure should be 25 cm H_2O or less to allow adequate capillary perfusion in the trachea. For patients with hypotension, the cuff pressure should be kept even lower to compensate for the reduced capillary flow due to hypotension. Figure 6-14 shows the use of a pressure manometer and syringe to adjust the ET tube cuff pressure. Figure 6-15 shows a photograph of the Posey Cufflator

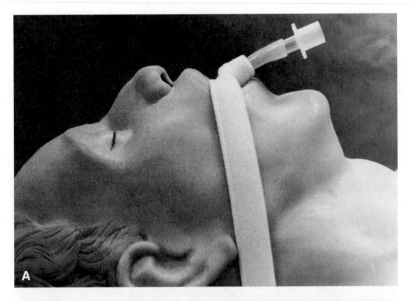

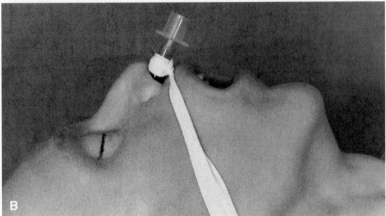

Figure 6-13 (A) Use of a commercially made harness to secure an oral endotracheal tube. (B) One method of securing the tube of a nasally intubated patient.

with a built-in manometer. Air may be added to the ET tube cuff by pumping the bulb on the Cufflator. Air may be removed from the ET tube cuff by opening the release valve on the Cufflator.

MINIMAL OCCLUSION VOLUME AND MINIMAL LEAK TECHNIQUE

If a cuff pressure manometer is not readily available, the minimal occlusion volume or minimal leak technique may be used to reduce

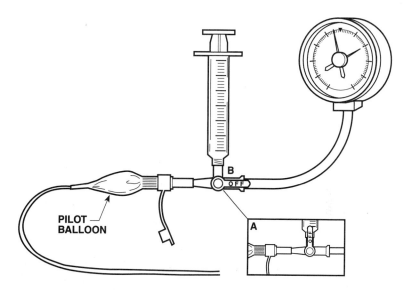

PILOT
BALLOON

Figure 6-14 (A) When the stop cock points toward the syringe, the manometer measures the cuff pressure. (B) When the stop cock points toward the manometer, the syringe may be used to fill or withdraw air from the cuff.

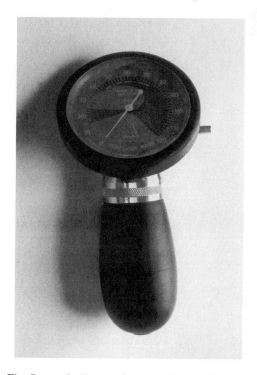

Figure 6-15 The Posey Cufflator. (Courtesy Delmar Thomson Learning)

✓ The minimal occlusion volume is obtained by inflating the cuff to a point at which no air leak is heard at end-inspiration.

✓ The minimal leak technique is done by inflating the cuff until the leak stops and then removing a small amount of air until a *slight* audible leak can be heard at end-inspiration.

the likelihood of pressure-induced injuries to the trachea caused by excessive cuff pressure.

The minimal occlusion volume is obtained by inflating the cuff to a point at which no air leak is heard at end-inspiration. The air leak around the cuff can be heard by placing the stethoscope diaphragm on the trachea, as close to the location of the cuff as possible. The end-inspiration point is used because the trachea reaches its maximal diameter at end-inspiration.

The minimal leak technique is done by inflating the cuff until the leak stops and then removing a small amount of air until a *slight* audible leak can be heard at end-inspiration (Chang, 1995).

IRRIGATION AND SUCTION

Intubated patients are at risk for secretion retention because the ET tube and ventilator attachments form a closed system and do not allow removal of secretions. Secretions must be removed by way of ET suctioning. However, frequent and inappropriate ET suctioning can cause mucosal damage and increase the incidence of suction-induced hypoxemia and arrhythmias. Therefore, ET suctioning should not be done on a preset sechedule, it should be done only when indicated.

The level of vacuum pressure should be kept below 100 mm Hg (Figure 6-16). The effectiveness of suction (based on the amount of secretion removed) is optimal at this vacuum pressure. Pressures higher than 100 mm Hg are not more effective but more likely to cause damage to the tracheal wall (Kuzenski, 1978).

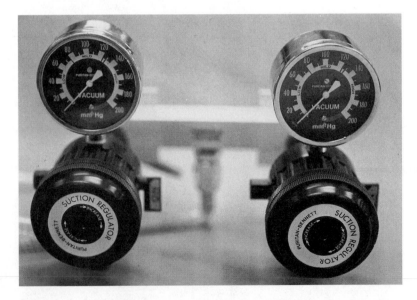

Figure 6-16 A Puritan-Bennett suction regulator with vacuum pressures ranging from 0 to 200 mm Hg.

✓ To avoid suction-induced hypoxemia, preoxygenate the patient and keep the duration of suction to less than 15 seconds.

Suction-induced hypoxemia may be avoided by preoxygenating the patient with 100% oxygen and limiting the duration of suctioning to less than 15 seconds (Belknap et al., 1980; Stone et al., 1989).

The sequence outlined in Table 6-6 provides a general procedure for ET suctioning. It should be modified to suit individual situations and to comply with existing protocols. For example, irrigation of the ET tube and lungs with saline solution before suctioning is a controversial practice (Bostick et al., 1987; Shekleton et al., 1987).

EXTUBATION

Extubation should be done as soon as feasible. Early extubation not only provides immediate relief to the patient, it shortens the duration of a hospital stay, reduces health care costs and conserves resources (Cheng, 1995; Lichtenthal et al., 1995; Velasco, 1995). In one study of patients undergoing coronary artery bypass grafting, the average saving per patient was $6,000 in the early extubation group (Arom, 1995).

PREDICTORS OF SUCCESSFUL EXTUBATION

A patient is ready for extubation after regaining airway reflexes and showing no signs of cardiopulmonary distress. The general criteria for assessing a patient's readiness to be extubated may include the rapid breathing index, occlusion pressure/maximal inspiratory pressure ratio, blood gases, muscle strength, and general cardiopulmonary signs.

✓ The patient should be allowed to breathe spontaneously for about three minutes before taking measurements. Otherwise, the f/VT index may not reflect the patient's actual condition.

Rapid Breathing Index.   The rapid breathing (f/VT) index can be obtained easily by measuring the breathing frequency and minute volume during one minute of spontaneous breathing (Epstein, 1995; Yang et al., 1991). The f/VT index is calculated by dividing the spontaneous breathing frequency per minute by the average tidal volume in liters. A value of less than 100/min/L is highly predictive of successful extubation outcome.

Other Common Indicators.   Acceptable blood gases, ventilatory reserve, and general cardiopulmonary signs are other useful indicators that may be used to guide the extubation decision. These criteria and the rapid breathing index are very simple and easy to use. They are summarized in Table 6-7 along with their respective methods of assessment.

P0.1/MIP Ratio.   The occlusion pressure at 0.1 sec to maximal inspiratory pressure (P0.1/MIP) ratio is a more complicated procedure than the preceding criteria. A special manometer is needed to measure the airway occlusion pressure at 0.1 second from the onset of inspiration, with the airway occluded at the functional residual capacity

TABLE 6-6   Endotracheal Suctioning

PROCEDURE	RATIONALE
Wash hands and gather all suction supplies (catheter, sterile gloves, water, water container, and saline solution).	Avoid need to obtain other supplies once sterile gloves have been put on hands.
Explain procedure to patient.	Assure patient understanding and cooperation.
Adjust vacuum to 100 mm Hg.	Prevent excessive vacuum and mucosal damage.
Put sterile water in container.	For testing suction device and flushing secretions inside catheter.
Put on sterile gloves using aseptic technique.	Minimize nosocomial infection.
Designate "sterile" and "contaminated" hands.	Use "sterile" hand to handle all supplies requiring asceptic technique (i.e., suction catheter). Use "contaminated" hand to handle all other supplies (e.g., ET tube adapter, suction tubing).
Attach suction catheter ("sterile" hand) to suction tubing ("contaminated" hand).	Ensure sterile and asceptic techniques.
Test vacuum and suction with sterile water.	Ensure proper function of suction setup.
Remove ET tube adapter and irrigate with 5 cc of sterile saline if necessary ("contaminated" hand).	Loosen secretions.
Manually hyperinflate the patient's lungs with resuscitation bag.	Ensure adequate ventilation and oxygenation. Seek help if neccessary.
Insert catheter into ET tube ("sterile" hand) and advance until resistance is met. Withdraw catheter slightly.	Avoid suctioning the tracheal wall and minimize mucosal damage.
Activate suction ("contaminated" hand) and withdraw catheter ("sterile" hand) by rotating the catheter.	Increase removal of secretions.
Limit the duration of suction to less than 15 seconds.	Prevent suction-induced hypoxia and arrhythmias.
Auscultate chest and repeat suction if necessary.	Avoid unnecessary suctioning.

(Data from Barnes, 1986; Belknap et al., 1980; Chulay, 1988; Stone, et al.,1989.)

TABLE 6-7   **General Criteria for Extubation**

CRITERIA	METHODS OF ASSESSMENT
Rapid breathing index	f/VT less than 100/min/L
Blood gases	Acceptable blood gases on F_IO_2 less than 40% and spontaneous minute ventilation less than 10 L/min PaO_2/F_IO_2 more than 250 mm Hg
Ventilatory reserve	Maximal inspiratory pressure >−20 cm H_2O Vital capacity >15 ml/kg
Cardiopulmonary assessment	Absence of cardiopulmonary problems (e.g., CHF, pulmonary edema, pneumonia, tachycardia, arrhythmia, chest retractions, distended stomach)

(Data from Capdevila et al., 1995; Epstein, 1995; Listello et al., 1994; Whelan et al., 1994; White, 1998; Whitten, 1997.)

✓ P0.1/MIP ratio of 0.9 or lower is predictive of successful extubation outcome.

(Capdevila et al., 1995; Whitelaw et al., 1993). Since P0.1 is measured at zero flow, it is independent of the compliance and resistance characteristics of the respiratory system. P0.1 reflects the neuromuscular drive to breathe—a prerequisite for successful extubation and adequate spontaneous breathing. The MIP reflects the respiratory muscle strength and ventilatory reserve. A P0.1/MIP ratio of 0.9 or lower has great predictive value of successful extubation (Capdevila et al., 1995).

PROCEDURE

✓ Competent personnel and intubation supplies must be readily available during extubation.

There should be no disagreement that extubation is easier than intubation. Nevertheless, the person who is doing the extubation must be proficient in intubation as well. Since the criteria used for the extubation decision cannot predict a successful outcome every time, one must anticipate the need for reintubation on short notice. Intubation supplies must also be readily available during extubation.

Before extubation, the procedure is explained to the patient and the patient is positioned in a Fowler's (semisitting) position. Hyperinflation and oxygenation are provided to the patient with a manual resuscitator via the ET tube. The ET tube is then suctioned.

✓ The cuff must be deflated before extubation.

If the patient has an adequate vital capacity and cough reflex, the cuff is deflated completely and the ET tube is removed. Encourage the patient to breathe deeply and cough, and use a Yankaur (rigid tonsil tip) suction device to remove excess secretions in the patient's oropharynx.

If the patient does not have an adequate vital capacity and cough reflex, the suction catheter may be left extending from the distal end of the ET tube and continuous suction is applied while the ET tube is being removed. An alternate method is to leave the suction catheter

☑ Aspiration,
laryngospasm,
hoarseness, laryn-
geal and subglottic
edema are some
complications
immediately after
extubation.

unplanned extuba-
tion: Unexpected
removal of an endo-
tracheal or trache-
ostomy tube before
the patient is ready
for extubation.

in the oropharynx with continuous suction while the ET tube is being removed. Either method may be used to remove secretions from the patient's airway or oropharynx (Figure 6-17).

Vital signs, blood gases, and signs of tissue damage should be assessed carefully after extubation. Some immediate postextubation complications include aspiration, laryngospasm, hoarseness, laryngeal and subglottic edema. Other more severe complications that may not be immediately apparent are mucosal injuries, laryngeal stenosis, tracheal inflammation, dilation or stenosis, and vocal cord paralysis (Young et al., 1995).

UNPLANNED EXTUBATION

Unplanned extubation (self-inflicted or accidental) accounts for about 8 to 10 percent of all extubations in ICU patients (Listello et al., 1994). Most of these patients tolerate the unplanned removal of an ET tube well and are not reintubated. Whether or not to reintubate the patient can be a difficult decision. Delayed reintubation may lead to adverse outcomes such as hypoventilation, hypoxemia, and hypoxia. In general, the decision to reintubate may be based on clinical observations and the criteria for extubation (i.e., rapid breathing index, blood gases, ventilatory reserve, and general cardiopulmonary signs). However, these measurements may not have been done immediately before extubation since the extubation is not planned.

To avoid this problem, other criteria based on routinely available patient information have been identified and used for the reintubation

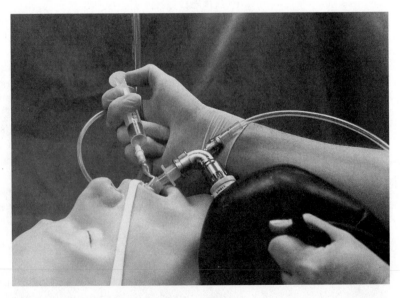

Figure 6-17 Use of a flow-inflating manual resuscitator, suction catheter, and a syringe during extubation.

TABLE 6-8 Clinical Predictors for Reintubation

UNFAVORABLE CLINICAL PREDICTOR*	RATIONALES
(1) SIMV or AC rate >6/min	Patient is dependent on the ventilator
(2) Most recent pH ≥7.45	Oxyhemoglobin saturation curve shifts to right ($\uparrow O_2$ affinity and $\downarrow O_2$ release to tissues)
(3) Most recent PaO_2 / F_IO_2 <250 mm Hg	Poor oxygenation status
(4) Highest heart rate in the past 24° >120/min	Cardiac compensation for poor perfusion or oxygenation
(5) Presence of ≥3 medical disorders	Potential of medical complications
(6) Not alert	Poor mental status; Blunted drive for breathing
(7) Reason for intubation other than preoperative	Presence of medical problems and potential complications

* Presence of four or more predictors favors reintubation. Presence of three or less predictors indicates no need for reintubation.

decision. They are summarized in Table 6-8. In the model set, the presence of 4 or more factors indicates the need for reintubation and the presence of 3 or fewer factors reflects a satisfactory patient outcome without reintubation (Listello et al., 1994).

COMPLICATIONS OF ENDOTRACHEAL INTUBATION

Endotracheal intubation is an extremely useful procedure in the establishment of an artificial airway but it also carries many potential complications. As shown in Table 6-9, complications may develop at different stages of intubation and extubation. Some conditions are life-threatening (e.g., esophageal intubation, bradycardia) while others are minor and often reversible (e.g., pressure sores, hoarseness). It is essential to understand and recognize the potential complications so that appropriate steps may be taken to avert harmful outcomes.

DURING INTUBATION

☑ Trauma to the teeth and soft tissues can occur during intubation.

Trauma to the teeth and soft tissues can occur during intubation since ET intubation is often done in emergency situations. Difficult intubations compound the problem and lead to injuries when the patient has one or more of these conditions: obesity, receding chin, overbite, rigid or short neck, or blood or vomitus in oropharynx.

TABLE 6-9   **Complications Related to Use of Endotracheal Tube**

SEQUENCE OF EVENTS	COMPLICATIONS
During intubation	Trauma to teeth and soft tissues Esophageal intubation Vomiting and aspiration Hypoxia due to prolonged intubation attempt Arrhythmias Bradycardia due to vagal stimulation
While intubated	Obstruction by secretions Pneumonia and atelectasis Kinking of ET tube Aspiration (from feeding and ineffective cuff) Mucosal injuries Improper tube position (too high, too low) Pressure sores around ET tube Inadvertent extubation Sinusitis (nasal intubation)
Immediately after extubation	Aspiration Laryngospasm Hoarseness Laryngeal and subglottic edema
Following extubation	Mucosal injuries Laryngeal stenosis Tracheal inflammation, dilation, stenosis Vocal cord paralysis

(Data from Chang, 1995; White, 1998; Whitten, 1997; Young et al., 1995.)

☑ Esophageal intubation is commonly done by inexperienced practitioners.

vagus nerve: *The pneumogastric or 10th cranial nerve. Its superior and recurrent laryngeal nerves and their branches adjoin the upper end of trachea and are sensitive to stimulation by the endotracheal tube or suction catheter.*

Esophageal intubation is the most dangerous complication. It may occur when it is performed by an inexperienced practitioner or under awkward patient positions (e.g., patient lies on the floor). Esophageal intubation frequently leads to vomiting and aspiration, thus making subsequent intubation attempts more difficult or nearly impossible.

Prolonged intubation attempt leads to hypoxia and if uncorrected, dangerous arrhythmias may occur. Excessive stimulation of the **vagus nerve** can cause bradycardia. Arrhythmias induced by hypoxia and bradycardia caused by vagal stimulation may be reversed by removing the ET tube and oxygenating the patient until a normal sinus rhythm returns.

WHILE INTUBATED

Complications that occur while the patient is intubated vary greatly according to the duration of ET tube placement and the airway management techniques. As a general rule, the longer an ET tube is in place, the more likely that complications will occur while the patient is intubated.

✓ Failure to re-
move retained
secretions could lead
to pneumonia and
atelectasis.

Since normal mucocillary functions of the mucosal membrane and
the cough reflex are lost with an ET tube in place, retention of secretions must be removed promptly. If secretions are thick, irrigation
with saline solution or acetylcysteine (Mucomyst®) should be done
before suctioning. Failure to remove retained secretions may lead to
pneumonia and atelectasis (Chang, 1995).

✓ The distance
marking on the
ET tube is made in
reference to the pa-
tient's lips or nares
(e.g., 22 cm at the
lips).

Kinking of an ET tube may be easily corrected by repositioning the
connection between the ET tube and the ventilator circuit. Inadvertent
extubation may be prevented by properly sedating the patient or by
using restraints on the extremities.

The position of the ET tube should be checked frequently by chest
auscultation and concurrently when a routine chest radiograph is
done. Once the ET tube is properly placed, the distance marking on
the ET tube (centimeter mark) should be noted on the ventilator flow
sheet. This reference number provides a quick reference point but
should not be used as a substitute for routine assessment of the ET
tube position.

✓ Extubation of a
semiconscious
patient may stimu-
late the vocal cords
and lead to reflex
spasm.

IMMEDIATELY AFTER EXTUBATION

Laryngospasm usually occurs as a result of extubation when the
patient is semiconscious. Extubation during this excitement stage
tends to stimulate the vocal cords and lead to reflex protective
spasm. For this reason, extubation should be done when the patient
is either deeply anesthetized or preferably, fully awake (Whitten,
1997).

✓ Stridor is the
harsh or high-
pitched sound heard
during spontaneous
respiration.

Stridor is heard when laryngospasm or laryngeal and subglottic
edema occur. In minor cases of stridor, use of cool aerosol and 0.25 to
0.5 cc of 2.25% racemic epinephrine in 5 cc of saline may be helpful.
Dexamethasone at 0.15 mg/kg may help prevent worsening laryngeal
and subglottic edema. In severe cases of laryngospasm, airway obstruction may have developed and reintubation is often required
(Whitten, 1997).

FOLLOWING EXTUBATION

Mucosal injuries, laryngeal stenosis, tracheal damages (inflammation, dilation, and stenosis), and vocal cord paralysis are some long-
term complications following extubation. The best way to avoid
these complications is to practice proper airway care while the patient is intubated.

SUMMARY

The most important element of airway management is intubation. Esophageal intubation can be deadly and it must not be done under any circumstance (e.g., secretions in the airway, poor view, or awkward patient position). The golden rule for endotracheal intubation is "If you don't see it (the vocal cords or related structures), don't do it."

Use of artificial airways also requires proper and routine maintenance to prevent complications. Humidification, suctioning, cuff pressure, and unplanned extubation are some important aspects in airway management during mechanical ventilation. Since the artificial airway is inside the patient's mouth and trachea and is not readily visible, practitioners must have a keen sense of observation and timely clinical judgement to detect any complications or potential troubles.

Self-Assessment Questions

1. The decision to intubate a patient is based on all of the following indications with the *exception* of:

    A. airway obstruction.   C. mechanical ventilation.
    B. hypoxemia.   D. removal of secretions.

2–5. Match the indications for using an artificial airway with the respective examples.

Indication	Examples
2. Relief of airway obstruction	A. Absence of coordinated swallow
3. Protection of the airway	B. Ventilatory failure
4. Facilitation of suctioning	C. Excessive secretions
5. Support of ventilation	D. Epiglottitis

6. As you are preparing to intubate a 49-year-old, 60-kg (132-lb) patient, you notice that there are two endotracheal tubes, size 7 and size 8. You would use the _____ tube because it offers _____ than the other ET tube.

    A. size 8, lower air flow resistance   C. size 7, lower air flow resistance
    B. size 8, higher air flow resistance   D. size 7, higher air flow resistance

7. You are called to intubate a patient in the dialysis unit. Since there are no crash cart and intubation equipment nearby, you are asked to bring along the minimal supplies needed for intubation. In addition to the laryngoscope handle, blade, and endotracheal tube, which of the following supplies is the most essential item for intubation and ventilation?

A. water-soluble lubricant
B. tape

C. stylet
D. 10-cc syringe

8. You are getting ready to perform an elective intubation on a 32-year-old, 78-kg (172-lb), 5'-2" patient in the intensive care unit. Based on the patient's physical character-istics, you would ask for a size _____, _____ laryngoscope blade.

A. 2, Miller
B. 3, Miller

C. 4, MacIntosh
D. 5, MacIntosh

9. When you intubate the patient in the preceding question, you would place the tip of the blade just under the _____ and use the laryngoscope handle to _____.

A. tongue, pry the mouth open.
B. tongue, lift up anteriorly.

C. epiglottis, pry the mouth open.
D. epiglottis, lift up anteriorly.

10. As you are intubating an apneic patient, you notice on the cardiac monitor that the pa-tient has developed arrhythmias during the procedure. You would remove the blade and endotracheal tube immediately and provide:

A. cardiac defibrillation and ventilation.

B. 100% oxygen via a nonrebreathing mask.

C. 100% oxygen via manual resuscita-tion bag/mask system.
D. chest compression and ventilation.

11. The best approach to avoid esophageal intubation is to ensure that the endotracheal tube goes through the _____ under direct vision.

A. underside of tongue
B. pharynx

C. vocal cords
D. epiglottis

12. Trauma done to the teeth of a patient undergoing an intubation procedure is most likely caused by using:

A. a straight blade.
B. a curved blade.

C. an oversized endotracheal tube.
D. pivoting action to lift blade and tongue.

13. After intubating a spontaneously breathing 40-kg (88-lb) patient, all of the following signs may be used to assess correct placement of the endotracheal tube *except*:

   A. presence of breath sounds at the sternum.
   B. loss of speech.

   C. air movement over the ET tube opening.
   D. formation of moisture inside the ET tube.

14. In order to avoid mucosal injuries of the trachea, the cuff of an endotracheal tube may be managed by any one of the following techniques *except*:

   A. minimal occlusion volume.
   B. periodic deflation for 20 minutes q 4°.

   C. cuff pressure less than 25 cm H_2O.
   D. minimal leak technique.

15. A physician asks you to evaluate Mr. King, a postabdominal surgical patient, for possible extubation. Based on the information below, you would recommend to the physician that the patient be a candidate for extubation because he meets all criteria for extubation with the *exception* of:

   A. rapid breathing (f/V_T) index of 150/min/L.
   B. PaO_2/F_IO_2 of 280 mm Hg.

   C. maximal inspiratory pressure of -38 cm H_2O.
   D. F_IO_2 of 35%.

16. A 25-year-old postappendectomy patient extubated herself and you are asked by the physician to evaluate this patient for possible reintubation. Based on the following list of clinical predictors for reintubation, you would recommend that the patient _____ since she has met _____ of the predictors.

Unfavorable Clinical Predictor

---

(1) SIMV rate = 8/min
(2) Most recent pH = 7.42
(3) Most recent PaO_2/F_IO_2 = 210 mm Hg
(4) Highest heart rate in the past 24° = 110/min
(5) Patient diagnosis is appendicitis
(6) Patient is alert
(7) Patient is in postoperative recovery

   A. be reintubated, 2
   B. be reintubated, 4

   C. not be reintubated, 2
   D. not be reintubated, 4

17. A patient develops bradycardia during an intubation attempt. You would stop intubation immediately and _____ the patient since this condition is likely caused by _____.

   A. rest, vagal stimulation.
   B. ventilate, hypoventilation.

   C. oxygenate, hypoxia.
   D. defibrillate, impending cardiac arrest.

18. Several hours after endotracheal intubation, a 35-year-old patient becomes restless in spite of using sedatives and analgesics. The physician is concerned that the ET tube may move down the main bronchus because of excessive head movement. You would recommend that _____ be done and the tip of the ET tube be positioned about _____ inch(es) from the carina.

    A. auscultation, 0.5   C. chest radiograph, 0.5
    B. auscultation, 1.5   D. chest radiograph, 1.5

References

Arom, K. V. (1995). Cost-effectiveness and predictors of early extubation. *Ann of Thorac Surg, 60*(1), 127–132.

Barnes, C. A. (1986). Minimizing hypoxemia due to endotracheal suctioning: A review of the literature. *Heart Lung, 15*, 164–172.

Belknap, J. D. et al. (1980). The effects of preoxygenation technique on arterial blood gases in the mechanically ventilated patient. *Am Rev Respir Dis, 121*(Suppl.), 210.

Bostick, J. et al. (1987). Normal saline installation as part of the suctioning procedure: Effects on PaO_2 and amount of secretions. *Heart Lung, 16*, 532–537.

Capdevila, X. J. et al. (1995). Occlusion pressure and its ratio to maximum inspiratory pressure are useful predictors for successful extubation following T-piece weaning trail. *Chest, 108*, 482–489.

Chang, V. M. (1995). Protocol for prevention of complications of endotracheal intubation. *Crit Care Nurse, 15*, 19–27.

Cheng, D. C. H. (1995). Pro-Early extubation after cardiac-surgery decreases intensive-care unit stay and cost. *J Cardiothorac Vas Anes, 9*(4), 460–464.

Chulay, M. (1988). Arterial blood gas changes with a hyperinflation and hyperoxygenation suctioning intervention in critically ill patients. *Heart Lung, 17*, 654–661.

Conrady, P. A. et al. (1976). Alteration of endotracheal tube position: flexion and extension of the neck. *Crit Care Med, 4*, 7–12.

Coppolo, D. P. et al. (1990). Self-extubation: a twelve-month experience. *Chest, 98*, 165–169.

Epstein, S. K. (1995). Etiology of extubation failure and the predictive value of the rapid breathing index. *Am J Respir Crit Care Med, 152*, 545–549.

Kasper, C. L., & Deem, S. (1998). The self-inflating bulb to detect esophageal intubation during emergency airway management. *Anesthesiology, 88*(4):898–902.

Kuzenski, B. M. (1978). Effect of negative pressure on tracheobronchial trauma. *Nurs Res, 28,* 260–273.

Lichtenthal, P. R. et al. (1995). Perioperative cardiac anesthesia and early extubation keys to decreasing costs in the cardiac-surgery ICU. *Anesthesiology, 83*(3A), A1093.

Listello, D. et al. (1994). Unplanned extubation—Clinical predictors for reintubation. *Chest, 105,* 1496–1503.

Scanlan, C. L., Wilkins, R. L., & Stoller, J. K. (1999). *Egan's fundamentals of respiratory care* (7th ed.). St. Louis: Mosby.

Shapiro, B. A. et al. (1991). *Clinical application of respiratory care* (4th ed.). St. Louis: Mosby-Year Book.

Shekleton, M. E. et al. (1987). Ineffective airway clearance related to artificial airway. *Nurs Clin North Am, 22,* 167–178.

Stone, K. S. et al. (1989). Endotracheal suctioning. *Annu Res Nur Res, 7,* 27–47.

Tasota, F. J. et al. (1987). Evaluation of two methods used to stabilize oral endotracheal tubes. *Heart Lung, 16,* 140–145.

Velasco, F. T. (1995). Economic rationale for early extubation. *J Cardiothorac Vas Anes, 9*(5), 2–9.

Whelan, J. et al. (1994). Unplanned extubation—Predictors of successful termination of mechanical ventilatory support. *Chest, 105,* 1808–1812.

White, G. C. (1998). *Basic clinical lab competencies for respiratory care—An integrated approach* (2nd ed.). Albany, N.Y.: Delmar Publishers.

Whitelaw, W. A. et al. (1993). Airway occlusion pressure. *J Appl Physiol, 74,* 1475–1483.

Whitten, C. E. (1997). *Anyone can intubate—A practical, step-by-step guide for health professionals* (3rd ed.). San Diego: KWP Publications.

Yang, K. L. et al. (1991). A prospective study of indexes predicting the outcome of trials of weaning from mechanical ventilation. *N Engl J Med, 324,* 1445–1450.

Young, A. et al. (1995). Laryngospasm following extubation in children. *Anesthesia, 50*(9), 827.

Suggested Reading

Whelan, J. et al. (1994). Unplanned extubation—Predictors of successful termination of mechanical ventilatory support. *Chest, 105,* 1808–1812.

CHAPTER SEVEN

NONINVASIVE POSITIVE PRESSURE VENTILATION

David W. Chang

OUTLINE

KEY TERMS

- **bilevel positive airway pressure (bilevel PAP)**
- **BiPAP™**
- **continuous positive airway pressure (CPAP)**
- **expiratory positive airway pressure (EPAP)**
- **facial mask**

- **inspiratory positive airway pressure (IPAP)**
- **nasal mask**
- **Nasal Pillows™**
- **noninvasive positive pressure ventilation (NPPV)**
- **obstructive sleep apnea (OSA)**
- **positive end-expiratory pressure (PEEP)**

INTRODUCTION

Noninvasive positive pressure ventilation (NPPV) is a technique of providing ventilation without the use of an artificial airway. It has been used successfully in the management of airflow obstruction in sleep apnea (Guilleminault, Philip & Robinson, 1998) and in the reduction of respiratory workload in gross obesity (Pankow, Hijjeh & Schuttler et al., 1997). More recently NPPV has been used in the management of acute respiratory failure. In selected patients with acute ventilatory failure, NPPV is as effective as conventional mechanical ventilation in improving gas exchange (Abou-Shala & Meduri, 1996). Since an artificial airway is not required in the use of NPPV, fewer complications and a shorter stay in an acute care setting are two additional benefits of NPPV (Antonelli, Conti & Rocco et al., 1998).

noninvasive positive pressure ventilation (NPPV): NPPV provides assisted ventilation without an artificial airway.

✓ NPPV may be used to assist patients with obstructive sleep apnea and acute ventilatory failure.

During the polio epidemics, negative pressure ventilators (i.e., iron lungs) were used to provide ventilation by generating a pressure gradient between the atmosphere and lungs. Air flows into the lungs and ventilation occurs when the pressure in the lungs becomes subatmospheric. Disadvantages of negative pressure ventilators include upper airway obstruction and lack of access for patient care. Modern ventilators generate the pressure gradient between the atmosphere and lungs by positive pressure. With positive pressure ventilation, the pressure in the airway opening is higher than that in the lungs. Some of the disadvantages of positive pressure ventilators are tracheal injury, infection, ventilator-associated pneumonia, barotrauma, and prolonged hospital stay (Antonelli, Conti & Rocco et al. 1998; Diaz, Iglesia & Ferrer et al., 1997; Keenan, Kernerman & Cook et al., 1997; Kramer, Myer & Meharg et al., 1995).

NPPV provides ventilation via the patient's nose or mouth without an artificial airway. For this reason, many complications of negative and positive pressure ventilation are minimized or eliminated.

TERMINOLOGY

In noninvasive positive pressure ventilation, the meanings of some terms are slightly different from traditional usage. These terms, abbreviations, and a brief description for each term are outlined in Table 7-1.

PHYSIOLOGICAL EFFECTS OF NPPV

inspiratory positive airway pressure (IPAP): level of airway pressure during inspiratory phase only.

As in traditional positive pressure ventilation, NPPV has two primary pressure settings. One pressure setting is used during the inspiratory phase and the other during the expiratory phase.

During the inspiratory phase, the **inspiratory positive airway pressure (IPAP)** works like any other positive pressure breathing

TABLE 7-1 Terms Used in NPPV

ABBREVIATION	TERM	NOTES
NPPV	Noninvasive positive pressure ventilation	(1) Ventilation without an artificial airway (2) May be used as CPAP or bilevel PAP
CPAP	Continuous positive airway pressure	(1) Positive airway pressure during spontaneous breaths (2) No mechanical breaths (3) CPAP is active when IPAP = EPAP
Bilevel PAP	Bilevel positive airway pressure	(1) Provides IPAP and EPAP (2) CPAP is active when IPAP = EPAP (3) Also known as BiPAP
IPAP	Inspiratory positive airway pressure	(1) Controls peak airway pressure during inspiration
EPAP	Expiratory positive airway pressure	(1) Controls end-expiratory pressure (2) Used as CPAP when IPAP = EPAP (3) Used as PEEP when IPAP > EPAP
PEEP	Positive end-expiratory pressure	(1) Positive airway pressure at end-expiratory phase (2) With mechanical breaths

expiratory positive airway pressure (EPAP): level of airway pressure during expiratory phase only.

(ventilation) device. The IPAP level is similar to the peak airway pressure in traditional mechanical ventilation. In general, the degree of ventilation is directly related to the IPAP level. A higher IPAP level would result in a larger tidal volume and minute ventilation. The **expiratory positive airway pressure (EPAP)** is the same as PEEP during mechanical ventilation or CPAP during spontaneous breathing. In addition to its ability to improve oxygenation by increasing the functional residual capacity, EPAP also relieves upper airway obstruction with its splinting action.

☑ PaO_2, $PaCO_2$, SpO_2, and $P_{ET}CO_2$ may be used for titration of IPAP and EPAP.

The level of IPAP and EPAP can be titrated according to a patient's oxygenation and ventilation needs. Since two benefits of NPPV are improvement of PO_2 and PCO_2, (Brown, Meecham Jones & Mikelsons et al., 1998; Nicholson, Tiep & Jones et al., 1998), these two parameters can be used as titration endpoints. If arterial blood gas results are available, oxygenation (PaO_2) and ventilation ($PaCO_2$) endpoints can be easily assessed. Alternatively, pulse oximetry (SpO_2) and capnography ($P_{ET}CO_2$) may be used for the titration of appropriate IPAP and EPAP levels.

USE OF CONTINUOUS POSITIVE AIRWAY PRESSURE (CPAP)

continuous positive airway pressure (CPAP): CPAP does not include any mechanical breaths.

Continuous positive airway pressure (CPAP) provides positive airway pressure during the entire spontaneous breath and it does not include any mechanical breaths. For this reason, the work of breathing is entirely assumed by the patient. CPAP is discussed in this chapter because it shares many similar characteristics with other strategies of NPPV (e.g., lack of artificial airway, use of nasal or facial mask, use of airway pressures). In fact, when the inspiratory pressure and expiratory pressure of a bilevel positive airway pressure device are set at the same level, the effect is similar to that of CPAP.

☑ CPAP is the treatment of choice for obstructive sleep apnea without significant CO_2 retention.

CPAP is the treatment of choice for obstructive sleep apnea without significant carbon dioxide retention (Henderson & Strollo, 1999; Rosenthal, Nykamp & Guido et al., 1998). CPAP should be used with care and close monitoring of the patient as it is not effective in apnea due to neuromuscular causes. Table 7-2 outlines the indication and contraindications for CPAP therapy.

OBSTRUCTIVE SLEEP APNEA

Sleep apnea is defined as a temporary pause in breathing that lasts at least 10 seconds during sleep (Wilkins & Dexter, 1998). Sleep apnea may be caused by air flow obstruction (obstructive sleep apnea), loss

TABLE 7-2   Indication and Contraindications for Continuous Positive Airway Pressure

INDICATION	CONTRAINDICATION
Obstructive sleep apnea	Apnea due to neuromuscular causes
	Progressive hypoventilation
	Fatigue of respiratory muscles
	Facial trauma
	Claustrophobia

obstructive sleep apnea (OSA): OSA is caused by severe air flow obstruction during sleep.

of neurological breathing effort (central sleep apnea), or a combination of these two conditions (mixed sleep apnea). **Obstructive sleep apnea (OSA)** is diagnosed by nocturnal polysomnography and the severity is determined by the apnea and desaturation index (Arai, Furuta & Kosaka et al., 1998; Redline & Strohl, 1998; Waite, 1998). Approximately 40 million Americans have chronic sleep disorders and the number of persons affected by OSA ranges from 2% to 4% of middle-aged adults. The distribution between genders is 4% to 9% in men and 1% to 2% in women. The incidence of OSA among morbidly obese patients is 12 to 30 times higher (Kyzer & Chaaruzi, 1998; Piccirillo, Gates & White et al., 1998; Skomro & Kryger, 1999).

Risk factors for OSA include history of snoring and witnessed apneas, obesity, increased neck circumference, hypertension, and family history of OSA (Skomro & Kryger, 1999). In patients with OSA, the major clinical signs and symptoms are snoring, daytime sleepiness, restless sleep, morning fatigue, and headaches. If untreated, OSA can lead to hypertension, left and right ventricular hypertrophy, sudden cardiovascular death, and increased risk for brain infarction (Kyzer & Charuzi, 1998).

Treatments for OSA include oral applications such as prosthetic mandibular advancement (Ishida, Inoue & Suto et al., 1998; Millman, Rosenberg & Kramer, 1998), surgical interventions such as tonsillectomy and uvulopalatopharyngoplasty for upper obstructions (Miyazaki, Itasaka & Tada et al., 1998; Powell, Riley & Robinson, 1998), and weight reduction gastric surgery for morbidly obese patients (Kyzer & Charuzi, 1998). Conservative therapies such as weight loss and patient positioning have been disappointing. CPAP has become the treatment of choice for the vast majority of patients with moderate to severe OSA (Henderson & Strollo, 1999; Rosenthal, Nykamp & Guido et al., 1998; Wilkins & Dexter, 1998). The procedure to titrate CPAP level is discussed later in this chapter.

USE OF BILEVEL POSITIVE AIRWAY PRESSURE (BILEVEL PAP)

bilevel positive airway pressure (bilevel PAP): Bilevel PAP has two pressure levels, whereas CPAP has only one.

positive end-expiratory pressure: An airway pressure that is above 0 cm H₂O at end-expiration.

☑ Two indications for bilevel PAP are acute respiratory failure and acute hypercapnic exacerbations of COPD.

Bilevel positive airway pressure (Bilevel PAP) differs from CPAP in that Bilevel PAP has two pressure levels, whereas CPAP has only one. Bilevel PAP has an inspiratory positive airway pressure (IPAP) setting that provides mechanical breaths and an expiratory positive airway pressure (EPAP) level that functions as **positive end-expiratory pressure (PEEP)**. When Bilevel PAP is used as an adjunct to provide mechanical ventilation, the two major indications are acute respiratory failure (Abou-Shala & Meduri, 1996; Jasmer, Luce & Matthay, 1997; Keenan, Kernerman & Cook et al., 1997; Kramer, Myer & Meharg et al., 1995; Wysocki, Tric & Wolff et al., 1995) and acute hypercapnic exacerbations of COPD (Diaz, Iglesia & Ferrer et al., 1997; Girault, Richard & Chevron et al., 1997). The most common criteria for the determination of acute respiratory failure are blood gas results. Typical results may show partially compensated respiratory acidosis with moderate hypoxemia (e.g., pH < 7.35, $PaCO_2$ > 50 mm Hg, PO_2 < 55 mm Hg). For patients with hypoxemic respiratory failure, refractory hypoxemia may be present in addition to increasing PCO_2. PaO_2/F_IO_2 ratio of less than 200 suggests presence of refractory hypoxemia (low PaO_2 at high F_IO_2).

Patients who are unable to use or tolerate a nasal or facial mask are not candidates for NPPV (CPAP or bilevel PAP). These patients include those with facial trauma and claustrophobia. Inability to handle secretions is also a contraindication for NPPV. NPPV should not be used in apneic patients. For apneic patients, traditional mechanical ventilation is indicated. Furthermore, patients who have acute respiratory distress requiring hospital admission should not be treated with NPPV, as this strategy may delay endotracheal intubation and initiation of mechanical ventilation and may lead to poor patient outcome (Wood, Lewis & Von Harz, et al., 1998). Table 7-3 outlines the common indications and contraindications for NPPV.

TABLE 7-3 Indications and Contraindications for Noninvasive Positive Pressure Ventilation

INDICATION	CONTRAINDICATION
Reduction of respiratory workload in obesity	Apnea
Acute respiratory failure	Unable to handle secretions
Acute hypercapnic exacerbations of COPD	Facial trauma Claustrophobia

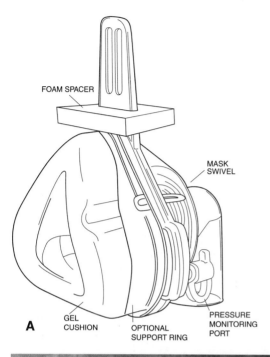

FOAM SPACER

MASK
SWIVEL

GEL
CUSHION

OPTIONAL
SUPPORT
RING

PRESSURE
MONITORING
PORT

A

Figure 7-1 (A) Structure of a nasal mask. (B) Nasal mask in use. (Courtesy of Respironics, Inc., Pittsburgh, Pa.)

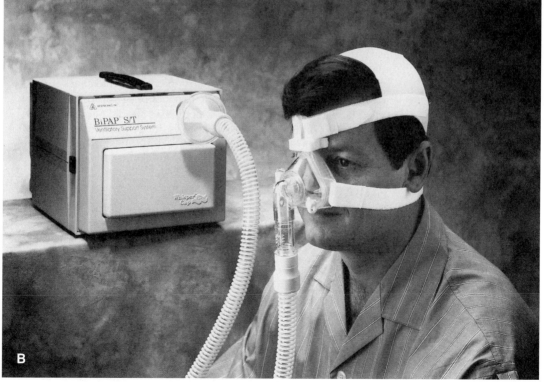

B

COMMON INTERFACES FOR CPAP AND BILEVEL PAP

☑ Nasal mask, facial mask, and nasal pillows are interfaces for NPPV.

Since CPAP or NPPV is done without an artificial airway, the interface between the patient and ventilator is typically an external device connecting the ventilator tubing to the patient's nose, mouth, or face. Some common NPPV devices are nasal mask, facial mask, and nasal pillows.

NASAL MASK

nasal mask: A mask that covers only the nose. It is used in noninvasive positive pressure ventilation.

The **nasal mask** is the most common interface used in NPPV. A typical nasal mask has a soft cushion that surrounds and makes contact with the patient's nasal area. The soft cushion provides comfort to the patient while maintaining a seal to keep gas from leaking. While a tight seal is desirable, a minor leak is acceptable as it is not likely to compromise the effectiveness of NPPV. A common error is selecting a nasal mask that is too large for the patient. There are many nasal masks available. For patient comfort and compliance, it is a good practice to let the patient try out different sizes for maximal comfort and minimal leakage. Figure 7-1 shows the structure of a typical nasal mask and when it is in use.

☑ A minor leak is acceptable when using a nasal mask. A facial mask should be considered when the leak is significant.

Since a nasal mask does not cover the mouth, leakage through the mouth is a common problem. This is particularly true when PPV is provided at high positive pressures. A minor leak is acceptable as long as ventilation and oxygenation are not hindered. However, a facial mask should be considered when the leak is significant. During initial set up of a nasal mask, pulse oximetry may be used to check for improvement in oxygenation and adequacy of oxygen saturation. Soon after stabilization of the patient, blood gases should be done to fine tune settings on the ventilator so as to verify proper oxygenation, ventilation, and acid-base balance. Table 7-4 shows the advantages and disadvantages of the nasal mask.

FACIAL MASK

facial mask: A mask that covers the nose and mouth. It is used in noninvasive positive pressure ventilation.

The function of a **facial mask** (Figure 7-2) is essentially the same as a nasal mask. It has a soft cushion that surrounds and makes contact with the patient's nasal and oral area. As does the nasal mask, the soft

TABLE 7-4 **Advantages and Disadvantages of the Nasal Mask**

ADVANTAGE	DISADVANTAGE
Comfort	Gas leaks
Patient compliance	Nasal dryness or drainage

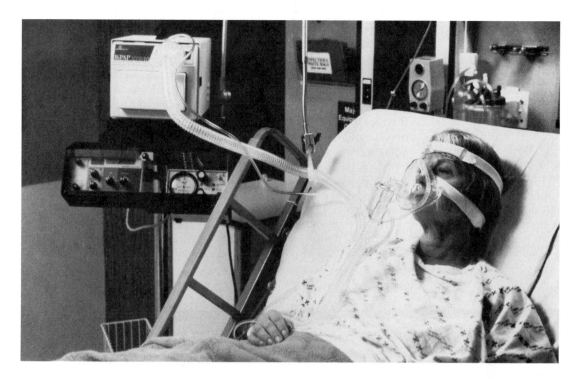

Figure 7-2   A facial mask in use. (Courtesy of Respironics, Inc., Pittsburgh, Pa.)

☑ Regurgitation and aspiration can be a potential problem when a facial mask is used.

☑ With a facial mask, asphyxiation can also be a problem in the event of ventilator failure, or electrical or gas source disconnection.

cushion provides comfort to the patient while maintaining a seal to keep gas from leaking. With a facial mask, a tight seal is easier to maintain than with a nasal mask because both the nose and mouth are covered. However, because the mouth is covered, regurgitation and aspiration can be potential problems with the use of a facial mask. Asphyxiation can also occur in the event of ventilator failure, or electrical or gas source disconnection. Proper disconnection alarms and patient monitors must be functional during use of NPPV via a facial mask. Table 7-5 shows the advantages and disadvantages of the facial mask.

TABLE 7-5   Advantages and Disadvantages of the Facial Mask

ADVANTAGE	DISADVANTAGE
Good seal	Claustrophobia
	Patient noncompliance
	Regurgitation and aspiration
	Asphyxiation in power or gas outage
	Alarm and monitor may be necessary

NASAL PILLOWS™

Nasal pillows™ resemble nasal masks but are smaller. Nasal pillows are more commonly used during continuous positive airway pressure (CPAP) therapy. This interface consists of two small cushions that fit under the nose. Since it has a pressure range of 3 to 20 cm H$_2$O, nasal pillows are not as effective as the larger nasal and facial masks when they are used in the bilevel PAP mode. Figure 7-3 shows the structure of nasal pillows and Figure 7-4 shows the insertion, placement, and adjustment of this interface.

Nasal Pillows™ are more comfortable than facial masks but gas leak is a potential problem. If significant gas leaks occur through the mouth, a chin strap may be used to close the mouth or a facial mask should be considered.

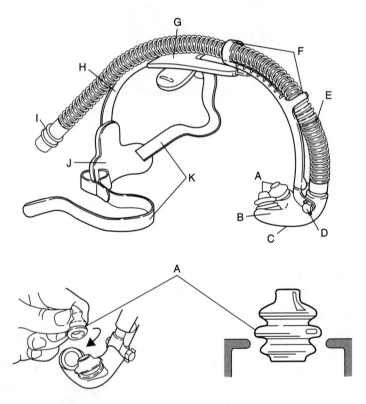

Figure 7-3 Structure of a nasal pillows interface. (a) Nasal Pillows™; (b) plenum shell; (c) vent-hole insert; (d) wing knob (to adjust the angle of plenum shell); (e) hose; (f) hose guide; (g) outrigger; (h) spine; (i) swivel adapter; (j) cradle; (k) side straps. (Reprinted by permission of Mallinckrodt, Inc., Pleasanton, Calif.)

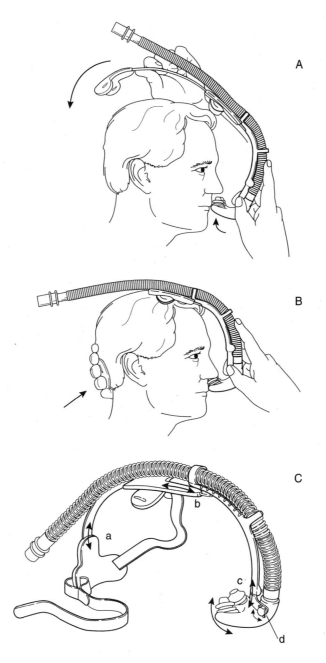

Figure 7-4 Use of a nasal pillows interface. (A) Insert the Nasal Pillows™ into nostrils; (B) Place the cradle (back pad) below the curve at the back of head; (C) For a comfortable fit, adjust the following points: (a) height of the cradle; (b) length of unit; (c) height of plenum shell; (d) angle of plenum shell. (Reprinted by permission of Mallinckrodt, Inc., Pleasanton, Calif.)

POTENTIAL PROBLEMS WITH INTERFACES

Since patients are different in size and facial structure, the selection of an interface must be done on an individual basis. Following selection of an interface, a trial period usually is required for the patient to get used to the interface and to identify problems with it. Table 7-6 outlines the potential problems with CPAP/NPPV interface and the possible solutions.

TABLE 7-6 Troubleshooting Potential Problems with Interfaces

POTENTIAL PROBLEM	SUGGESTED SOLUTIONS
Air leaks	Adjust headgear
	Try chin strap
	Try spacers or foam pads
	Try another size or a different mask
Pressure points	Adjust headgear
	Change spacers or foam pads
	Try another size or a different mask
Nasal congestion/discharge	Adjust positive pressure setting
	Add filter
	Add humidity
Nasal airway drying	Increase fluid intake
	Try nasal saline or water-based lubricant
Skin breakdown/irritation	Adjust or try another headgear
	Use spacers, foam pads, or topical ointments
	Try another size or a different mask
	Resize mask
	Change to a different cleaning solution
Sensitive front teeth	Adjust headgear
	Try smaller or different mask
Headgear problem	Try disposable headgear with more stretch
	Try different or larger headgear

(Modified from An interface for every face, from Mallinckrodt, Inc. Used with permission.)

inspiratory positive airway pressure:
An airway pressure that is above 0 cm H_2O during inspiration.

expiratory positive airway pressure:
An airway pressure that is above 0 cm H_2O at end-expiration.

☑ The initial CPAP is started at 4 cm H_2O, and titrated to a desired endpoint.

☑ The initial bilevel positive airway pressures are started at 8 cm H_2O (inspiratory) and 4 cm H_2O (expiratory) and titrated to a desired endpoint.

TITRATION OF CONTINUOUS POSITIVE AIRWAY PRESSURE

When positive airway pressure is used to treat or relieve OSA, the appropriate CPAP level is done by setting the **inspiratory positive airway pressure (IPAP)** and **expiratory positive airway pressure (EPAP)** at the same level, initially at 4 cm H_2O. After setting up the machine and placing the interface on the patient, pulse oximetry readings and number of apnea episodes during polysomnography are used to fine tune the CPAP level.

TITRATION OF BILEVEL POSITIVE AIRWAY PRESSURES

When positive airway pressure is used to treat acute respiratory failure, the IPAP and EPAP levels are set independently. Bilevel refers to the inspiratory and expiratory positive airway pressure settings. For example, a bilevel positive airway pressure setting of 8 and 4 means that the IPAP is 8 cm H_2O and the EPAP is 4 cm H_2O. The procedure for titration of IPAP and EPAP (ResMed Corp., 1998a) is outlined in Table 7-7.

TABLE 7-7   Procedure to Titrate Bilevel Positive Airway Pressure

1. Set mode: spontaneous/timed.
2. Start the IPAP at 8 cm H_2O and the EPAP at 4 cm H_2O.
3. Set IPAP maximum time 0.15 to 0.25 sec. longer than the patient's actual inspiratory time. IPAP maximum time should not be set longer than 50% of the respiratory cycle.
4. Attach mask to patient, ensure proper fit, and start machine.
5. Increase IPAP in 1 to 2 cm H_2O increments to provide more ventilatory assistance and larger tidal volume.
6. Increase EPAP in 1 to 2 cm H_2O increments to improve oxygenation or to relieve upper airway obstruction.
7. If poor synchronization occurs, check for leaks or alter IPAP maximum time to improve synchronization.
8. Use supplemental oxygen if baseline saturation remains low with appropriate IPAP and EPAP settings.
9. Do not increase IPAP or EPAP level beyond patient tolerance.

(*Modified from* ResMed VPAP II S/T Clinical Guide.)

SUMMARY

Noninvasive strategies of assisted breathing have been used successfully in providing suffi-cient ventilation and oxygenation to patients with obstructive sleep apnea (CPAP), acute ven-tilatory failure and impending ventilatory failure (bilevel positive airway pressure). The two advantages of NPPV are (1) an artificial airway is not necessary, (2) reduced risks associated with endotracheal intubation and traditional mechanical ventilation.

As with other noninvasive procedures applied to a potentially critical condition, close monitoring of the patient is an absolute requirement. Use of accessory muscles, changes in vital signs, and signs of hypoxia are some indications that the patient's condition is deteriorating. The patient must be assessed in a timely manner. If indicated, the patient should be intubated and mechanically ventilated if NPPV fails to stabilize or improve the patient's condition.

Self-Assessment Questions

1. Which of the following is *not* true in regard to noninvasive positive pressure ventilation (NPPV)?

   A. NPPV provides assisted ventilation with an artificial airway.
   B. NPPV can provide positive end-expiratory pressure (PEEP).

   C. NPPV may be used to assist patients with obstructive sleep apnea.
   D. NPPV may be used to assist patients with acute ventilatory failure.

2. The titration endpoints of IPAP and EPAP during bilevel PAP may include all of the following measurements *except*:

   A. SpO_2
   B. PaO_2

   C. PvO_2
   D. $P_{ET}CO_2$

3. Continuous positive airway pressure (CPAP) provides positive airway pressure during the _____ spontaneous breath, and it _____ mechanical breaths.

   A. entire, includes
   B. entire, does not include

   C. inspiratory phase of, includes
   D. inspiratory phase of, does not include

4. When CPAP is in use, the total amount of work of breathing is provided by the:

   A. patient
   B. ventilator

   C. patient and ventilator
   D. pressure level of CPAP

5. CPAP is the treatment of choice for _____ sleep apnea without significant _____.

   A. central, hypoxemia
   B. central, carbon dioxide retention

   C. obstructive, hypoxemia
   D. obstructive, carbon dioxide retention

6. All of the following clinical conditions are contraindications for CPAP *except*:

   A. fatigue of respiratory muscles.
   B. progressive hypercapnia.

   C. obesity.
   D. hypoventilation due to neuro-
      muscular causes.

7. Sleep apnea is defined as a temporary pause in breathing that lasts at least _____ during sleep

   A. 5 seconds
   B. 10 seconds

   C. 30 seconds
   D. 60 seconds

8. During NPPV, mechanical breaths are provided by the _____ setting whereas the end-expiratory pressure is determined by the _____ setting.

   A. IPAP, EPAP
   B. EPAP, IPAP

   C. PEEP, IPAP
   D. PEEP, EPAP

9. The interfaces for NPPV include all of the following devices *except*:

   A. nasal mask
   B. endotracheal tube

   C. nasal pillows
   D. facial mask

10. Which of the following interfaces is *least* likely to develop a significant air leak during NPPV?

    A. nasal mask
    B. simple mask

    C. nasal pillows
    D. facial mask

11. The facial mask is the only NPPV interface that has all of the following inherited risks *except*:

    A. aspiration
    B. asphyxiation

    C. regurgitation
    D. hyperventilation

12. The initial CPAP level is started at _____ cm H_2O and titrated to a desired endpoint.

    A. 2
    B. 4

    C. 6
    D. 8

13. The initial bilevel positive airway pressures are started at _____ cm H_2O (inspiratory) and _____ cm H_2O (expiratory) and subsequently titrated to a desired endpoint.

   A. 2, 6
   B. 4, 8

   C. 6, 2
   D. 8, 4

14. During titration of bilevel positive airway pressure, the _____ is increased in 1 to 2 cm H_2O increments to provide more ventilatory assistance and larger tidal volume.

   A. PEEP
   B. CPAP

   C. IPAP
   D. EPAP

15. During titration of bilevel positive airway pressure, the _____ is increased in 1 to 2 cm H_2O increments to improve oxygenation or to relieve upper airway obstruction.

   A. IPAP
   B. EPAP

   C. peak airway pressure
   D. plateau pressure

References

Abou-Shala, N., & Meduri, G. U. (1996). Noninvasive mechanical ventilation in patients with acute respiratory failure. *Crit Care Med, 24*(4), 705–715.

Antonelli, M., Conti, G., & Rocco, M. et al. (1998). A comparison of noninvasive positive-pressure ventilation and conventional mechanical ventilation in patients with acute respiratory failure. *N Engl J Med, 339*(7):429–435.

Arai, H, Furuta, H., & Kosaka, K. et al. (1998). Changes in work performances in obstructive sleep apnea patients after dental appliance therapy. *Psychiatry Clin Neurosci, 52*(2):224–225.

Brown, J. S., Meecham Jones, D. J., & Mikelsons, C. et al. (1998). Using nasal intermittent positive pressure ventilation on a general respiratory ward. *J R Coll Physicians Lond, 32*(3):219–224.

Diaz, O., Iglesia, R., & Ferrer, M. et al. (1997). Effects of noninvasive ventilation on pulmonary gas exchange and hemodynamics during acute hypercapnic exacerbations of chronic obstructive pulmonary disease. *Am J Respir Crit Care Med, 156*, 1840–1845.

Girault, C., Richard, J. C., & Chevron, V. et al. (1997) Comparative physiologic effects of non-invasive assist-control and pressure support ventilation in acute hypercapnic respiratory failure. *Chest, 111*(6), 1639–1648.

Guilleminault, C., Philip, P., & Robinson, A. (1998). Sleep and neuromuscular disease: Bilevel positive airway pressure by nasal mask as a treatment for sleep disordered breathing in patients with neuromuscular disease. *J Neurol Neurosurg Psychiatry, 65*(2):225–232.

Henderson, J. H., & Strollo, P. J. Jr. (1999). Medical management of obstructive sleep apnea. *Prog Cardiovasc Dis, 41*(5):377–386.

Ishida, M., Inoue, Y., & Suto, Y. et al. (1998). Mechanism of action and therapeutic indication of prosthetic mandibular advancement in obstructive sleep apnea syndrome. *Psychiatry Clin Neurosci, 52*(2):227–229.

Jasmer, R. M., Luce, J. M., & Matthay, M. A. (1997). Noninvasive positive pressure ventilation for acute respiratory failure—underutilized or overrated? *Chest, 111*(6), 1672–1678.

Keenan, S. P., Kernerman, P. D., & Cook, D. J. et al. (1997). Effects of noninvasive positive pressure ventilation on mortality in patients admitted with acute respiratory failure: A meta-analysis. *Crit Care Med, 25*(10), 1685–1692.

Kramer, N., Myer, T. J., & Meharg, J. et al. (1995). Randomized, prospective trial of non-invasive positive pressure ventilation in acute respiratory failure. *Am J Respir Crit Care Med, 151*, 1799–1806.

Kyzer, S., & Charuzi, I. (1998). Obstructive sleep apnea in the obese. *World J Surg, 22*(9):998–1001.

Millman, R. P., Rosenberg, C. L., & Kramer, N. R. (1998). Oral appliances in the treatment of snoring and sleep apnea. *Clin Chest Med, 19*(1):69–75.

Miyazaki, S., Itasaka, Y., & Tada, H. et al. (1998). Effectiveness of tonsillectomy in adult sleep apnea syndrome. *Psychiatry Clin Neurosci, 52*(2):222–223.

Nicholson, D., Tiep, B., & Jones, R. et al. (1998). Noninvasive positive-pressure ventilation in chronic obstructive pulmonary disease. *Curr Opin Pulm Med, 4*(2):66–75.

Pankow, W., Hijjeh, N., Schuttler, F. et al. (1997). Influence of noninvasive positive pressure ventilation on inspiratory muscle activity in obese subjects. *Eur Respir J, 10*(12):2847–2852.

Piccirillo, J. F., Gates, G. A., & White, D. L. et al. (1998). Obstructive sleep apnea treatment outcomes pilot study. *Otolaryngol Head Neck Surg, 118*(6):833–844.

Powell, N. B., Riley, R. W., Robinson, A. (1998). Surgical management of obstructive sleep apnea syndrome. *Clin Chest Med, 19*(1):77–86.

Redline, S. & Strohl, K. P. (1998). Recognition and consequences of obstructive sleep apnea hypopnea syndrome. *Clin Chest Med, 19*(1):1–19.

ResMed Corp. (1998a). *ResMed VPAP II S/T Clinical Guide*, North Ryde, Australia.

ResMed Corp. (1998b). *ResMed VPAP II S/T Clinical Manual*, North Ryde, Australia.

Rosenthal, L., Nykamp, K., & Guido, P. et al. (1998). Daytime CPAP titration: A viable alternative for patients with severe obstructive sleep apnea. *Chest, 114*(4):1056–1060.

Skomro, R. P., & Kryger, M. H. (1999). Clinical presentations of obstructive sleep apnea syndrome. *Prog Cardiovasc Dis, 41*(5):331–340.

Waite, P. D. (1998). Obstructive sleep apnea: A review of the pathophysiology and surgical management. *Oral Surg Oral Med Oral Pathol Oral Radiol Endod, 85*(4):352–361.

Wilkins, R. L., & Dexter, J. R. (1998). *Respiratory Disease A Case Study Approach to Patient Care* (2nd ed.). Philadelphia: F.A. Davis Company.

Wood, K. A., Lewis, L., & Von Harz, B. et al. (1998). The use of noninvasive positive pressure ventilation in the emergency department: Results of a randomized clinical trial. *Chest, 113*(5):1339–1346.

Wysocki, M., Tric, L., & Wolff, M.A. et al. (1995). Noninvasive pressure support ventilation in patients with acute respiratory failure. *Chest, 107*(3), 761–768.

CHAPTER EIGHT

INITIATION OF MECHANICAL VENTILATION

James H. Hiers

OUTLINE

KEY TERMS

- acute ventilatory failure
- alveolar-arterial oxygen pressure gradient [P(A–a)O_2]
- circuit compressible volume
- flow rate

- I:E ratio
- impending ventilatory failure
- maximum inspiratory pressure (MIP)
- medical futility
- prophylactic ventilatory support

INTRODUCTION

This chapter covers the indications, contraindications, and strategies for the initiation of mechanical ventilation. Once a decision is made to implement mechanical ventilation, the initial settings on the ventilator must be made using a systematic approach. It is important to realize that these initial settings are subject to change according to patient condition. Frequent intensive monitoring of the patient is necessary to use the ventilator properly and to improve the patient outcome.

INDICATIONS

acute ventilatory failure: An increase of $PaCO_2$ (> 50 mm Hg) with a concurrent decrease of arterial pH (< 7.30).

impending ventilatory failure: A gradual increase of $PaCO_2$ (> 50 mm Hg) caused by decreasing lung functions.

prophylactic ventilatory support: Early intervention of potential ventilatory failure by means of mechanical ventilation.

Mechanical ventilation is indicated when the patient cannot maintain spontaneous ventilation to provide adequate oxygenation or carbon dioxide removal. The clinical conditions leading to mechanical ventilation can be grouped into four areas: (1) **acute ventilatory failure;** (2) **impending ventilatory failure;** (3) severe hypoxemia; and (4) **prophylactic ventilatory support** (Brown, 1994; Otto, 1986). Table 8-1 outlines the indications of mechanical ventilation.

ACUTE VENTILATORY FAILURE

The primary indication of mechanical ventilation is acute ventilatory failure. This is defined as a sudden increase in the $PaCO_2$ to greater than 50 mm Hg with an accompanying respiratory acidosis (pH < 7.30). In the COPD patient, mechanical ventilatory support is indicated by an acute increase in the $PaCO_2$ above the patient's normal baseline $PaCO_2$ accompanied by a decompensating respiratory acidosis (Brown, 1994; Otto, 1986).

Other signs that may be useful in the assessment of acute ventilatory failure include apnea and severe cyanosis. However, mild to moderate hypoxemia (PaO_2 = 50 to 60 mm Hg or SaO_2 = 85 to 90%) does not by itself indicate the presence of acute ventilatory failure or the need for ventilatory support. If a hypoxemic patient is able to

TABLE 8-1   Indications for Mechanical Ventilation

INDICATION	EXAMPLES
1. Acute ventilatory failure	pH < 7.30, $PaCO_2$ > 50 mm Hg
2. Impending ventilatory failure	Progressive acidosis and hypoventilation to pH < 7.30 and $PaCO_2$ > 50 mm Hg
3. Severe hypoxemia	PaO_2 < 40 mm Hg, SaO_2 < 75%
4. Prophylactic ventilatory support	Postanesthesia recovery

☑ Mechanical ventilation is indicated when the patient cannot maintain spontaneous ventilation to provide adequate oxygenation or carbon dioxide removal.

☑ Acute ventilatory failure is defined as a sudden increase in the $PaCO_2$ to greater than 50 mm Hg with an accompanying respiratory acidosis (pH < 7.30).

☑ Assessment of impending ventilatory failure relies on the measurements related to the lung functions (i.e., V_T, RR, V_E, VC, MIP).

maintain adequate ventilation as documented by the $PaCO_2$, then the patient may be supported with supplemental oxygen or continuous positive airway pressure (CPAP). Table 8-2 shows some common methods to assess the presence of acute ventilatory failure.

IMPENDING VENTILATORY FAILURE

Impending ventilatory failure occurs when a patient can maintain or marginally normal blood gases, but only at the expense of a significantly increased work of breathing. Depending on the pulmonary reserve and lung function of a patient, the $PaCO_2$ value may be normal or low at the beginning of impending ventilatory failure. This is because of an increase in minute ventilation in an attempt to compensate for the gas exchange deficiencies. However, if the underlying pathology is not corrected in time, ventilatory failure will ensue when muscle fatigue occurs as a result of prolonged, excessive work of breathing. At this time, the $PaCO_2$ will rise and the pH will fall.

If the early clinical signs indicate that a patient is in impending ventilatory failure, it is appropriate to initiate mechanical ventilation. Early intervention is done to correct hypoxemia and acidosis imposed on the major organs and to reduce the stress placed on the cardiopulmonary system. There are several objective measurements that can be used to determine whether the patient is in impending ventilatory failure. These measurements are discussed below.

Assessment of Impending Ventilatory Failure.   Development of impending ventilatory failure is dependent on the balance of

TABLE 8-2   Assessment of Acute Ventilatory Failure in Non-COPD Patient

PARAMETER	LIMIT
$PaCO_2$	> 50 mm Hg (higher for COPD patients)
pH	< 7.30

metabolic needs and work of breathing. When metabolic needs cause excessive work of breathing, impending ventilatory failure is likely. Since the work of breathing is carried out entirely by the respiratory system, assessment of impending ventilatory failure relies solely on the measurements related to the lung functions (i.e., tidal volume, respiratory rate, minute volume, vital capacity, and maximal inspiratory pressure). Table 8-3 shows the factors for the assessment of impending ventilatory failure.

Tidal volume. A spontaneous tidal volume of less than 3 to 5 ml/kg is indicative of impending ventilatory failure.

Respiratory rate. A spontaneous respiratory rate of greater than 25 to 35 breaths per minute signifies impending ventilatory failure.

Minute volume. If the patient's spontaneous minute volume is greater than 10 liters/min, then impending ventilatory failure is likely. Although it may appear that an increasing minute volume is a sign of improving lung functions, in actuality the patient may not be able to sustain the increased work of breathing. Muscle fatigue can occur over time and lead to eventual ventilatory failure. In addition, an increase in minute volume achieved by an increased respiratory rate and a decreased tidal volume lead to a larger percentage of deadspace (wasted) ventilation. This condition increases the oxygen cost of breathing and carbon dioxide production, progressive hypercapnia, and hypoxemia.

Vital capacity. If the patient's vital capacity is less than 15 ml/kg, then impending ventilatory failure is likely. An accurate measurement of vital capacity requires patient cooperation, which may be difficult to achieve during impending ventilatory failure. The maximum inspiratory pressure measurement can be used as its alternative if the patient is unable to perform the vital capacity maneuver.

Maximum Inspiratory Pressure. The **maximum inspiratory pressure (MIP)** is a measure of the inspiratory muscle strength reflecting the patient's pulmonary reserves. Patients with an MIP of better than

maximum inspiratory pressure (MIP): *Also called negative inspiratory force (NIF). MIP reflects a patient's respiratory muscle strength. MIP of less than -20 cm H_2O (e.g., –10 cm H_2O) is one of the indications of impending ventilatory failure. It is obtained by measuring the maximum negative pressure during a forced inspiratory maneuver against a closed manometer.*

TABLE 8-3   **Assessment of Impending Ventilatory Failure**

PARAMETER	LIMIT
Tidal volume	< 3 to 5 ml/kg
Respiratory rate and pattern	> 25 to 35/min Labored or irregular respiratory pattern
Minute ventilation	> 10 l/min
Vital capacity	< 15 ml/kg
Maximum inspiratory pressure (MIP)	< –20 cm H_2O
PaCO$_2$ trend	Increasing to over 50 mm Hg
Vital signs	Increase in heart rate, blood pressure

−25 cm H_2O obtained within 20 seconds can be assumed to have a vital capacity of 15 ml/kg (Shapiro et al., 1991). When MIP is less than −20 cm H_2O, it is one of the signs of impending ventilatory failure.

The MIP is obtained by measuring the maximum negative pressure that the patient can generate with a forced *inspiratory* maneuver against a negative manometer (pressure measuring device). Although the MIP maneuver can be performed using a face mask, it is easier to obtain with an endotracheal or tracheostomy tube.

MIP can be measured by using a T-piece with one port attached to the endotracheal or tracheostomy tube, one port attached to the negative pressure manometer, and one port attached to a special unidirectional valve that allows exhalation only. The patient is encouraged to exhale to residual volume and then inhale as forcefully as possible. The unidirectional valve allows the patient to exhale so that the subsequent MIP maneuvers can be performed from the residual volume level (Caruso, 1999).

PaCO_2 trend. A gradual but persistent increase of the $PaCO_2$ to more than 50 mm Hg is indicative of impending ventilatory failure. The $PaCO_2$ measurements should be done over a period of time and on an as needed basis. The $PaCO_2$ should be interpreted along with the patient's breathing pattern since progressive tachypnea is common during impending ventilatory failure.

Vital signs. Any clinical indicators that show a patient is under distress or is tiring must also be considered when asssessing impending ventilatory failure. These indicators include tachycardia, arrhythmias, hypertension, tachypnea, use of accessory respiratory muscles, diaphoresis, and cyanosis.

SEVERE HYPOXEMIA

Hypoxemia is a common finding of lung diseases. When hypoxemia is severe, mechanical ventilation may be necessary to support the oxygenation requirement of the body. ARDS, pulmonary edema, and carbon monoxide poisoning are some clinical conditions that often require ventilatory support for the primary purpose of oxygenation.

Hypoxemia can be assessed by measuring the PaO_2, or the **alveolar-arterial oxygen pressure gradient [P(A-a)O_2]**. Severe hypoxemia is present when the PaO_2 is less than 60 mm Hg on 50% or more of oxygen or less than 40 mm Hg at any F_IO_2 (Shapiro et al., 1994). $P(A-a)O_2$ is the difference of PAO_2 and PaO_2. The normal $P(A-a)O_2$ at 21% F_IO_2 should be less than 4 mm Hg for every 10 years of age. On 100% oxygen, every 50 mm Hg difference in $P(A-a)O_2$ approximates 2% shunt.

$$P(A-a)O_2 = PAO_2 - PaO_2$$

PaO_2 is obtained from arterial blood gas analysis and PAO_2 can be calculated as follows:

Margin notes:

✓ Severe hypoxemia is present when the PaO_2 is less than 60 mm Hg on 50% or more of oxygen or less than 40 mm Hg at any F_IO_2.

alveolar-arterial oxygen pressure gradient [P(A−a)O_2]: *The difference of PAO_2 and PaO_2. A gradient over 450 mm Hg while on 100% oxygen indicates severe hypoxemia or intrapulmonary shunting.*

✓ See Appendix 1 for example.

TABLE 8-4   Indications for Prophylactic Ventilatory Support

INDICATION	EXAMPLES
Reduce risk of pulmonary complications	Prolonged shock Head injury Smoke inhalation
Reduce hypoxia of major body organs	Hypoxic brain Hypoxia of heart muscles
Reduce cardiopulmonary stress	Prolonged shock Coronary artery bypass surgery Other thoracic or abdominal surgeries

☑ $PaCO_2/0.8$ may be changed to $PaCO_2 \times 1.25$

A simplified alveolar air equation:

$PAO_2 = (P_B-PH_2O) \times F_IO_2 - (PaCO_2/R)$, where as P_B = Barometric Pressure, PH_2O = water vapor pressure (47 mm Hg at 37 °C), and R = Respiratory Quotient (estimated to be 0.8). PAO_2 is mainly affected by changes of F_IO_2, $PaCO_2$, and P_B.

☑ Prophylactic ventilatory support is provided in clinical conditions in which the risk of pulmonary complications, ventilatory failure, or oxygenation failure is high.

PROPHYLACTIC VENTILATORY SUPPORT

Prophylactic ventilatory support is provided in clinical conditions in which the risk of pulmonary complications, ventilatory failure, or oxygenation failure is high. In addition, prophylactic or early commitment of patient to the ventilator can minimize hypoxia of the major body organs. It can also reduce the work of breathing and oxygen consumption and thus preserve and rest the cardiopulmonary system, and promote patient recovery (Otto, 1986). Indications for prophylactic ventilatory support are outlined in Table 8-4.

☑ Untreated tension pneumothorax is an absolute contraindication to mechanical ventilation.

CONTRAINDICATIONS

Since positive pressure ventilation is contraindicated in untreated tension pneumothorax, mechanical ventilation at any positive pressure level must not be done without a functional chest tube to relieve the pleural pressure. Other contraindications to mechanical ventilation are relative in nature and deal with the condition and prognosis of the patient.

medical futility: A condition in which medical interventions are useless based on past experience.

There are three considerations in which mechanical ventilation should be terminated or should not be started (Campbell et al., 1992). They are based on (1) patient's informed request; (2) **medical futility;** and (3) reduction or termination of patient pain and suffering.

A patient's informed request carries with it many legal, ethical, medical, and economical concerns. The health care facilities and professionals should be prepared to work with the patient and his family on this type of request. A protocol should be established to serve as a guide before a hasty decision is needed concerning whether ventilatory support should be started or discontinued.

Schneiderman et al. (1990) suggested that medical intervention may be futile if the physicians have concluded that intervention was useless in the last 100 similar cases. It is reasonable to infer that if medical intervention will not be effective in all *probability*, life support measures including mechanical ventilation should not be started. In this case, the physician must establish an open, honest discussion with the patient and the concerned parties about the potential outcomes for withholding ventilatory support.

Another relative contraindication to mechanical ventilation is to reduce or terminate patient pain and suffering. In probable terminal cases such as metastatic cancer and multiorgan failure, the benefit of mechanical ventilation must be weighed against the degree of pain and expected length of suffering that a patient may be subjected to. Physical restraints, painful and uncomfortable medical procedures, and psychological trauma are just a few problems that may not be completely alleviated by sedatives and analgesics (Campbell et al., 1992). Of course, medical futility would be a concurrent concern in dealing with this question.

Withdrawing ventilatory support from a patient poses a greater challenge than withholding mechanical ventilation. But this difficult decision should be based on the fact that mechanical ventilation is a supportive measure, rather than a curative procedure.

I:E ratio: A time ratio comparing the inspiratory time and expiratory time, normally between 1:2 and 1:4 in mechanical ventilation. This ratio is regulated by the inspiratory flow rate, I time, or E time and is affected by the tidal volume and respiratory rate.

✓ Full ventilatory support may be necesssary if the patient is not breathing spontaneously between mechanical breaths.

INITIAL VENTILATOR SETTINGS

When it becomes necessary to provide mechanical ventilatory support for a patient, the following basic ventilator settings must be determined: mode, respiratory rate, tidal volume, F_IO_2, inspiratory:expiratory ratio (**I:E ratio**), inspiratory flow pattern, and various alarm limits.

These initial ventilator settings are mainly based on a patient's body size, diagnosis, pathophysiology, and laboratory results. These settings only serve as a starting point and they should be adjusted according to changes in the patient's condition and requirements.

MODE

The first step in selecting the ventilator mode is to decide whether the patient should receive full ventilatory support (FVS) or partial ventilatory support (PVS). Full ventilatory support is achieved by any mode that assumes essentially all of the work of breathing. The majority of ventilator patients initially require full support, with the control mode or the assist/control mode. The synchronized intermittent mandatory ventilation (SIMV) mode also provides full ventilatory support if the patient is not breathing spontaneously between mechanical breaths, and the mandatory respiratory rate is set at 12 BPM or higher.

✓ Partial ventilatory support is achieved by any mode that provides less than the total amount of the work of breathing.

Partial ventilatory support is achieved by any mode that provides less than the total amount of the work of breathing. Partial support would be inappropriate initially for patients with ventilatory failure, and they are more commonly used during the weaning process. Some examples are bi-level positive airway pressure (BiPAP), and pressure support ventilation (PSV). These topics are discussed elsewhere in this text.

RESPIRATORY RATE

The initial respiratory rate (frequency) is the number of breaths per minute that is intended to provide eucapneic ventilation ($PaCO_2$ at patient's normal). It is usually between 10 to 12 breaths per minute. This rate, coupled with a 10 to 15 ml/kg tidal volume, usually produces a minute volume that is sufficient to normalize the patient's $PaCO_2$. Respiratory rates of 20 or more breaths/min. during pressure support ventilation are associated with *auto-PEEP* and should be avoided (Shapiro et al., 1994).

✓ Air trapping and low inspiratory flow are also contributing factors of *auto-PEEP*.

An alternative method of selecting the initial respiratory rate is to estimate the patient's minute volume requirement and divide the estimated minute volume by the tidal volume.

$$\text{Respiratory rate} = \frac{\text{Estimated minute volume}}{\text{Tidal volume}}$$

The estimated minute volume for males is equal to 4.0 multiplied by the body surface area (BSA) and for females is equal to 3.5 multiplied by the BSA. The BSA (in square meters) can be obtained from a nomogram such as the Dubois body surface area chart (Appendix 2).

Minute volume (male) = (4)(BSA)

Minute volume (female) = (3.5)(BSA)

Changing the Respiratory Rate. Both of these methods of selecting the initial respiratory rate assume that both CO_2 production and physiologic deadspace are normal. If the CO_2 production is elevated (due to an increase of metabolic rate) or the physiologic deadspace is increased (due to a decrease of pulmonary perfusion), the minute volume required to normalize the $PaCO_2$ will need to be increased. Since increasing the tidal volume results in higher airway pressures on a volume-limited ventilator, it is usually more appropriate to increase the minute volume by raising the respiratory rate.

✔️ RR is the primary control to alter the $PaCO_2$.

✔️ ↑ RR if the $PaCO_2$ is too high; ↓ RR if the $PaCO_2$ is too low.

After placing the patient on a ventilator, blood gases should be obtained within 15 to 30 minutes after the patient has stabilized to assess both ventilation and oxygenation. Since the $PaCO_2$ varies inversely with the alveolar minute ventilation, a higher than normal $PaCO_2$ (e.g., > 45 mm Hg or > 50 mm Hg for patients with chronic CO_2 retention) means the patient's minute volume should be increased, usually by increasing the respiratory rate. On the other hand, a lower than normal $PaCO_2$ (e.g., < 35 mm Hg or < 40 mm Hg for patients with CO_2 retention) indicates that the minute volume should be decreased, usually by decreasing the respiratory rate.

TIDAL VOLUME

The initial tidal volume is usually set between 10 to 15 ml/kg of ideal body weight. Usually the patient's actual weight can be used for selecting the tidal volume unless the patient is significantly underweight or overweight. Table 8-5 shows a method to calculate the patient's ideal body weight.

The lower end of the acceptable tidal volume range (i.e., about 10 ml/kg) may be appropriate for certain patients. Tidal volumes as low as 6 ml/kg have been recommended for ARDS patients (Hall et al., 1987). The primary reason for using lower tidal volumes (i.e., permissive hypercapnia) is to minimize the airway pressures and the risk of barotrauma (Feihl et al., 1994).

✔️ Decreasing the tidal volume by 100 to 200 ml in COPD patients reduces the expiratory time requirements and helps to prevent air trapping.

COPD patients may also benefit from a reduced tidal volume setting. These patients have reduced expiratory flow rates due to decreased alveolar elastic recoil. For this reason, a longer expiratory time is needed for complete exhalation. If there is not enough time for complete exhalation, air trapping, V/Q mismatch, hypoxemia, and hypercapnia may result. Decreasing the tidal volume by 100 to 200 ml in COPD patients reduces the expiratory time requirements and helps to prevent air trapping. A higher **flow rate** may also be used to shorten the inspiratory time and lengthen the expiratory time for COPD patients.

flow rate: *Peak flow during the inspiratory phase. It determines how fast the tidal volume is delivered to the patient.*

For patients with a reduction of lung volumes due to lung resection, lower tidal volumes may also become necessary. Table 8-6 lists examples of clinical conditions where lower tidal volume settings may be beneficial or necessary for the patient.

TABLE 8-5   Calculation of Ideal Body Weight

The ideal body weight (IBW) in pounds (lb) and kilograms (kg) can be calculated as follows:

Male IBW in lb = 106 + [6 x (height in inches – 60)]
Female IBW in lb = 105 + [5 x (height in inches – 60)]

Convert the patient's body weight from lbs to kg by dividing lb by 2.2.

TABLE 8-6 Conditions That May Require Lower Tidal Volumes

CONDITION	EXAMPLES
Increase of airway pressure requirement	ARDS Pulmonary edema
Increase of lung compliance	Emphysema
Decrease of lung volumes	Pneumonectomy

circuit compressible volume: Expansion of the ventilator circuits during inspiration leading to a small "lost" volume of gas that does not reach the patient, but is recorded as part of the expired tidal volume.

Gas Leakage and Circuit Compressible Volume. The tidal volume actually delivered to the patient's lungs is usually lower than the ventilator delivered tidal volume. This is mainly due to (1) gas leakage in the ventilator circuitry; (2) gas leakage at the endotracheal tube cuff; and (3) **circuit compressible volume** loss.

When significant gas leakage (>5% of ventilator tidal volume) occurs, the cause must be identified and corrected. Minor gas leakage and circuit compressible volume loss can be compensated by using a larger tidal volume. Some ventilators (e.g., Puritan-Bennett 7200) automatically compensate for the compressible volume loss and thus maintain a stable tidal volume. Other ventilators (e.g., Hamilton Veolar) measure the volume delivered to the patient at the airway opening. This allows detection of significant volume loss due to circuit compression factor or gas leakage.

Ventilator circuits are compliant and expand during a positive pressure breath. The amount of circuit expansion results in a volume that does not reach the patient but is recorded as part of the expired tidal volume. This volume "lost" in the ventilator circuit is called the circuit compressible volume and it may be calculated by following the steps in Table 8-7 (Barnes et al., 1993; Scanlan, 1999).

Once the circuit compressible volume is known, the patient's corrected tidal volume can be calculated by:

☑ See Appendix 1 for example.

Corrected tidal volume = expired tidal volume
– circuit compressible volume

F_IO_2

For patients with severe hypoxemia or abnormal cardiopulmonary functions (e.g., postresuscitation, smoke inhalation, ARDS), the *initial* F_IO_2 may be set at 100%. The F_IO_2 should be evaluated by means of arterial blood gas analyses after stabilization of the patient. It should be adjusted accordingly to maintain a PaO_2 between 80 and 100 mm Hg (lower for patients with chronic CO_2 retention). After stabilization of the patient, the F_IO_2 is best kept below 50% to avoid oxygen-induced lung injuries (Shapiro, 1994).

☑ After stabilization of the patient, the F_IO_2 is best kept below 50% to avoid oxygen-induced lung injuries.

For patients with mild hypoxemia or patients with normal cardiopulmonary functions (e.g., drug overdose, uncomplicated postoperative

TABLE 8-7 Determination of Circuit Compressible Volume

(1) With the circuit warmed to an operating temperature, set the respiratory rate at 10 to 16/min and the tidal volume between 100 to 200 ml with minimal flow rate and maximum high pressure limit.

(2) Completely occlude the patient Y-connection of the ventilator circuit.

(3) Record the expired volume (ml) and the peak inspiratory pressure during Y occlusion (cm H_2O).

(4) Divide the expired volume (ml) by the peak inspiratory pressure during Y occlusion (cm H_2O); this is the circuit compression factor.

(5) Multiply the circuit compression factor (ml/cm H_2O) by the peak inspiratory pressure during mechanical ventilation (cm H_2O), or (peak inspiratory pressure–PEEP) if PEEP is used.

Example:
Expired volume = 150 ml; Peak inspiratory pressure (Y occlusion) = 50 cm H_2O;
Peak inspiratory pressure (mechanical ventilation) = 60 cm H_2O; PEEP = 10 cm H_2O.

Circuit compression factor = 150 ml / 50 cm H_2O = 3 ml/cm H_2O
Circuit compression volume = 3 ml/cm H_2O × (60 − 10) cm H_2O = 3 × 50 = 150 ml

recovery), the initial F_IO_2 may be set at 40% or at the patient's F_IO_2 prior to mechanical ventilation. It must also be evaluated and changed accordingly by means of subsequent blood gas analyses and correlated with pulse oximetry trending.

PEEP

☑ Set the initial PEEP at 5 cm H_2O and make changes based on the patient's blood gas results, F_IO_2 requirement, tolerance of PEEP, and cardiovascular responses.

Positive end-expiratory pressure (PEEP) increases the functional residual capacity and is useful to treat refractory hypoxemia (low PaO_2 not responding to high F_IO_2). The initial PEEP level may be set at 5 cm H_2O. Subsequent changes of PEEP should be based on the patient's blood gas results, F_IO_2 requirement, tolerance of PEEP, and cardiovascular responses.

I:E RATIO

☑ Auto-PEEP is present when the end-expiratory pressure does not return to baseline pressure at the end of expiration.

The I:E ratio is the ratio of inspiratory time to expiratory time. It is usually kept in the range between 1:2 to 1:4. A larger I:E ratio (longer E ratio) may be used on patients needing additional time for exhalation because of the possibility of air trapping and auto-PEEP. Occurrence of air trapping during mechanical ventilation may be checked by occluding the expiratory port of the ventilator circuit at the end of exhalation. Auto-PEEP is present when the end-expiratory pressure does not return to baseline pressure (i.e., 0 cm H_2O or the PEEP level when PEEP is in use) at the end of expiration. This unintended end-expiratory pressure caused by incomplete exhalation is called auto-PEEP.

TABLE 8-8   Effects of Flow Rate on I Time and I:E Ratio

PARAMETER CHANGE	I TIME	E TIME	I:E RATIO
Increase flow rate	Decrease	Increase	Increase
Decrease flow rate	Increase	Decrease	Decrease

Inverse I:E ratios have been used to correct refractory hypoxemia in ARDS patients with very low compliance. But it should not be the initial I:E setting since reverse I:E ratio has its inherent cardiovascular complications. Inverse I:E ratio should be tried only after traditional strategies have failed to improve a patient's ventilation and oxygenation status.

Depending on the features available on the ventilator, the I:E ratio may be altered by manipulating any one or a combination of the following controls: (1) flow rate, (2) inspiratory time, (3) inspiratory time %, (4) respiratory rate, and (5) minute volume (tidal volume and respiratory rate).

Effects of Flow Rate on I:E Ratio.   Adjusting the flow rate is the most common method to change an I:E ratio because the flow rate control is a feature available on almost all ventilators. Table 8-8 shows the effects of a changing flow rate on the I Time and I:E ratio when the V_T and RR are kept unchanged. Note that the I time and I:E ratio are inversely related. A higher I time leads to a lower I:E ratio (Tejeda, Boix & Alvarez et al., 1997).

Other Ventilator Controls That Affect the I:E Ratio.   Besides the flow rate control, other settings available on some ventilators may also alter the I:E ratio. Table 8-9 shows the effect of changing the tidal volume on the I:E ratio, and Table 8-10 shows the effect of changing the RR on the I:E ratio.

TABLE 8-9   Effects of V_T on I:E Ratio

PARAMETER CHANGE	I TIME	E TIME	I:E RATIO
Increase tidal volume	Increase	Decrease	Decrease
Decrease tidal volume	Decrease	Increase	Increase

TABLE 8-10   Effects of RR on I:E Ratio

PARAMETER CHANGE	I TIME	E TIME	I:E RATIO
Increase RR	Minimal change	Decrease	Decrease
Decrease RR	Minimal change	Increase	Increase

Changing the I:E Ratio. Since the I:E ratio may be changed by altering different settings available on selected ventilators, different methods to obtain a desired I:E ratio are provided as follows (Chang, 1999).

☑ The calculated flow in Example 1 is the *minimum* flow rate required for this I:E ratio. It is usually set 10 l/min. higher to meet changing minute volume requirements.

Example 1 Using Flow to Change the I:E Ratio

Given: Minute Volume = 12 l/min
Desired I:E Ratio = 1:3

Calculate: The flow rate for an I:E ratio of 1:3

Solution: Flow = Minute Volume × Sum of I:E Ratio
= 12 l/min × (1+3)
= 12 l/min × 4
= 48 l/min

☑ At RR of 16/min, the I time needed for an I:E ratio of 1:4 is 0.75 sec. The E time is (3.75 – 0.75) sec = 3 sec.

Example 2 Using I Time to Change the I:E Ratio

Given: RR = 16/min
Desired I:E Ratio = 1:4

Calculate: The I time needed for an I:E ratio of 1:4

Solution: Since RR = 16/min, time for each breath = 60 sec/16 or 3.75 sec

I Time = Time for each breath x [I ratio / Sum of I:E ratio]
= 3.75 sec × [1 / (1+4)]
= 3.75 sec × [1 / 5]
= 3.75 sec / 5
= 0.75 sec

I Time % and I:E Ratio. Some ventilators (e.g., Hamilton Veolar) permit the I:E ratio to be preset, usually by setting an I time % (percent inspiratory time). In these ventilators, the flow rate is automatically adjusted by the ventilator to maintain a constant I:E ratio regardless of changes in tidal volume or respiratory rate.

The I time % and I:E ratio equivalent are listed in Table 8-11. For other I:E ratios not listed in the table, they may be calculated by following Example 3:

Example 3   Using I Time % to Set the I:E Ratio

Given: Desired I:E Ratio = 1:3.5

☑ The I time %
needed for an
I:E ratio of 1:3.5 is
22.2%.

Calculate: The I time % needed for an I:E ratio of 1:3.5

Solution: I Time % = $\dfrac{\text{I ratio}}{\text{Sum of I:E ratio}}$

$= \dfrac{1}{(1 + 3.5)}$

$= \dfrac{1}{4.5}$

$= 22.2\%$

FLOW PATTERN

Most modern ventilators offer different inspiratory flow patterns. Although there are subtle variations, the principle flow patterns are (1) square (constant) flow pattern, (2) accelerating (ascending) flow pattern, (3) decelerating (descending) flow pattern, and (4) sine wave flow pattern. The waveforms for each of these flow patterns are shown in Figure 8-1.

The square flow pattern may be used initially upon setting up the ventilator. This flow pattern provides an even, constant peak flow during the entire inspiratory phase. The initial peak flow at the very beginning of the inspiratory phase should help to overcome the airway resistance and parenchymal elastance, and the remaining peak flow throughout the inspiratory phase should enhance gas distribution in the lungs. Adjustment of the flow pattern may be made after stabilization of the patient. Note that the constant flow pattern is the only flow pattern in which the peak flow rate equals the mean flow rate. All other flow patterns will produce a mean flow rate that is less than the peak flow.

TABLE 8-11   I Time % and I:E Ratio Equivalent

I TIME %	I:E RATIO
14.3%	1:6
16.7%	1:5
20%	1:4
25%	1:3
33.3%	1:2
50%	1:1
60%	1.5:1
66.7%	2:1

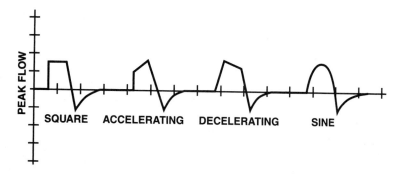

Figure 8-1   Normal flow tracing of four different flow patterns: square, accelerating, decelerating, and sine. (Courtesy of Novametrix Medical Systems, Inc.)

With its increasing flow throughout the respiratory cycle, the accelerating waveform may improve the distribution of ventilation in patients with partial airway obstruction. The decelerating flow pattern typically produces a high initial inspiratory pressure and the decrease in flow may help improve distribution of tidal volume and gas exchange (Sullivan et al., 1977). The sine wave is considered more physiologic because it is similar to the normal spontaneous breathing inspiratory flow pattern. The sine wave may also improve the distribution of ventilation and therefore improve gas exchange.

For ventilators that do not permit a preset inspiratory time (e.g., Puritan-Bennett 7200), the inspiratory time may increase if the patient's peak inspiratory pressure increases. This is because as the PIP increases, the pressure gradient between the ventilator and the patient's airway opening increases, resulting in an increased inspiratory time. However, on ventilators in which the inspiratory time is preset, such as the Hamilton Veolar, the inspiratory time is held constant for any flow pattern selected.

In performing calculations that involve the inspiratory flow as a variable (e.g., Resistance = Pressure / Flow), the mean inspiratory flow should be used. Since the only flow pattern in which the peak flow equals the mean inspiratory flow is the square wave pattern, the ventilator should be switched to a constant flow pattern prior to measurement.

VENTILATOR ALARM SETTINGS

Although different ventilators have different alarm systems, the following alarms should be basic to any ventilator: low exhaled volume alarm, low inspiratory pressure alarm, high inspiratory pressure alarm, apnea alarm, high respiratory rate alarm, and F_1O_2 alarm. These alarms should be backed up by a battery source to prevent malfunction in the event of electrical failure.

LOW EXHALED VOLUME ALARM

The *low* exhaled volume alarm (low volume alarm) should be set at about 100 ml *lower* than the expired mechanical tidal volume. This alarm is triggered if the patient does not exhale an adequate tidal volume. This alarm is typically used to detect a system leak or circuit disconnection.

LOW INSPIRATORY PRESSURE ALARM

The *low* inspiratory pressure alarm (low pressure alarm) should be set at 10 to 15 cm H_2O *below* the observed peak inspiratory pressure. This alarm is triggered if the peak airway pressure is less than the alarm setting. The low inspiratory pressure alarm complements the low exhaled volume alarm and is also used to detect system leaks or circuit disconnection.

HIGH INSPIRATORY PRESSURE ALARM

The *high* inspiratory pressure alarm (high pressure limit alarm) should be set at 10 to 15 cm H_2O *above* the observed peak inspiratory pressure. This alarm is triggered when the peak airway pressure is equal to or higher than the high pressure limit. Once the alarm is triggered, inspiration is immediately terminated and the ventilator goes into expiratory cycle.

The patient must be evaluated to determine the cause of the alarm. Common causes that trigger the high inspiratory pressure alarm include water in the ventilator circuit, kinking or biting of the endotracheal tube, secretions in the airway, bronchospasm, tension pneumothorax, decreases in lung compliance, increases in airway resistance, and coughing.

APNEA ALARM

The apnea alarm should be set with a 15- to 20-second time delay, with less time delay at higher respiratory rate. On some ventilators such as the Puritan-Bennett 7200, the apnea alarm also triggers an apnea ventilation mode in which the ventilator provides full ventilatory support until the alarm condition no longer exists.

HIGH RESPIRATORY RATE ALARM

The *high* respiratory rate alarm (high rate alarm) should be set at 10 to 15 breaths per minute *over* the observed respiratory rate. This alarm is especially important in the MMV mode. The high respiratory rate alarm indicates that the patient is becoming tachypneic—a sign of respiratory distress.

✓ The *low* exhaled volume alarm (low volume alarm) should be set at about 100 ml *lower* than the expired mechanical tidal volume.

✓ The *low* inspiratory pressure alarm (low pressure alarm) should be set at 10 to 15 cm H_2O *below* the observed peak inspiratory pressure.

✓ The *high* inspiratory pressure alarm (high pressure limit alarm) should be set at 10 to 15 cm H_2O *above* the observed peak inspiratory pressure.

✓ The apnea alarm should be set with a 15- to 20-second time delay.

✓ The *high* respiratory rate alarm (high rate alarm) should be set at 10 to 15 breaths per minute *over* the observed respiratory rate.

☑ **Set the low and high F_IO_2 alarms at 40% and 50%, respectively for an F_IO_2 of 45%.**

HIGH AND LOW F_IO_2 ALARMS

The high F_IO_2 alarm should be set at 5 to 10% over the analyzed F_IO_2 and the low F_IO_2 alarm should be set at 5 to 10% below the analyzed F_IO_2.

HAZARDS AND COMPLICATIONS

Mechanical ventilation has many potential hazards (e.g., ventilator disconnection, nosocomial infection) and complications (e.g., barotrauma, hypotension). The frequency of occurrence is directly related to the length of mechanical ventilation (Liu et al., 1991; Pierson, 1990). Patients who require mechanical ventilation for longer periods are likely to develop more complications.

This section summarizes the common hazards and complications of mechanical ventilation based on several prospective studies. Special emphasis is provided for barotrauma and decrease in cardiac output and blood pressure since the effects of these complications are more urgent to the patient's progress and outcome.

TYPES OF HAZARDS AND COMPLICATIONS

Prospective studies of patient outcome during mechanical ventilation indicate that hazards and complications are related to: (1) positive pressure ventilation (e.g., barotrauma, impedance of cardiac output) (2) patient condition (e.g., organ failure), (3) ventilator and artificial airway (accidental extubation), and (4) medical professionals (e.g., nosocomial infection). Examples for each of these four areas are shown in Table 8-12.

BAROTRAUMA

☑ **Risk of barotrauma is high when: PIP > 50 cm H_2O, plateau pressure > 35 cm H_2O, MAWP > 30 cm H_2O, and PEEP > 10 cm H_2O.**

Barotrauma is the term used to describe lung tissue injury or rupture that results from alveolar overdistention. General agreement is that in most cases, peak inspiratory pressures greater than 50 cm H_2O, plateau pressures greater than 35 cm H_2O, mean airway pressure greater than 30 cm H_2O, and PEEP greater than 10 cm H_2O may induce the development of barotrauma (Bezzant et al., 1994; Slutsky, 1994). The risk of barotrauma also increases with the duration of positive pressure ventilation.

Barotrauma can occur at mean airway pressures lower than 30 cm H_2O either due to patient susceptibility or to an uneven distribution of ventilation. COPD patients are more susceptible to barotrauma presumably due to air trapping and weakened parenchymal areas (e.g., lung blebs and bullae). Uneven distribution of ventilation may result in patients with significant airway obstruction and lung parenchymal changes. A mechanical tidal volume tends to preferentially distribute to areas of low resistance and high compliance during the early por-

TABLE 8-12 Hazards and Complications of Mechanical Ventilation

CONDITION	EXAMPLES
Related to positive pressure ventilation	Barotrauma (pneumothorax, mediastinal air leak, subcutaneous air leak) Hypotension, decrease in cardiac output Arrhythmia Oxygen toxicity Bronchopleural fistula Bronchopulmonary dysplasia (in infants) Upper gastrointestinal hemorrhage
Related to patient condition	Infection (due to reduced immunity) Physical and psychologic trauma Multiple organ failure (may be preexisting)
Related to equipment (ventilator and artificial airway)	Ventilator and alarm malfunction Ventilator circuit disconnection Accidental extubation Main bronchus intubation Postintubation stridor Endotracheal tube blockage Tissue damage Atelectasis (due to inadequate tidal volume)
Related to medical professionals	Nosocomial pneumonia (due to cross-contamination) Inappropriate ventilator settings Misadventures (due to lapses of understanding and communication)

(Data from Ventilator alarm failures, *Bourke et al., 1987; Brunner et al., 1989; Milligan, 1992; Pottie et al., 1993; Pryn et al., 1989; Slee et al., 1988; and* Other hazards and complications, *Bezzant et al., 1994; Cox et al., 1991; Liu et al., 1991; Pierson, 1990; Rivera et al., 1992.)*

tion of inspiration. This may result in transient elevated alveolar pressures with resultant overdistention and rupture despite what would normally be accepted as a "safe" pressure.

Other lung injuries that may occur as a result of positive pressure ventilation include pulmonary interstitial emphysema, pneumomediastinum, pneumoperitoneum, pneumothorax, tension pneumothorax, and subcutaneous emphysema.

DECREASE IN CARDIAC OUTPUT AND BLOOD PRESSURE

Positive pressure ventilation has been implicated in the development of decreased cardiac output and arterial blood pressure (Bezzant et al., 1994; Franklin et al., 1994). The reason for this is that positive airway and alveolar pressures may potentially increase the normally subatmospheric pleural pressures that surround the heart and vena

☑ Since positive pressure ventilation increases the CVP, the pressure gradient between the right atrium and the venous drainage will be decreased with a resultant decreased venous return to the right atrium.

☑ A competent cardiovascular system can compensate for a small drop in venous return by an increased heart rate and arterial vasoconstriction.

☑ High airway pressures are more detrimental to the cardiac output in patients with high lung compliance than those with low compliance.

cava. The increased pleural pressure tends to compress the right atrium and vena cava, increasing the intravascular resistance and pressures associated with these structures. The pressures in the vena cava and right atrium are approximately equal and are collectively known as the central venous pressure (CVP). The usually low central venous pressure creates an intravascular pressure gradient between the right atrium and the systemic venous drainage that augments venous blood return to the right atrium. If positive pressure ventilation increases the CVP, the pressure gradient between the right atrium and the venous drainage will be decreased with a resultant decreased venous return to the right atrium. If the venous return is significantly reduced, this can result in a decreased cardiac output and arterial hypotension.

If the patient has no preexisting cardiovascular disease and is not hypovolemic, a competent cardiovascular system can compensate for a small drop in venous return and thus maintain cardiac output and blood pressure. The two primary compensatory mechanisms include an increased heart rate and arterial vasoconstriction initiated by the cardiac baroreceptors.

The magnitude of the increase in the CVP and the resultant decrease in venous return depends on several factors, including the airway pressure, lung compliance and chest wall compliance. Higher airway pressures will more likely result in higher pleural and central venous pressures. It is important to note that increases of the mean airway pressures tend to depress venous return more than increases of the peak inspiratory pressures.

The degree of increased pleural pressure for a given airway pressure is further affected by the patient's lung and chest wall compliance. If the patient's lung compliance is low (stiff lungs), then airway pressures are less readily transmitted into the pleural space. Therefore in patients with low lung compliance, a given airway pressure will result in a smaller increase in pleural pressure and a less dramatic decrease in venous return. This does not mean that patients with low lung compliance cannot have significant decreases in cardiac output due to positive pressure ventilation. These patients must also be closely monitored for potentially significant decreases in cardiac output and blood pressure.

Patients with more compliant lungs, such as COPD patients, tend to more readily transmit a higher airway pressure into the pleural space. Therefore in these patients, a given airway pressure will tend to result in a more dramatic decrease in venous return and cardiac output.

The effects of chest wall compliance on the transmission of airway pressure into the pleural space are exactly opposite to the effects of lung compliance. A low chest wall compliance (stiff chest wall) will tend to increase the pleural pressure more significantly for a given airway pressure than a normal chest wall compliance. Conditions in which the chest wall would be less compliant than normal include the application of tight chest wall bandages that encircle the thorax and extensive chest wall burn injuries.

All ventilator patients must be monitored for signs of cardiovascular instability. However, because ventilator patients with suspected or known preexisting cardiovascular disease are more likely to suffer clinically significant decreases in cardiac output and blood pressure, these patients must be monitored with an extra measure of vigilance.

SUMMARY

Initiation of mechanical ventilation requires many decisions, ranging from the mode of ventilation to the level of PEEP. Nevertheless, this process can be simplified by following a set of established guidelines. Under most clinical conditions, the initial settings on the ventilator will satisfy the immediate requirement of most patients.

It is essential to remember that the initial settings are just that; subsequent changes to these settings must be made based on the ever-changing condition of the patient. In summary, Table 8-13 outlines the indications of mechanical ventilation and Table 8-14 provides an overview of the initial ventilator settings for an adult patient.

TABLE 8-13　**Indications for Mechanical Ventilation**

INDICATION	PARAMETERS
Acute ventilatory failure	$PaCO_2$ > 50 mm Hg (Higher for COPD) pH < 7.30 Apnea
Impending ventilatory failure	Tidal volume < 3 to 5 ml/kg Respiratory rate > 25 to 35/min Minute ventilation > 10 l/min Vital capacity < 15 ml/kg MIP < −20 cm H_2O Rising $PaCO_2$ > 50 mm Hg
Severe hypoxemia	PaO_2 < 60 mm Hg at F_IO_2 > 50%, or PaO_2 < 40 mm Hg at any F_IO_2 Severe cyanosis
Prophylatic ventilatory support	Reduce risk of pulmonary complications 　Prolonged shock 　Head injury 　Smoke inhalation Reduce hypoxia of major body organs 　Hypoxic brain 　Hypoxia of heart muscles Reduce cardiopulmonary stress 　Prolonged shock 　Coronary artery bypass surgery 　Other thoracic or abdominal surgeries

TABLE 8-14   **Initial Ventilator Settings**

PARAMETER	SETTING	NOTES
Mode	Assist/Control or SIMV	Provide ventilatory support.
RR	10 to 12/min	Primary control to alter ventilation and $PaCO_2$.
V_T	10 to 15 ml/kg	Peak airway pressure is *directly* related to the V_T setting. Use lower V_T to reduce risk of pressure-related lung injuries.
F_IO_2	100% for severe hypoxemia or compromised cardiopulmonary status	40% for mild hypoxemia or normal cardiopulmonary status.
PEEP	5 cm H_2O for refractory hypoxemia	Monitor patient and note cardio-vascular adverse effects.
I:E	1:2 to 1:4	1:4 for patients needing longer E time due to air trapping.
Flow pattern	Square	Other flow patterns for a lower peak airway pressure (manometer) and better gas distribution (breath sounds).

Self-Assessment Questions

1. Which of the following is *not* an indication for mechanical ventilation?

    A. acute ventilatory failure
    B. impending ventilatory failure

    C. severe hypoxemia
    D. airway obstruction

2. A patient has an admitting diagnosis of acute ventilatory failure. This condition is characterized by a $PaCO_2$ of _____ mm Hg or greater with an accompanying respiratory _____.

    A. 20, acidosis
    B. 20, alkalosis

    C. 50, acidosis
    D. 50, alkalosis

3. Impending ventilatory failure may be confirmed by trending a patient's:

    A. lung functions.
    B. PaO_2.

    C. $PaCO_2$.
    D. pH.

4. Among other criteria of assessment, impending ventilatory failure may be present when the patient's minute ventilation is _____ 10 l/min and maximum inspiratory pressure is less than _____.

    A. more than, 20 cm H_2O C. less than, 20 cm H_2O
    B. more than, -20 cm H_2O D. less than, -20 cm H_2O

5. The primary purposes of prophylactic mechanical ventilation include all of the following *except*:

    A. to minimize the risk of pulmonary complications.   C. to reduce the work of the cardio-pulmonary system.
    B. to reduce prolonged hypoxia of major body organs.   D. to monitor the arterial blood gases and vital signs.

6. A physician asks you to set up a volume-limited ventilator for a 35-year-old postoperative male patient who weighs 132 lb (60 kg). You would select an initial tidal volume of _____ and respiratory rate of _____.

    A. 500 ml, 12/min   C. 500 ml, 20/min
    B. 800 ml, 20/min   D. 800 ml, 12/min

7. As you are measuring the compressible volume of a new ventilator circuit, you notice that the observed expired volume (ml) and peak inspiratory pressure (cm H_2O) are 150 ml and 30 cm H_2O, respectively. The circuit compressible volume is therefore:

    A. 2 ml/cm H_2O.   C. 4.5 ml/cm H_2O.
    B. 3 ml/cm H_2O.   D. 5 ml/cm H_2O.

8. With a circuit compressible volume of 3 ml/cm H_2O, what would be the actual tidal volume delivered to the patient if the expired tidal volume is 800 ml and the peak inspiratory pressure is 50 cm H_2O?

    A. 500 ml   C. 750 ml
    B. 650 ml   D. 950 ml

9. Positive end-expiratory pressure (PEEP) is indicated in patients who have a decreased _____ and _____.

    A. tidal volume, chronic hypercapnia   C. vital capacity, acute hypercapnia
    B. functional residual capacity, refractory hypoxemia   D. tidal volume, refractory hypoxemia

10. At constant tidal volume and respiratory rate, increasing the inspiratory flow rate will lead to a _____ inspiratory time (I time) and _____ expiratory time (E time).

    A. longer, longer   C. shorter, longer
    B. longer, shorter   D. shorter, shorter

11. What should be the *minimum* flow rate for a minute volume of 12 l/min. and an I:E ratio of 1:4?

    A. 40 l/min   C. 60 l/min
    B. 50 l/min   D. 70 l/min

12. If the desired I:E ratio is 1:2.5, what should be the I time %?

    A. 29%   C. 45%
    B. 40%   D. 60%

13. The _____ and _____ are two alarms that are useful to detect circuit disconnection.

    A. low pressure, high pressure   C. low volume, low PEEP
    B. high PEEP, high volume   D. low pressure, low volume

14. Which of the following is *not* a common potential complication of positive pressure ventilation?

    A. hypertension   C. accidental patient disconnection
    B. decrease in cardiac output   D. barotrauma

15 to 18. Match the conditions of mechanical ventilation with the examples of the hazards and complications that might occur during mechanical ventilation.

CONDITION	EXAMPLES
15. Related to positive pressure ventilation	A. Ventilator circuit disconnect
16. Related to patient condition	B. Barotrauma
17. Related to equipment	C. Inappropriate ventilator settings
18. Related to medical professionals	D. Physical and psychological trauma

References

Barnes, T. A. et al. (1993). *Core textbook of respiratory care practice.* St. Louis: Mosby-Year Book.

Bezzant, T. B. et al. (1994). Risks and hazards of mechanical ventilation: A collective review of published literature. *Dis Mon, 40*(11), 581–638.

Bourke, A. E. et al. (1987). Failure of a ventilator alarm to detect patient disconnection. *J Med Eng Technol, 11*(2), 65–67.

Brown, B. R. (1994). Understanding mechanical ventilation: Indications for and initiation of therapy. *J Okla State Med Assoc, 87,* 353–357.

Brunner, J. X. et al. (1989). Prototype ventilator and alarm algorithm for the NASA Space Station. *J Clin Monit, 5*(2), 90–99.

Campbell, M. L. et al. (1992). Terminal weaning from mechanical ventilation: Ethical and practical considerations for patient management. *Amer J Crit Care, 1*(3), 52–56.

Caruso, P., Friedrich, C., & Denari, S. D. et al. (1999). The unidirectional valve is the best method to determine maximal respiratory pressure during weaning. *Chest, 115*(4): 1096–1101.

Chang, D. W. (1999). *Respiratory care calculations* (2nd ed.). Albany, NY: Delmar Publishers, Inc.

Cox, R. G. et al. (1991). Efficacy, results, and complications of mechanical ventilation in children with status asthmaticus. *Pediatr Pulmonol, 11*(2), 120–126.

Feihl, F. et al. (1994). Permissive hypercapnia. How permissive should we be? *Am J Respir Crit Care Med, 150*(6 Pt. 1), 1722–1737.

Franklin, C. et al. (1994). Life-threatening hypotension associated with emergency intubation and the initiation of mechanical ventilation. *Amer J Emerg Med, 12*(4), 425–428.

Hall, J. B. et al. (1987). Liberation of the patient from mechanical ventilation. *JAMA, 257,* 1621–1628.

Liu, Y. N. et al. (1991). Complications of mechanical ventilation: A clinical analysis of 82 cases. *Chung Hua Nei Ko Tsa Chih, 30*(11), 692–694.

Milligan, K. A. (1992). Disablement of a ventilator disconnect alarm by a heat and moisture exchanger [letter]. *Anaesthesia, 47*(3), 279.

Otto, C. W. (1986). Ventilatory management in the critically ill. *Emerg Med Clin North Am, 4*(4), 635–654.

Pierson, D. J. (1990). Complications associated with mechanical ventilation. *Crit Care Med, 6*(3), 711–724.

Pottie, J. C. et al. (1993). Alarm failure in the oxygen-air mixture. *Ann Fr Anesth Reanim, 12*(6), 607–608.

Pryn, S. J. et al. (1989). Ventilator disconnection alarm failures. The role of ventilator and breathing accessories. *Anaesthesia, 44*(12), 978–981.

Rivera, R. et al. (1992). Complications of endotracheal intubation and mechanical ventilation in infants and children. *Crit Care Med, 20*(2), 193–199.

Scanlan, C. L. (1999). *Egan's fundamentals of respiratory care* (7th ed.). St. Louis: Mosby-Year Book.

Schneiderman, L. J. et al. (1990). Medical futility: Its meaning and ethical implications. *Ann Intern Med, 112,* 949–954.

Shapiro, B. A. (1994). A historical perspective on ventilator management. *New Horiz, 2*(1), 8–18.

Shapiro, B. A. et al. (1991). *Clinical application of respiratory care* (4th ed.). St. Louis: Mosby-Year Book.

Shapiro, B. A. et al. (1994). *Clinical application of blood gases* (5th ed.). St. Louis: Mosby-Year Book.

Slee, T. A. et al. (1988). Failure of low pressure alarm associated with the use of a humidifier. *Anesthesiology, 69*(5), 791–793.

Slutsky, A. S. (1994). Consensus conference on mechanical ventilation—January 28–30, 1993 at Northbrook, IL, USA, Part I. *Int Care Med, 20,* 64–79.

Sullivan, M. et al. (1977). Relationship between ventilator waveform and tidal-volume distribution. *Respir Care, 22*(4), 386–393.

Tejeda, M., Boix, J. H., & Alvarez, F. et al. (1997). Comparison of pressure support ventilation and assist-cointrol ventilation in the treatment of respiratory failure. *Chest, 111*(5): 1322–1325.

CHAPTER NINE

MONITORING IN MECHANICAL VENTILATION

Walter C. Chop

OUTLINE

KEY TERMS

- anion gap
- diffusion defect
- dyshemoglobins
- end-tidal carbon dioxide monitoring
- hypoventilation
- hypoxemia
- hypoxia

- intrapulmonary shunting
- oliguria
- pulse oximeter
- transcutaneous $PtcCO_2$
- transcutaneous $PtcO_2$
- ventilation/perfusion (V/Q) mismatch

INTRODUCTION

Monitoring a patient's clinical condition during mechanical ventilation is vital because clinical status often changes rapidly and unpredictably. A patient's clinical status may be affected by the underlying illness, medications, organ failure, and even the settings on the ventilator.

There are four reasons for monitoring a patient on a continuous basis: (1) baseline measurements can be used to establish the initial treatment plan and serve as a reference point for future measurements; (2) a trend can be established to document the progress or regression of a patient's condition; (3) treatment plans can be added, altered, or discontinued according to the measurements obtained; and (4) high-limit and low-limit alarms can be set on most monitors to safeguard a patient's safety.

This chapter provides an overview of monitoring techniques pertinent to ventilatory care.

VITAL SIGNS

Vital signs (heart rate, blood pressure, respiratory rate, and temperature) can provide very useful information on the overall condition of a patient. During mechanical ventilation, changes in vital signs often indicate changes in the patient's cardiopulmonary status.

HEART RATE

In the intensive care unit, heart rate assessment is readily available on the electrocardiograph (ECG) monitor. High and low alarms can be set on the monitor to warn of tachycardia and bradycardia.

Tachycardia. During mechanical ventilation, some conditions that may increase a patient's heart rate are **hypoxemia,** pain, anxiety and stress, fever, drug reactions, and myocardial infarction. Tachycardia can alert the clinician to blood volume or cardiac output deficits.

☑ Normal adult heart rate is between 60 and 100/min.

hypoxemia: Deficiency of oxygen in blood; low PaO₂.

✓ Tachycardia
may be caused
by hypoxemia, pain,
anxiety and stress,
fever, drug reactions, and myocardial infarction.

*hypoxia: Deficiency
of oxygen in tissues.*

Increase in heart rate must be looked at as part of the larger picture as it can be secondary to extreme conditions ranging from hypovolemia to anxiety.

Bradycardia.   Bradycardia and arrhythmias often occur during prolonged suctioning of the airways. Preoxygenation is necessary to minimize the occurrence of arterial desaturation during suctioning. Since arterial desaturation occurs in as little as 5 seconds during suctioning, **hypoxia** and cardiac complications can happen rather rapidly. When arrhythmia or bradycardia occurs, endotracheal suctioning must be stopped and 100% oxygen should be provided to the patient immediately (Burton et al., 1997).

Bradycardia, if it appears together with a low cardiac output, can be ominous and may suggest a decrease in coronary blood flow. Table 9-1 outlines the conditions that affect the heart rate.

BLOOD PRESSURE

Continuous blood pressure monitoring in the critical patient is usually done via an indwelling arterial catheter interfaced with a pressure monitor. The most common insertion site for the catheter is the radial artery. Other sites include the brachial, femoral, popliteal, and dorsalis pedis arteries.

✓ Fluid overload,
vasoconstriction, stress, anxiety,
and pain may lead to
hypertension.

Hypertension.   Hypertension, higher than normal blood pressure, may be caused by acute or chronic patient conditions. Acute conditions such as fluid overload, vasoconstriction, stress, anxiety, and pain may lead to hypertension. Patients who have a history of congestive heart failure, cardiovascular disease, or polycythemia may develop hypertension, which can become a complicating factor during mechanical ventilation.

TABLE 9-1   Conditions That Affect the Heart Rate

CONDITIONS THAT MAY CAUSE TACHYCARDIA	CONDITIONS THAT MAY CAUSE BRADYCARDIA
Hypoxemia	Sudden hypoxia and/or vagal stimulation during endotracheal suctioning
Hypovolemia	Inadequate coronary blood flow
Pain	Heart block
Anxiety and stress	Abnormal SA node function
Fever	Hypothermia
Drug reaction (e.g., epinephrine)	Drug reaction (e.g., morphine sulfate)
Myocardial infarction	

Hypotension. Hypotension, lower than normal blood pressure, may be due to absolute hypovolemia (blood loss), relative hypovolemia (shock), or pump failure (CHF). When hypotension occurs during mechanical ventilation, it is often associated with excessive intrathoracic pressure, peak airway pressure, and lung volume. Hypotension is one of the complications of positive pressure ventilation or positive end-expiratory pressure. Table 9-2 outlines the conditions that affect the blood pressure.

RESPIRATORY RATE

hypoventilation:
Below normal level of alveolar ventilation characterized by an elevated $PaCO_2$.

The normal spontaneous respiratory rate for adults is 10 to 16 breaths per minute. An increased respiratory rate (tachypnea) may be an early warning sign of **hypoventilation** or hypoxemia (Bone, 1985). If the rate exceeds 20 breaths per minute and rising, the patient should be monitored closely for an impending crisis. A sudden increase in respiratory rate may indicate acute events such as pulmonary embolism or tension pneumothorax. Rates in excess of 30 breaths per minute generally indicate respiratory distress and may lead to severe hypoxia (Bone, 1985).

☑ Rapid shallow breathing is a reliable sign of ventilatory insufficiency.

Tachypnea may precede the development of respiratory failure and use of mechanical ventilation (Krieger & Ershowshy, 1994). During mechanical ventilation, tachypnea is indicative of respiratory dysfunction (Gravelyn & Weg, 1980). When tachypnea and low tidal volume are observed in a patient, successful weaning from mechanical ventilation is not likely (Tobin & Perez et al., 1986).

Routine monitoring of a patient's spontaneous respiratory rate is a simple but very useful method to assess the pulmonary status of a ventilator patient. This is especially true during the weaning process. A sudden increase in spontaneous respiratory rate during weaning attempt is indicative of moderate or severe respiratory insufficiency or hypoxia.

TABLE 9-2 Conditions That Affect the Blood Pressure

CONDITIONS THAT MAY CAUSE HYPERTENSION	CONDITIONS THAT MAY CAUSE HYPOTENSION
Fluid overload	Decreased venous return due to positive pressure ventilation
Stress	Absolute hypovolemia (e.g., blood loss, dehydration)
Anxiety	Relative hypovolemia (e.g., sepsis, shock)
Pain	Pump failure (e.g., CHF)
Congestive heart failure	
Cardiovascular disease	
Polycythemia (↑ blood viscosity)	

TEMPERATURE

In the intensive care unit, a patient's temperature may be measured routinely at regular intervals or monitored continuously via a rectal, esophageal, or pulmonary artery catheter probe.

Hyperthermia.   Hyperthermia can occur as a result of infection, tissue necrosis, leukemia, or other conditions that increase a patient's metabolic rate and oxygen utilization. Hyperthermia also shifts the oxyhemoglobin dissociation curve to the right causing a lower oxygen saturation level at any PaO_2. This oxygen desaturation occurs because increased temperature promotes unloading of oxygen from hemoglobin to the tissues.

☑ Hyperthermia causes a lower oxygen saturation at any PaO_2.

Hypothermia.   Hypothermia, though seen less commonly in the critically ill patient, can occur as a result of central nervous system (CNS) problems, metabolic disorders, and from certain drugs or toxins. Hypothermia is sometimes induced in head trauma patients as a means of decreasing the patient's basal metabolic rate.

☑ Hypothermia lowers a person's basal metabolic rate.

Hypothermia is also induced in patients undergoing coronary artery bypass (CAB) surgery. At this extreme low temperature, the hypothermic condition must be taken into account during management of the ventilator and patient. For example, the measured PaO_2 and $PaCO_2$ values are higher than the actual values when the sample is collected under hypothermic conditions and is analyzed at body temperature. In order to have blood gas values that accurately reflect a patient's true ventilatory and oxygenation status, corrections to the patient's core temperature must be done during blood gas analysis.

In other nonextreme hypothermic conditions ($+/-2°$ C), temperature corrections are not necessary as long as the uncorrected PaO_2 is above 60 mm Hg (Malley, 1990).

☑ Excessive cooling of the phrenic nerve during CAB surgery may cause paralysis of the hemidiaphragms.

Excessive cooling of the phrenic nerve during CAB surgery may cause paralysis of the hemidiaphragms. This condition, though temporary, may take months to resolve completely (Wilkins & Dexter, 1998). Table 9-3 outlines the conditions that affect the body temperature.

TABLE 9-3   Conditions That Affect the Body Temperature

CONDITIONS THAT MAY CAUSE HYPERTHERMIA	CONDITIONS THAT MAY CAUSE HYPOTHERMIA
Infection	CNS problem
Tissue necrosis	Metabolic disorders
Leukemia	Drugs and toxins

Increased metabolic rate	Induced
	    Coronary bypass surgery
	    Head injury

CHEST INSPECTION AND AUSCULTATION

Since the lungs are protected by the thoracic cage, they are not readily accessible for direct examination. Chest inspection and auscultation are two indirect methods that are useful in evaluating the condition of the lungs.

CHEST MOVEMENT

During mechanical ventilation it is important to observe the overall chest movement. One should observe the symmetrical movement of the chest with each inspiration as well as the depth and rhythm of each tidal volume cycle.

Asymmetrical movement can occur in conditions such as right bronchial intubation, atelectasis, or tension pneumothorax (Figure 9-1) (Bone, 1985). If dysynchronous motion of the chest and abdomen is noted, the patient should be evaluated for diaphragmatic fatigue or underlying pathology.

AUSCULTATION

Auscultation of a patient's breath sounds should be performed each time the practitioner assesses the patient/ventilator system. Diminished or absent breath sounds or the presence of wheezes and crackles are signs of ventilatory problems and should be recognized as causes of respiratory distress (Wilkins & Dexter, 1998). Table 9-4 shows these abnormal breath sounds and their related clinical conditions.

Figures 9-2 through 9-4 show the surface projections of lung segments and they are helpful for the correct placement of the stethoscope diaphragm. Proper identification of the lung segments involved in the disease process is essential for consistent charting and reporting, and

TABLE 9-4 Abnormal Breath Sounds and Related Conditions

BREATH SOUND	CONDITIONS
Diminished or absent	Airway obstruction Atelectasis Main-stem intubation Pleural effusion Pneumothorax
Wheezes	Airway narrowing
Inspiratory crackles	Lung consolidation Pulmonary edema
Coarse crackles	Excessive secretions

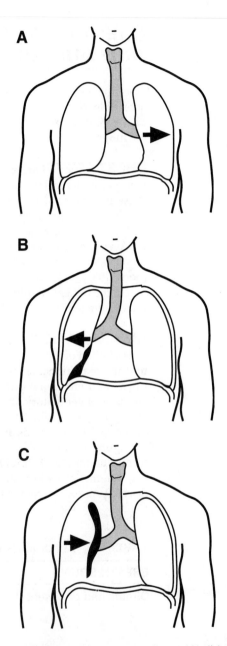

Figure 9-1 Asymmetrical chest movement due to (A) right bronchial intubation; note overinflation of the right lung and underinflation of the left lung; (B) atelectasis, the trachea and mediastinum are shifted to the affected side; (C) tension pneumothorax, the trachea and mediastinum are shifted to the opposite side.

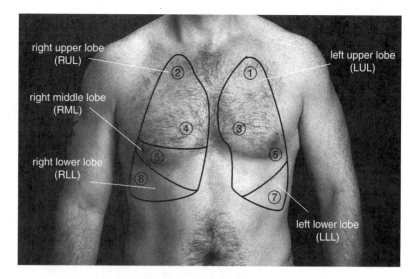

Figure 9-2 Anterior surface projection of the lung lobes and segments. Left lung: 1 LUL apical segment, 3 LUL anterior segment, 5 LUL lingula inferior and superior segments, 7 LLL anterior segment. Right lung: 2 RUL apical segment, 4 RUL anterior, 6 RML medial and lateral segments, 8 RLL anterior segment.

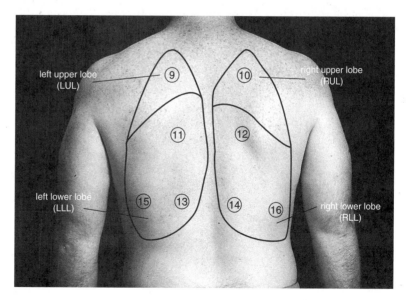

Figure 9-3 Posterior surface projection of the lung lobes and segments. Left lung: 9 LUL posterior segment, 11 LLL superior segment, 13 LLL posterior segment, 15 LLL lateral segment. Right lung: 10 RUL posterior segment, 12 RLL superior segment, 14 RLL posterior segment, 16 RLL lateral segment.

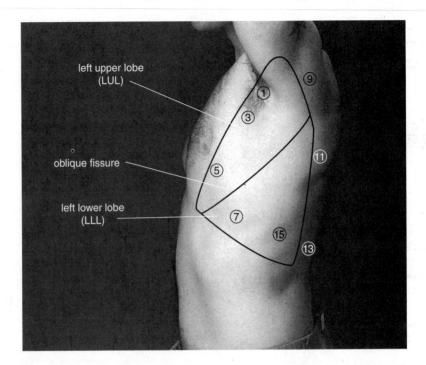

Figure 9-4 Left lateral surface projection of the lung lobes and segments. Left upper lobe: 1 LUL apical segment, 3 LUL anterior segment, 5 LUL lingula inferior and superior segments, 9 LUL posterior segment. Left lower lobe: 7 LLL anterior segment, 11 LLL superior segment, 13 LLL posterior segment, 15 LLL lateral segment.

for performing the correct chest percussion and postural drainage procedure.

The stethoscope can also be used for detection of a leaky cuff on an endotracheal or tracheostomy tube, as well as for right main-stem (bronchial) intubation. A cuff leak may be detected by placing the stethoscope diaphragm over the trachea and on top of the cuff's location. The cuff is leaking if distinct air movement can be heard toward the end of a mechanical breath. Uneven bilateral breath sounds in the absence of lung pathology (e.g., atelectasis, tension pneumothorax) may indicate main-stem intubation. The placement of an endotracheal tube should be confirmed by chest radiograph.

FLUID BALANCE AND ANION GAP

Mechanical ventilation may affect a patient's renal function and fluid balance. Since fluid balance and electrolyte concentration are related, the **anion gap** may also be affected as a result of positive

anion gap: *The difference between cations (positive ions) and anions (negative ions) in the plasma. The normal range is 15 to 20 when K+ is included in the calculation (10 to 14 mEq/L when K+ is excluded).*

pressure ventilation. Proper fluid and electrolyte maintenance should be an integral part of mechanical ventilation to prevent these adverse outcomes.

FLUID BALANCE

Positive pressure ventilation reduces cardiac output and thus renal perfusion. Urine output is decreased due to hypoperfusion of the kidneys. Mechanical ventilation also reduces urine output as a result of an increase in antidiuretic hormone (ADH) and reduction of atrial natriuretic factor (ANF). The end result of these changes is decreased fluid output and fluid retention.

For these reasons, the fluid level of a ventilator patient must be monitored closely because positive pressure ventilation affects fluid balance (intake and output). Fluid intake is recorded by adding all fluids received by the patient to include fluids provided via the intravenous, oral, and nasogastric routes. Fluid output is commonly done by measuring the urine output. **Oliguria** indicates fluid inadequacy and may occur as a result of system malfunctions, decreased renal perfusion, decreased fluid intake and decreased cardiac output. Normal urine output is 50 to 60 ml/hr. Urine output of below 20 ml/hr (or 400 ml in a 24-hour period or 160 ml in 8 hours) is indicative of fluid inadequacy (Kraus et al., 1993).

Reduction in cardiac output can be directly attributed to decreased venous return secondary to positive pressure ventilation and increased intrathoracic pressure. Positive pressure ventilation also causes an increase in the production of antidiuretic hormone (ADH) which further reduces the urine output.

oliguria: Below normal urine output.

☑ Oliguria may be seen after bleeding, diarrhea, renal failure, shock, drug poisoning, deep coma, or hypertrophy of the prostate.

☑ Normal urine output is 50 to 60 ml/hr.

ANION GAP

Table 9-5 shows a typical set of electrolyte parameters with their normal results. Using some of these parameters, the anion gap may be calculated and used to assess a patient's overall electrolyte balance. Anion gap is the relationship of the cations (sodium [Na^+] and potassium [K^+]) to the

TABLE 9-5 Normal Serum Electrolytes

CATION	CONCENTRATION (mEq/L)	ANION	CONCENTRATION (mEq/L)
Na^+	140 (138 to 142)	Cl^-	103 (101 to 105)
K^+	4 (3 to 5)	HCO_3^-	25 (23 to 27)
Ca^{++}	5 (4.5 to 5.5)	Protein	16 (14 to 18)
Mg^{++}	2 (1.5 to 2.5)	HPO_4^{--}, $H_2PO_4^-$	2 (1.5 to 2.5)
		SO_4^{--}	1 (0.8 to 1.2)
		Organic acids	4 (3.5 to 4.5)
Total cations	151	Total Anions	151

anions (chloride [Cl^-] and bicarbonate [HCO_3^-]). The anion gap may be determined as follows:

$$Anion\ gap = Na^+ - Cl^- - HCO_3^-$$
Normal range: 10 to 14 mEq/L

or

$$Anion\ gap = Na^+ + K^+ - Cl^- - HCO_3^-$$
Normal range: 15 to 20 mEq/L

✓ See Appendix 1 for example.

✓ Metabolic acidosis in the presence of a normal anion gap is usually caused by a loss of base.

✓ Metabolic acidosis in the presence of an increased anion gap is usually due to increased fixed acids.

Metabolic Acidosis and Anion Gap. Metabolic acidosis in the presence of a normal anion gap is usually caused by a loss of base. This condition is called hyperchloremic metabolic acidosis because it is usually related to excessive chloride ions in the plasma (Chang, 1999).

Metabolic acidosis in the presence of an increased anion gap is usually due to increased fixed acids. These acids may be produced biologically (e.g., renal failure, diabetic ketoacidosis, lactic acidosis), or they may be added from an external source (e.g., poisoning by salicylates and alcohol) (Chang, 1999).

Respiratory Compensation for Metabolic Acidosis. In ventilator patients with adequate lung function, respiratory compensation of metabolic acidosis in the form of hyperventilation may occur. For this reason, one should not assume that respiratory insufficiency (primary alveolar hyperventilation) is present. The cause of metabolic acidosis must be identified and corrected. Furthermore, the ventilator rate must not be reduced under this condition because persistent hyperventilation by the patient will likely continue (Rooth, 1974).

✓ Severe K^+ depletion can lead to metabolic alkalosis and compensatory hypoventilation.

Metabolic Alkalosis. It is also important to monitor a patient's potassium level during mechanical ventilation. Severe K^+ depletion can lead to metabolic alkalosis and compensatory hypoventilation (Adams & Hahn, 1982). This may prolong the weaning process when mechanical ventilation is needed to supplement the decreasing spontaneous ventilation.

ARTERIAL BLOOD GASES

Arterial blood gas (ABG) analysis provides useful information about a patient's ventilation ($PaCO_2$), oxygenation (PaO_2), and acid-base (pH) status. It is therefore an essential monitoring tool for patients receiving mechanical ventilation as these patients often have gas exchange and acid-base abnormalities. Table 9-6 shows the normal ABG values for adult patients.

TABLE 9-6   Blood Gas Parameters and Normal Range for Adult

MONITORING FUNCTION	PARAMETER	NORMAL (P_B 760 mm Hg)	(P_B 630 mm Hg)
Ventilation	$PaCO_2$	35 to 45 mm Hg	32 to 42 mm Hg
Oxygenation	PaO_2	80 to 100 mm Hg	60 to 80 mm Hg
Acid-Base	pH	7.35 to 7.45	7.32 to 7.42
	HCO_3^-	22 to 26 mEq/L	
	B.E.	−2 to 2 mEq/L	

ASSESSMENT OF VENTILATORY STATUS

Direct measurement of arterial carbon dioxide tension ($PaCO_2$) via arterial puncture or indwelling catheter is the most accurate method of assessing a patient's ventilatory status. Hypoventilation and respiratory acidosis are present when the $PaCO_2$ is increased with a concurrent decrease in pH. This condition may be corrected by increasing the rate or tidal volume on the ventilator. On the other hand, the rate or tidal volume should be reduced when hyperventilation and respiratory alkalosis occur.

When the acid-base imbalance is caused by metabolic acidosis or alkalosis, it calls for a different ventilator management strategy. The underlying metabolic problem must be corrected before changing the ventilator settings. Ventilator tidal volume or rate adjustment should not be made to "correct" metabolic acid-base abnormalities during mechanical ventilation.

Respiratory Fatigue.   The ventilator patient who develops hypercapnic respiratory failure secondary to increased carbon dioxide - production (VCO_2) should be monitored closely. The VCO_2 may be increased due to a hypermetabolic state. This condition may lead to increased minute ventilation in an attempt to keep up with the increasing CO_2 production. A prolonged increase in the work of breathing may lead to respiratory muscle fatigue and ventilatory failure. It has been documented that excessive work of breathing (minute ventilation in excess of 10 L/min.) is often associated with poor outcomes when trying to wean the patient from mechanical ventilation (Stoller, 1991).

Patients with depressed central respiratory drive, elevated V_D/V_T, diminished compliance, or respiratory muscle weakness may also develop respiratory fatigue as they are unable to maintain an increased minute ventilation over an extended period of time.

ASSESSMENT OF OXYGENATION STATUS

Changes in the patient's oxygen status are commonly assessed by: (1) arterial oxygen tension (PaO_2), (2) alveolar-arterial oxygen tension gradient [P(A-a)O$_2$ or (A-a)DO$_2$], and (3) arterial to alveolar oxygen tension ratio (PaO$_2$/PAO$_2$). A decreased PaO$_2$, an increased P(A-a)O$_2$, or a decreased PaO$_2$/PAO$_2$ reflects tissue hypoxia. Table 9-7 outlines the guideline for interpretation of a patient's oxygenation status.

In general, a decrease in PaO$_2$ with concurrent increase in P(A-a)O$_2$ is indicative of hypoxemia due to **diffusion defect**, V/Q mismatch or shunt. A decrease in PaO$_2$ with little or no increase in P(A-a)O$_2$ is probably due to hypoventilation and this can be confirmed by an elevated PaCO$_2$ (Tobin, 1990).

P(A-a)O$_2$ is the difference of PAO$_2$ and PaO$_2$. It can be calculated as follows:

$$P(A-a)O_2 = PAO_2 - PaO_2$$

PaO$_2$ is obtained from arterial blood gas analysis and PAO$_2$ can be calculated by the simplified alveolar air equation, as follows:

$$PAO_2 = (P_B - PH_2O) \times F_IO_2 - (PaCO_2/R)$$

P$_B$ = Barometric Pressure, PH$_2$O = water vapor pressure (generally 47 mm Hg at 37 °C), and R = Respiratory Quotient (estimated to be 0.8 and it may be deleted from equation when the F$_I$O$_2$ is greater than 60%). PAO$_2$ is mainly affected by changes of F$_I$O$_2$, PaCO$_2$ and P$_B$.

Hypoventilation. Acute hypoventilation causes CO$_2$ retention (increased PaCO$_2$) and respiratory acidosis. Without supplemental oxygen, hypoventilation leads to hypoxemia as well. This type of hypoxemia should not be treated with oxygen alone as the underlying condition can only be corrected by improving the alveolar ventilation.

diffusion defect: *Pathologic condition leading to impaired gas exchange through the alveolar-capillary membrane. An example is interstitial or pulmonary edema.*

✓ Acute hypoventilation causes respiratory acidosis.

TABLE 9-7 Interpretation of Oxygenation Status

PARAMETERS	CRITERIA	INTERPRETATION
PaO$_2$	80-100 mm Hg	Normal
	60-79 mm Hg	Mild hypoxemia
	40-59 mm Hg	Moderate hypoxemia
	< 40 mm Hg	Severe hypoxemia
P(A-a)O$_2$	Room air	Should be less than 4 mm Hg for every 10 years of age, otherwise hypoxemia
	100% O$_2$	Every 50 mm Hg difference approximates 2% shunt
PaO$_2$/PAO$_2$	F$_I$O$_2 \geq$ 30%	> 75% Normal
		< 75% Hypoxemia

(Data from Malley, 1990; Shapiro et al., 1994.)

ventilation/perfusion (V/Q) mismatch: An abnormal distribution of ventilation and pulmonary blood flow. High V/Q is related to dead-space ventilation, whereas low V/Q is associated with intrapulmonary shunting.

intrapulmonary shunting: Pulmonary circulation that does not come in contact with ventilated alveoli.

☑ When the PaO_2 is decreased with little or no change in $PaCO_2$, V/Q mismatch or intrapulmonary shunt should be suspected.

☑ Hypoxemia caused by intrapulmonary shunting does not respond well to high concentrations of oxygen.

☑ PEEP and oxygen are usually required to correct hypoxemia caused by intrapulmonary shunting.

Ventilation/Perfusion Mismatch.   When PaO_2 is decreased with little or no change in $PaCO_2$, **ventilation/perfusion (V/Q) mismatch** or intrapulmonary shunt should be suspected. Hypoxemia caused by ventilation/perfusion (V/Q) mismatch is characterized by a normal or low $PaCO_2$, and this type of hypoxemia responds well to moderate levels of supplemental oxygen.

Intrapulmonary Shunting.   Hypoxemia caused by **intrapulmonary shunting** does not respond well to high concentrations of oxygen. This is because shunted blood does not come in contact with ventilated (oxygenated) alveoli. The $PaCO_2$ is usually normal or low because the peripheral chemoreceptors respond readily to hypoxemia by increasing the minute ventilation (Bone, 1985).

   Positive end-expiratory pressure (PEEP) in conjunction with oxygen are usually required to correct hypoxemia caused by intrapulmonary shunting. If hypoventilation is present as documented by an increased $PaCO_2$, ventilatory assistance may also be necessary.

Diffusion Defects.   Diffusion abnormalities can cause hypoxemia by three mechanisms: (1) low oxygen pressure gradient, (2) increased alveolar-capillary thickness, and (3) decreased alveolar surface area.

   Low alveolar-arterial oxygen tension gradient is usually due to reduction in alveolar PO_2. Oxygen therapy increases the alveolar PO_2 and alveolar-arterial PO_2 tension gradient. It is therefore very effective in correcting hypoxemia caused by uncomplicated diffusion defect.

   Increased alveolar-capillary thickness can be seen in conditions such as pneumonia, and pulmonary and interstitial edema. In mild and uncomplicated cases, hypoxemia may be corrected by oxygen therapy.

   Decreased alveolar surface area can be seen in emphysema due to destruction of the lung tissues (Tobin, 1990). This type of structural defect is not reversible, but the diffusion problem may be partially managed by oxygen therapy.

LIMITATIONS OF BLOOD GASES

Blood gas analysis and monitoring is not without its limitations. Arterial blood sampling is an invasive procedure requiring the puncture of an artery or placement of an arterial catheter. Inaccurate results can occur with introduction of air bubbles, dilution with excessive heparin, or with faulty handling of the sample itself. It is also important to keep in mind that blood gas values reflect an isolated moment in time rather than a trend. They should be used to correlate and document trends established by noninvasive monitoring devices such as pulse oximetry. Finally, arterial blood gas measurements are generally a late indicator of respiratory failure and of limited use as an early warning sign (Tobin, 1990). Nevertheless, arterial blood gases can still provide very useful information when used in conjunction with other monitoring techniques.

OXYGEN SATURATION MONITORING

Oxygen saturation is traditionally measured by arterial blood gases. The arterial oxygen saturation (SaO_2) is not always readily available. A simple and noninvasive method to monitor the oxygen saturation is by using a **pulse oximeter.** The pulse oximetry oxygen saturation (SpO_2) is less accurate than SaO_2 but it can provide quick spot checks or a trend reflecting a patient's oxygenation status.

pulse oximeter: A device that estimates arterial oxygen saturation (SpO_2) by emitting dual wavelengths of light through a pulsating vascular bed.

PULSE OXIMETRY

Pulse oximetry has become perhaps the most frequently used method of assessing a patient's oxygenation status. This noninvasive method measures the approximate oxyhemoglobin saturation (SpO_2). It is safe and easy to use. Pulse oximeters may be used intermittently to "spot check" the SpO_2 or continuously to monitor the patient's SpO_2 trend. Figures 9-5A and B show two portable pulse oximeters and Figure 9-6 illustrates a stationary unit.

The pulse oximeter works by emitting dual wavelengths of light through a pulsating vascular field (Figure 9-7). Proper placement of the probe is necessary to obtain an accurate reading (Figure 9-8). The heart rate is also measured as the oximeter evaluates each arterial pulse (Figure 9-9). If the heart rate on the oximeter varies significantly from the actual pulse as measured by palpation or cardiac monitor, one should verify the accuracy of the SpO_2 reading. It should however be noted that a good match of actual and oximetry heart rates does not necessarily indicate an accurate SpO_2 reading. The accuracy of the SpO_2 reading should be verified by periodic arterial blood gases.

ACCURACY AND CLINICAL USE OF PULSE OXIMETRY

Pulse oximetry has been used as a reliable noninvasive means of monitoring oxygenation in ventilator patients. Figure 9-10 shows a saturation >95% by pulse oximeter correlates with a PaO_2 >70 mm Hg with a sensitivity of 100% (Niehoff, Delguercio & LaMorte et al., 1988).

SpO_2 can be used to facilitate F_IO_2 weaning of a ventilator patient. The F_IO_2 may be reduced to an appropriate level by use of a single arterial blood gas measurement followed by multiple pulse oximetry measurements (Rotello, Warren & Jastremski et al., 1992). Oxygenation of the ventilator-dependent patient can be assured when the SpO_2 is kept above 92% to 95% as this level correlates with a PaO_2 above

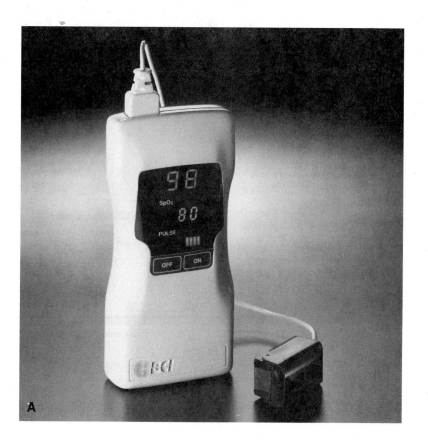

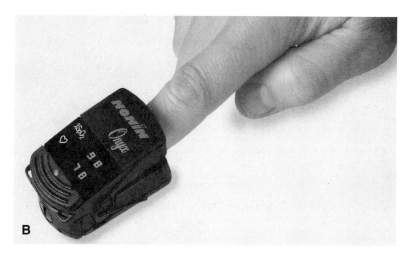

Figure 9-5 Portable pulse oximeters. [(A) Courtesy of BCI International (B) Courtesy of Nonin Medical, Inc., Plymouth, Minn.]

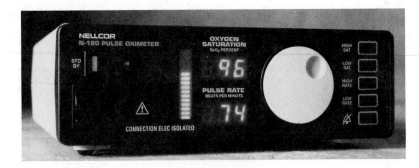

Figure 9-6 Stationary pulse oximeter. (Courtesy of Nellcor Incorporated, Pleasanton, Calif.)

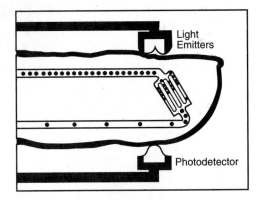

Figure 9-7 Functional view of a pulse oximeter sensor. The light source passes through the pulsating capillary bed to a photodetector. (Courtesy of Nellcor Incorporated, Pleasanton, Calif.)

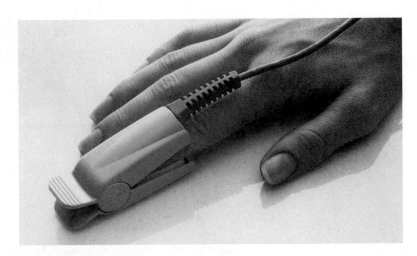

Figure 9-8 Proper placement of a pulse oximeter sensor. (Courtesy of Nellcor Incorporated, Pleasanton, Calif.)

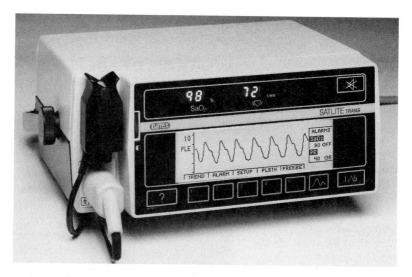

Figure 9-9 A pulse oximeter capable of monitoring SpO_2 and heart rate. (Courtesy of Datex Medical Instrumentation, Inc., Tewksbury, Mass.)

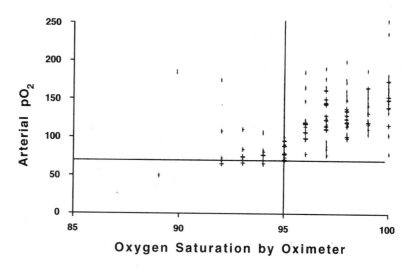

Figure 9-10 Comparison between PaO_2 by ABG measurement and O_2 Sat by pulse oximetry. The relationship is best described as a logarithmic function: $\ln(PaO_2) = 0.088\ (O_2\ Sat) - 3.736\ (r = 0.65, p < 0.0001)$. Note that a saturation >95% by pulse oximetry correlated with a $PaO_2 > 70$ mm Hg with a sensitivity of 100%. From J. Niehoff et al. "Efficacy of pulse oximetry and capnometry in postoperative ventilatory weaning." *Crit Care Med* *16*(7): 701–705, 1988. Used with permission of Williams and Wilkins.

60 mm Hg (Jubran & Tobin, 1990). Table 9-8 outlines other clinical applications of pulse oximeter.

LIMITATIONS OF PULSE OXIMETRY

SpO_2 has good correlation with arterial oxygen saturation (SaO_2) when the SaO_2 is 95% or greater (Niehoff, Delguercio & LaMorte et al., 1988). SpO_2 becomes less accurate as SaO_2 decreases and overestimation of a patient's oxygenation status may result.

The accuracy of pulse oximetry can be affected by factors such as artifact and underlying patient conditions. Artifact due to motion remains a cause of inaccurate measurement despite corrective efforts (Pologe, 1987). Sunlight has been reported to give a falsely high SpO_2 measurement (Abbott, 1986). Nail polish (primarily blue, green, and black), and intravascular dyes can also give a falsely low SpO_2 reading (Welch, DeCesare & Hess, 1990). Improper placement of the oximeter probe can give a faulty SpO_2 reading as well. If a patient is wearing nail polish, the probe may be placed sideways (White, 1989).

Pathologic factors such as low perfusion states and presence of **dyshemoglobins** may lead to SpO_2 measurements that are higher than the actual SaO_2 (Schnapp & Cohen, 1990). Table 9-9 shows the factors that affect the accuracy of pulse oximetry.

dyshemoglobins:
Hemoglobins that do not carry oxygen (e.g., carboxyhemoglobin, methemoglobin). In the presence of dyshemoglobins, pulse oximeter reads higher than actual SaO_2.

TABLE 9-8   Clinical Applications of Pulse Oximetry

CLINICAL APPLICATION	EXAMPLES
Monitor oxygenation status	Mechanical ventilation Intubation Surgery
Titrate F_IO_2	Increase F_IO_2 in hypoxemia Decrease F_IO_2 in weaning
Verify ABG accuracy	Compare O_2 saturation readings to rule out venous sample

TABLE 9-9   Factors That Affect the Accuracy of Pulse Oximetry

FACTORS	TYPE OF INACCURACY
Sunlight Nail polish Fluorescent light Intravenous dyes	SpO_2 measures lower than actual SaO_2.
Dyshemoglobins (methemoglobin, sulfahemoglobin, carboxyhemoglobin) Low perfusion states	SpO_2 measures higher than actual SaO_2.

INNOVATIONS IN PULSE OXIMETRY

A new technology for pulse oximetry has been developed to counter-act common problems such as motion artifacts and low perfusion states (Barker, Novak & Morgan, 1997). This new innovation uses an adaptive filtering technology to separate the arterial pulse signal from nonarterial interference. Laboratory and clinical tests have shown that this new technology can provide accurate pulse oximetry readings during patient motion, low blood flow to the extremities in adults and neonates, unfavorable ambient lights, and electrical noises. These new pulse oximeters are marketed by several manufacturers (Rushworth, 1999).

END-TIDAL CARBON DIOXIDE MONITORING

end-tidal carbon dioxide monitoring: *The CO_2 level measured at the end of exhalation; measured in mm Hg pressure units.*

End-tidal carbon dioxide monitoring is done to monitor a patient's ventilatory status. Once a good correlation is established between $PaCO_2$ and end-tidal PCO_2 ($PetCO_2$), the number of routine blood gases may be reduced. In addition, changes of the $PetCO_2$ values and waveforms may also be obtained and interpreted for additional information about the patient/ventilator system.

CAPNOGRAPHY

Capnography is a measurement of the partial pressure of carbon dioxide in a gas sample. When the sample is collected at the end of inspiration, it is called end-tidal partial pressure of carbon dioxide ($PetCO_2$). $PetCO_2$ monitoring provides real time, noninvasive analysis of a patient's expired CO_2 trend during mechanical ventilation. See Figures 9-11 and 9-12 for examples of end-tidal CO_2 monitors.

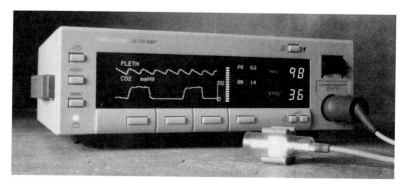

Figure 9-11 End-tidal CO_2 monitor with pulse oximetry capability. (Courtesy of Nellcor Incorporated, Pleasanton, Calif.)

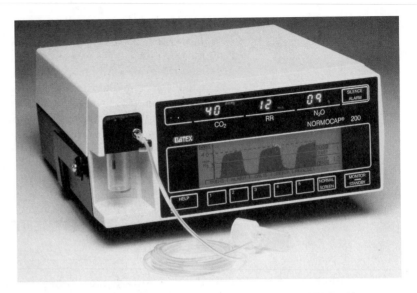

Figure 9-12 End-tidal CO_2 monitor. (Courtesy of Datex Medical Instrumentation, Inc., Tewksbury, Mass.)

The exhaled CO_2 from the patient ventilator circuit is collected and measured by the infrared absorption technique (Hess, 1990). A mainstream sensor is placed directly onto the ventilator circuit, usually attached to an adaptor on the endotracheal tube. A sidestream sensor aspirates a sample of gas via a small tube connected to the endotracheal tube adapter. Figure 9-13 illustrates these two types of sensors.

The major advantage of mainstream analysis is the fast response time between actual CO_2 sampling and the display update. The disadvantage of the mainstream adapter is its excessive weight on the endotracheal tube as well as the additional deadspace in the ventilator/patient circuit. With mainstream sampling, water condensation does not affect analysis; however, secretion buildup on the cell windows can affect the accuracy. A mainstream analyzer also tends to be more frequently handled than the sidestream sensor as the clinician must disconnect it manually to suction the patient (Shelley, 1989).

A sidestream analyzer (aspirating analyzer) places the analyzing mechanism safely within the monitor and draws a sample via a tubing connected at the patient's airway (e.g., endotracheal tube). The major advantage with sidestream analysis is the ease of handling and it can be attached to other patient devices (e.g., cannula, mask). The major disadvantage is that with periodic aspiration of air samples, secretions and water can be drawn into the sampling tube and cause an occlusion. Lag time for CO_2 display is slightly (a few tenths of a second) longer than the mainstream analyzer but it is negligible. Equipment contamination may be a problem with the sidestream analyzer (Shelley, 1989).

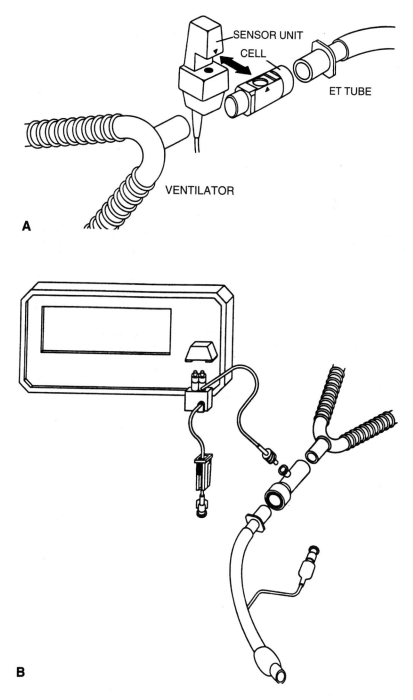

Figure 9-13 (A) Mainstream capnography sensor; (B) Sidestream capnography sensor. (Courtesy of Criticare Systems, Inc. Waukesha, Wisc.)

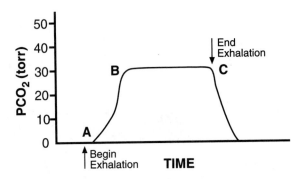

Figure 9-14 The normal capnogram. (A, phase I) PCO$_2$ remains zero as gas exits from the anatomic deadspace; (A to B, phase II) PCO$_2$ rises rapidly as alveolar gas mixes with deadspace gas; (B to C, phase III) alveolar plateau shows gas flow from alveoli; Point (C) is called the end-tidal PCO$_2$ (PetCO$_2$). (From D. Hess, "Capnometry and capnography: technical aspects, physiologic aspects, and clinical applications." *Respir Care 35*(6):557–576, 1990. (Used with permission.)

CAPNOGRAPHY WAVEFORMS AND CLINICAL APPLICATIONS

A capnogram (Figure 9-14) shows the changes in P$_E$CO$_2$ during a complete respiratory cycle. The P$_E$CO$_2$ remains at zero during inspiration. At the beginning of expiration, the P$_E$CO$_2$ remains at zero as anatomic deadspace volume and exits the airways. The P$_E$CO$_2$ then increases dramatically as alveolar gas begins mixing with deadspace gas. Then, for the larger part of expiration, the curve plateaus, reflecting alveolar gas. The end of the "alveolar plateau" is called the end-tidal PCO$_2$.

Transitory events can be examined by review of the capnographic tracing. The capnogram can be useful in determining accidental esophageal intubations, endotracheal tube cuff leaks, and airway obstructions. It can also be used to determine the synchronization of respiratory rates between the patient and ventilator. Some other clinical applications for capnography include use during weaning, cardiopulmonary resuscitation, intubation, bronchoscopy, and hypocapnic management of patients with head trauma (Carlon, Ray & Mordownik et al., 1988; Hess, 1990). The capnographs do not provide absolute measurements but they can be used to follow the PCO$_2$ changes in hemodynamically stable trauma patients (Hess, 1990). Figure 9-15 shows the representative capnograms that correlate with some common clinical conditions.

P(a-et)CO$_2$ GRADIENT

Figure 9-16 shows that the correlation between PaCO$_2$ and PetCO$_2$ is excellent (Niehoff, Delguercio & LaMorte et al., 1988). The P(a-et)CO$_2$ gradient (difference) between these two measurements is about 2 mm Hg

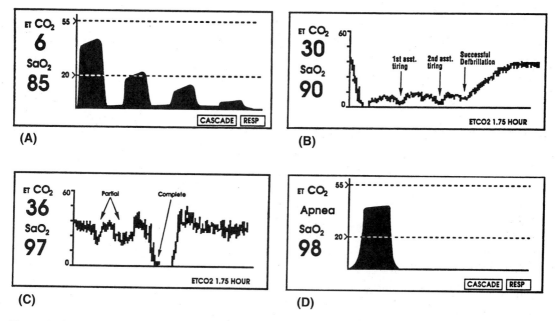

Figure 9-15 Abnormal capnograms monitored via real time or trend screen. (A) Cardiac arrest (real time). The PetCO₂ values drop suddenly and proportionally. This condition indicates lung perfusion is inadequate due to a decreased cardiac output. (B) Effectiveness of external compressions can be monitored by the resultant rise in PetCO₂ as shown in the trend screen. (C) Kinked ET tube (trend screen). As the ET tube is obstructed (partially or completely), the PetCO₂ values reflect the degree of obstruction. With complete obstruction, zero PetCO₂ is seen. (D) Disconnection. Immediate disappearance of the PetCO₂ values and waveform are observed. (Courtesy of Criticare Systems, Inc. Waukesha, Wisc.)

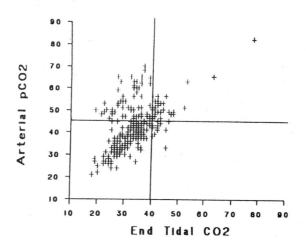

Figure 9-16 Comparison between PaCO₂ by ABG measurement and PetCO₂ by capnometry. The relationship is best described as linear: $PaCO_2 = 0.72 (PetCO_2) + 18.5$ (r = 0.52 p < 0.0001). From J. Niehoff et al. "Efficacy of pulse oximetry and capnometry in postoperative ventilatory weaning." *Crit Care Med 16*(7): 701–705, 1988. Used with permission of Williams and Wilkins.

TABLE 9-10   Factors That Increase the P(a-et)CO$_2$ Gradient

CLINICAL CONDITION	FACTORS
Ventilation	Increased deadspace ventilation
	Positive pressure ventilation
Perfusion	Decreased cardiac output
	Decreased pulmonary perfusion
	Cardiac arrest
	Pulmonary embolic disease
Temperature	Hyperthermia
	Hypothermia

in normal individuals. For critical patients, a gradient of 5 mm Hg is considered acceptable.

The P(a-et)CO$_2$ gradient is primarily affected by alveolar deadspace ventilation (Perel & Stock, 1992), old age, presence of pulmonary disease, and changes in mechanical volume and modality. Table 9-10 lists some specific conditions that increase the P(a-et)CO$_2$ gradient.

Disposable ETCO$_2$ Detector.   Capnography can also be estimated via a low cost, disposable, plastic, CO$_2$ (pH) sensitive device (Figure 9-17). With this device attached to the endotracheal tube, one can quickly differentiate tracheal from esophageal intubation (Hess, 1990). This occurs when the pH-sensitive device on the material senses the changes in CO$_2$ concentration.

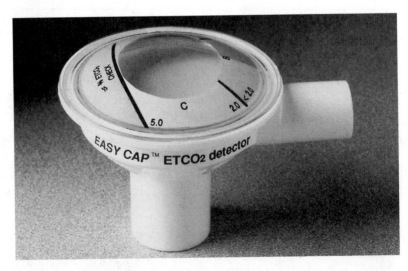

Figure 9-17   Disposable EASY CAP™ ETCO$_2$ detector. (Courtesy of Nellcor Incorporated, Pleasanton, Calif.)

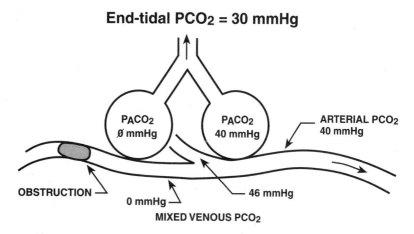

End-tidal PCO2 = 30 mmHg

Figure 9-18   Deadspace ventilation induced by blockage of a portion of the pulmonary blood flow (e.g., pulmonary embolism). This condition leads to a reduced PetCO$_2$ reading.

✓ Capnography readings reflect only changes in a patient's ventilatory status, rather than improvement or deterioration of the patient.

✓ Decreased PetCO$_2$ may not be indicative of improvement in gas exchange.

LIMITATIONS OF CAPNOGRAPHY MONITORING

Capnography readings reflect only changes in a patient's ventilatory status, rather than improvement or deterioration of the patient (Whitaker, 1997). An example of this is deadspace ventilation as seen in pulmonary embolism (Figure 9-18). A decrease in PetCO$_2$ due to physiological deadspace ventilation does not mean that the patient's ventilatory status has improved. Lowering the ventilator rate in this situation could lead to grave consequences.

Other conditions leading to an increase in deadspace ventilation (thus a decrease in PetCO$_2$) are hypotension and high intrathoracic pressure secondary to mechanical ventilation (Whitaker, 1997). This could cause the practitioner to incorrectly assume that the decreased PetCO$_2$ indicates an improvement in gas exchange.

TRANSCUTANEOUS BLOOD GAS MONITORING

Transcutaneous blood gas monitoring involves placement of a miniature Clark (PO$_2$) or a Severinghaus (PCO$_2$) electrode on the skin via a double-sided adhesive disk. A heating coil in the electrode increases the permeability of the epidermis thus facilitating diffusion of gas from the underlying capillaries to the electrode. Transcutaneous blood gas monitoring has been used more often in neonates than in adults (Eberhard, Mint & Schafer, 1981). Figures 9-19 and 9-20 show two examples of transcutaneous O$_2$ and CO$_2$ monitors.

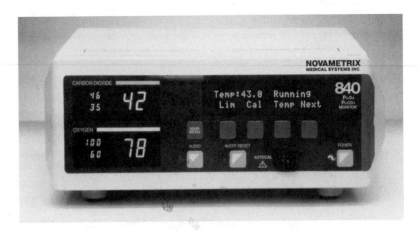

Figure 9-19 Transcutaneous PCO₂ and PO₂ monitor. (Courtesy of Novametrix Medical Systems, Inc., Wallingford, Conn.)

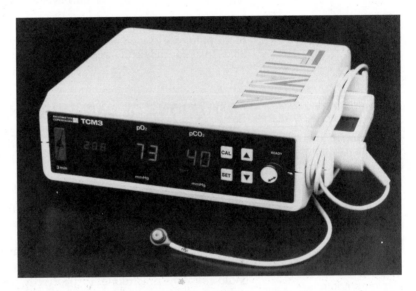

Figure 9-20 Transcutaneous PCO₂ and PO₂ monitor. (Courtesy of Radiometer America, Inc., Westlake, Ohio.)

TRANSCUTANEOUS PO₂ (PtcO₂)

transcutaneous PtcO₂: *Measurement of PO₂ through the skin by means of a miniature Clark (PO₂) electrode.*

In neonates, the **transcutaneous PO₂ (PtcO₂)** closely approximates the PaO₂. But in adults, the PtcO₂ measures lower than the actual PO₂ due to thicker skin in adults. For this reason, pulse oximetry has become the preferred method to monitor the oxygenation status of adult patients.

PtcO₂ also approximates the central organ PO₂ (Tremper, Waxman & Shoemaker, 1979). It has a good correlation with the cardiac output changes in a ventilator patient (Shapiro et al., 1989). In addition, a fall in PtcO₂ can be associated with a need for suctioning, misplaced endotracheal tube, pneumothorax, or other causes of hypoxemia (Pilbeam, 1999).

✓ Accuracy of the PtcO$_2$ electrode is affected by skin edema, hypothermia, and capillary perfusion status.

Limitations. Accuracy of the PtcO$_2$ electrode is affected by skin edema, hypothermia, and capillary perfusion status. PtcO$_2$ is a better predictor of PaO$_2$ when it falls below 80 mm Hg. However, the PtcO$_2$ becomes less accurate when the PaO$_2$ is greater than 80 mm Hg (Figure 9-21) (Palmisano & Severinghaus, 1990). When cardiac output decreases, as with the patient in shock, a disproportionate fall in PtcO$_2$ occurs.

Two other disadvantages of transcutaneous monitors are the need for frequent site changes (every three to four hours) to prevent heat damage to skin and long equilibration times after each site change.

TRANSCUTANEOUS PCO$_2$ (PtcCO$_2$)

transcutaneous PtcCO$_2$: Measurement of PCO$_2$ through the skin by means of a miniature Severinghaus (PCO$_2$) electrode.

Transcutaneous PCO$_2$ (PtcCO$_2$) monitoring is done to provide a means of continuous ventilatory assessment. The PtcCO$_2$ is measured by heating the underlying skin to 44°C (40 to 42°C in neonates), which facilitates CO$_2$ diffusion across the skin to the CO$_2$ electrode.

The correlation between PtcCO$_2$ and PaCO$_2$ is good in neonates as long as perfusion is normal. This correlation in adults shows mixed results, but in general the PtcCO$_2$ may be useful as a monitoring tool once the trend has been established.

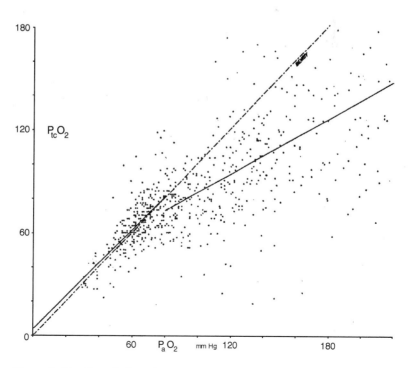

Figure 9-21 Correlation of PaO$_2$ to PtcO$_2$. [Reprinted with permission from *J Clin Monit* (1990, July), *6*(3), 192.]

Limitations. It should be noted that $PtcCO_2$ values are usually higher than $PaCO_2$ values. This is due to increased CO_2 production as underlying tissues are heated (Marini, 1988). In addition, during shock or low perfusion states, the $PtcCO_2$ measures higher than the actual $PaCO_2$ due to increased accumulation of tissue CO_2 (Tremper & Shoemaker, 1981).

SUMMARY

Monitoring in mechanical ventilation is done to provide information about the condition of the patient and the overall effectiveness of a treatment plan. The results obtained from different monitoring techniques should be used and interpreted together and should not be treated as isolated measurements. For example, a decrease in end-tidal CO_2 may indicate the presence of deadspace ventilation. But this assumption must be confirmed with other supporting evidence such as a concurrent decrease in perfusion (decrease in cardiac output or other hemodynamic values). Trending or interpreting a series of measurements is also more meaningful since the overall condition of a patient is a dynamic process, not a set of separated events.

Finally, the condition of the patient should be assessed in conjunction with the monitoring results. This is because the patient may temporarily compensate for abnormal conditions under extremely stressful settings. This erroneous "normal" measurement may not be apparent by reviewing the laboratory results alone. Therefore, careful examination of the patient should always be a vital part of monitoring in mechanical ventilation.

Self-Assessment Questions

1. A patient in the intensive care unit suddenly develops shortness of breath and the SpO_2 drops to 87%. You would anticipate all of the following vital sign measurements to increase with the *exception* of:

   A. heart rate.
   B. minute ventilation.
   C. respiratory rate.
   D. temperature.

2. Prolonged suctioning of the lungs via the endotracheal tube is not advised because this can induce:

   A. hypovolemia and shock.
   B. bradycardia and arrhythmia.
   C. hyperventilation.
   D. productive coughs.

3. One of the complications of positive pressure ventilation is that it can cause a(n) _____ venous return and _____.

   A. increased, hypertension
   B. increased, hypotension
   C. decreased, hypertension
   D. decreased, hypotension

4. A blood gas sample was collected from a hypothermic patient whose core temperature was 24°C. If the sample was analyzed at 37°C with a PO_2 of 90 mm Hg, the temperature corrected PO_2 (to patient's 24°C) would be:

   A. negligible or almost 90 mm Hg.
   B. much higher than 90 mm Hg.

   C. much lower than 90 mm Hg.
   D. dependent on the position of the oxyhemoglobin curve.

5. A physician asks you to evaluate the breath sounds of a patient who has an admitting diagnosis of pneumonia. By placing the stethoscope diaphragm next to the side of the spine below the scapula, you are listening to the breath sounds of the _____ segments of the _____ lobes.

   A. posterior, upper
   B. superior, middle

   C. posterior, middle
   D. superior, lower

6 to 9. Match the breath sounds with the conditions that may be the cause of these abnormalities. Use each answer only once.

Breath Sound	Condition
6. Diminished or absent	A. Lung consolidation
7. Wheezes	B. Airway obstruction
8. Inspiratory crackles	C. Excessive secretions
9. Coarse crackles	D. Airway narrowing

10. Excessive positive pressure or volume during mechanical ventilation may _____ the intrathoracic pressure and _____ the cardiac and urine outputs.

    A. increase, increase
    B. increase, decrease

    C. decrease, increase
    D. decrease, decrease

11. Metabolic acidosis (low bicarbonate) with a(n) _____ anion gap is called hyperchloremic metabolic acidosis because the excessive chloride (Cl^-) ions _____ the deficiency of bicarbonate (HCO_3^-) ions in the plasma.

    A. normal, offset
    B. normal, aggravate

    C. abnormal, offset
    D. abnormal, aggravate

12. A patient who has been undergoing the weaning process for mechanical ventilation suddenly stops breathing spontaneously. You would expect to see the following changes on the next set of blood gas results *except:*

    A. increase in PO_2.
    B. increase in PCO_2.

    C. decrease in pH.
    D. decrease in HCO_3^-.

13. In blood gas interpretation, the $PaCO_2$ is primarily used to assess a patient's _____ status and the PO_2 is useful for the _____ status.

A. ventilatory, acid-base
B. ventilatory, oxygenation

C. acid-base, oxygenation
D. acid-base, ventilatory

14 to 16. Match the causes of hypoxemia with the characteristics that may be used to distinguish these abnormalities. Use each answer only once.

Cause of Hypoxemia	Characteristics
14. Hypoventilation	A. Normal or low $PaCO_2$; hypoxemia does not respond to high levels of oxygen.
15. V/Q mismatch or diffusion defects	B. High $PaCO_2$; hypoxemia improves with ventilation and low levels of oxygen.
16. Intrapulmonary shunt	C. Normal or low $PaCO_2$; hypoxemia responds very well to moderate levels of oxygen.

17. A patient rescued from a house fire has an admitting diagnosis of severe smoke inhalation. She is breathing spontaneously and receiving 100% oxygen via a nonrebreathing mask. Due to her condition, pulse oximetry _____ be done because _____.

A. should, of cost savings

B. should, continuous monitoring is required

C. should not, the SpO_2 reading will be higher than actual SaO_2
D. should not, the SpO_2 reading will be lower than actual SaO_2

18. In metabolic acidosis, patients with adequate lung function are capable of compensating for this condition by _____. This would cause the end-tidal CO_2 readings to be _____ than normal.

A. hyperventilation, higher
B. hyperventilation, lower

C. hypoventilation, higher
D. hypoventilation, lower

19. Which of the following statements is *not* true regarding transcutaneous oxygen and carbon dioxide monitors?

A. Site changes are required every 3 to 4 hours.
B. Long equilibration time for calibration.

C. Accurate PO_2 and PCO_2 measurements.
D. More accurate in neonatal use.

References

Abbott, M. A. (1986). Monitoring oxygen saturation levels in the early recovery phase of general anesthesia. In T. P. Payne, J. W. Severinghaus (Eds.), *Pulse oximetry* (pp. 165–172). Dorchester: Springer-Verlag.

Adams, A. P., & Hahn, C. E. W. (1982). *Principles and practice of blood gas analysis.* Edinburgh: Churchill Livingstone.

Barker, S. J., & Shah, N. K. (1997). The effects of motion on the performance of pulse oximeters in volunteers. *Anesthesiology, 86,* 101–108.

Bone, R. C. (1985). Monitoring respiratory and hemodynamic function in the patient with respiratory failure. From *Mechanical ventilation.* New York: Churchill Livingstone.

Burton, G. G. et al. (1991). Respiratory care: A guide to clinical practice (4th ed.). Philadelphia: J.B. Lippincott.

Carlon, G., Ray, C., & Mordownik, S. et al. (1988). Capnography in mechanically ventilated patients. *Crit Care Med, 16,* 550–556.

Chang, D. W. (1999). *Respiratory care calculations* (2nd ed.). Albany, NY: Delmar Publishers, Inc.

Eberhard, P., Mindt, W., & Schafer, R. (1981). Cutaneous blood gas monitoring in the adult. *Crit Care Med, 9,* 702–705.

Gravelyn, T. R., & Weg, J. R. (1980). Respiratory rate as an indicator of acute respiratory dysfunction. *JAMA, 244,* 1123–1125.

Hess, D. (1990). Capnometry and capnography: Technical aspects, physiologic aspects, and clinical applications. *Resp Care, 35,* 557–573.

Jubran, A., & Tobin, M. J. (1990). Reliability for pulse oximetry in titrating supplemental oxygen therapy in ventilator-dependent patients. *Chest, 97,* 1420–1425.

Kraus, P. A. et al. (1993). Acute lung injury at Baragwanath ICU—An eight-month audit and call for consensus for other organ failure in the adult respiratory distress syndrome. *Chest, 103*(6), 1832–1836.

Krieger, B. P., & Ershowshy, P. (1994). Noninvasive detection of respiratory failure in the intensive care unit. *Chest, 2,* 254–261.

Malley, W. J. (1990). *Clinical blood gases.* Philadelphia: W.B. Saunders Co.

Marini, J. J. (1988). Monitoring during mechanical ventilation. *Clinics in Chest Med, 9*(1), 73–100.

Niehoff, J., Delguercio, C., & LaMorte, W. et al. (1988). Efficacy of pulse oximetry and capnometry in postoperative ventilatory weaning. *Crit Care Med, 16*(7), 701–705.

Novametrix Medical Systems, Inc. (1991). *Capnograph Monitor Model 1260 User's Manual.* Wallingford, CT.

Palmisano, B. W., & Severinghaus, J. W. (1990). Transcutaneous PCO_2 and PO_2: A multicenter study of accuracy. *J Clin Monit, 6,* 189–195.

Perel, A., & Stock, M. C. (1992). *Handbook of mechanical ventilatory support.* Baltimore: Williams & Wilkins.

Pilbeam, S. P. (1999). *Mechanical ventilation: Physiological and clinical applications* (3rd ed). St. Louis: Mosby-Year Book.

Pologe, J. A. (1987). Pulse oximetry: Technical aspects. *Int Anesthiol Clin, 25,* 137–154.

Rooth, G. (1974). *Acid-base and electrolyte balance.* Chicago: Year Book Med Pub Inc.

Rotello, L. C., Warren, J., & Jastremski, M. S. et al. (1992). A nurse-directed protocol using pulse oximetry to wean mechanically ventilated patients from toxic oxygen concentrations. *Chest, 102,* 1833–1835.

Rushworth, G. T. (1999). Pulse oximetry: Past, present, and future. *RT, 12*(5), 53–56.

Schnapp, L. M., & Cohen, N. H. (1990). Pulse oximetry uses and abuses. *Chest, 98,* 1244–1250.

Shapiro, B. A. et al. (1989). Blood gas monitoring: Yesterday, today, and tomorrow. *Crit Care Med, 17,* 573–581.

Shapiro, B. A. et al. (1994). *Clinical application of blood gases* (5th ed.). St. Louis: Mosby-Year Book.

Shelley, E. J. (1989). *CSI capnography training manual.* Waukesha, WI: Criticare Systems, Inc.

Stoller, J. K. (1991). Establishing clinical unweanability. *Respir Care, 36,* 186–198.

Tobin, M. J. (1990). Respiratory monitoring during mechanical ventilation. *Crit Care Clinics, 6*(3), 679–707.

Tobin, M. J., & Perez, W. et al. (1986). The pattern of breathing during successful and unsuccessful trails of weaning from mechanical ventilation. *Am Rev Respir Dis, 134,* 1111–1118.

Tremper, K., & Shoemaker, W. C. (1981). Transcutaneous oxygen monitoring of critically ill adults with and without low flow shock. *Crit Care Med, 9,* 706–709.

Tremper, K., Waxman, K., & Shoemaker, W. C. (1979). Effects of hypoxia and shock on transcutaneous PO_2 values in dogs. *Crit Care Med, 7,* 526.

Welch, J. P., DeCesare, R., & Hess, D. (1990). Pulse oximetry: Instrumentation and clinical applications. *Respir Care, 35,* 584–601.

Whitaker, K. B. (1997). *Comprehensive perinatal and pediatric respiratory care* (2nd ed.). Albany, NY: Delmar Publishers, Inc.

White, P. F. et al. (1989). Nail polish and oximetry. *Anesth Analg, 68,* 546–547.

Wilkins, R. L., & Dexter, J. R. (1998). *Respiratory Disease—Principles of Patient Care* (2nd ed.). Philadelphia: F.A. Davis Co.

Suggested Reading

Rozycki, H. J., Sysyn, G. D., & Marshall, M. K. et al. (1998). Mainstream end-tidal carbon dioxide monitoring in the neonatal intensive care unit. *Pediatrics, 101*(4 Pt 1), 648–653.

CHAPTER TEN

HEMODYNAMIC WAVEFORM ANALYSIS

David W. Chang
Gary Hamelin

OUTLINE

KEY TERMS

- afterload
- cardiac index
- cardiac output
- central venous pressure
- contractility
- hemodynamic monitoring
- mean arterial pressure

- preload
- pulmonary vascular resistance
- stroke volume
- systemic vascular resistance
- transducer
- venous return

INTRODUCTION

A recent advance in the management of mechanical ventilation is the use of invasive hemodynamic monitoring. This monitoring technology is not intended for every patient who requires mechanical ventilation. But for many critically ill patients, hemodynamic measurements can add valuable information to the clinical management of the patient.

In the most basic sense, hemodynamic monitoring is the measurement of the force (pressure) exerted by the blood in the blood vessels or heart chambers during systole (i.e., contraction and pumping) and diastole (i.e., relaxation and filling).

In addition to systolic and diastolic pressures in both the systemic and pulmonary circulations, hemodynamic monitoring equipment also measures cardiac output and mixed venous oxygen saturation. These and other direct measurements gathered through hemodynamic monitoring can be used to obtain other calculated values.

HEMODYNAMIC MONITORING

hemodynamic monitoring: Measurement of the blood pressure in the vessels or heart chambers during contraction (systole) and relaxation (diastole).

Complete **hemodynamic monitoring** requires the use of the central venous and pulmonary artery catheters. The central venous catheter measures the **central venous pressure** (right ventricular **preload**), and the pulmonary artery catheter measures the pulmonary artery pressure (right ventricular **afterload**) and the pulmonary capillary wedge pressure (left ventricular preload).

TECHNICAL BACKGROUND

Measurement of hemodynamic pressures is based on the principle that liquids are noncompressible and that pressures at any given point within a liquid are transmitted equally. When a closed system is filled with liquid, the pressure exerted at one point can be measured accurately at any other point on the same level. For example, if a catheter

central venous pressure: *Pressure measured in the vena cava or right atrium. It reflects the status of blood volume in the systemic circulation.*

preload: *The end-diastolic stretch of the muscle fiber*

afterload: *The resistance of the blood vessels into which the ventricle is pumping blood. Expressed in pressure units.*

transducer: *A device that converts one type of energy signal into another type of energy signal (e.g., a pressure signal converted into an electronic signal).*

is placed into the radial artery facing the flow of blood and then connected directly to a tubing that is filled with liquid, the pressure exerted by the blood at the tip of the catheter will be accurately transmitted to the liquid-filled tubing. This pressure signal can then be changed to an electronic signal by a **transducer** and amplified and displayed on a monitor as both a waveform and digital display.

Hemodynamic monitoring is generally done by using a combination of arterial catheter, central venous catheter, and pulmonary artery catheter. One or more of these catheters are introduced into the blood vessel, advanced to a suitable location, and then connected to a monitor at the patient's bedside. The display on the monitor is made possible by using a transducer and an amplifier between the catheter and monitor. In hemodynamic monitoring, the transducer converts a pressure signal (in the catheter) to an electronic signal (on the monitor).

To ensure accurate measurements, the transducer, catheter, and measurement site should all be at the same level. Otherwise, the force of gravity will alter the actual readings. For example, a higher reading may be obtained if the transducer and catheter are located lower than the measurement site.

As with other invasive procedures, hemodynamic monitoring should only be used when truly indicated since infection, dysrhythmia, bleeding, and trauma to blood vessels are potential complications.

UNITS OF MEASUREMENT

Hemodynamic pressure readings are measured in units of millimeters of mercury (mm Hg) in the United States and in kilopascals (kPa) in other countries using Systeme International (SI) units. The conversion factors in Table 10-1 may be used to change between mm Hg and kPa pressure units. Hemodynamic readings begin with the atmospheric pressure as the zero point. Since changes in atmospheric pressure are slow and insignificant, adjustments are not necessary in trending a series of measurements.

TYPES OF CATHETERS

Three different catheters are used in hemodynamic monitoring: arterial catheter, central venous catheter, and pulmonary artery catheter. The arterial catheter is used to monitor systemic arterial pressure. Venous pressure is measured by a central venous catheter in the superior vena cava or right atrium. A pulmonary artery

TABLE 10-1   Conversions of mm Hg and kilopascal (kPa)

FROM mm Hg TO pKa	FROM pKa TO mm Hg
mm Hg × 0.133 = pKa	pKa × 7.502 = mm Hg

TABLE 10-2 Insertion Sites, Location, and Uses of Hemodynamic Catheters

CATHETER	INSERTION SITES	LOCATION	COMMON USES
Arterial	Radial (first choice), brachial, femoral, or dorsalis pedis artery	Within systemic artery near insertion site	(1) Measure systemic artery pressure. (2) Collect arterial blood gas samples.
Central venous	Subclavian or internal jugular vein	Superior vena cava near right atrium or within right atrium	(1) Measure central venous pressure. (2) Administer fluid or medication.
Pulmonary artery	Subclavian or internal jugular vein	Branch of pulmonary artery	(1) Measure CVP, PAP, and PCWP. (2) Collect mixed venous blood gas samples. (3) Monitor mixed venous O_2 saturation. (4) Measure cardiac output. (5) Provide cardiac pacing.

☑ The proximal opening in the pulmonary artery catheter can also measure the right atrial pressure (i.e., CVP).

catheter (commonly known as the Swan-Ganz catheter) is used to measure the pulmonary arterial pressure and pulmonary capillary wedge pressure. The proximal opening in the pulmonary artery catheter can also measure the pressure in the right atrium. The insertion sites, location, and uses of hemodynamic catheters are summarized in Table 10-2.

ARTERIAL CATHETER

In hemodynamically unstable patients who are receiving fluid infusion or drugs to improve circulation, heart function and blood vessel caliber, continuous and accurate blood pressure readings are essential. With an arterial catheter, most bedside monitors will display a graphic waveform as well as a digital readout of systolic pressure, diastolic pressure, and **mean arterial pressure.**

mean arterial pressure: The average blood pressure in the arterial circulation. Normal is >60 mm Hg.

INSERTION OF ARTERIAL CATHETER

Systemic arterial pressure is measured by placing an arterial catheter into the radial artery. The brachial, femoral, or dorsalis pedis arteries may also be used, but the radial artery remains the first choice because of the collateral circulation to the hand provided by the ulnar artery. The femoral artery is sometimes used to monitor left atrial pressures during cardiac surgery.

✓ Collateral circulation to the hand must be confirmed by doing the Allen test before radial artery puncture.

Correct placement of the arterial catheter may be assessed by the appearance of an arterial waveform on the monitor (Figure 10-1). Once in place, an arterial line allows for continuous, direct measurement of systemic blood pressure as well as for convenient access to arterial blood samples for repeated blood gas analysis. Although this invasive procedure has potential risks such as bleeding, blood clot, and infection, it has advantages over noninvasive monitoring of blood pressure. Use of a sphygmomanometer (blood pressure cuff) can be simpler and safer but inaccuracies may occur in conditions of increased vascular tone and vasoconstriction (Keckeisen, 1991).

Figure 10-1 shows a normal arterial pressure waveform. The systolic upstroke (C to A) reflects the rapid increase of arterial pressure in the blood vessel during systole (ventricular contraction). The downslope or dicrotic limb (A to C) is caused by the declining pressure that occurs during diastole (ventricular relaxation). The dicrotic notch (B) is caused by the closure of the semilunar valves during diastole. The lowest point (C) of the tracing represents the arterial end-diastolic pressure.

NORMAL ARTERIAL PRESSURE AND MEAN ARTERIAL PRESSURE

The normal arterial pressure values are in the range of 100 to 140 mm Hg systolic and 60 to 90 mm Hg diastolic in most adults. From the systolic and diastolic pressures, the mean arterial pressure may be calculated as follows:

$$MAP = \frac{(P_{systolic} + 2 \times P_{diastolic})}{3}$$

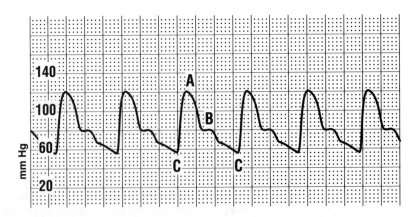

Figure 10-1 Normal arterial pressure waveform. The systolic and diastolic pressures are about 120 mm Hg and 60 mm Hg, respectively. (A) systolic peak; (B) dicrotic notch.

A normal MAP of 60 mm Hg is considered the minimum pressure needed to maintain adequate tissue perfusion (Bustin, 1986). The diastolic value receives greater weight in this formula because the diastolic phase is about twice as long as the systolic phase. Accuracy of blood pressure readings depends on proper setup and calibration of the monitoring system.

Since arterial pressure is the product of **stroke volume** (i.e., blood flow) and vascular resistance, changes in either parameter can affect the arterial pressure. Opposing changes of these two parameters (e.g., increase in stroke volume and decrease in vascular resistance) may present an unchanged arterial pressure or mean arterial pressure. Therefore, interpretation of arterial pressure measurements should take these two factors into consideration.

stroke volume:
Blood volume
pumped by the
ventricles in one
contraction.

PULSE PRESSURE

Pulse pressure is the difference between arterial systolic and diastolic pressure. Since the arterial systolic and diastolic pressures are affected by stroke volume and vascular compliance, pulse pressure can be used to assess the gross changes in stroke volume and/or blood vessel compliance. High pulse pressure may occur in conditions where the stroke volume is high, blood vessel compliance is low, or heart rate is low. Low pulse pressure may occur in conditions where the stroke volume is low, blood vessel compliance is high, or heart rate is high (Christensen, 1992).

High Pulse Pressure. When the stroke volume is increased or the blood vessel compliance is decreased, there is a corresponding increase in systolic pressure. As long as the diastolic pressure does not increase by the same proportion, a high pulse pressure results. Bradycardia may also lead to a higher pulse pressure as a slow heart rate allows the blood volume more time for diastolic runoff and causes a lower diastolic pressure. The conditions that may lead to a high pulse pressure are summarized in Table 10-3.

Low Pulse Pressure. By the same mechanism, a decreased stroke volume or an increased blood vessel compliance leads to a corresponding decrease in systolic pressure. A low pulse pressure is seen as long as the diastolic pressure does not decrease by the same proportion.

TABLE 10-3 Conditions Leading to High Pulse Pressure

CONDITION	EXAMPLE
High stroke volume	Hypervolemia
Noncompliant blood vessel	Arteriosclerosis
Abnormal heart rate	Bradycardia

TABLE 10-4 Conditions Leading to Low Pulse Pressure

CONDITION	EXAMPLE
Low stroke volume	Hypovolemia
High compliance blood vessel	Shock
Abnormal heart rate	Tachycardia

Tachycardia may also lead to a lower pulse pressure because a high heart rate allows the blood volume less time for diastolic runoff and causes a higher diastolic pressure. The conditions leading to a low pulse pressure are summarized in Table 10-4.

POTENTIAL PROBLEMS WITH ARTERIAL CATHETER

Air bubbles and loose tubing connections can "dampen" the pressure signal. Improper leveling of the transducer and catheter can cause false high or false low readings. Inadequate pressure applied to the heparin solution bag can result in backup of blood in the tubing when the arterial pressure becomes higher than the heparin line pressure. Clotting of blood at the catheter tip or blockage of the catheter tip by the wall of the artery can interfere with the hemodynamic signal. The potential problems that are related to the arterial catheter are shown in Table 10-5.

Most intensive care units have standard procedures in place to ensure that such problems are kept to a minimum. Careful adherence to proper setup and calibration of hemodynamic monitoring equipment is essential.

TABLE 10-5 Potential Problems with Arterial Catheter

FACTORS	PROBLEM
Air bubbles in tubing, Loose tubing connections	Dampens the pressure signal
Transducer and catheter placed higher than measurement site	Measurement lower than actual
Transducer and catheter placed lower than measurement site	Measurement higher than actual
Inadequate pressure applied to the heparin solution bag	Backup of blood in the tubing
Blood clot at catheter tip, catheter tip blocked by wall of artery	Inaccurate reading, signal interference

CENTRAL VENOUS CATHETER

> ☑ The CVP can also be monitored via the proximal port of a pulmonary artery catheter.

The central venous pressure (CVP) can be monitored through a central venous catheter placed either in the superior vena cava near the right atrium or in the right atrium. The pressure measured in the right atrium is correctly called right atrial pressure or RAP, but it is commonly called CVP.

The major advantage of the CVP in hemodynamic monitoring is to measure filling pressures in the right heart. The CVP is helpful in assessing fluid status and right heart function. However, it is often late to reflect changes in the left heart. The central venous catheter can also be used to collect "mixed" venous blood samples and for administration of medications and fluids. (Note: A true mixed venous blood sample should be obtained from the pulmonary artery via a pulmonary artery catheter). Figure 10-2 shows the position of the catheter tip of a central venous catheter.

INSERTION OF CENTRAL VENOUS CATHETER

The central venous catheter is commonly inserted through the subclavian vein or the internal jugular vein. Correct placement of the central venous catheter may be assessed by the proper appearance of a venous pressure tracing on the monitor (Figure 10-3). Infection, bleeding, and pneumothorax are potential complications of CVP line insertion.

COMPONENTS OF CENTRAL VENOUS PRESSURE WAVEFORM

Figure 10-3 shows the tracing of a central venous (right atrial) pressure waveform and the corresponding ECG tracing. The upstroke *a* wave reflects right atrial contraction (follows the p wave on the ECG); *c* wave

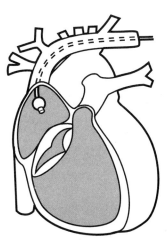

Figure 10-2 Position of a central venous (right atrial) catheter.

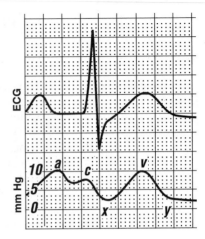

Figure 10-3 Tracing of a central venous pressure waveform and its relationship to the electrocardiogram (ECG).

reflects closure of the tricuspid valve during systole (appears within the QRS complex on the ECG); x downslope occurs as the right atrium relaxes; v wave is caused by right ventricular contraction (appears at the T wave on the ECG); and y downslope reflects ventricular relaxation and rapid filling of blood from the right atrium to the right ventricle.

Abnormal Right Atrial Pressure Waveform. Since each wave or downslope on the right atrial waveform coincides with an event during systole or diastole, changes in the hemodynamic status of the heart will cause changes to certain components of the waveform, particularly the a and v waves (Schriner, 1989).

The a wave on the right atrial waveform may be elevated in conditions in which the resistance to right ventricular filling is increased. Examples include tricuspid valve stenosis, decreased right ventricular compliance due to ischemia or infarction, right ventricular volume overload or failure, pulmonic valve stenosis, and primary pulmonary hypertension. The a wave may be absent if atrial activity is absent or extremely weak.

Reflux of blood into the right atrium during contraction due to an incompetent triscupid valve will cause an elevated v wave. Elevation of a and v waves may be seen in conditions such as cardiac tamponade, volume overload, or left ventricular failure.

NORMAL CVP MEASUREMENT

venous return:
Blood flow from the systemic venous circulation to the right heart.

CVP is reported as a mean pressure and its normal range in the vena cava is from 0 to 6 mm Hg. When the measurement is taken in the right atrium, the normal value range is from 2 to 7 mm Hg, slightly higher than the CVP reading (Christensen, 1992).

TABLE 10-6 Conditions That Affect the Central Venous Pressure

CHANGE	EXAMPLES
Decrease in CVP	Absolute hypovolemia (blood loss, dehydration)
	Relative hypovolemia (shock, vasodilation)
Increase in CVP	Positive pressure ventilation
	Increased **pulmonary vascular resistance**
	Hypervolemia
	Right ventricular failure
	Left ventricular failure (late change in CVP)

pulmonary vascular resistance: Resistance of the arterial system into which the right heart is pumping. Normal range is 50 to 150 dynes.sec/cm5.

CHANGES IN CVP MEASUREMENT

Since **venous return** is determined by the pressure gradient between the mean arterial pressure and CVP, an increased CVP leads to a smaller pressure gradient and a lower blood return to the right heart. This condition is observed during positive pressure ventilation or as a result of right ventricular failure (e.g., reduced compliance of the ventricle after right-sided myocardial infarction). The conditions that may affect the CVP measurements are summarized in Table 10-6.

PULMONARY ARTERY CATHETER

The first pulmonary artery catheter was developed in 1953 and used in dogs by United States physiologists Michael Lategola and Hermann Rahn. In the late 1960s, a more refined pulmonary artery catheter was developed and used in humans by United States physicians Harold James Swan and William Ganz (Swan et al., 1970). The new pulmonary artery catheter (commonly called the Swan-Ganz catheter) is a flow-directed, balloon-tipped catheter. The addition of thermistor (for **cardiac output** measurement), and light reflective fiberoptic element (for mixed venous oxygen saturation measurement) to the catheter greatly expanded the scope and capability of hemodynamic monitoring.

cardiac output: Blood volume pumped by the heart in one minute. Normal range is 4 to 8 L/min.

The pulmonary artery catheter is placed within the pulmonary artery, and it can measure the pulmonary arterial pressure (PAP) and the pulmonary capillary wedge pressure (PCWP). Since it is inserted at the same site as the CVP catheter, it has similar complications as well as additional ones related to balloon inflation, such as pulmonary artery hemorrhage and pulmonary infarction.

The pulmonary artery catheter (Figure 10-4) has a number of variations but typically it is 110 cm in length with three lumens (interior

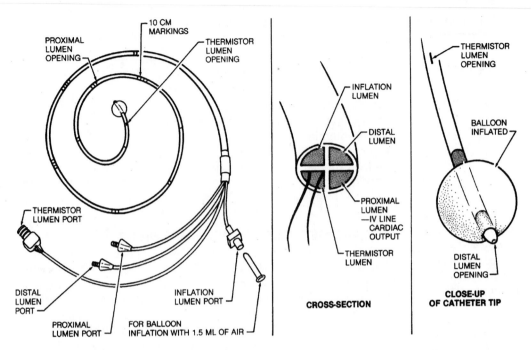

Figure 10-4 A diagram identifying the components of a Swan-Ganz catheter.

channels). The exterior of the catheter is marked off in 10 cm segments by thin and thick black lines to estimate the catheter tip location upon insertion. At the tip of the catheter there is an opening (PA distal lumen or port) connected with one lumen. About 30 cm back from the catheter tip there is another opening (proximal injectate port) connected to another lumen. When properly inserted, this proximal port is in the right atrium. Near the catheter tip is a small (1.5 cc maximum inflation volume) balloon connected to a lumen that allows for inflation of the balloon with a syringe. Also at the catheter tip is a thermistor (temperature sensing device) connected to a wire.

INSERTION OF PULMONARY ARTERY CATHETER

The pulmonary artery catheter is usually inserted into either the subclavian or internal jugular vein. From there, it is advanced to the superior vena cava and right atrium. The balloon is then inflated and the blood flow moves the catheter with its inflated balloon just as the wind moves a sail. The catheter proceeds to the right ventricle and into the pulmonary artery where it will eventually "wedge" in a smaller branch of the pulmonary artery. The balloon is then deflated and the catheter stabilized in place (Figure 10-5).

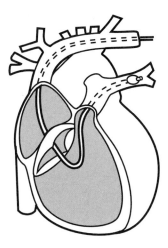

Figure 10-5 Position of a pulmonary artery catheter.

As the pulmonary artery catheter is being inserted, its movement can be followed on the bedside monitor by observing the various pressure waveforms as the catheter passes freely from the right atrium (RA) to a wedged position in the pulmonary artery (Figure 10-6).

The balloon stays deflated and the PAP tracing remains on the monitor at all times. The balloon is inflated only when the pulmonary capillary wedge pressure is being taken.

COMPONENTS OF PULMONARY ARTERIAL PRESSURE WAVEFORM

The pulmonary arterial pressure waveform has three components: systolic phase, diastolic phase, and dicrotic notch. The dicrotic notch on the PAP waveform reflects closure of the semilunar valves at the end of contraction and prior to refilling of the ventricles. The slight elevation seen at the dicrotic notch represents the transient increase in pulmonary artery pressure due to backup of blood flow immediately following closure of the semilunar valves (Figure 10-7).

Abnormal Pulmonary Artery Waveform.   The systolic component of the pulmonary artery pressure waveform may be increased in conditions in which the pulmonary vascular resistance or pulmonary blood flow is increased. Obstruction in the left heart may also cause backup of blood flow in the pulmonary artery and an increase in pulmonary artery pressure (Schriner, 1989). An irregular pressure tracing on the pulmonary artery pressure waveform may be seen in arrhythmias due to changes in diastolic filling time and volume.

ABNORMAL PULMONARY ARTERIAL PRESSURE

Pulmonary arterial pressure (PAP) is measured when the pulmonary artery (Swan-Ganz) catheter is inside the pulmonary artery with the

☑ The dicrotic notch reflects closure of the semilunar valves at the end of contraction and prior to refilling of the ventricles.

☑ The systolic component of the PAP waveform may be increased in conditions in which the pulmonary vascular resistance or pulmonary blood flow is increased.

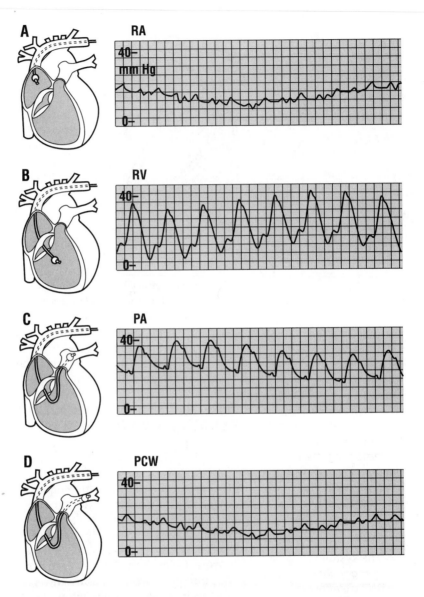

Figure 10-6 Waveform characteristics during advancement of pulmonary artery catheter. (A) right atrium (RA) and right atrial (central venous) waveform; (B) right ventricle (RV) and right ventricular waveform; (C) pulmonary artery (PA) and pulmonary arterial waveform; and (D) pulmonary capillary wedge (PCW) and pulmonary capillary wedge pressure waveform.

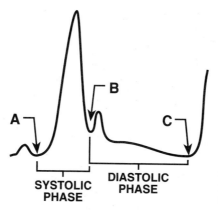

Figure 10-7 Pulmonary arterial pressure (PAP) waveform. (A) beginning systole; (B) dicrotic notch (closure of aortic valve); and (C) end-diastole.

✓ The normal systolic PAP ranges from 15 to 25 mm Hg. The diastolic PAP normal range is from 6 to 12 mm Hg.

balloon deflated. The normal systolic PAP is about the same as the right ventricular systolic pressure and ranges from 15 to 25 mm Hg. The normal diastolic PAP range is from 6 to 12 mm Hg.

Positive end-expiratory pressure (PEEP) can increase the PAP because overdistension of the alveoli compresses the surrounding capillaries and raises the capillary and arterial pressures (Versprille, 1990). Increase in pulmonary vascular resistance or pulmonary blood flow can also lead to an increased PAP, because the pressure measurement is directly related to the resistance and blood flow.

A higher than normal PAP may also be seen in left ventricular dysfunction such as left ventricular failure and mitral valve disease. This is because obstruction or backup of blood flow in the left heart leads to congestion in the pulmonary circulation. This is reflected as an elevated PAP.

On the other hand, the PAP may be decreased in conditions of hypovolemia or use of mechanical ventilation. When positive pressure ventilation is used on patients who have unstable hemodynamic status, it may lead to a depressed cardiac output, venous return, pulmonary circulating volume, and PAP (Versprille, 1990). The conditions that may affect the PAP are summarized in Table 10-7.

✓ Positive pressure ventilation causes a decrease in the pulmonary arterial pressure.

Effects of Positive Pressure Ventilation. Positive pressure ventilation causes a decrease of the pulmonary arterial pressure (Figure 10-8). This condition is due to the resultant decreased venous return to the right ventricle, lower right ventricular output, and lower blood volume (pressure) in the pulmonary arteries (Perkins et al., 1989; Versprille, 1990). In the absence of compensation by increasing the heart rate, decrease of right and left ventricular stroke volumes generally leads to a decreased cardiac output.

TABLE 10-7   Conditions That Affect the Pulmonary Arterial Pressure

PAP	CONDITIONS	EXAMPLES
Increase	Mechanical ventilation*	PEEP
	Increase in pulmonary vascular resistance	Pulmonary embolism Hypoxic vasoconstriction Primary pulmonary hypertension
	Increase in pulmonary blood flow	Hypervolemia Left to right shunt
	Left heart pathology	Left ventricular failure Mitral valve disease
Decrease	Mechanical ventilation*	Positive pressure ventilation
	Decrease in pulmonary blood flow	Hypovolemia

*The effects of mechanical ventilation on the PAP are highly variable, depending on the interaction between the peak airway pressure, PEEP, and patient's compliance and hemodynamic status.

PULMONARY CAPILLARY WEDGE PRESSURE

☑ PCWP reflects the left ventricular preload.

The pulmonary artery catheter is also used to measure the pulmonary capillary wedge pressure (PCWP). PCWP is measured by slowly inflating the balloon via the balloon inflation port on the pulmonary artery catheter. As the balloon inflates, the pulmonary arterial waveform on the monitor will change to the wedged pressure waveform (Figure 10-6D). Proper inflation of the balloon usually requires no more than 1.5 cc (0.75 to 1.5 cc depending on balloon size) of air. The balloon is deflated as soon as the reading of PCWP is made.

Positive pressure ventilation (without PEEP)
↓
Increase in intrathoracic pressure
↓
Decreased venous return
↓
Lower right ventricular output
↓
Lower blood volume (pressure) in the pulmonary artery

NOTE: When PEEP is used in conjunction with positive pressure ventilation, the PAP may not show a decrease because PEEP tends to increase the PAP by compressing the pulmonary vessels.

Figure 10-8   Effects of positive pressure ventilation.

The PCWP reading is typically taken at end-expiration for both spontaneous breathing and mechanically ventilated patients (Ahrens, 1991; Campbell et al., 1988). This practice should be done consistently for valid PCWP measurements and meaningful interpretation of hemodynamic data.

COMPONENTS OF PULMONARY CAPILLARY WEDGE PRESSURE WAVEFORM

The components of the PCWP waveform are similar to the CVP or right atrial waveform. When all of the components are present, the *a* wave of the PCWP waveform reflects left atrial contraction and *x* downslope represents the decrease in left atrial pressure following contraction. The *c* wave, if present, is seen along the *x* downslope and it occurs during closure of the mitral valve. The *v* wave indicates left ventricular contraction and passive atrial filling. The *y* downslope is due to the decrease in blood volume and pressure following the opening of the mitral valve (Figure 10-9).

Abnormal Pulmonary Capillary Wedge Pressure Waveform. Increased PCWP measurements are often observed in conditions where partial obstruction or excessive blood flow is present in the left heart (Schriner, 1989). Two common changes in the PCWP waveform are the *a* and *v* waves.

The *a* wave of the PCWP waveform may be increased in conditions leading to higher resistance to left ventricular filling. Some examples are mitral valve stenosis, left ventricular hypervolemia or failure, and decreased left ventricular compliance.

The *v* wave of the PCWP waveform may be increased due to mitral valve insufficiency. This condition leads to regurgitation (backward flow) of blood from the left ventricle to the left atrium through the incompetent mitral valve.

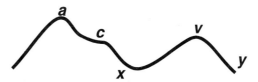

Figure 10-9 Pulmonary capillary wedge pressure (PCWP) waveform. *a* wave: left atrial contraction; *c* wave (may be absent): closure of mitral valve; *x* downslope: decreased left atrial pressure following atrial contraction; *v* wave: left ventricular contraction and passive atrial filling; *y* downslope: decrease of blood volume (pressure) following the opening of mitral valve.

ABNORMAL PULMONARY CAPILLARY WEDGE PRESSURE

☑ The normal PCWP ranges from 8 to 12 mm Hg.

The normal range for PCWP is from 8 to 12 mm Hg. Positive pressure ventilation or PEEP can affect wedge pressure readings since overdistension of the alveoli compresses the surrounding capillaries and raises the capillary and arterial pressures. A higher than normal wedge pressure may also be seen in left ventricular dysfunction. This is because left ventricular failure causes backup of blood flow in the left heart and pulmonary circulation. This is reflected as an elevated PCWP.

☑ The PCWP may be increased during positive pressure ventilation or in left ventricular dysfunction.

The PCWP measurement may be used to distinguish cardiogenic and noncardiogenic pulmonary edema. In pulmonary edema that is caused by left ventricular failure, the PCWP is usually elevated. When pulmonary edema occurs with a normal PCWP, it is probably due to an increase in capillary permeability as seen in ARDS. The conditions that may affect the PCWP measurements are outlined in Table 10-8.

VERIFICATION OF THE WEDGED POSITION

Since artifact or dampened waveform may occur during inflation of the balloon, and it resembles that of a wedged pressure tracing, using the PCWP tracing alone on the monitor to verify the wedged position may not be always reliable. Three methods are available to confirm a properly wedged pulmonary artery catheter.

☑ Three methods may be used to confirm a properly wedged pulmonary artery catheter: PAP diastolic-PCWP gradient; postcapillary-mixed venous PO₂ gradient; and post-capillary-mixed venous O₂ saturation gradient.

PAP Diastolic-PCWP Gradient. Under normal conditions, the PAP diastolic value is about 1 to 4 mm Hg higher than the average wedge pressure of the same individual (Daily et al., 1985). However, the PAP diastolic value may be lower than actual with forceful spontaneous inspiratory efforts. The PCWP may be higher than actual if there is significant downstream obstruction such as mitral valve disease (McGrath, 1986). These factors must be taken into account when evaluating the pressure gradient between PAP diastolic pressure and PCWP.

TABLE 10-8 Conditions That Affect the Pulmonary Capillary Wedge Pressure

PCWP	CONDITIONS	EXAMPLES
Increase	Increase in pulmonary blood flow	Hypervolemia
	Left heart pathology	Left ventricular failure; Mitral valve disease
	Mechanical factor	Overwedging of balloon
Decrease	Mechanical ventilation	PEEP
	Decrease in pulmonary blood flow	Hypovolemia

Postcapillary-Mixed Venous PO₂ Gradient. The PO_2 of a blood gas sample from the distal opening of a properly wedged catheter should be at least 19 mm Hg higher than that from a systemic artery. The PCO_2 should be at least 11 mm Hg lower. These differences are expected because a properly wedged catheter does not allow mixing of shunted venous blood with the postcapillary blood. This procedure may not be feasible for a hypovolemic patient because up to 40 cc of waste (mixed venous) blood sample may be required before reaching the postcapillary blood sample (Morris et al., 1985).

Postcapillary-Mixed Venous O₂ Saturation Gradient. If the pulmonary artery catheter is capable of monitoring oxygen saturation by the oximetry method, the oxygen saturation value of a properly wedged catheter should be about 20% higher than the one recorded with the balloon deflated (Morris et al., 1985).

CARDIAC OUTPUT AND CARDIAC INDEX

✓ The normal cardiac output for an adult is from 4 to 8 L/min.

Another important value of the pulmonary artery catheter is its ability to measure cardiac output by the thermodilution technique. During cardiac output measurement, a small amount (10 ml) of iced or room temperature fluid (usually 5% dextrose in water, D5W) is injected into the proximal port of the pulmonary artery catheter. The temperature change of the blood flow is recorded as the flow passes by the thermistor at the catheter tip. This and other measurements are computed and the flow rate through the heart is displayed as cardiac output. The normal cardiac output for an adult is from 4 to 8 L/min.

Since cardiac output normally varies from person to person depending on the size of the individual, it is common to "index" the value by dividing cardiac output (C.O.) by body surface area (BSA). The **cardiac index** (C.I.) is normally 2.5 to 3.5 L/min/m² and it is calculated as follows:

cardiac index: A cardiac output measurement relative to a person's body size.

$$C.I. = C.O. / BSA$$

✓ The cardiac index is normally 2.5 to 3.5 L/min/m².

SUMMARY OF PRELOADS AND AFTERLOADS

Each ventricle has its own preload and afterload measurements. Their meaning and common pathological implications are shown in Table 10-9.

TABLE 10-9   Ventricular Preloads and Afterloads

DEVICE (MEASUREMENT)	MAIN IMPLICATION	EXAMPLES
Arterial catheter (Left ventricular afterload)	Condition of systemic arterial pressure	Arterial pressure is increased in systemic hypertension or fluid overload. Arterial pressure is decreased in systemic hypotension or fluid depletion.
Central venous catheter (Right ventricular preload)	Condition of systemic venous return	Central venous pressure (CVP) is increased in systemic hypertension or hypervolemia. Central venous pressure (CVP) is decreased in systemic hypotension or hypovolemia.
Pulmonary artery catheter (Right ventricular afterload)	Condition of pulmonary artery	Pulmonary artery pressure (PAP) is increased in pulmonary hypertension or blood flow obstruction in left heart. Pulmonary artery pressure (PAP) is decreased in pulmonary hypotension.
Pulmonary artery catheter (balloon inflated) (Left ventricular preload)	Condition of left heart	Pulmonary capillary wedge pressure (PCWP) is increased in left heart blood flow obstruction. PCWP is decreased in severe hypotension or dehydration.

CALCULATED HEMODYNAMIC VALUES

From the CVP, PAP, and other related measurements, the following parameters may be calculated: stroke volume and stroke volume index, oxygen consumption and oxygen consumption index, pulmonary vascular resistance, and **systemic vascular resistance.**

systemic vascular resistance: Resistance of the arterial system into which the left heart is pumping. Normal range is 800 to 1,500 dynes.sec/cm[5].

STROKE VOLUME AND STROKE VOLUME INDEX

Stroke volume (S.V.) is calculated by dividing the cardiac output (C.O.) by the heart rate (HR). The stroke volume index is calculated by dividing the stroke volume by the body surface area (BSA).

$$S.V. = C.O. / HR$$

$$S.V.I. = S.V. / BSA$$

The stroke volume is determined by three factors: **contractility,** preload, and afterload. Contractility is the pumping strength of the heart. Some conditions that may lower the contractility of the heart include extremes of myocardial compliance (too high or too low), and excessive end-diastolic volume. Preload is the end-diastolic stretch of cardiac muscle fiber, expressed in pressure units (mm Hg or cm H_2O). Hypovolemia and shock are two conditions that usually cause a decreased preload. Afterload is the tension or pressure that develops in the ventricle during systole (contraction), expressed in pressure units (mm Hg or cm H_2O). Afterload is usually increased in conditions of downstream flow obstruction or excessive volume.

OXYGEN CONSUMPTION AND OXYGEN CONSUMPTION INDEX

The oxygen consumption reflects the amount of oxygen consumed in one minute. The oxygen consumption index is used to reflect the amount of oxygen used relative to the body size. They are calculated as follows:

$$VO_2 = Q_T \times C(a-\dot{v})O_2$$

$$VO_2 \text{ index} = VO_2 / BSA$$

PULMONARY VASCULAR RESISTANCE

The pulmonary vascular resistance (PVR) measures the blood vessel resistance to blood flow in the pulmonary circulation. For example, PVR is elevated in pulmonary hypertension or left heart obstruction (e.g., mitral valve stenosis).

$$PVR = (PAP - PCWP) \times 80/C.O.$$

SYSTEMIC VASCULAR RESISTANCE

The systemic vascular resistance (SVR) measures the blood vessel resistance to blood flow in the systemic circulation. For example, SVR is elevated in systemic hypertension.

$$SVR = (MAP - RAP) \times 80/C.O.$$

MONITORING OF MIXED VENOUS OXYGEN SATURATION

A special version of the pulmonary artery catheter uses fiberoptic technology to enable monitoring of mixed venous oxygen saturation ($S\dot{v}O_2$). The fiberoptic central venous catheter measures the $S\dot{v}O_2$

accurately well within the clinical range (between 50% to 80%) (Fletcher, 1988). $S\dot{v}O_2$ had been used to reflect a patient's cardiac output and cardiac index status even before thermodilution cardiac output became common practice (Muir, 1970; Waller, 1982). When $S\dot{v}O_2$ is used with other monitoring capabilities of the pulmonary artery catheter, it can provide valuable data concerning oxygen delivery and consumption.

DECREASE IN MIXED VENOUS OXYGEN SATURATION

✓ The normal $S\dot{v}O_2$ is about 75%. $S\dot{v}O_2$ of less than 60% is indicative of hypoxemia, decrease in cardiac output, or increase in peripheral oxygen consumption.

For normal individuals, the measured $S\dot{v}O_2$ is between 68% to 77% with an average of 75% (McMichan, 1983). $S\dot{v}O_2$ of less than 60% is indicative of hypoxemia, decrease in cardiac output, or increase in peripheral oxygen consumption (McMichan, 1983). It reflects an imbalance between oxygen supply, oxygen demand, and use of venous oxygen reserve (Mims, 1989).

Common causes of decreased $S\dot{v}O_2$ due to poor oxygen supply include inadequate cardiac output, anemia, and hypoxic hypoxia. Causes of decreased $S\dot{v}O_2$ due to excessive oxygen use include fever, seizures, increased physical activity or work of breathing. Some conditions that may lead to a decreased $S\dot{v}O_2$ are summarized in Table 10-10.

TABLE 10-10   Conditions That Affect the $S\dot{v}O_2$ Measurement

$S\dot{v}O_2$	CONDITIONS	EXAMPLES
Decrease	Poor oxygen supply	Inadequate cardiac output Anemia Hypoxic hypoxia
	Excessive oxygen demand	Fever Seizures Increased metabolic rate Increased physical activity
	Depletion of venous oxygen reserve	Severe and prolonged hypoxia
Increase	Technical problem	Improperly wedged catheter
	Impaired oxygen utilization	Sepsis Cyanide poisoning
	Decrease in oxygen demand	Hypothermia Postanesthesia Pharmacologic paralysis

INCREASE IN MIXED VENOUS OXYGEN SATURATION

Increases in $S\dot{v}O_2$ above 75% are uncommon but may occur when the tip of the pulmonary artery catheter is improperly wedged. Once in this abnormal position, the forward mixed venous blood flow is obstructed while the catheter tip senses the blood from an area with a high ventilation/perfusion ratio, and therefore a high oxygen level (Briones, 1988).

An increased $S\dot{v}O_2$ may also be observed in patients with sepsis or cyanide poisoning in which the tissues become unable to utilize oxygen (White, 1987). The mechanism of hypoxia for sepsis is due to peripheral shunting. Cyanide poisoning causes histotoxic hypoxia that renders the tissues unable to carry out aerobic metabolism. These patients may have normal PaO_2, SaO_2, CaO_2, and oxygen transport but they are often hypoxic. Lactic acidosis is a common event for these patients (Mims, 1989). Some conditions that may lead to an increased $S\dot{v}O_2$ are summarized in Table 10-10.

☑ Increases in $S\dot{v}O_2$ above 75% are uncommon but may occur when the tip of the pulmonary artery catheter is improperly wedged.

SUMMARY

In order to monitor and use hemodynamic waveforms efficiently, one must remember the normal values and recognize the characteristics of normal waveforms. It is only with constant clinical practice that one may learn the intricacies and interactions of those variables that affect hemodynamic waveforms.

It is also essential to realize that monitoring of hemodynamic waveforms should be done on a continuing basis. Isolated and independent observations are of limited value since they do not provide a trend of changing events or patient conditions.

Self-Assessment Questions

1. In hemodynamic monitoring, the pressure measurement made inside a blood vessel is dependent on all of the following factors *except* the:

    A. blood volume.
    B. blood flow.
    C. size of blood vessel.
    D. barometric pressure.

2. During hemodynamic monitoring, the transducer, catheter, and measurement site are usually aligned at the same level. This is done to ensure that the measurements are not affected by the effect of:

    A. barometric pressure.
    B. gravity.
    C. fluid level.
    D. transducer sensitivity.

3. In the arterial pressure waveform shown, the dicrotic notch is labeled as _____ and it is caused by the _____. (See Figure 10-10.)

A. A, opening of the aortic valve

B. B, closure of the semilunar valves

C. B, opening of the pulmonic valve

D. C, closure of the semilunar valves

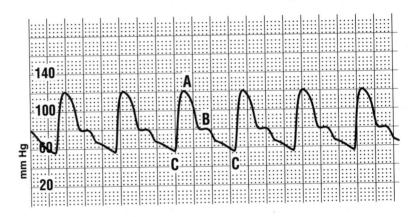

Figure 10-10   Arterial pressure waveform.

4. As you are caring for a ventilator patient, the arterial pressure waveform shows a decreasing systolic pressure and a stable diastolic pressure. Based on these two pressure measurements, the pulse pressure is _____. This condition may be caused by _____.

A. increasing, shock

B. increasing, hypervolemia

C. decreasing, bradycardia

D. decreasing, arteriosclerosis

5 to 7. Matching: Refer to the central venous pressure waveform (Figure 10-11) and match the wave or slope with the proper events during a cardiac cycle. Use only three of the five answers provided.

Wave or Slope	Corresponding Event
5. *a*	A. ventricular relaxation
6. *c*	B. atrial contraction
7. *v*	C. ventricular contraction
	D. relaxation of right atrium
	E. closure of tricuspid valve during systole

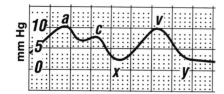

Figure 10-11   Central venous pressure waveform.

8. As you review a patient's chart, you notice that the central venous pressure readings have been decreasing from an average of 6 mm Hg to 2 mm Hg. This condition may be caused by all of the following conditions *except*:

   A. positive pressure ventilation.
   B. blood or fluid depletion.

   C. shock.
   D. vasodilation.

9. Which of the following outlines the proper sequence for the placement of a Swan-Ganz catheter?

   A. femoral vein, left atrium, left ventri-
      cle, pulmonary artery.
   B. internal jugular vein, left atrium, left
      ventricle, pulmonary artery.

   C. femoral artery, right atrium, right
      ventricle, pulmonary artery.
   D. subclavian vein, right atrium, right
      ventricle, pulmonary artery.

10 to 13. Matching: Match the type of catheter with the intended hemodynamic measurements.

Catheter	Hemodynamic Measurement
10. Arterial catheter	A. left ventricular preload
11. Central venous catheter	B. left ventricular afterload
12. Pulmonary artery catheter with bal- loon deflated	C. right ventricular preload
13. Pulmonary artery catheter with bal- loon inflated	D. right ventricular afterload

14. Mr. Jones, a patient in the coronary care unit being treated for congestive heart failure, has a pulmonary artery catheter in place and the SvO_2 is 55%. This SvO_2 value is _____ and it may be caused by _____.

   A. too high, increase in cardiac output
   B. too high, increase in peripheral
      oxygen consumption

   C. too low, decrease in cardiac output
   D. too low, decrease in peripheral
      oxygen consumption

References

Ahrens, T. S. (1991). Effects of mechanical ventilation on hemodynamic waveforms. *Crit Care Nurs Clin North Am, 3,* 629–639.

Briones, T. L. (1988). SvO$_2$ monitoring: Part I. Clinical case application. *Dim Crit Care Nurs, 7,* 70–78.

Bustin, D. (1986). *Hemodynamic monitoring for critical care.* Norwalk, CT: Appleton-Century-Crofts.

Campbell, M. L. et al. (1988). Reading pulmonary artery wedge pressure at end-expiration. *Focus Crit Care, 15,* 60–63.

Christensen, B. (1992). Hemodynamic monitoring: What it tells you and what it doesn't, Part I. *J Post Anesth Nurs, 7*(5), 330–337.

Christensen, B. (1992). Hemodynamic monitoring: What it tells you and what it doesn't, Part II. *J Post Anesth Nurs, 7*(5), 338–345.

Daily, E. K. et al. (1985). *Techniques in bedside hemodynamic monitoring.* St. Louis: Mosby-Year Book.

Fletcher, E. C. (1988). Accuracy of fiberoptic central venous saturation catheter below 50%. *J Appl Physiol, 64*(5), 2220–2223.

Keckeisen, M. (1991). Techniques for measuring arterial pressure in the postoperative cardiac surgery patient. *Crit Care Nurs Clin North Am, 3,* 699–708.

McGrath, R. B. (1986). Invasive bedside hemodynamic monitoring. *Prog Cardiovasc Dis, 29,* 129–144.

McMichan, J. C. (1983). Continuous monitoring of mixed venous oxygen saturation. In J. F. Schweiss (Ed.), *Continuous measurement of blood oxygen saturation in the high risk patient.* Beach International.

Mims, B. C. (1989). Physiologic rationale of SvO$_2$ monitoring. *Crit Care Nurs Clin North Am, 1,* 619–628.

Morris, A. H. et al. (1985). Wedge pressure confirmation by aspiration of pulmonary capillary blood. *Crit Care Med, 13,* 756–759.

Muir, A. L. (1970). Mixed venous oxygen saturation in relation to cardiac output in myocardial infarction. *Br Med J, 4,* 276.

Perkins, M. W. et al. (1989). Physiologic implications of mechanical ventilation on pharmacokinetics. *DICP, The annals of pharmacotherapy, 23,* 316–323.

Schriner, D. K. (1989). Using hemodynamic waveforms to assess cardiopulmonary pathologies. *Crit Care Nurs Clin North Am, 1,* 563–575.

Swan, H. J. et al. (1970). Catheterization of the heart in man with the use of a flow directed balloon-tipped catheter. *N Engl J Med, 283,* 447–451.

Versprille, V. (1990). The pulmonary circulation during mechanical ventilation. *Acta Anaesthesiol Scand, 34, Supplementum 94,* 51–62.

Waller, J. L. (1982). Clinical evaluation of a new fiberoptic catheter during cardiac surgery. *Anesth Analg, 61,* 676.

White, K. M. (1987). Continuous monitoring of mixed venous oxygen saturation (SvO_2): A new assessment tool in critical care nursing—Part II. *Cardiovasc Nurs, 23,* 7–12.

CHAPTER ELEVEN

BASIC VENTILATOR WAVEFORM ANALYSIS

Frank Dennison

OUTLINE

KEY TERMS

- **airway opening pressure (P_{AO})**
- **alveolar pressure (P_{ALV})**
- **dyssynchrony**
- **flow-time waveform**
- **flow volume loop (FVL)**

- **lung–thorax compliance (C_{LT})**
- **peak inspiratory pressure (PIP)**
- **pressure-time waveform**
- **pressure volume curve (PVC)**
- **transairway pressure (P_{TA})**

INTRODUCTION

The advent of waveform analysis marked the beginning of a new and exciting era in ventilator–patient management for respiratory care professionals. Waveforms give us the capacity to observe and document real-time measurements of patient–ventilator interactions. In the past, many problematic interactions between the patient and ventilator that were suspected could not be confirmed without sophisticated equipment and time-consuming effort. Someone skilled at analyzing waveforms can now determine such matters as the level of patient–ventilator synchrony, appropriateness of adjustments to improve synchrony, sensitivity of equipment in meeting various patient demands, changes in pulmonary status, and presence of autoPEEP within a few seconds. And when respiratory therapists implement appropriate ventilator adjustments or therapy, they can observe and document improvements in ventilator–patient management. Once it is normal practice to use waveforms to assist in ventilator–patient assessment, you are left with a sense of total inadequacy in their absence. You may suspect that some type of dyssynchrony or malfunction is occurring, but you lack the tools to confirm and quickly change it.

Waveform analysis requires an in-depth understanding of the basic principles that govern the shape of waveforms, and the characteristics of flow, pressure, and volume that vary over time during respiration. Skill in analysis can be developed through math and lab exercises and implementing adjustments to ventilator settings at the bedside while observing the results. It is very helpful to observe graphics while simulating patient–ventilator interactions under varied conditions of lung compliance and circuit/airway resistance via training test lungs. It is also valuable experience to breathe through an endotracheal tube and ventilator circuit on different ventilators set in different modes while observing graphics. In doing so, clinicians can get a feel for the patient's experience, and to what extent ventilators are able to respond to variations in effort, flow, and volume demand, and observe how those demands affect waveforms. In this chapter, I give the reader an appreciation for the basics involved with waveform analysis, and the use of graphics for improved ventilator–patient management.

☑ Waveform analysis requires an in-depth understanding of the basic principles that govern the shape of waveforms, and the characteristics of flow, pressure, and volume that vary over time during respiration.

☑ The square flow wave can present a convex pattern (dashed line) if the rise to peak flow is slowed or tapered by the manufacturer (i.e., PB7200) for patient comfort during volume-limited or pressure-limited ventilation. The decelerating flow wave is also called a descending or ramp waveform.

FLOW WAVES USED FOR POSITIVE PRESSURE VENTILATION

During positive pressure ventilation with computerized ventilators that incorporate graphics, flow, pressure, and volume are the three variables measured and graphically displayed in real time. Flow-volume curves or loops and pressure-volume curves are also available. Depending on conditions, modes, or manufacturers, six distinct flow patterns can be considered to be set or to develop in delivering gas to patients: the rectangular or square, the convex rise (dashed line); the decelerating, or exponential decay (dashed line); the accelerating, and sine flow patterns (Figure 11-1). The square flow wave can present a convex pattern (dashed line) if the rise to peak flow is slowed or tapered by the manufacturer (i.e., PB7200) for patient comfort during volume-limited. The decelerating flow wave is also called a descending or ramp waveform. Depending on the manufacturer, ventilators offer waveforms that decelerate from the initial peak flow to zero end flow as presented in Figure 11-1; to decelerate to some partial end flow level (e.g., 5 L/min); or to decelerate to 50% of the initial peak flow level. During pressure-limited ventilation, decelerating flow waves may present an exponential decay pattern (dashed line) depending on lung characteristics and patient demand.

The accelerating (also called ascending or ramp) and sine (also called sinusoidal) flow waveforms are seldom used for positive

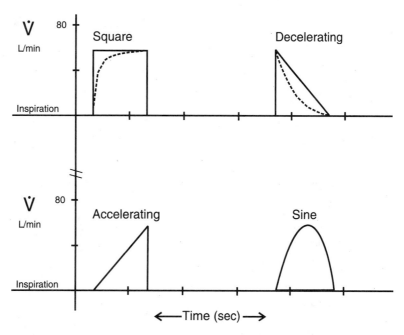

Figure 11-1 Six flow waveforms available for positive pressure ventilation: the rectangular or square, the convex pattern (dashed line); the decelerating or exponential decay pattern (dashed line), the accelerating, and sine flow pattern.

☑ The accelerating (also called ascending or ramp) and sine (also called sinusoidal) flow waveforms are seldom used for positive pressure ventilation because the initial flow rate is not sufficient to accommodate synchronized assisted ventilation for most patients. These two waveforms may be appropriate for controlled ventilation where initial flow demand is not an issue.

pressure ventilation because the initial flow rate is not sufficient to accommodate synchronized assisted ventilation for most patients. The fast rise to peak flow offered by the square and decelerating flow patterns has proven to be superior in meeting patient flow demands in clinic and research.

The use of the sine or accelerating flow waveforms may be appropriate for controlled ventilation where initial flow demand is not an issue. When a patient is heavily sedated and there is no demand for flow, the slow rise to peak flow levels may improve lung gas distribution. When there is variable resistance in diseased airways throughout the lungs, gas follows the path of least resistance, preferentially ventilating normal lung parenchyma. Utilizing slower flow rates or rise time to peak flow levels may reduce flow resistance and improve gas distribution to the poorly ventilated areas of the lung. During assisted ventilation, however, there is a time lag between patient demand for flow (patient-effort) because of ventilator inspiratory valve opening response time and time for gas to accelerate to the flow level demanded. When the initial flow level is set higher than demanded, it will compensate for the time lag (Marini et al., 1985). Thus, during assisted ventilation, the flow level demand is commonly too high for

☑ (Flow waveform of Figure 11-2) *a* represents the end of expiration and the beginning of the inspiration where flow is ventilator or time triggered and always a positive upward stroke on ventilator graphics; *b* marks the peak and constant flow (60 L/min) sustained during inspiration; *c* marks the change from inspiration to expiration where the breath is volume or time cycled into expiration; *d* marks the beginning of the expiratory flow and phase of breathing, which is always to the negative side or slope from baseline or zero flow (*x*-axis); *e* represents the peak expiratory flow attained (60 L/min), which is assigned a negative value on graphics; *f* represents the end of a patient's flow as it returns to baseline; *g* is the passive expiratory pause time in flow until the next breath.

the slower rise to peak flow pattern characteristics of the sine or accelerating flow waveforms to facilitate ventilator–patient synchrony.

EFFECTS OF CONSTANT FLOW DURING VOLUME-CONTROLLED VENTILATION

Figure 11-2 displays two theoretical sets of waveforms, a set of ideal flow and pressure (*y*-axis) waveforms contiguous in time (*x*-axis), and another set of waves with characteristic changes made for comparison. Both sets of waveforms represent mandatory breaths, which are started (triggered), volume- or flow-controlled (limited), and ended (cycled) by the ventilator. The letters represent the various components and

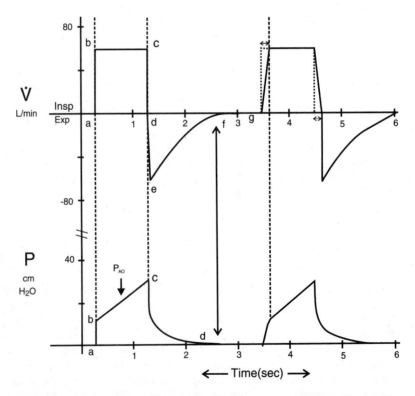

Figure 11-2 Two sets of flow- and pressure-time waveforms. The letters in the first set of waveforms mark the various phases of the respiratory cycle (see text). The second set of waveforms demonstrate pattern changes that result when there is a delay in time in rise to peak flow.

phases of breathing (Chatburn, 1991) recorded by flow and pressure-time graphics.

FLOW-TIME WAVEFORM

flow-time waveform: A graphic display showing the relationship between flow (vertical axis) and time (horizontal axis).

pressure-time waveform: A graphic display showing the relationship between pressure (vertical axis) and time (horizontal axis).

For the square flow waveform, *a* represents the end of expiration and the beginning of the inspiration where flow is ventilator or time triggered and always a positive upward stroke on ventilator graphics; *b* marks the peak and constant flow (60 L/min) sustained during inspiration; and *c* marks the change from inspiration to expiration where the breath is volume or time cycled into expiration. This inspiratory flow waveform represents a conceptual or idealized waveform. The initial flow cannot reach the peak flow level instantaneously. Gas, obviously, does not travel at the speed of light. The same is true at the end of the inspiratory phase where flow appears to have dropped from peak flow to zero instantaneously. No ventilator can "square off" flow and pressure waveforms as they are presented in textbooks. Realistic waveforms will have more rounded or slightly jagged corners and angles (noise) with transitive changes in flow rate and pressure. Attention to such details for realistic representation of each waveform would require meticulous, time-consuming work that is not necessary for learning the concepts and major principles involved with waveform analysis. Thus, minor details have been omitted for ease of presentation as well as mathematical analysis. Clinically relevant exceptions will be presented and explained.

☑ (Pressure waveform of Figure 11-2) *a* indicates the beginning of inspiration; *b* represents the change in slope on a pressure waveform that occurs once peak flow is attained and then sustained (constant flow) throughout inspiration; *c* marks the PIP, the end of inspiration, and the beginning of expiration where the ventilator is time cycled into expiration; *d* marks the end of expiratory pressure being sensed by the pressure manometer.

Letter *d* marks the beginning of the expiratory flow and phase of breathing, which is always to the negative side or slope from baseline or zero flow (*x*-axis). Letter *e* represents the peak expiratory flow attained (60 L/min), which is assigned a negative value on graphics. The expiratory flow from peak to end flow is normally an exponential decay pattern under passive conditions (Nunn, 1977). Letter *f* represents the end of a patient's flow as it returns to baseline, and *g* is the passive expiratory pause time in flow until the next breath.

PRESSURE-TIME WAVEFORM

It is important to realize that it is the **flow-time waveform** that dictates the pressure-time and pressure-volume graphics displayed. The ideal **pressure-time waveform** that is created under passive conditions of square flow wave ventilation is called a trapezoid pattern (Marini et al., 1986). Letter *a* on the pressure waveform indicates the beginning of inspiration, and corresponds in time to the flow waveform as indicated by the dashed line connecting the two waveforms. The beginning of the pressure waveform provides information about the triggering variable of the inspiratory phase of ventilation. There is no negative deflection in pressure to indicate patient effort to trigger an assist breath (Figure 11-27), indicating that the breath is ventilator or time triggered. The initial flow delivered from the ventilator pushes

*airway opening
pressure (P$_{AO}$): The
pressure measure-
ments in the airway
during the inspira-
tory phase.*

*peak inspiratory
pressure (PIP): The
maximal pressure
reading during the
inspiratory phase,
usually at end-
inspiration.*

gas from the circuit into the patient's lungs as it accelerates to peak
flow level. Little volume is actually delivered to the lungs during this
initial time period. Some volume is lost because of large bore tubing
compliance (tubing expansion) and compression of gas. The rise
in pressure is mostly the result of resistance to flow through the ventilator circuit and endotracheal tube (Tobin, 1994). Back pressure resulting from impedance to ventilation (flow resistance, tubing, and lung
tissue recoil) is graphically recorded by a pressure manometer at the
inspiratory valve of the ventilator. Letter *b* represents the change in
slope on a pressure waveform that occurs once peak flow is attained
and then sustained (constant flow) throughout inspiration. Once flow
delivery from the ventilator becomes constant, there is a relatively linear rise in the dynamic or **airway opening pressure (P$_{AO}$)**, which par-
allels the linear rise in lung pressure until **peak inspiratory pressure
(PIP)** is reached at end inspiration. Flow cannot be constant at both
ends of a ventilator circuit because volume is lost per unit pressure as
a result of tubing compliance (expansion) and gas compression. A loss
in volume equates to a loss in flow (flow = volume per time). There
has to be some reduction in flow from the ventilator end of the circuit
to the patient's end, depending on the level of pressure exerted on the
circuit gas (PIP), tubing compliance, and gas compression. However,
flow is presented throughout this chapter as constant during square
flow wave ventilation for educational and conceptual purposes. Flow
appears relatively constant on graphics because it is measured only at
one end of the ventilator circuit. For square flow ventilation, pressure
will rise throughout inspiration. Letter *c* marks the PIP, the end of inspiration, and the beginning of expiration where the ventilator is time
cycled into expiration. The second dashed line shows that the end of
inspiratory flow and PIP are contiguous in time. As flow exits through
the expiratory limb of the circuit, pressure is created by the resistance
to flow through the circuit and measured by a manometer at the expiratory valve. Pressure subsides as gas is released into the atmosphere.
Letter *d* marks the end of expiratory pressure being sensed by the
pressure manometer. The bold, double-headed arrow shows that flow
is still being recorded as gas is passing through the pneumotachome-
ter at the expiratory valve. Apparently there is often insufficient back
pressure from resistance to flow or the manometer is not sufficiently
sensitive or appropriately placed at the expiratory valve for pressure
to be continuously recorded until end expiration is reached on some
ventilators. It is a common characteristic of ventilator graphics for
pressure-time recordings.

   In the second flow wave, the time involved (upper double-headed
arrow) for the rise to peak flow may be a little exaggerated to clearly
demonstrate that there is a lag in time between the beginning of inspiration and attainment of peak flow. This delay in time corresponds to
a loss in flow and, therefore, volume in the initial phase of inspiration.
At the end of inspiration, the volume lost initially is regained as the

☑ **(Figure 11-3)**
The area under a flow-time curve equals volume.

☑ **(Figure 11-3)**
Since patients exhale what they inhale, area *b* enclosed under the expiratory flow wave should equal area *a* under the square flow graphic. If the volume enclosed by area *b* during mechanical ventilation is less than area *a*, circuit leak or gas trapping may be present.

flow slows to zero over the same delay in time and area under the flow pattern (lower double-headed arrow). Thus, flow-controlled ventilation equates to volume-controlled ventilation. The concept concerning volume and the area under the flow pattern is explained in more detail in Figure 11-3. The dashed line from peak flow to the recorded pressure demonstrates that once peak flow is reached and flow remains constant, the initial rise in predominantly flow-resistive pressure changes slope and rises linearly to PIP as in the preceding example. The slope of the initial rise in pressure is lower than in the preceding vertical example because of the slower rise to peak flow.

The basic mathematical principle demonstrated in Figure 11-3 is that area, under a flow-time curve or pattern, equals volume. We know from geometry that the area of a rectangle equals length times width ($A = L \times W$). On the flow graph, the length of the flow side of the waveform (y-axis) is 60 L/min or 1 L/s (60 L/min $\times$ 1 min/60 s = 1 L/s). Flow is constant for 1 second, therefore, the width of the rectangle (x-axis) is 1 second and, since length times width equals area, 1 L/s $\times$ 1s = 1 liter tidal volume (V_T) delivered. Also, constant flow means there is a constant delivery of volume per unit time. For example,

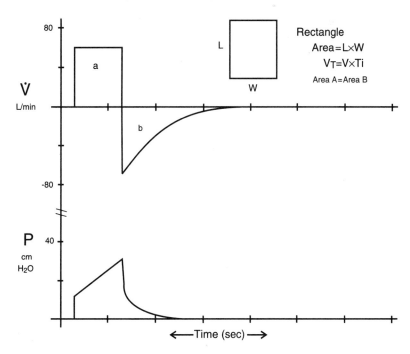

Figure 11-3 Flow waveform to demonstrate that area under a flow curve or rectangle equals volume. Tidal volume (V_T) is the product of constant flow and inspiratory time (Ti) (V_T = flow $\times$ time).

if 0.25s is used as the unit of time, a 0.25-liter of gas is delivered every 0.25s (Volume = 1 L/s × 0.25s = 0.25 L).

Since patients exhale what they inhale, it can be stated that area *b* enclosed under the expiratory flow wave equals area *a* under the square flow graphic. If the volume enclosed by area *b* during mechanical ventilation is less than area *a*, then there must either be a leak in the circuit, some gas has not been expired or has been trapped in the patient's lungs momentarily, or the patient had insufficient time to exhale before the next mechanical breath was triggered (autoPEEP). The pressure pattern shows a constant rise in lung pressure during the constant flow period as discussed in Figure 11-2.

Figure 11-4 depicts the ideal pressure waveform with details that correspond to the enclosed square flow wave presented above it. In this example, a 0.5s pause in delivery of flow from the ventilator has been set at the end of inspiration (prolonging inspiratory time). The pause in flow delivery results in a static pressure measurement being maintained at the same level for 0.5s, creating a plateau or pause pressure at the end of the waveform. For the flow waveform, the double-headed arrow shows that no flow is being delivered from the ventilator for 0.5s. During this time period, the inspiratory and expiratory valves of

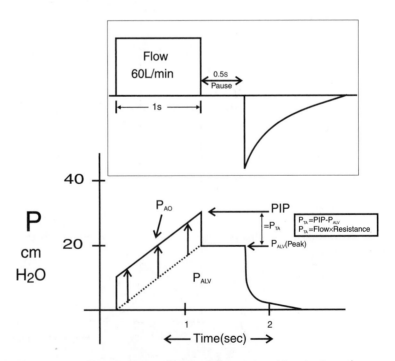

Figure 11-4 Use of a pause in flow delivery at end inspiration to measure peak alveolar pressure (P_{ALV}) and transairway pressure (P_{TA}) to determine static compliance and circuit/airway resistance.

alveolar pressure (P$_{ALV}$): The pressure in the alveoli; an indirect measurement.

lung-thorax compliance (C$_{LT}$): The volume/pressure relationship that is affected by the characteristics of the lungs and chest wall.

transairway pressure (P$_{TA}$): The pressure affected by the non-elastic characteristics of airways, difference of PIP and P$_{ALV}$.

☑ Once P$_{ALV}$ is known, circuit and airway resistance can be determined [Resistance = (PIP – P$_{ALV}$)/Flow].

☑ Measuring P$_{ALV}$ under static conditions allows for total static lung-thorax compliance (C$_{LT}$) to be calculated (C$_{LT}$ = volume/pressure).

the ventilator are closed to hold gas volume constant in the patient's lungs, allowing clinicians to measure lung pressure or, more important, **alveolar pressure (P$_{ALV}$).** Since there is no flow, the corresponding pressure created by resistance to flow dissipates immediately. Pressure drops to the P$_{ALV}$ level, which can be measured because of the open communication in the ventilator circuit between the alveoli and the pressure manometer at the ventilator. All lung pressure, not just P$_{ALV}$, is monitored during this pause in flow. However, P$_{ALV}$ is used for emphasis throughout this chapter. The extremely thin type 1 pneumocytes lining alveoli are more sensitive to pressure and trauma than the progressively thicker airway. P$_{ALV}$ is a major concern and reason for performing the plateau pressure measurement during ventilator management. Once P$_{ALV}$ is known, circuit and airway resistance can be determined [Resistance = (PIP – P$_{ALV}$)/Flow], providing a constant flow pattern is present. Measuring P$_{ALV}$ under static conditions allows for total static **lung–thorax compliance (C$_{LT}$)** to be calculated (e.g., C$_{LT}$ = volume/pressure, observing the graphic it can be determined that C$_{LT}$ = 1L/20 cm H$_2$O = 0.50 L/cm H$_2$O). The pressure-time waveform in Figure 11-4 shows, as noted earlier, that the dynamic pressure pattern represents two distinct pressures involved during inspiration with flow: the pressure caused by resistance to flow through the circuit and airway, and the elastic recoil pressure created by the airway and alveoli (P$_{ALV}$). Under ideal conditions (no change in C$_{LT}$ and no loss of volume or a proportionate loss of volume per unit pressure because of tubing compliance and gas compression), there is a linear rise in P$_{ALV}$ (dotted line) during the inspiratory cycle since there is a constant rise in volume per unit time with constant flow delivery. Flow-resistive pressure (arrows above dotted line) is also constant, assuming flow through the ventilator circuit is constant. Flow-resistive pressure will rise parallel to the rise in P$_{ALV}$ during constant flow. The airway opening pressure (P$_{AO}$) is the dynamic pressure recorded by the pressure manometer that clinicians observe at the ventilator as gas is being forced into lungs. Thus, the P$_{AO}$ is equal to the summation of the two distinct pressures during inspiration: flow-resistive pressure and P$_{ALV}$. Another term for flow-resistive pressure during inspiration is **transairway pressure (P$_{TA}$),** which is the difference between P$_{AO}$ and P$_{ALV}$ (P$_{TA}$ = P$_{AO}$ – P$_{ALV}$). P$_{TA}$ at end inspiration equals the difference between the PIP and the peak P$_{ALV}$ (P$_{TA}$ = PIP – P$_{ALV}$). Also, P$_{TA}$ equals flow times resistance (P$_{TA}$ = Flow × Resistance), and the dynamic or P$_{AO}$ is the sum of P$_{TA}$ and P$_{ALV}$ (P$_{AO}$ = P$_{TA}$ + P$_{ALV}$).

CONTROLLED MECHANICAL VENTILATION

Figure 11-5 is an example of the volume-controlled mechanical or mandatory mode of ventilation (CMV) with a 1:3 inspiratory to expiratory (I:E) ratio: 1 second for inspiration and 3 seconds for expiration.

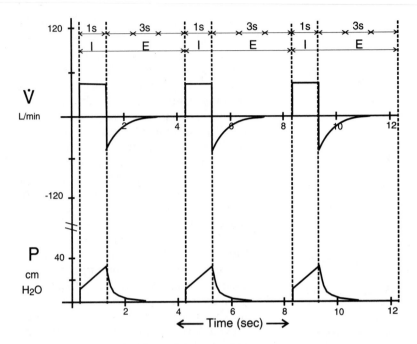

Figure 11-5 Square flow and corresponding pressure-time waveforms used to demonstrate the controlled mechanical mode (CMV) of ventilation.

☑ TCT = I + E

☑ b/min = 60s/TCT

Total respiratory cycle time (TCT = I + E) is 4s. The rate is set at 15 breaths per minute (b/min), (b/min = 60s/TCT = 60s/4s = 15). Thus, this graph is consistent with the definition of volume-controlled ventilation. Each breath is a time-triggered mechanical breath. The flow pattern has been set and is the same each breath, so the same volume is being delivered (controlled) each breath.

ASSIST MECHANICAL VENTILATION

☑ (Figure 11-6)
As soon as the negative pressure created by patient effort reaches the sensitivity threshold level set (e.g., –2 cm H₂O), the ventilator responds immediately by providing flow.

Figure 11-6 shows ideal response to patient-triggered breaths during the assist mandatory or mechanical mode of ventilation (AMV). As soon as the negative pressure created by patient effort reaches the sensitivity threshold level set (–2 cm H_2O [dashed line]), the ventilator responds by providing flow. In each example, patient effort is assisted by the ventilator. The dotted line connecting the first set of waveforms demonstrates that as soon as flow begins, the negative deflection in pressure is reversed and pressure in the ventilator circuit begins to build as gas is forced into the circuit and patient's lungs. The breath is then very similar to a controlled breath with the exception that there is some reduction in the P_{AO} during inspiration as the patient actively breathes in response to positive pressure building in his or her lungs during assisted ventilation (Dick et al., 1996). When patients expand

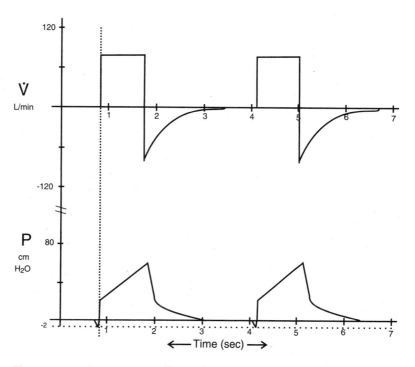

Figure 11-6 Square flow and corresponding pressure-time waveforms used to demonstrate assist mechanical mode (AMV) of ventilation.

their thorax in synchrony with gas delivery from the ventilator, it relieves some of the inspiratory pressure that would build up in the circuit compared with a patient (sedated and paralyzed) being passively ventilated under the same conditions of volume and flow delivery. Under optimal conditions of patient–ventilator synchrony, the pressure-time waveform will appear synchronous or relatively ideal. Slight reductions or alterations in the P_{AO} pattern are unremarkable. Patients commonly perform 33% to 50% of the work of ventilation during optimal AMV (Marini et al., 1985).

ASSIST CONTROL MODE OF MECHANICAL VENTILATION

☑ (Figure 11-7) In assist/control mode, the I:E ratio is variable because the E time of a breath is dependent on the timing of the following breath.

Figure 11-7 describes the assist-control (AC) mode of ventilation with ideal flow and pressure patterns. The I:E ratios are 1:3 for the second and third mechanical breaths as the patient expires and relaxes after the second assist breath and allows the ventilator to take control. The expiratory pause time for the first breath is cut short because the patient triggers a second assist breath. The I:E ratio is less than 1:3 for the first breath because the patient triggers the second breath before the controlled 3s expiratory time (Te) has elapsed. The third and fourth

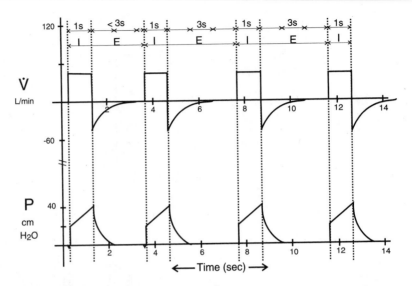

Figure 11-7 Square flow and corresponding pressure-time waveforms demonstrate assist/control mode (AC) of ventilation.

breaths are time triggered. The backup rate (control mode rate) is set at 15 b/min (TCT = 4 seconds, 60s/4s = 15 b/min). Through observation a therapist can estimate that inspiratory time is one second and peak flow is approximately 50 L/min (0.83 L/s). The set V_T is 0.83 L [V_T = flow (L/s) × time (s)]. Thus, as defined in the AC mode, flow, V_T, and rate (backup) are set as in the control mode, but the patient is allowed to trigger as many breaths as desired. *Actual* CMV is no longer available on ventilators, since patients' attempts to breathe should always be complimented. The CMV and AC modes are now used interchangeably, and CMV is used for the rest of this chapter to mean AC mode, where the rate is set as a backup. Setting CMV on a microprocessor ventilator, means AC is set unless the sensitivity is set so low that the patient cannot reach the threshold level, which is contraindicated. CMV ensures that if a patient does not breathe, flow, V_T and rate are set, and the patient will be ventilated regardless of effort.

ASSIST CONTROL, PEEP, AND VOLUME WAVEFORMS

In Figure 11-8, volume-time graphics and positive end-expiratory pressure (PEEP) have been added to the example of CMV that was presented in Figure 11-7. The y-axis measures volume in liters during inspiration and expiration over time (x-axis). For a square flow wave, volume rises linearly over time once flow is constant as demonstrated. During expiration, volume demonstrates an exponential decay pattern in correspondence with the expiratory flow pattern (normal lungs)

☑ (Figure 11-8, pressure waveform) PEEP is present when the positive end-expiratory pressure rests above 0 cm H_2O.

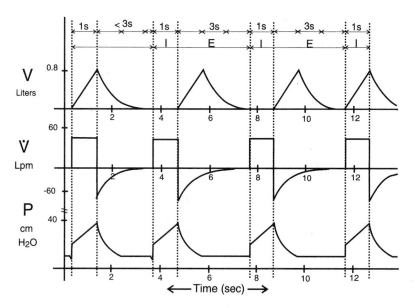

Figure 11-8 Volume, square flow, and corresponding pressure-time waveforms demonstrate assist/control ventilation.

over the same time period. The baseline pressure for the pressure-time waveforms is approximately 10 cm H_2O PEEP. For the assist breaths, it can be seen that pressure drops to 8 cm H_2O or 2 cm H_2O below PEEP level to trigger the first two breaths. The ventilator compensates for the adjustment in baseline pressure, and sensitivity is considered to be PEEP compensated.

SPONTANEOUS VENTILATION DURING MECHANICAL VENTILATION

SYNCHRONIZED INTERMITTENT MECHANICAL VENTILATION MODE

Figure 11-9 shows the three types of breaths (controlled, spontaneous, and assist) offered during synchronized intermittent mandatory ventilation (SIMV). The first set of waveforms is ideal flow and pressure-time patterns for a volume- or flow-controlled mechanical breath. Letter *a* (arrow) beneath the first pressure waveform indicates that the breath is ventilator initiated (time triggered and controlled). The patient did not attempt to breathe within the window of time (SIMV period) set up for synchronized (assist) mechanical breaths. Two sets of flow- and pressure-time waveforms depicting ideal spontaneous

☑ Figure 11-9 shows three types of breaths during SIMV: controlled (1st set of waveform does not show assist effort on the pressure tracing); spontaneous (2nd and 3rd waveforms show that mechanical breaths are absent); assist (4th waveform shows assist effort on the pressure tracing).

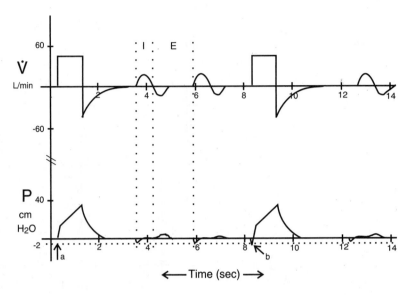

Figure 11-9 Synchronized intermittent mechanical ventilation (SIMV).

breaths are recorded next during the time (spontaneous period) allotted for spontaneous breaths. Relative sine waves are created during rested spontaneous ventilation. Spontaneous breathing is accommodated on ventilators in SIMV and continuous positive airway pressure (CPAP) modes. During spontaneous ventilation, the patient controls flow, volume, inspiratory time, and expiratory time. The ventilator responds to patient effort by supplying the flow demanded. The spontaneous breaths show that the patient created a peak inspiratory flow of about 20 L/min and peak expiratory flows of about 15 L/min. The pressure waves during spontaneous breathing show a negative pressure to trigger demand flow and some positive pressure recorded in the circuit during expiration. Spontaneous breaths are explained in more detail in Figure 11-10. The next breath in this graphic is an assist mechanical breath. Letter *b* (arrow) indicates that patient effort occurred to trigger the breath during the SIMV period. The manufacturer determines the amount of time allotted for synchronized mechanical and spontaneous breaths. For the next breath in the graphic, sufficient time has not elapsed for a mechanical breath to be synchronized with the patient's effort, so flow delivery is based on demand and another spontaneous breath is provided. An SIMV rate of 6 b/min has probably been set for the patient in this graphic with 5 to 6 seconds allotted for the spontaneous breaths and 4 to 5 seconds allotted for the SIMV breaths.

CONTINUOUS POSITIVE AIRWAY PRESSURE MODE

☑ (Figure 11-10)
In CPAP mode, there are no mechanical breaths and the airway pressure is always above 0 cm H₂O.

Figure 11-10 is an example of spontaneous ventilation in the continuous positive airway pressure (CPAP) mode. CPAP has been set at 5 cm H_2O. In the flow graphic, a labels the end of expiration and start of inspiration (arrow); b marks the peak flow reached (20 L/min) for an idealized sine flow wave created by the patient during spontaneous breathing; c indicates the change from inspiration to expiration; d indicates the peak expiratory flow attained (20 L/min); e indicates the end of expiratory flow; and f indicates the pause following expiratory flow. The patient creates an inspiratory flow time of approximately 0.75s, an expiratory flow time of 1.25s and an expiratory pause time of 0.75s. The dotted lines connecting the flow and pressure recordings in time delineate the total respiratory time into the inspiratory and total expiratory time periods. As with mechanical breaths, inspiratory effort (negative pressure recorded) triggers flow on demand (demand CPAP) once the negative pressure reaches the sensitivity threshold (–1 cm H_2O, dotted line), or the pressure drops during a continuous flow (continuous flow CPAP). Ideally, gas is delivered to the patient according to his or her flow demands, which means that pressure will be maintained at zero throughout the inspiratory phase of ventilation. In this example, the pressure recorded during inspiration is kept near

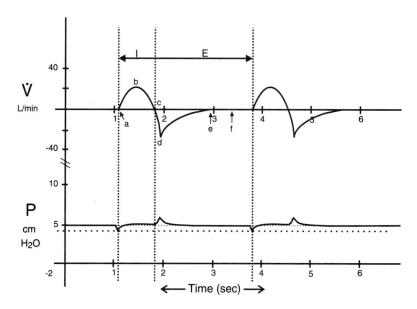

Figure 11-10 Ideal flow- and pressure-time waveforms during spontaneous ventilation with CPAP/PEEP set at 5 cm H₂O.

zero indicating patient flow demand is being met. During expiration, as gas is expired into the circuit, a positive pressure is momentarily recorded until the expiratory flow is too slow or the expiratory circuit and valve resistance is so low that near baseline pressure is recorded.

EFFECTS OF FLOW, CIRCUIT, AND LUNG CHARACTERISTICS ON PRESSURE-TIME WAVEFORMS

☑ Figure 11-11 shows un-changed P_{ALV} but increased PIP and P_{TA}. This observation reflects increase in airflow resistance. P_{ALV} remains con-stant because neither the C_{LT} nor the lung volume is changed.

FLOW AND TRANSAIRWAY PRESSURE (P_{TA})

A pause has been set in Figure 11-11 to delineate the dynamic pressure curve into the two distinct pressures, P_{TA} and P_{ALV} (double-headed arrows) generated during gas flow through a ventilator circuit into a patient's lungs. For waveform analysis, it is important to know how each of these pressures is affected by changes in flow and lung charac-teristics. Figure 11-11 demonstrates the effects of increased flow rate on a pressure-time waveform, which can be compared to the effects

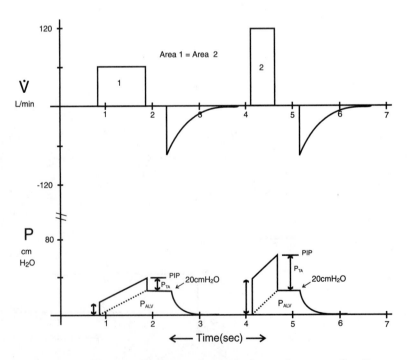

Figure 11-11   Flow- and pressure-time waveforms demonstrating the effects of flow rate on P_{TA}, P_{ALV}, and expiratory flow pattern.

on them created by decreased compliance (Figure 11-12). The pressure-time graphics in Figure 11-11 depict (double-headed arrows) that there has been a rise in the P_{TA} from beginning to end in the second pressure waveform because of an increase in turbulence when the constant flow was doubled from 60 to 120 L/min in the second flow wave. As gas flows through a circuit system with different twists and turns, and varied lumen sizes such as large bore tubing, humidifiers, and endotracheal tubes, turbulent flow results, which causes an exponential rise in *circuit* pressure with increments in flow. Conversely, an exponential decay in pressure is observed when flow is reduced (Dennison et al., 1989). Thus, the area depicting the P_{TA} gradient ($P_{AO} - P_{ALV}$) has been more than doubled in the second pressure wave. Note, however, that the remarkable change in P_{AO} and PIP did not affect the *peak* P_{ALV} because neither the C_{LT} nor lung volume was changed. Only the rise time to peak P_{ALV} was affected because Ti was cut in half. In this example, resistance was increased by an increase in flow. An increase in airway resistance from various lung pathologies causing bronchoconstriction and obstruction will also increase the area depicting the P_{AO} and P_{TA} gradient without a change in flow, but P_{ALV} will not be affected. Airway obstruction and bronchoconstriction will affect waveforms in other ways, but these are dealt with during discussion of using expiratory waveforms as a diagnostic tool.

COMPLIANCE AND ALVEOLAR PRESSURE (P_{ALV})

Figure 11-12 demonstrates a similar comparison between flow and pressure waveforms. Neither flow nor airway resistance has changed, but the PIP has substantially increased in the second example as in Figure 11-11. If there is no change in flow or V_T to explain the increase in PIP, a plateau needs to be set to analyze the cause. P_{TA} remains the same for each waveform, but P_{ALV} has substantially increased in the second waveform. Given the information presented in the graphic, a decrease in total C_{LT} is the only explanation for the increase in P_{ALV} and PIP. The same peak flow, flow pattern, and volume (Area 1 = Area 2) are being used for volume delivery in each example, which would create the same P_{ALV} and pattern in each example. One can estimate total C_{LT} by observing the information provided in such graphics and determine that total C_{LT} has decreased by half according to the second waveform. The area under the flow curve is 1 Liter or 1000 mL (1 L/s × 1 s), and total C_{LT} = 1000 mL/20 cm H_2O or 50 mL/cm H_2O versus total C_{LT} = 1000 mL/40 cm H_2O or 25 mL/cm H_2O. Thus, in the first example total C_{LT} equals 50 mL/cm H_2O, and in the second example C_{LT} has been reduced to half its original value, from 50 to 25 mL/cm H_2O.

✔ Figure 11-12 shows unchanged P_{TA} but increased PIP and P_{ALV}. This observation reflects a decrease in total C_{LT}.

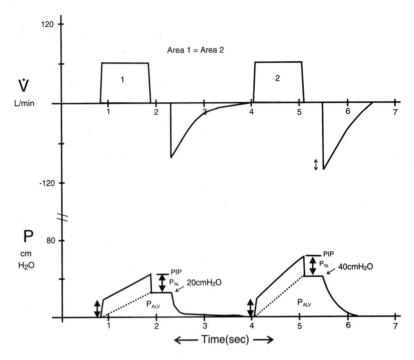

Figure 11-12 Flow- and pressure-time waveforms demonstrating the effects of lung–thorax compliance on P_{TA}, P_{ALV}, and expiratory flow pattern.

EFFECTS OF DECELERATING FLOW DURING VOLUME-CONTROLLED VENTILATION

☑ (Figure 11-13, first example) With time-limited ventilation, the inspiratory time does not change when the flow waveform selection is changed from square to decelerating. The same volume can only be delivered if the peak flow of the decelerating pattern is increased.

TIME-LIMITED AND FLOW-LIMITED VENTILATION

Figure 11-13 demonstrates the changes that occur when the flow pattern is switched from a constant to decelerating flow for a time-limited ventilator (first example) compared to a flow-limited ventilator (second example). These examples show a decelerating flow pattern (solid lines) that descends from the initially high peak flow level to zero end flow. The decelerating wave *end flows* available for selection in the CMV and SIMV modes may vary depending on the ventilator. For example, the Puritan Bennett (PB) 7200 uses an end flow of 5 L/min and the Hamilton Medical Veolar provides the option to select an end flow of zero or 50% of the initial peak flow (e.g., the second example in Figure 11-16). The concepts presented here are the same for the various types of decelerating flow patterns. In the first example, a decelerating flow wave is superimposed over a square wave pattern (dashed lines)

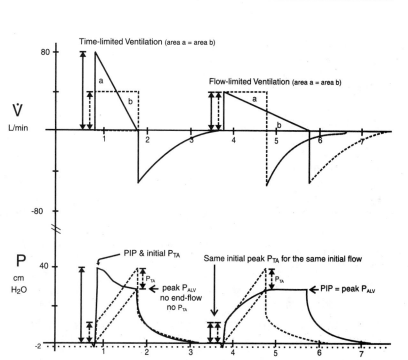

Figure 11-13 Characteristic changes to the dynamic pressure pattern created by decelerating flow during time-limited and flow-limited ventilation.

☑ (Figure 11-13, second example) With flow-limited ventilation, the inspiratory peak flow does not change when the flow waveform selection is changed from square to decelerating. The same volume can only be delivered if the inspiratory time of the decelerating pattern is increased.

for a time-limited ventilator (Veolar) during CMV. Inspiratory time does not change (time-limited) when the flow waveform selection is changed from square to decelerating, so the same volume can only be delivered if the peak flow and area under the flow wave of the decelerating pattern are increased. As demonstrated in the first flow example, the area enclosed by the solid and dashed line labeled *a* on the decelerating flow wave replaces the same area and, therefore, volume that was truncated from the square flow wave area labeled *b*. Thus, the same volume is being delivered by either flow pattern within the same time period. Transition from a square to a zero-end-flow decelerating flow wave on a time-limited ventilator requires peak flow to be doubled to deliver the same volume. For example, the square flow wave delivered a V_T of 0.67 liter ($V_T = 40$ L/min/60s/min × 1 s = 0.67 L) and doubling the peak flow, the decelerating flow wave delivered the same V_T ($V_T = (80$ L/min)/2/60s/min × 1 s = 0.67 L). In general, when employing decelerating flow waves, peak flow has to be proportionately greater as end flow is reduced if the same volume is to be delivered in the same time period. The second example of superimposed flow wave

✔ (Figure 11-13, pressure waveform in first example) With time-limited ventilation, the higher *initial* peak flow for the decelerating flow wave creates a higher initial flow-resistive pressure (P_{TA}) than the P_{TA} created by the square flow.

✔ (Figure 11-13, pressure waveform in second example) With flow-limited ventilation, the initial flow-resistive pressure (P_{TA}) is the same for the square and decelerating flow waves. The *initial* peak flow level stays the same for square and decelerating flow during flow-limited ventilation.

patterns demonstrates the results of switching from a square to a decelerating pattern during flow (peak) limited ventilation. The ventilator's peak flow does not change when the decelerating flow is selected, and as the flow decelerates, it eliminates the volume that was enclosed under area *a*. Time has to be extended until the same volume eliminated is replaced (i.e., area *b*). Given flow-limited ventilation, time fluctuates rather than peak flow to deliver the same V_T. Thus, depending on ventilator type, when flow is changed during CMV or SIMV from a square to a zero-end-flow decelerating flow pattern, either the peak flow has to be doubled (time-limited ventilation) or the inspiratory time has to be doubled (flow-limited ventilation) for the same V_T to be delivered.

The pattern and level of pressure developed (Figure 11-13) during decelerating flow ventilation depend, as for square flow ventilation, on the peak to end-flow pattern, circuit/lung resistance, and C_{LT}. The pressure waveform examples (solid lines) for the time- and flow-limited decelerating flow patterns are superimposed over the trapezoid pressure waveforms (dashed lines) created by square flow waveforms. Pressure during decelerating flow wave ventilation, depending on the peak flow level set (80 versus 40 L/min for these examples), tends to "square-off" compared to rising linearly as it does for square flow ventilation. Assuming the same circuit and lung characteristics for the comparison, the higher initial peak flow for the decelerating flow wave in the first example (80 L/min) creates a higher peak flow-resistive pressure or P_{TA} (40 cm H_2O) at the beginning of inspiration on the pressure waveform compared to flow-resistive pressure (10 cm H_2O) for the square flow. And as demonstrated, the flow-resistive pressure for decelerating flow decreases over time with reduction in flow, whereas the flow-resistive pressure stays constant (dashed line, double-headed arrows) for the constant or square flow pattern. Since the same volume is being delivered in each decelerating flow example and zero flow occurs at end inspiration, the pressure at end inspiration for both examples is the patient's P_{ALV}. There is no flow at end inspiration, so no flow-resistive pressure (P_{TA}) is being created. Flow-resistive pressure steadily drops to zero during inspiration for zero-end-flow ventilation. Note that PIP and P_{ALV} are the same for the second pressure waveform example. In the first example, PIP is greater than the peak P_{ALV} and comes at the beginning of inspiration because of the very high initial flow rate (80 L/min). During square flow ventilation, PIP is always the highest pressure and always at the end of inspiration because flow resistive pressure (P_{TA}) is "stacked" on top of the P_{ALV} at end inspiration (double-headed arrows). Note, also, in the second example, that initial flow-resistive pressure is the same for the square and decelerating flow waves because the initial peak flow level stays the same when switching from square to decelerating flow for flow-limited ventilation. Pressure rises after the initial flow period because volume accumulates in the lung and flow-resistive pressure is stacked on top of P_{ALV}.

☑ In square and decelerating flow ventilation, the rise in alveolar pressure (P_{ALV}) is directly related to volume delivery and inversely related to compliance.

Volume Delivery. Figure 11-14 delineates the decelerating flow pressure patterns (solid lines) into their component parts of flow-resistive pressure (open arrows) and P_{ALV} superimposed for comparison over the flow-resistive and P_{ALV} areas for square flow waves (dotted lines). The P_{TA} and P_{ALV} for the square flow waves rise linearly as discussed in Figure 11-4. Like square flow ventilation, the rise in P_{ALV} during decelerating flow wave ventilation is dependent on volume delivered and C_{LT}. Volume delivery (area under the flow wave) for decelerating flow is obviously different. For example, calculation of the volume under the zero-end-flow decelerating flow wave shows that 75% of the volume is delivered during the first half of inspiration. The flow waveforms in Figure 11-14 are the same as in Figure 11-13. The V_T for the square flow wave is 0.67 L (see calculation, Figure 11-13), and, therefore, 0.333 L is delivered the first half of inspiration. The volume delivered in the first half of inspiration for the decelerating flow wave is 0.5 L {V_T = ½ [(peak flow L/min + end flow L/min)/60s/min] × Ti} = ½ [(80 L/min + 40 L/min)/60s/min] × 0.5s = 0.5 L, which is 75% of the V_T (0.5L/0.67L = 75%). For time-limited ventilation, greater volume being delivered the first half of inspiration

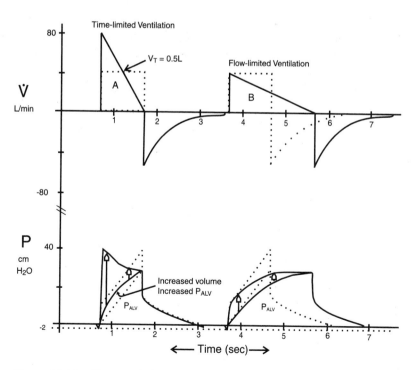

Figure 11-14 Characteristic changes to the dynamic and alveolar pressure (P_{ALV}) patterns created by decelerating flow during time-limited and flow-limited ventilation.

equates to a faster rise or slope in P_{ALV} in the first half of inspiration compared to the square flow P_{ALV} slope, which is noted in the first pressure wave. The slope in P_{ALV} for the decelerating wave is lower than the square flow wave P_{ALV} slope for the second half of inspiration because only 25% of the V_T is delivered compared to 50% of the V_T being delivered during square flow ventilation.

The same concepts explored above can be applied to the P_{ALV} pattern for the decelerating flow wave in the second pressure waveform in Figure 11-14, but the comparison with the square flow pattern is a little more complicated. In this example, the comparison between flow and pressure waves is made during flow-limited ventilation, and time for V_T delivery via decelerating wave ventilation has been doubled. For the decelerating flow in the first example, there is a proportionate reduction in the slope or rise to peak P_{ALV} throughout inspiration. In this second example, the P_{ALV} slope for the square flow is higher throughout inspiration compared to the decelerating flow wave. That is because the *entire* V_T is delivered by the square flow wave within the time period for which only 75% of the V_T is delivered via decelerating flow. Because of volume delivery, the decelerating flow pattern generates a curvilinear P_{ALV} pattern. During ideal square flow ventilation constant volume is delivered and, therefore, a constant rise (linear) in P_{ALV} per unit time from beginning to end inspiration (assuming no change in C_{LT}). But during deceleration in flow to zero, there is a proportionate *decrease* in volume delivered per unit time and, although the summative P_{ALV} steadily rises, the P_{ALV} generated per unit time steadily drops from beginning to end inspiration. For example, 75% of the V_T is delivered and 75% of the *peak* P_{ALV} is generated the first half of inspiration. The second half of inspiration, 25% of the V_T is delivered with only a 25% increase in P_{ALV}, which is a substantial reduction in P_{ALV} per unit time compared to the first half of inspiration. Thus, Figure 11-14 demonstrates that the slope for the P_{ALV} curve generated during decelerating flow ventilation proportionately decreases per unit time as summative P_{ALV} increases, and a convex (decay) pattern is created from beginning to end inspiration consistent with the pattern of volume delivery. This issue is discussed in more detail in Figure 11-17. Note also that in Figure 11-14 as in Figure 11-13 the initial P_{TA} is higher (open arrows) when initial flow is higher. P_{TA} is the same for square and decelerating flow waves when the initial peak flow is the same, but the P_{TA} for the decelerating flows proportionately drop to zero by end inspiration with reduction in flow to zero, as P_{ALV} proportionately increases to the peak level at zero-end-flow.

PEAK FLOW AND TIDAL VOLUME RELATIONSHIP IN TIME-LIMITED VENTILATION

Figure 11-15 demonstrates decelerating flow ventilation where Ti is maintained but flow is reduced. The first example shows the flow-resistive pressure is high for the set flow rate (80 L/min). Given the

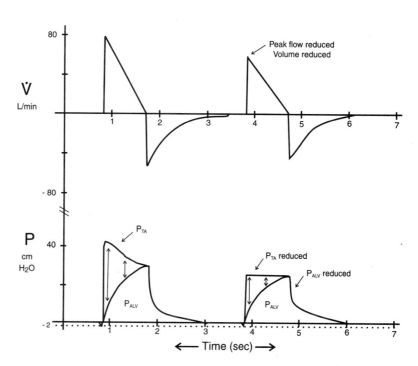

Figure 11-15 Characteristic changes to transairway (P_{TA}) and alveolar pressure (P_{ALV}) created by changes in peak decelerating flow during time-limited ventilation.

☑ At constant Ti, a decreased flow leads to lower V_T, P_{TA}, and P_{ALV}.

same lung and circuit characteristics for each set of waveforms, the second example shows the results to the pressure pattern if Ti is maintained (time-limited ventilation), but flow is reduced. Given the same Ti and a reduction in flow, the V_T is reduced (V_T = average flow × Ti). The consequence of the reduction in flow is that V_T is reduced as is the P_{TA} and P_{ALV}.

EFFECTS OF END FLOW ON TIDAL VOLUME

Figure 11-16 demonstrates the changes in P_{TA} patterns that could be expected when *end* flows for decelerating flow waves are increased. In the first example, the end flow is 5 L/min (PB7200). The pressure pattern shows a slight increase in the flow-resistive pressure above the P_{ALV} at end inspiration as a consequence of end flow being above baseline at end inspiration. The second set of waveforms shows a 50% decelerating flow wave where end flow is 50% of the initial peak flow set. The initial flow set is very high (100 L/min), which causes a high initial P_{TA} (40 cm H_2O) because of circuit/airway resistance. The end P_{TA} is also relatively high from flow-resistive pressure above the peak P_{ALV} compared to the first example since end flow is 50 L/min compared to 5 L/min. These flow and pressure patterns do not represent

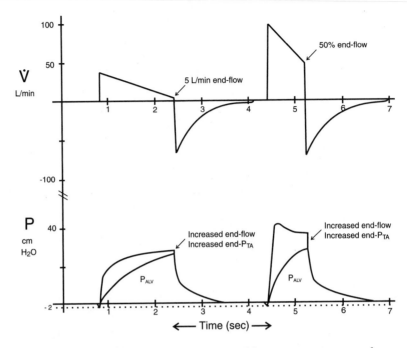

Figure 11-16 The effects of variation in end flow on pressure waveforms during decelerating flow ventilation.

✓ A higher end flow leads to a larger V_T.

ventilation of the same patient. Peak P_{ALV} is at the same level, but V_T delivered is much greater for the second flow wave example compared to the first.

DISTRIBUTION OF DELIVERED TIDAL VOLUME

In Figure 11-17 volume-time waveforms have been added for comparison with decelerating flow and pressure-time waveforms. Some ventilator computer software programs allow monitoring of three or more waveforms as presented in this example. Since flow rate is highest in the beginning of inspiration for decelerating flow, the slope in rise to peak volume, like P_{ALV}, is initially fast and becomes proportionately reduced over time as flow descends. In the first example, peak flow is set at 60 L/min and Ti is 1 second, the volume delivered is 0.5 liter [1/2 (60 L/min)/60s/min × 1s = 0.5 L]. The volume delivered in the first half of inspiration is 0.375 L [1/2 (60 L/min peak flow + 30 L/min end flow)/2/60s/min x 0.5s (Ti) = 0.375 L], which is 75% of 0.5 L (0.75 × 0.5 L = 0.375 L). The volume delivered in the second half of inspiration is 0.125 L (0.5 L − 0.375 L = 0.125 L), which is 25% of the V_T (0.25 × 0.5 L = 0.125 L).

The pressure-time pattern in the first example in Figure 11-17 shows the development of P_{ALV} in correspondence with delivery of the V_T. Determining the P_{ALV} curve requires knowing the volume delivered

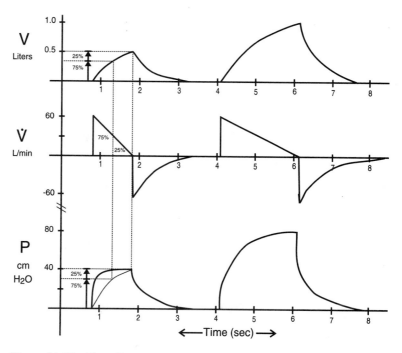

Figure 11-17 The effects the decelerating flow pattern has on the volume and alveolar pressure (P_{ALV}) waveforms.

per time and the total C_{LT}. According to the flow and pressure-time curve, peak P_{ALV} is 40 cm H_2O because there is no flow at end inspiration. Total C_{LT} is 0.0125 L/cm H_2O or 12.5 mL/cm H_2O (C_{LT} = volume/ P_{ALV} = 0.5 L/40 cm H_2O = 0.0125 L/cm H_2O). If there is no change in C_{LT} during V_T delivery, P_{ALV} half way through inspiration will depend on the volume delivered by that time. The example shows as discussed earlier that 75% of the V_T is delivered the first half of inspiration, consequently 75% of the peak P_{ALV} will be attained, which is 30 cm H_2O (0.75 × 40 cm H_2O = 30 cm H_2O), or P_{ALV} is equal to volume calculated for that time divided by total C_{LT} (P_{ALV} = 0.375 L/0.0125 L/cm H_2O = 30 cm H_2O). The remaining 25% of the P_{ALV} is developed the second half of inspiration (P_{ALV} = 0.25 × 40 cm H_2O = 10 cm H_2O, or P_{ALV} = 0.125 L/0.0125 L/cm H_2O = 10 cm H_2O). Thus, any point along the P_{ALV} curve can be predicted and plotted by calculating the volume delivered per time provided total C_{LT} is known.

In the second example, peak flow is maintained at 60 L/min, but V_T is doubled [1/2 (60 L/min)/60s/min × 2s = 1 L], which increases Ti to 2 seconds. As a result of doubling V_T, peak P_{ALV} is doubled (P_{ALV} = 1.0 L/0.0125 L/cm H_2O = 80 cm H_2O). Note that the initial flow-resistive pressure is sustained in the second pressure waveform since the initial flow has not changed.

☑ When peak flow is kept unchanged, V_T, Ti, and P_{ALV} are directly related.

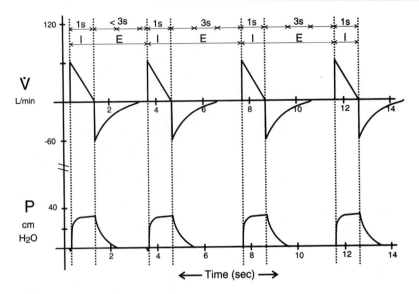

Figure 11-18 Assist/control mechanical ventilation during decelerating flow ventilation.

CMV DURING DECELERATING FLOW VENTILATION

✓ With zero-end-flow decelerating flow ventilation, P_{ALV} equals end pressure.

Figure 11-18 is an example of CMV during decelerating flow ventilation, where the patient initiates the first two breaths and then relaxes and the ventilator triggers the next two breaths. A benefit of the decelerating flow wave being used in this example is that the P_{ALV} and C_{LT} can be determined without a pause being set. P_{ALV} equals end pressure so C_{LT} is 14.3 mL/cm H_2O (C_{LT} = 500 mL/35 cm H_2O = 14.3 mL/cm H_2O).

WAVEFORMS DEVELOPED DURING PRESSURE-LIMITED VENTILATION

PRESSURE CONTROL VENTILATION

✓ In PCV, pressure level, rate, and I:E ratio are set by the operator. The V_T delivered is not set. The flow level and V_T are dependent on the pressure level set, patient effort, and lung characteristics.

Figure 11-19 is an example of pressure control ventilation (PCV), which is an AC or CMV mode where pressure is maintained (controlled or limited). There are no assist breaths attempted by the patient in this example to simplify mode description. In PCV, pressure level, rate, and I:E ratio are set by the operator. The V_T delivered is not set. The flow level and V_T are dependent on the pressure level set, patient effort, and lung characteristics. The ventilator is time or

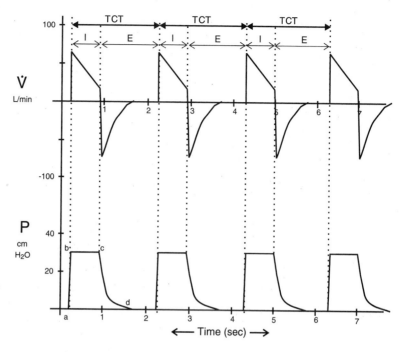

Figure 11-19   Characteristics of pressure control ventilation (PCV).

☑ Under normal conditions, the area under the inspiratory *or* expiratory flow waveforms determines the V$_T$ delivered.

patient triggered and the ventilator delivers flow in a manner that will reach and maintain the set pressure level as in this example, unless the manufacturer opts to establish a slow rise (convex pattern) to gradually reach the pressure limit (PB7200) for patient comfort. If flow demand is increased, the ventilator will increase flow sufficiently to maintain the set pressure limit. If flow demand drops, flow rate will be slowed to maintain the set pressure limit. If flow demand drops to zero before end inspiration, the ventilator will maintain the set pressure level by closing the expiratory valve if necessary to maintain circuit and lung pressure at the set level. In this example, the pressure level set for ventilation is 30 cm H$_2$O, and the area under the inspiratory flow (*or* expiratory flow providing there is no circuit leak or air trapping) waveforms determines the V$_T$ delivered. For the letters on the pressure-time wave *a* marks the end expiration and beginning inspiration; *b* indicates the PIP level set; *c* is the end inspiration and pressure level sustained and change from inspiration to expiration; and *d* is end expiration. Total cycle time (TCT) is 2 seconds and frequency is 30 b/min (60s/2s/breath = 30 b/min). Te is twice Ti. The I:E ratio set is 1:2. Thus, TCT is composed of three parts and Ti is 0.67s and Te is 1.33s (TCT/3 parts = Ti, 2s/3 = 0.67s, TCT – Ti = Te, 2s – 0.67s = 1.33s).

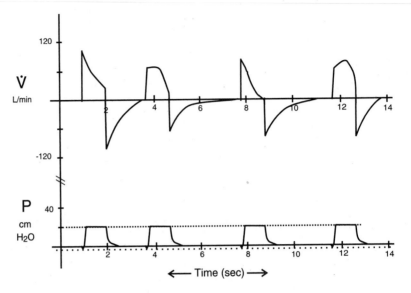

Figure 11-20 Variations in flow and volume during pressure control ventilation (PCV).

✓ During PCV the flow pattern may fluctuate with each breath and the delivered V_T depends on patient effort and lung characteristics.

dyssynchrony: A breathing pattern that is out of synchronization with the ventilator.

✓ IRPCV is typically used under conditions of severe hypoxia and lung injury (ARDS).

Assisted Breaths during PCV. Figure 11-20 is an example of a patient who is not relaxed and is triggering all the breaths during PCV. Since the flow pattern fluctuates with each breath, the delivered V_T depends on patient effort and lung characteristics. In Figure 11-20, the PIP is set at 20 cm H_2O, and this pressure level is sustained (dashed line) by the ventilator. One of the major advantages of pressure control ventilation is that the patient can vary the flow and volume at any time. Pressure control ventilation differs from volume control ventilation in that the latter forces a set flow pattern onto the patients and they have to adapt to it or be in **dyssynchrony** with the ventilator.

INVERSE RATIO PCV

Figure 11-21 demonstrates inverse ratio pressure control ventilation (IRPCV) set at 20 cm H_2O with 10 cm H_2O PEEP administered (PIP = 30 cm H_2O). IRPCV is only used under conditions of severe hypoxia and lung injury (ARDS). Since an inverse ratio respiratory pattern is abnormal and uncomfortable, patients are sedated and paralyzed to prevent them from "fighting" the ventilator. In this example, inspiratory flow drops to zero (bold arrow) since Ti is prolonged and there is no flow demand by the patient. As stated earlier, if there is no flow demand the ventilator will maintain set pressure level by curtailing flow and closing the expiratory valve. This process holds gas in the patient's lungs under conditions of no flow and consequently the circuit

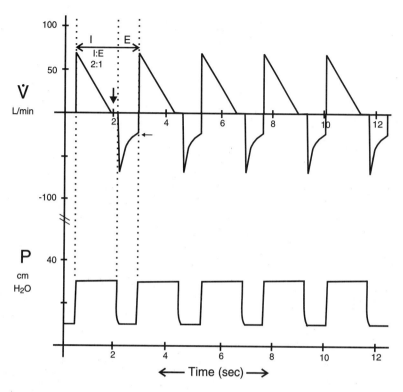

Figure 11-21 AutoPEEP created during inverse-ratio pressure control ventilation (IRPCV).

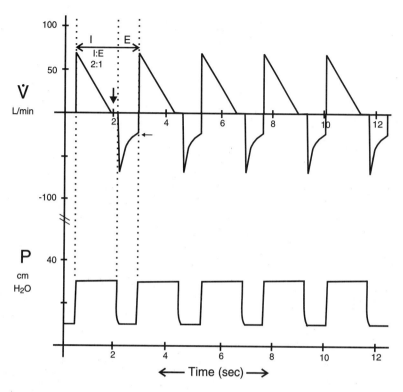 Since an inverse ratio respiratory pattern is abnormal and uncomfortable, patients are sedated and paralyzed to prevent dyssynchrony with the ventilator.

pressure is the same as P_{ALV}. The volume held in the patient's lungs depends on the patient's C_{LT}. If the V_T expired is monitored, the patient's lung compliance can be measured [$C_{LT} = V_T/(P_{CL} - PEEP)$]. Total PEEP includes PEEP set plus intrinsic or autoPEEP. The arrow at the first expiratory flow wave shows that autoPEEP is being created because the ventilator time triggers successive breaths before the patient's expiratory flow is able to descend to baseline, trapping gas in the patient's lungs and raising the patient's functional residual capacity. This level of IRV used to be common practice, but it is recommended now to avoid autoPEEP, if possible, and use applied PEEP instead to raise mean airway pressure to sustain a minimal level of oxygenation. A valuable advantage of having graphics is that autoPEEP can be readily observed and prevented whenever lung conditions have changed or ventilator settings have been altered. Also, graphics can be observed as Ti is increased in small steps to a level that allows exactly enough time for expiration to prevent autoPEEP, which serves to maximize mean P_{ALV} and oxygenation as a result, but avoids high peak P_{ALV} (> 35 cm H_2O) as long as possible.

PRESSURE SUPPORT AND SPONTANEOUS MODES OF VENTILATION

PRESSURE SUPPORT VENTILATION

☑ For the PSV mode, only the pressure support level is set and all breaths are patient triggered.

☑ Under normal conditions, flow, volume, and inspiratory time are primarily under the patient's control.

Figure 11-22 is an example of the various features of pressure support ventilation (PSV). The first set of waveforms shows the patterns that develop for a relaxed patient breathing synchronously with the ventilator, a concave flow and a square pressure-time pattern. For the PSV mode, only the pressure support level is set and all pressure support breaths are patient triggered. PSV is considered a spontaneous mode of ventilation, because in the pressure support mode, although each breath is mechanically supported by pressure, each breath requires a spontaneous "effort" by the patient throughout most of inspiration to sustain flow delivery above cycling level. Under normal conditions, flow, volume, and inspiratory time are primarily under the patient's control. For that reason, the mode is defined as a spontaneous mode of ventilation. However, the pressure can be set high enough to limit virtually all effort by the patient except for triggering the breath. If the

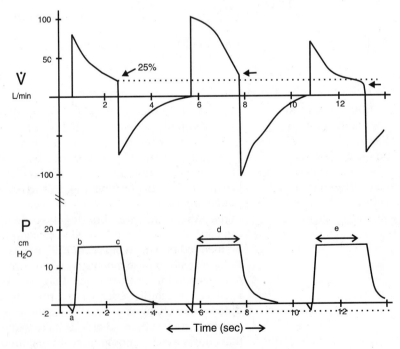

Figure 11-22 Characteristics of pressure support ventilation (PSV).

patient inspires in a relaxed manner as presented here, the flow accelerates to peak flow but then slows quickly (decays) and cycles into expiration at 25% of the initial peak flow level attained, or some manufacturer set level (i.e., 5 L/min for the PB7200). For the first pressure waveform example, *a* indicates it is an assist, pressure/patient-triggered breath; *b* indicates that the pressure level set, 15 cm H_2O, has been quickly reached; and *c* shows that the pressure limit has been sustained throughout inspiration and the transition to expiration. The flow wave demonstrates that the ventilator provides flow at a high level initially to *overcome* or outpace the patient's flow demands in order to reach the set pressure level. Initial flow has to be delivered to surpass the patient's flow demands to reach and sustain the set pressure support level. The flow waves and dotted line show that each wave is flow cycled into expiration at 25% (arrows) of the initial peak flow rate, which may vary with each breath. The second flow wave demonstrates that increased patient flow and volume demands are supplied as the set pressure level is maintained. The third flow wave shows a low, but sustained demand until 25% of the initial flow is reached. The double-headed arrows indicate the same time length, which shows that the inspiratory time for pressure waves *d* and *e* varies. Thus, flow, volume, and time can all vary and depend on lung characteristics and patient demand.

ADJUSTING RISE TIME DURING PSV

Figure 11-23 demonstrates PSV at 10 cm H_2O with a PEEP of 5 cm H_2O administered. The first two sets of waveforms are ideal with instantaneous rise to peak flow and set pressure limit. Letters *a* and *b* label flow waves that demonstrate a feature called rise percent (%) time, which is available on some ventilators (i.e., SV300). The dotted lines on the third and fourth pressure waveforms show that the slope or rise to the set pressure limit is progressively slower compared to the ideal pressure waveforms. Flow wave *a* shows a faster rise to peak flow than flow *b*. Perpendicular dashed lines are drawn so the lapse in time in rise to peak flow can be compared. The faster the initial rise to peak flow level, the sooner the set pressure limit is reached. Thus, the corresponding slope of the pressure wave is higher for flow wave *a* versus flow wave *b*. The pressure wave for flow wave *b* demonstrates that less flow-resistive pressure, and to a lesser extent, elastic recoil pressure per unit time is generated when there is a slower rise to peak flow. An advantage of slow rise to set pressure levels is that greater comfort is provided for some patients during PSV. An excessively fast rise to peak flow may cause the ventilator to overshoot the initial pressure limit and create a pressure spike at the beginning of inspiration, which can cause patient discomfort and increased work of breathing (Dick et al., 1996).

☑ The faster the initial rise to peak flow level, the sooner the set pressure limit is reached.

☑ A slow rise to set pressure level is more comfortable for the patient.

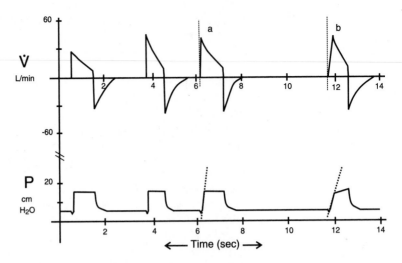

Figure 11-23 This graphic demonstrates an increase in rise percent (%) time and the change in the slope of the pressure-time waveforms (dotted lines *a* and *b*) during PSV.

SIMV (SQUARE FLOW) AND PSV

Figure 11-24 exemplifies the combination mode, SIMV + PSV. Two ideal square flow patterns and corresponding trapezoid pressure patterns, *a* and *d*, depict volume-controlled breaths, the first mandatory and the other an assist breath. Also, three ideal pressure-supported breaths, *b*, *c*, and *e*, displaying ideal decelerating flow, patient-triggered, pressure-

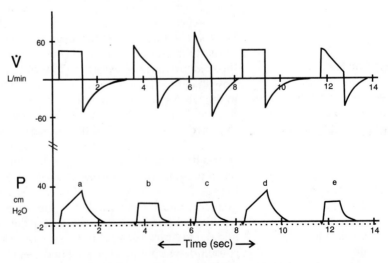

Figure 11-24 Synchronized intermittent mechanical ventilation (SIMV) plus pressure support ventilation (PSV) during square flow ventilation.

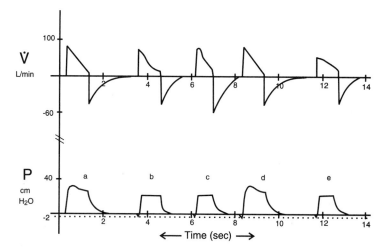

Figure 11-25 Synchronized intermittent mechanical ventilation (SIMV) plus pressure support ventilation (PSV) during decelerating flow ventilation.

limited (20 cm H_2O) breaths of varied flow, volume, and respiratory time are displayed.

SIMV (DECELERATING FLOW) AND PSV

Figure 11-25 also depicts the combination mode, SIMV + PSV, except that decelerating flow waves (end flows at 5 L/min) have replaced the square flow waves used in Figure 11-24. The ideal decelerating flow patterns show that the initial flows have been set high (80 L/min) so that the PIP for the pressure patterns, *a* and *d*, are created at the beginning of inspiration. Three ideal pressure-supported breaths, *b*, *c*, and *e*, are displayed again.

EFFECTS OF LUNG CHARACTERISTICS ON PRESSURE-LIMITED WAVEFORMS

Figure 11-26 exemplifies the effect that changes in circuit/airway resistance and C_{LT} can have on waveforms and volume delivered during pressure-limited ventilation. For each breath, the pressure-time waveform is the same (dotted line) regardless of changes in lung characteristics during pressure-limited ventilation. Two sets of flow and pressure waveforms under the dotted lines labeled *A* and *B* characterize different lung conditions. The peak flow and area under the inspiratory curve of the first flow wave is comparatively greater than the second in examples *A* and *B*. Thus, greater volume is being delivered

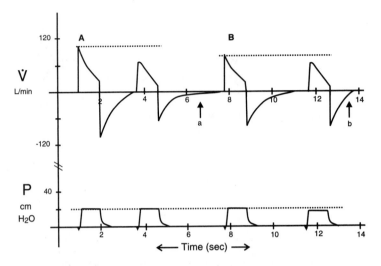

Figure 11-26 The effects of airway resistance and lung–thorax compliance changes on flow- and pressure-time waveforms during pressure limited ventilation.

by the first flow wave in each example. For example *A*, given no change in C_{LT} or effort, greater airway/circuit resistance could cause the observed reduction in flow and, therefore, V_T in the second flow wave. Greater flow resistive pressure (P_{TA}) causes the set pressure limit to be reached at a lower flow rate, and thus, a reduction in delivered V_T. Example *B* presents a similar pattern during inspiration for analysis. Given the same patient effort, a lower lung or chest wall compliance (i.e., ascites) produces the same results as in example *A*. Given lower C_{LT}, more pressure will be created per unit volume. Consequently, less volume is delivered in the second flow wave in example *B* to attain the same pressure level. Thus, during pressure-limited ventilation in contrast to volume-limited ventilation, the V_T delivered is altered rather than pressure with changes in lung status. Letters *a* and *b* are discussed in the section on using expiratory flow waves as diagnostic tools.

☑ During pressure-limited ventilation, an increased airflow resistance or decreased compliance would reduce the delivered flow and tidal volume.

USING WAVEFORMS FOR PATIENT AND VENTILATOR-SYSTEM ASSESSMENT

Understanding the basic characteristics of ideal waveforms corresponding to the major conventional modes of mechanical ventilation, AC, SIMV, PCV, and PSV, has been covered. The next objective is to use waveforms to improve or benefit ventilator–patient assessment and ventilator management. Positive pressure in the lungs is not natural. Too much volume under pressure is detrimental (volutrauma). Too little volume or not enough positive end-expiratory pressure (PEEP) to keep alveoli from collapsing (derecruitment) and then re-opening (recruitment) during tidal ventilation is also considered detrimental. Too little respiratory muscle use (disuse atrophy) leads to respiratory muscle weakness, and excessive imposed work of breathing (WOB) leads to respiratory muscle weakness or fatigue. Either way, mechanical ventilation is prolonged. No research to date suggests that patients triggering all the volume- or pressure-limited breaths in synchrony with the ventilator (appearance of normal patient-triggered waveforms) will develop respiratory muscle weakness from either too little or too much WOB. Conversely, volumes of research suggest that dyssychrony during ventilator management may impose too much WOB and prolong mechanical ventilation (Dick et al., 1996). Research suggests lack of assist ventilation (patient-triggered breaths) from prolonged paralysis or sedation as a reason for prolonged mechanical ventilation from respiratory muscle disuse. Thus, observation of graphics to ensure patient–ventilator synchrony plays an important role in mechanical ventilation. The best oxygenation and ventilation should be derived at the lowest volume and least lung pressure if patients are breathing in synchrony with the ventilator, which obviates excess WOB and mitigates the potential for excess lung pressures. AutoPEEP can be easily observed and corrected using graphics, which reduces the potential for volume trauma. And the level of synchrony can be controlled to ensure adequate use of the patient's respiratory muscles.

> ☑ Dyssychrony during ventilator management may impose too much WOB and prolong mechanical ventilation.

PATIENT–VENTILATOR DYSSYNCHRONY

Dyssynchrony requires greater WOB, oxygen consumption, minute ventilation, and work by the heart. It can begin with the assist or pressure-triggered breath. Figure 11-27 depicts a detailed analysis of assist (patient-triggered) ventilation. The pressure-time waveforms (above baseline) depict ideal trapezoid patterns. Thus, a square flow pattern must have been set for these pressure waveforms to be produced. The minus 2 cm H_2O value below baseline (zero) represents the sensitivity threshold level setting. In the first waveform, patient effort to trigger the breath is exaggerated to analyze the negative pressure deflection in greater detail. The negative pressure deflection crosses the set sensitivity threshold level descending to about minus 4 cm H_2O before the ventilator is able to respond (deliver gas). How fast the ventilator reacts to a patient's efforts depends on the patient's respiratory drive, sensitivity level set, inspiratory valve response time, and peak flow level set. The response time is measured from the time the sensitivity threshold setting is reached to the time flow is initiated by the ventilator (short, double-headed arrow). Once flow is initiated, pressure changes course

> ☑ Dyssynchrony requires greater WOB, oxygen consumption, minute ventilation, and work by the heart.

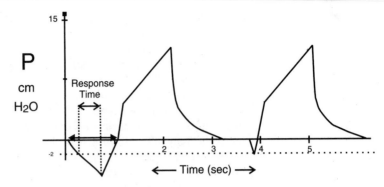

Figure 11-27   Pressure-time waveform demonstrates response time during assist (patient-triggered) ventilation.

☑ If a patient has a high ventilatory drive, a higher sensitivity setting (–0.5 cm H_2O versus –2 cm H_2O), a higher peak flow setting, or a ventilator manufactured with a faster response time should improve patient–ventilator synchrony.

from a negative to a positive direction. If a patient has a high ventilatory drive, a higher sensitivity setting (–0.5 cm H_2O versus –2 cm H_2O), a higher peak flow setting, or a ventilator manufactured with a faster response time should improve patient–ventilator synchrony.

When analyzing the patient-trigger phase of inspiratory effort, it is important to realize that the patient is always experiencing *higher* negative intrathoracic and intrapulmonary pressures than those recorded at the ventilator (Dick et al., 1996; Messinger et al., 1995). There is a time lag for the propagation of the pressure in the patient's airway to the pressure transducer in the ventilator. Research has shown that a –5 versus –2 cm H_2O sensitivity setting can increase WOB to intolerable levels (Marini et al., 1985). Thus, there can be substantial metabolic work to breathe required during the negative pressure time period recorded (long, double-headed arrow). Consider, for comparison, that for normal rested spontaneous breathing, approximately –1 cm H_2O P_{ALV} is incurred during inspiration and gas is flowing into the alveoli throughout the inspiratory effort and alveoli are expanding to aid in oxygenation and ventilation. There is no gas movement into the alveoli during the negative deflection time period depicted in example *A*. Gas is simply being decompressed and recompressed until positive pressure is recorded. Thus, during pressure triggering, since negative intrathoracic pressure is less than ventilator-recorded negative pressure (e.g., –10 cm H_2O intrathoracic vs. –2 cm H_2O at ventilator) metabolic work (O_2 consumption) can be greatly increased while oxygenation and ventilation are being compromised compared to normal spontaneous breathing, especially if sensitivity is set too low.

DYSSYNCHRONY DURING SQUARE FLOW VENTILATION

A lack of ventilator sensitivity to patient effort may set up the patient–ventilator dyssynchrony presented in the pressure waveform examples *a* and *b* in Figure 11-28, although these examples of dyssynchrony may

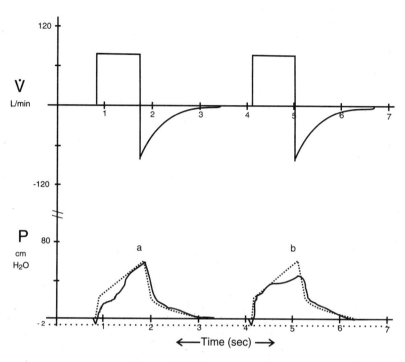

Figure 11-28 Square flow and pressure-time waveforms demonstrating dyssynchronous ventilation as a result of *a*, inadequate initial peak flow set, or *b*, inadequate V_T set to meet patient demand.

☑ Patient–ventilator dyssynchrony occurs when increased ventilatory demands are not met by a sufficient sensitivity flow or volume setting on the ventilator.

☑ Signs of patient–ventilator dyssynchrony include tachypnea, agitation, accessory muscle use, active expiration, paradoxical breathing and/or respiratory alternans.

occur irrespective of adequate ventilator sensitivity. Figure 11-28 shows that patient–ventilator dyssynchrony occurs when the increased ventilatory demands are not met by a sufficient flow or volume setting on the ventilator. Whether a particular pattern of dyssynchrony can be proven to be excessive or not is a complicated issue and beyond the scope of this chapter. Perfect waveforms are not necessary. When signs of patient–ventilator dyssynchrony are graphically displayed, decisions about ventilator management require a competent physical assessment. The first physical sign of increased WOB is tachypnea (> 20 b/min) and a general appearance of agitation. Some physical signs of respiratory muscle stress include accessory muscle use, supra- or substernal and/or intercostal retractions, and active expiration (use of abdominal muscles) accompany an agitated appearance and increased respiratory rate. In time, depending on a patient's strength reserve and nutritional status, signs of respiratory muscle weakness or fatigue can develop, that is, a paradoxical breathing pattern and/or respiratory alternans. Unfortunately, the last sign of respiratory muscle weakness or fatigue is blood gas results demonstrating respiratory failure (Tobin et al., 1986). So simply using arterial blood gas results as proof of competent

✔ Tachypnea and appearance of agitation may be caused by other factors such as pain and psychological stress.

ventilator management can be a serious mistake. Tachypnea and general appearance of agitation may be caused by other factors such as pain and psychological stress. So patient–ventilator synchrony may not be the problem. But if improvement in patient–ventilator synchrony eliminates the signs of physical and psychological distress, quality patient care has been enhanced. The right adjustment on the ventilator to improve synchrony is easily facilitated through waveform analysis.

The dotted line for the first pressure waveform, Figure 11-28 example *a*, exemplifies the ideal waveform for a passive patient being mechanically ventilated, that is, the ventilator is generating all the pressure necessary to expand the patient's lungs. The solid line depicts patient–ventilator dyssynchrony and the corresponding waveform actually created during mechanical ventilation. The greater the drop in pressure from the ideal pattern (dyssynchrony), the less the ventilator is assisting the patient with breathing. In fact, the dyssynchrony can impose more WOB onto the patient than that incurred by spontaneous breathing off the ventilator. Physical signs of distress indicate that the patient is enduring too much WOB. Dyssynchronous ventilation for patients with lung disease can require several times the energy required for normal work of breathing. If the patient is not on the ventilator because of respiratory failure, some dyssynchrony may not pose a serious problem. Research suggests that it will compromise oxygenation and ventilation compared to optimal and increase WOB, which may be uncomfortable for the patient. Morbidity and mortality outcomes, however, may be the same; the patient is simply doing more of the WOB. But research shows that if patients are recovering from respiratory muscle failure, dyssynchrony can sustain respiratory muscle weakness or fatigue, and it will prolong mechanical ventilation because recovery time to regain the strength for spontaneous breathing without mechanical support is compromised. The first pressure-time waveform presented indicates that the initial flow needs to be increased to keep pace with the patient's initial flow demands. The initial flow-resistive pressure is partially removed, so that the pressure to inflate the lungs has been transferred (imposed on) to the patient. The patient is drawing gas (flow demand) from the circuit almost as fast as the gas is entering the circuit from the ventilator, so less pressure is created. Increasing the flow rate to some level greater than the patient's demand will provide assistance (restore the appearance of a normal pressure pattern), which means synchrony with the ventilator has been improved. In the second waveform, Figure 11-28 example *b*, the initial flow demand appears to be met since the initial rise in pressure is relatively normal; the ventilator is accommodating the patient's flow demand sufficiently. The drop in pressure in this example is at end inspiration and suggests that the patient needs more flow than is being supplied. More flow delivery at the end of inspiration means more volume is being demanded than is being supplied. The ventilator, however, is time cycled into expiration before that demand is met.

✔ (Figure 11-28) Pressure tracing *a* shows that the *initial* flow is not high enough. Pressure tracing *b* shows that the *end-inspiratory* flow is not high enough.

Sometimes, increasing the peak flow will satisfy the patient's demands in this situation because more volume is provided sooner, and the patient relaxes and breathes in synchrony with the ventilator. Increasing the sensitivity may also make it easier to breathe initially, relaxing the patient and satisfying what appeared to be an inadequate peak flow setting. So experience suggests that all three methods should be attempted. No research shows that there is only one way to satisfy a particular dyssynchronous waveform pattern. These suggestions are based on knowledge and experience. Sometimes only a change in mode will provide patient–ventilator synchrony. Pressure-limited ventilation allows the patient to have more control over ventilation (flow delivery). Every breath does not have to be the same pattern (controlled). Thus, patient-limited ventilation may improve synchrony when volume ventilation will not. And sometimes, nothing works. Some patients' breathing patterns can be so erratic that no ventilator can provide synchronous ventilation. Pain, neurological damage, psychological stress, or unknown reasons may be causing erratic patterns of breathing that cannot be matched by today's ventilators. Patients may have to be sedated for periods of rest under such circumstances.

DYSSYNCHRONY DURING DECELERATING FLOW VENTILATION

Figure 11-29 presents the same dyssynchronous conditions depicted in Figure 11-28 except that decelerating flow waves are being utilized. The dashed lines show the ideal pressure-time waveforms. Example *a* suggests a higher peak flow setting to meet initially high flow demands, and example *b* suggests a need for increasing the V_T. In Figures 11-28 and 11-29, physical signs of respiratory distress would probably result unless the patient was being sedated and his normal response to dyssynchrony blunted.

CHANGES IN PRESSURE WAVEFORMS DUE TO DYSSYNCHRONOUS VENTILATION

Figure 11-30 demonstrates another important benefit of graphics: assurance that the respiratory mechanics are being accurately measured. These are the same waveforms depicted in Figure 11-4 except that the dotted lines pointed to in *a* and *b* (arrows) represent possible variations in P_{ALV} that could result during a pause in flow. Rather than pressure remaining constant during the pause, pressure either rises above relaxed P_{ALV} or descends below it. Pressure rising as in example *a* often occurs when a patient tries to expire during the pause time. The procedure (pause at end inspiration) is unnatural and patients do not always relax. Dyssynchronous ventilation may be occurring as well and the patient's pattern does not correspond to end inspiration in sync with the ventilator. There may be many reasons for an increase in pressure during this period of time. Any movement such as turning

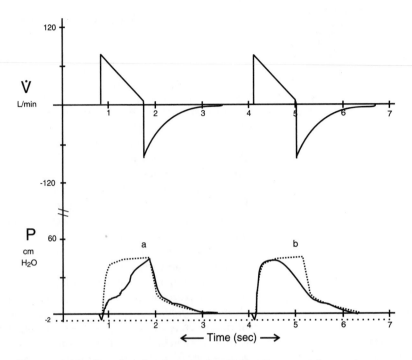

Figure 11-29 Decelerating flow- and pressure-time waveforms demonstrating dyssynchronous ventilation as a result of *a*, inadequate initial peak flow set, or *b*, inadequate V_T set to meet patient demand.

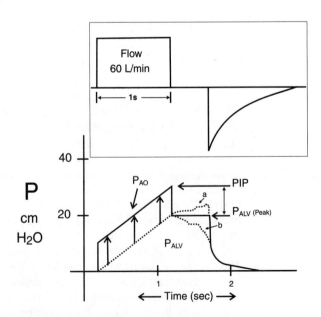

Figure 11-30 Measurements in P_{TA} and P_{ALV} can be affected by effort to breathe, exhale, or leaks (dotted lines *a* and *b*).

☑ Dyssynchronous ventilation with rising pressure may occur when the patient moves, talks, or coughs.

☑ Dyssynchronous ventilation with decreasing pressure may occur with a small leak in the circuit.

or twisting of the thorax can cause pressure to rise. Hands placed on the patient's chest while being attended to by a health care provider can increase thoracic and, therefore, peak P_{ALV}. The patient trying to talk or cough will increase P_{ALV}. In *b* the patient may be trying to continue to inspire, expanding thoracic volume, decompressing gas in the system, and dropping pressure. There may be a small leak in the circuit causing pressure to drop during a pause. Any movement of the thorax or abdomen done by or to the patient by attendants will change the pressure exerted on the lung. Using graphics, you will learn with experience that it is very difficult to obtain accurate respiratory mechanics measurements. Without graphics, errors cannot be observed and may be documented as fact. Patients have to be totally relaxed and passive during the static compliance measurement. Usually, only the CMV mode can be used during respiratory mechanics measurements. Often the minute ventilation has to be increased 10% to 15% to reduce the patient's $PaCO_2$ to apneic threshold (about 32 mm Hg) to eliminate patient's respiratory drive and induce relaxation, and to obtain valid measurements.

DYSSYNCHRONY DURING PRESSURE-LIMITED VENTILATION

Figure 11-31 demonstrates a pressure-support level that is set too low to comfortably satisfy patient flow or volume demand. The patient's rate has increased well above normal (approximately 28 b/min) with graphic display of dyssynchrony. Physical signs of discomfort and increased work of breathing would undoubtedly accompany such a

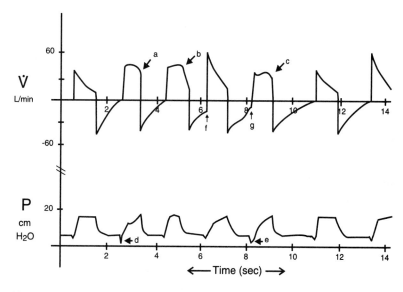

Figure 11-31 An example of pressure support ventilation (PSV) where patient demands are not being adequately met.

✓ **(Figure 11-31)** *a*, *b*, and *c* show that flow demand is high throughout inspiration, sustaining near square flow wave patterns, which are created under conditions of stress.

✓ **(Figure 11-31)** The expiratory flow does not return to baseline (*f* and *g*). Expiration is incomplete and this condition leads to gas trapping.

graphic display. The second, third, and fifth flow waves, *a*, *b*, and *c* (arrows), show that flow demand is high (35 to 45 L/min) throughout inspiration, sustaining near square flow wave patterns, which are created under conditions of stress. The flow waves do not show a relaxed pattern as in the first flow wave where flow gradually descends to cycle the ventilator into expiration at 25% of the initial flow. Instead, high flow demand is sustained at a high level and ends abruptly, dropping quickly to zero so another breath can be initiated. The more that flow appears to square off and drop perpendicularly to the 25% cycling level, the higher the flow demand, and the less the patient is relaxing during inspiration and pausing between breaths at that set level of pressure support. The patient's high respiratory drive is also evident by patient-triggering efforts *d* and *e* (arrows). The negative pressure is substantially below the sensitivity threshold level set below PEEP before the ventilator demand valve can open. Gas trapping is apparent in the graphic as well, which can be seen on the third and fourth expiratory flow waves, *f* and *g* (arrows). Thus, expiration is not complete before the patient triggers breaths four and five. Several of the pressure waveforms are not squared off, so obviously the pressure limit set is not being sustained because the patient's demands for flow are not being met. Increasing the pressure-support level to 15 to 20 cm H_2O would probably eliminate this patient's distress and provide adequate support for a normal level of WOB. If PCV were being demonstrated in this example at the same pressure-limit setting, similar patterns of dyssynchrony would be manifest and the pressure limit would have to be increased. The only difference is that a Ti would have been set and maintained consistent with the pressure-controlled mode of ventilation.

USING THE EXPIRATORY FLOW AND PRESSURE WAVES AS DIAGNOSTIC TOOLS

INCREASED AIRWAY RESISTANCE

Given physical assessment and comparison to the pressure waveforms, the expiratory flow wave can be used to determine whether a patient has excessive airway resistance (asthma), secretions, or obstructive or restrictive disease. The solid line expiratory flow wave in Figure 11-32 demonstrates excessive expiratory airway resistance. The dashed line represents a normal curve. Circuit and endotracheal tube (ETT) resistance (i.e., size 6 mm I.D. ETT) can complicate the assessment by creating a similar pattern, but respiratory therapists can easily measure circuit resistance and eliminate it as the cause for the abnormal expiratory flow curve. Typically, circuit resistance is about

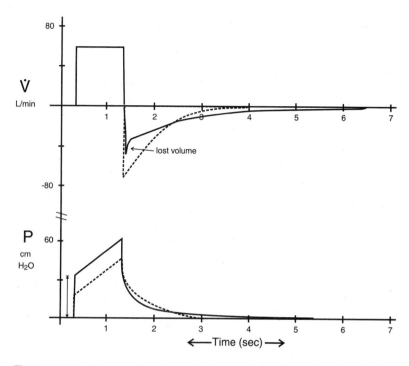

Figure 11-32 Flow- and pressure-time waveforms show the changes in expiratory flow patterns and pressure waveforms (solid lines) created by a severe increase in circuit/airway resistance compared to patient with relatively normal airway resistance (dashed lines).

✓ Decreased expiratory flow and increased expiratory time may be caused by excessive airway resistance.

8.5 cm H_2O/L/s at 60 L/min with an 8 mm I.D.ETT and humidifier in line (Dennison et al., 1989), which can be subtracted from clinical measurements of airway resistance. The low peak expiratory flow, the average flow level, and abnormally long expiratory time (> 5 seconds) compared to the normal curve are the obvious signs of severely elevated airway resistance in this example. High resistance will quickly reduce peak expiratory flow rate to low levels compared to normal expiratory flow waves given the same driving pressure (P_{ALV}). P_{ALV} is usually normal for mandatory V_T (5 to 12 mL/kg ideal body weight) for most obstructive diseases other than emphysema. The spiked peak flow (arrow) indicates the lost volume (compressed gas not delivered to the patient) being driven from the expiratory limb of the circuit ahead of lung volume (Nilsestuen et al., 1996) because it is under high ventilating pressures (PIP = 60 cm H_2O).

The solid line pressure-time waveform represents the pattern that should be expected for the abnormal expiratory flow waveform presented in this example. This is a typical pattern for exacerbated asthma or bronchitis. The initial P_{TA} (double-headed arrow) and PIP (60 cm H_2O) are well above typical levels of airway/circuit resistance and

PIP, which are represented by the dashed-line pressure pattern. The expiratory pressure measured in the expiratory limb of the circuit is lower than normal because the expiratory flow resistive pressure is decreased because the V_T is being slowly expired. Te is increased as a result. The dashed line depicts inspiratory pressure when airway resistance is relatively normal. The P_{TA} and PIP are lower, but circuit expiratory pressure is higher, since expiratory flow rate and consequent flow-resistive pressure is greater. Since Te is longer than normal for obstructive diseases, there is greater potential for volutrauma from autoPEEP, which will be readily apparent when graphics are available. Patients may have to be sedated so they can be mechanically controlled at low rates (6–8 b/min) and low V_T (5 mL/kg IBW) to prevent severe autoPEEP and lung damage.

☑ Since Te is longer than normal for obstructive diseases, there is greater potential for volutrauma from autoPEEP.

☑ For a patient with emphysema, the spiked peak expiratory flow is not present and the P_{ALV} is reduced.

LOSS OF ELASTIC RECOIL

Figure 11-33 displays graphics for a patient with emphysema. The expiratory flow wave is similar to the example in Figure 11-32 for the asthma/bronchitic patient, but with noted changes. First, the spiked peak expiratory flow is not present because ventilating pressures for emphysema patients are typically low as in this example, where PIP is 25 cm H_2O (solid-line pressure wave). Also, lung tissue recoil and

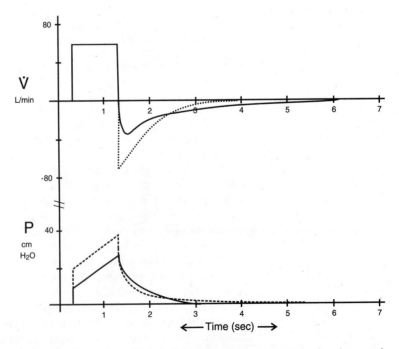

Figure 11-33 Flow- and pressure-time waveforms show the changes in expiratory flow patterns and pressure waveforms (solid lines) created by loss of elastic recoil compared to patient with relatively normal elastic recoil (dashed lines).

P_{ALV} are reduced (approximately 10 cm H_2O in this example) and as a result the peak expiratory flow pattern develops more slowly and is rounded, and Te is prolonged.

DECREASED C_{LT}

When C_{LT} is reduced (i.e., ARDS) and there is little change in total airway resistance, the peak expiratory flow generated will be higher and expiratory time will be shorter (Figure 11-34). The solid expiratory flow curve demonstrates low C_{LT} where peak flow is higher and expiratory time is shorter (arrow) compared to the dotted normal expiratory flow curve where, given the same expiratory resistance, peak flow is lower and expiratory flow time is longer.

The pressure waveform shows that the PIP (solid line) would increase as C_{LT} decreased. Note that since the flow rate is the same and airway resistance is unaffected, the initial flow resistive pressure (arrow) has not changed. Thus, the increase in PIP must be the result of a rise in P_{ALV}. The expiratory portion of the pressure curve shows that the pressure generated in the circuit on average is higher under conditions of low C_{LT} (solid line) and expiratory time is shorter compared to the dotted line. Reduction in C_{LT} creates higher recoil or driving pressure

> ✓ A decreased C_{LT} leads to a higher expiratory peak flow, a higher PIP, and a lower expiratory time.

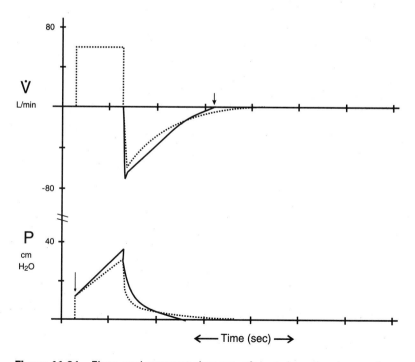

Figure 11-34 Flow- and pressure-time waveforms show the changes in expiratory flow patterns and pressure waveforms (dashed lines) created by decreased compliance.

(P_{ALV}) and, therefore, higher flow rates through the expiratory circuit. Higher expiratory flow causes greater flow-resistive pressure recorded in the circuit by the pressure manometer at the expiratory valve of the ventilator.

GAS TRAPPING AND UNCOUNTED EFFORT

In Figure 11-35, the expiratory flow in the first flow wave is similar to patterns often observed in clinic for patients with obstructive airway diseases from bronchoconstriction, lesions, or severe excess in airway secretions and loss of elastic recoil. The first double-headed arrow *a* indicates that the expiratory flow is dropping rapidly toward zero flow. This may indicate that the patient has a high drive to breathe and is actively trying to "inspire" during expiration and, hence, slowing the expiratory flow and reducing expiratory pressure as pointed to on the pressure wave below it. It could also indicate that airway obstruction is slowing flow. As a result of hyperinflation or trapped gas some patients cannot expand their thorax or lungs enough to create negative pres-

☑ **(Figure 11-35)** *a* indicates that the expiratory flow is dropping rapidly toward zero flow. This may indicate that the patient has a high drive to breathe and is actively trying to "inspire" during expiration and, hence, slowing the expiratory flow and reducing expiratory pressure.

☑ **(Figure 11-35)** *b* points to a sudden increase in flow and corresponding expiratory pressure. This can occur if the patient attempts to actively expire or the obstruction is momentarily relieved.

☑ **(Figure 11-35)** *c* points to an inspiratory effort during expiration since flow drops momentarily to zero and a negative pressure is recorded.

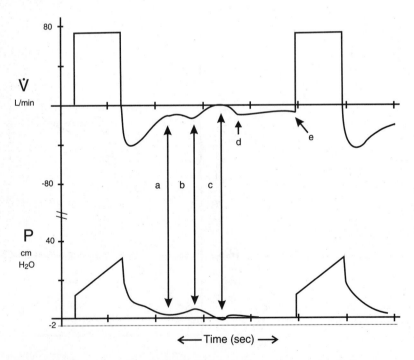

Figure 11-35 Expiratory flow and pressure pattern changes during volume-control ventilation showing obstruction to flow, inspiratory efforts, and autoPEEP during expiration.

sure at the mouth (subatmospheric P_{AO}). Their ineffective inspiratory efforts may only slow the flow of gas being released from areas of the lungs, which have longer time constants. They may be able to reduce the driving pressure (P_{ALV}), but may not be able to create sufficient negative P_{AO} to trigger a breath. The drop in flow or pressure may be obstruction to flow, which might be caused by excess secretions, structural damage to airway, or dynamic airway compression. Obstruction from a more homogeneous condition (bronchoconstriction) may present a different pattern (Figure 11-32). The second double-headed arrow b points to a sudden increase in flow and corresponding expiratory pressure. This can occur if the patient attempts to actively expire or the obstruction is momentarily relieved with a change in flow dynamics and time constants. A third double-headed arrow c points to an obvious inspiratory effort during expiration since flow drops momentarily to zero and an insufficient negative pressure (above sensitivity threshold) is recorded. The patient continues to expire more of the trapped gas (arrow d) and flow increases and some positive pressure is recorded. A controlled mechanical breath is then time triggered before the patient has completed expiration as indicated (arrow e). The patient needs to be physically assessed for respiratory movements whenever such patterns are observed. V_T and Ti may have to be reduced to allow more Te, and the sensitivity threshold may have to be increased (-0.5 versus -2 cm H_2O). The respiratory effort needs to be correctly documented during evaluation for weaning. Patients are often expending the energy to trigger two or three times as many breaths as recorded at the ventilator or pulse oximeter. Inspiratory efforts during expiration can be felt by placing a hand over the patient's abdomen. Contraction of the abdominal muscles can be felt during forced expirations. Visual signs of chest movement, supra- or subclavicular retractions, and interruption of expiratory flow can be heard on auscultation during inspiratory efforts. The graphics can be monitored at the same time in coordination with the physical signs of respiration.

Now that expiratory flow waves as a diagnostic tool has been discussed, refer back to Figure 11-26. Letters a and b and arrows indicate the cause for a reduction in V_T for the second flow waves in examples A and B. Can you correctly interpret the reason the change in the second flow waveforms compare to the first? In the first example, a indicates a prolonged Te and lower flow rate. Thus, increased airway resistance is responsible for the reduction in V_T delivery. In the second example, Te has been decreased. The peak flow is the same, but at a lower V_T expired. Thus, C_{LT} has to be decreased. Both evaluations assume the same patient effort as discussed when Figure 11-26 was presented.

☑ Dysfunction of the inspiratory valve or sensitivity setting would cause a delay of positive pressure waveform (i.e., lack of ventilator response) in spite of a normal negative pressure waveform (i.e., good patient effort).

☑ (Figure 11-36) *a* (arrow) demonstrates that a leak has developed since the expiratory volume never returns to the zero baseline.

☑ (Figure 11-36) *b* shows that a leak causes a decreased PIP and less volume is being delivered to the patient.

☑ (Figure 11-36) *c* shows a negative pressure is present. In circuit leak situations, more negative pressure must be generated in order to reduce the pressure to the sensitivity threshold.

TROUBLESHOOTING VENTILATOR FUNCTION

LACK OF VENTILATOR RESPONSE

Another use of graphics is to check proper ventilator function. For example, inspiratory valve dysfunction (i.e., a sticking valve) or an out-of-calibration sensitivity threshold can be readily observed when monitoring the pressure-time waveforms via graphics. (Refer back to Figure 11-27.)

CIRCUIT LEAKS

Figure 11-36 demonstrates another use of volume waveforms other than the primary use of ensuring accurate V_T delivery, that is, checking for circuit leaks. In the second volume waveform letter *a* (arrow) demonstrates that a leak has developed since the volume never returns to the zero baseline. The ventilator still delivers the same flow pattern, but the pressure waveforms show that the PIP for ventilation has been reduced, *b*, since less volume is being delivered to the patient's lungs. Also note that the expiratory flow waves have decreased volumes expired after the leak develops. The arrow, *c*, for the third pressure-time waveform is used to emphasize that the negative pressure to trigger inspiration may appear the same (although sometimes the descent to the sensitivity threshold may be prolonged), but since negative pressure in the circuit is dependent on gas decompression, it will be more difficult

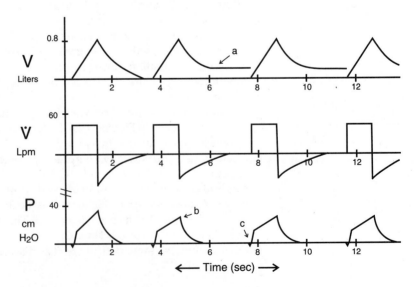

Figure 11-36 Changes to volume, flow, and pressure waveforms demonstrate the development of a circuit leak.

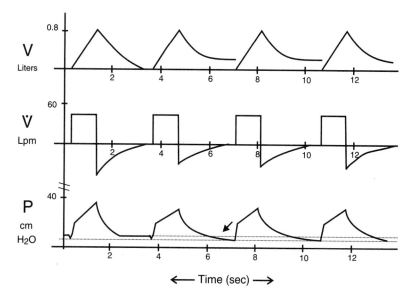

Figure 11-37 Changes to volume, flow, and pressure waveforms show the development of a circuit leak sufficient to cause autotriggering when positive end-expiratory pressure (PEEP) is being administered.

☑ **(Figure 11-37)**
When a circuit leak occurs in the presence of PEEP, pressure in the circuit drops to the sensitivity setting below the PEEP level (dotted lines). This leads to autotriggering and fast mechanical breaths.

pressure-volume curve (PVC): A graphic display showing the relationship between volume (vertical axis) and pressure (horizontal axis).

for the patient to reduce pressure to the sensitivity threshold if gas can be drawn from the atmosphere.

Figure 11-37 demonstrates the same leak problem as presented in Figure 11-36. However in this example, approximately 10 cm H_2O PEEP have been added to the circuit and patient's lungs. Again, volume does not return to zero. The PIPs and expiratory flow patterns have also been reduced for the waveforms depicted after the leak appeared. The arrow indicates that once the leak begins, pressure in the circuit starts dropping to the sensitivity setting below the PEEP level set (dotted lines). This leads to autotriggering and extremely fast mechanical breaths.

PRESSURE-VOLUME AND FLOW-VOLUME CURVES OR LOOPS

PRESSURE-VOLUME CURVE (PVC)
Another option offered by graphics software is the **pressure-volume curve (PVC)** or loop presented in Figure 11-38 for an assist breath during square flow wave ventilation. The negative pressure (arrow) indicates the negative pressure created to trigger the assist breath. P_{AO} and

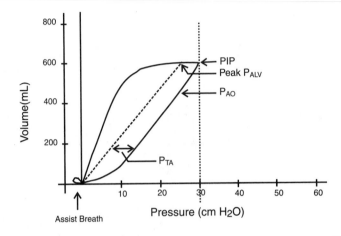

Figure 11-38   Characteristics of the pressure-volume curve (PVC).

(Figure 11-38)
☑ (Figure 11-38) The double-headed arrow indicates the flow-resistive pressure (P$_{TA}$) is the difference between P$_{ALV}$ (dashed line) and P$_{AO}$.

☑ It is assumed the C$_{LT}$ is unchanged in this example since P$_{ALV}$ rises linearly with increases in volume.

☑ (Figure 11-39) A reduction in C$_{LT}$ causes the PVC to move down and to the right.

☑ (Figure 11-39) A reduction in C$_{LT}$ will not change the P$_{TA}$ because the gradient between PIP and P$_{ALV}$ remains the same.

☑ In situations where resistance is increased, P$_{ALV}$ remains unchanged while P$_{TA}$, PIP, and P$_{AO}$ are increased.

PIP can be read from the x-axis and volume from the y-axis. The double-headed arrow indicates the flow-resistive pressure (P$_{TA}$) is the difference between P$_{ALV}$ (dashed line) and P$_{AO}$. P$_{TA}$ remains the same throughout inspiration as it does for the trapezoid pressure waveform once peak flow is reached and maintained during square flow wave ventilation. The PIP of 30 cm H$_2$O (dotted line) and *peak* P$_{ALV}$ of 25 cm H$_2$O are labeled. It is assumed that the C$_{LT}$ is unchanged in this example since P$_{ALV}$ rises linearly with increase in volume.

EFFECTS OF CHANGES IN C$_{LT}$ ON THE PVC

Figure 11-39 shows a control breath in which the negative pressure to trigger the observed mechanical breath is absent. This PVC illustrates how a reduction in C$_{LT}$ causes the PVC to move down and to the right. From PIP$_{(1)}$ and P$_{AO(1)}$ to PIP$_{(2)}$ and P$_{AO(2)}$, these pressure readings are increased proportionally as a result of increase in the P$_{ALV}$ due to the reduction in C$_{LT}$. The gradient between PIP and P$_{ALV}$ (or flow resistive pressure [P$_{TA}$]) stays the same because it is not affected by changes in C$_{LT}$.

EFFECT OF CHANGES IN RESISTANCE ON THE PVC

Figure 11-40 shows how the volume pressure curve is affected by an increase in resistance (double-headed arrows and dotted lines). P$_{ALV}$ remains unchanged in this example, while inspiratory and expiratory flow-resistive pressure (P$_{TA}$), PIP, and P$_{AO}$ are increased.

LOWER INFLECTION POINT ON THE PVC AND TITRATION OF PEEP

Figure 11-41 shows the effects on the PVC if C$_{LT}$ changes during tidal volume delivery. The dashed line indicates that the slope of the P$_{ALV}$

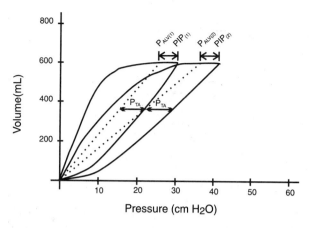

Figure 11-39 The effect of lung–thorax compliance changes on a pressure-volume curve (PVC) during volume-controlled, square flow ventilation.

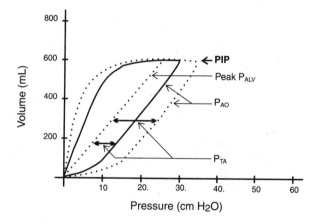

Figure 11-40 The effect of airway/circuit resistance changes on a pressure-volume curve (PVC) during volume-controlled, square flow ventilation.

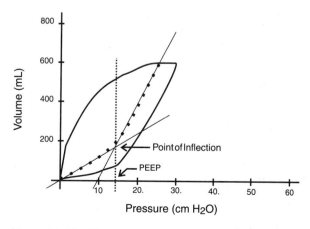

Figure 11-41 Alveolar pressure plotted (manually) at various volumes to determine the initial inflection point on a PVC created by alveolar recruitment.

☑ (Figure 11-41) Change in the slope from low to improved compliance is known as the initial point of inflection (Ipi). Ipi occurs when alveoli are recruited (opened) during inspiration.

☑ In the presence of Ipi, PEEP can be added at or slightly above the inflection point to prevent the alveoli from closing during expiration.

☑ C_{LT} changed later during V_T delivery because of overinflation of the alveoli. The reduction in C_{LT} late in the inspiratory cycle is called the Ipu.

during V_T delivery has changed. A line has been drawn through the initial slope and low C_{LT} and the change in the slope with a higher C_{LT}. This change in the slope from low to improved compliance is known as the initial point of inflection (Ipi) (Beydon et al., 1991). The Ipi occurs when alveoli are recruited (opened) during inspiration. In this example, P_{ALV} could have been measured by adding progressively larger volumes of gas (beginning at approximately 35 mL) to the patient's lung via a large volume syringe until the V_T was reached, and then plotting the plateau pressures acquired. Two or three P_{ALV} measurements can be made intermittently to a patient who is heavily sedated, or sedated and paralyzed, and, after allowing the patient to be ventilated normally for a couple of minutes, proceeding with the measurements until the compliance study is completed. In the presence of Ipi, PEEP can be added slightly above the inflection point to prevent the alveoli from closing during expiration. This is a useful strategy in the management of mechanical ventilation because studies suggest that the repeated opening and closing of alveoli during mechanical ventilation causes shearing of lung parenchyma and barotraumas, and may augment ARDs.

UPPER INFLECTION POINT ON THE PVC AND ADJUSTMENT OF V_T

Figure 11-42 presents a PVC where an upper inflection point (Ipu) exists. In this example, the P_{ALV} has been plotted as described for Figure 11-37. C_{LT} changed later during V_T delivery because of overinflation of

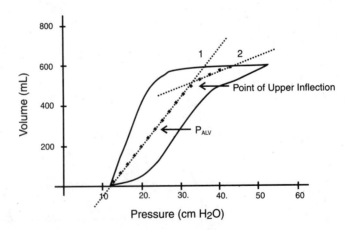

Figure 11-42 Alveolar pressure plotted (manually) at various volumes to determine the point of alveolar overdistension (upper inflection point) on a PVC.

the alveoli. The reduction in C_{LT} late in the inspiratory cycle is called the Ipu (Dambrosio et al., 1997). In this example, slope 1 for P_{ALV} (dotted line) is normal, and slope 2 (dotted line) shows a decrease in C_{LT} and the point of upper inflection is pointed out. The appearance of the upper shape of the P_{AO} curve indicating the presence of an Ipu is known as the duck bill PVC. When a duck bill occurs, the V_T can be reduced until the duck bill disappears (Roupe et al., 1995). A C_{LT} measurement should show improvement at that point.

EFFECTS OF AIRWAY STATUS ON FLOW-VOLUME LOOP (FVL)

Figure 11-43 shows another waveform option, the **flow-volume loop (FVL).** FVLs show flow measurements on the y-axis, and volume measurement on the x-axis. Inspiratory flow is above the volume measurement and expiratory flow is below. This example shows two superimposed waveforms during square flow wave ventilation at 40 L/min and results of pre- and postbronchodilator therapy. Following bronchodilator therapy, peak and average expiratory flow is typically improved (Gay, 1987).

☑ In the presence of Ipu, V_T can be reduced until the duck bill disappears.

flow-volume loop (FVL): *A graphic display showing the relationship between flow (vertical axis) and volume (horizontal axis).*

☑ (Figure 11-43) Inspiratory flow is above the horizontal axis (volume measurement) and expiratory flow is below.

☑ (Figure 11-43) Following bronchodilator therapy, peak and average expiratory flow was improved.

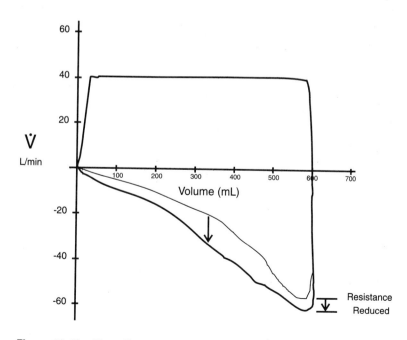

Figure 11-43 The effect of circuit/airway resistance changes on the flow-volume loop (FVL).

SUMMARY

In summary, if graphics of flow, volume- and pressure-time waveforms, PVCs, and FVLs are saved when patients are first placed on a ventilator, their initial condition can be compared to the progress in their condition and management. Follow-up graphics can be saved and superimposed over the initial copies for comparison as is done in the figures throughout this chapter. Disk files or printed copies of therapeutic interventions (i.e., bronchodilators, changes in mode of ventilation) and improvements based on intervention can be documented. Graphic analysis can be used to facilitate discussion with colleagues and physicians and often eliminates the guesswork regarding needed changes in management and therapy. Outcome assessments about the performance of therapists and respiratory care departments in the area of ventilator management can also be documented. At minimum, patient assessment and care is easier on a day-to-day basis through graphic analysis, and quality of care is greatly enhanced.

Self-Assessment Questions

1. The accelerating and sine flow waveforms are not used for positive pressure ventilation because the initial flow rate is _____ for most patients. These two waveforms may be appropriate for _____ ventilation.

   A. too high, control
   B. too high, intermittent mandatory

   C. not sufficient, control
   D. not sufficient, intermittent mandatory

2. In flow and pressure waveforms, time in seconds is displayed along the _____ axis.

   A. *x* or horizontal
   B. *x* or vertical

   C. *y* or horizontal
   D. *y* or vertical

3. Tidal volume can be calculated or determined by measuring the _____ under a _____ waveform.

   A. slope, flow/time
   B. slope, pressure/time

   C. area, flow/time
   D. area, pressure/time

4. The area enclosed under the expiratory flow waveform should _____ the area under the inspiratory flow waveform. If the expiratory volume is less than the inspiratory volume, _____ may be present.

   A. be greater than, airflow obstruction

   B. equal to, airflow obstruction

   C. be greater than, circuit leak or gas trapping

   D. equal circuit leak or gas trapping

5. In assist/control mode, the I:E ratio is variable because the _____ time of a breath is dependent on the timing of the _____ breath.

    A. inspiratory, preceding   C. expiratory, preceding
    B. inspiratory, following   D. expiratory, following

6. On a pressure waveform, PEEP is present when the end-expiratory pressure rests:

    A. at 0 cm H_2O.   C. above 0 cm H_2O.
    B. below 0 cm H_2O.   D. above 5 cm H_2O.

7. On the pressure waveform, assist effort is present when the trigger pressure reaches the _____ setting.

    A. tidal volume   C. pressure limit
    B. sensitivity   D. peak flow

8. In CPAP mode, there are no _____ breaths and the airway pressure is above _____ cm H_2O.

    A. mechanical, 0   C. spontaneous, 0
    B. mechanical, 5   D. spontaneous, 5

9. An increase in airflow resistance would show an unchanged _____ but increased _____. (See Figure 11-11.)

    A. P_{ALV}, PIP and P_{TA} C. P_{TA} and P_{ALV}, PIP
    B. P_{ALV} and PIP, P_{TA} D. P_{ALV}, P_{TA}

10. A decrease in total compliance (C_{LT}) would show an unchanged _____ but increased _____. (See Figure 11-12.)

    A. P_{ALV}, PIP and P_{TA} C. PIP, P_{ALV} and PIP
    B. P_{TA}, PIP, and P_{ALV} D. P_{ALV}, P_{TA}

11. When the flow waveform selection is changed from square to decelerating during *time-limited* ventilation, the same volume can only be maintained if the *peak flow* of the decelerating pattern is:

    A. increased.   C. halved.
    B. decreased.   D. doubled.

12. When the flow waveform selection is changed from square to decelerating during *flow-limited* ventilation, the same volume can only be maintained if the *inspiratory time* of the decelerating pattern is:

    A. increased.   C. halved.

    B. decreased.   D. doubled.

13. With time-limited ventilation, the higher *initial* peak flow for the decelerating flow wave creates a _____ initial flow resistive pressure (P_{TA}) than the P_{TA} created by the square flow. (See Figure 11-14.)

    A. higher   C. similar

    B. lower   D. constant

14. With flow limited ventilation, the initial flow resistive pressure (P_{TA}) is the same for the _____ flow waves. The *initial* peak flow level stays the same for _____ flow during flow limited ventilation. (See Figure 11-14.)

    A. square, square   C. decelerating, decelerating

    B. square, decelerating   D. square and decelerating, square and decelerating

15. In square and decelerating flow ventilation, the rise in alveolar pressure (P_{ALV}) is directly related to _____ and inversely related to _____.

    A. compliance, volume delivery   C. volume delivery, compliance

    B. compliance, airflow resistance   D. volume delivery, airflow resistance

16. At constant Ti, a decreased flow leads to _____.

    A. higher V_T, and P_{ALV} C. lower P_{TA}, and P_{ALV}

    B. higher V_T, P_{TA}, and P_{ALV} D. lower V_T, P_{TA}, and P_{ALV}

17. During decelerating flow ventilation, a higher end flow leads to a _____ V_T average flow rate and it _____ affect the P_{TA} and P_{ALV}.

    A. larger, does   C. smaller, does

    B. larger, does not   D. smaller, does not

18. When peak flow is constant (square), _____ are _____ related.

    A. V_T, and P_{ALV}; directly   C. V_T, and P_{ALV}; inversely

    B. V_T, Ti, and P_{ALV}; directly   D. V_T, Ti, and P_{ALV}; inversely

19. In pressure control ventilation, _____ are typically set by the operator.

    A. rate and I:E ratio
    B. pressure level and I:E ratio

    C. pressure level and rate
    D. pressure level, rate, and I:E ratio

20. In pressure control ventilation, the flow level and V_T delivered are dependent on the:

    A. pressure level set.

    B. pressure level set and patient effort.

    C. pressure level set and lung charac-
       teristics.
    D. pressure level set, patient effort, and
       lung characteristics.

21. During inverse ratio pressure control ventilation, the patients are usually sedated and paralyzed in order to prevent:

    A. barotrauma.
    B. dyssynchrony with the ventilator.

    C. hyperventilation.
    D. hypoxia.

22. In pressure support ventilation, only the _____ level is set and under normal condition, _____ are primarily under the patient's control.

    A. pressure support; flow, volume, and in-
       spiratory time
    B. tidal volume; flow, volume, and inspira-
       tory time

    C. peak inspiratory pressure; flow and
       volume
    D. plateau pressure; inspiratory time
       and volume

23. During pressure limited ventilation, a(n) _____ airflow resistance or _____ compliance would reduce the delivered flow and tidal volume.

    A. increased, increased
    B. increased, decreased

    C. decreased, increased
    D. decreased, decreased

24. Tachypnea, agitation, accessory muscle use, active expiration, muscle fatigue, and respiratory failure are signs of:

    A. patient–ventilator dyssynchrony.
    B. hyperventilation.

    C. anxiety.
    D. decreased metabolic rate.

25. On a flow waveform, failure of the expiratory flow to return to baseline is indicative of _____ and this condition may lead to _____ and possibly auto-PEEP.

    A. incomplete inspiration, gas trapping
    B. incomplete inspiration, hypoventilation

    C. incomplete expiration, gas trapping
    D. incomplete expiration, hypoventilation

26. In the presence of excessive airway resistance, the expiratory flow is _____ and the expiratory time is _____.

    A. increased, prolonged
    B. increased, shortened

    C. decreased, prolonged
    D. decreased, shortened

27. A decreased C_{LT} leads to a higher expiratory peak flow, a _____ PIP, and a _____ expiratory time.

    A. higher, longer
    B. higher, shorter

    C. lower, longer
    D. lower, shorter

28. A delay of positive pressure waveform (i.e., lack of ventilator response) in spite of a normal negative pressure waveform (i.e., good patient effort) is indicative of:

    A. inadequate line pressure.

    B. ventilator malfunction.

    C. dysfunction of the inspiratory valve or sensitivity setting.
    D. electrical malfunction.

29. Failure of the expiratory flow to return to the zero baseline is indicative of:

    A. gas leak.
    B. airflow obstruction.

    C. power failure.
    D. high lung compliance.

30. When circuit leak occurs in the presence of PEEP, pressure in the circuit drops to the sensitivity setting below the PEEP level and _____ develops and leads to extremely _____ mechanical breaths.

    A. auto-PEEP, slow
    B. auto-PEEP, fast

    C. autotriggering, slow
    D. autotriggering, fast

31. The difference between P_{ALV} and P_{AO} is: (See Figure 11-38.)

    A. PIP.
    B. P_{TA}.

    C. PEEP.
    D. C_{LT}.

32. On a volume pressure curve, the _____ is assumed to be stable and unchanged if P_{ALV} rises linearly with increases in volume. (See Figure 11-38.)

    A. C_{LT}
    B. PIP

    C. P_{TA}
    D. PEEP

33. On a volume pressure curve, a reduction in C_{LT} causes the PVC to move _____ and to the _____.

    A. up, right
    B. up, left

    C. down, right
    D. down, left

34. On a volume pressure curve, a reduction in C_{LT} will not change the P_{TA} because the gradient between _____ remains the same. (See Figure 11-39.)

    A. P_{TA} and P_{AO}
    B. P_{AO} and P_{ALV}

    C. PIP and P_{AO}
    D. PIP and P_{ALV}

35. On a volume pressure curve, an increase in resistance would not affect the _____ while the _____ are increased. (See Figure 11-40.)

    A. P_{ALV}; P_{TA} and PIP
    B. P_{ALV}; P_{TA}, PIP, and P_{AO}

    C. P_{TA}; PIP and P_{AO}
    D. P_{TA}; P_{AO}, PIP, and P_{ALV}

36. The initial point of inflection (Ipi) occurs when alveoli are recruited during _____. In the presence of Ipi, _____ can be added slightly above the inflection point to prevent the alveoli from closing during expiration.

    A. inspiration, PEEP
    B. inspiration, tidal volume

    C. expiration, PEEP
    D. expiration, tidal volume

37. Overinflation of the alveoli and _____ in C_{LT} leads to the appearance of an upper inflection point (Ipu). The Ipu can be minimized by reducing the _____.

    A. increase, PEEP
    B. increase, tidal volume

    C. decrease, PEEP
    D. decrease, tidal volume

38. On a flow-volume loop, the expiratory flow is _____ the horizontal axis (volume measurement) and it is usually _____ following bronchodilator therapy.

    A. above, increased
    B. above, decreased

    C. below, increased
    D. below, decreased

References

Beydon, L. et al. (1991). Lung mechanics in ARDS: Compliance and pressure-volume curves. In: Aapol, W. M. et al. *Adult respiratory distress syndrome.* New York: Marcel Dekker, 139–161.

Chatburn, R. L. (1991). A new system for understanding mechanical ventilators. *Respir Care, 36,* 1123.

Dambrosio, M. et al. (1997). Effects of positive end-expiratory pressure and different tidal volumes on alveolar recruitment and hyperinflation. *Anesthesiology, 87*(3), 495–503.

Dennison, F. H. et al. (1989). Analysis of resistance to gas flow in nine adult ventilator circuits. *Chest, 96,* 1374–1379.

Dick, C. R. et al. (1996). Patient–ventilator interactions. *Clinics in Chest Medicine, 17*(3), 423–438.

Gay, P. C. (1987). Evaluation of bronchodilator responsiveness in mechanically-ventilated patients. *Am Rev Respir Dis, 136,* 880–885.

Marini, J. J. et al. (1985). The inspiratory work of breathing during assisted mechanical ventilation. *Chest, 87*(5), 612–618.

Marini, J. J. et al. (1986). Bedside estimation of the inspiratory work of breathing during mechanical ventilation. *Chest, 89*(1), 56–63.

Messinger, G. et al. (1995). Using tracheal pressure to trigger the ventilator and control airway pressure during continuous positive airway pressure decreases work of breathing. *Chest, 108,* 509–514.

Nilsestuen, J. O. et al. (1996). Managing the patient–ventilator system using graphic analysis: An overview and introduction to graphics corner. *Resp Care, 41*(12), 1105–1120.

Nunn, J. F. (1977). *Applied respiratory physiology* (2nd ed). Boston: Butterworths.

Roupe, E. et al. (1995). Titration of tidal volume and induced hypercapnia in acute respiratory distress syndrome. *Am J Respir Crit Care, 152,* 121–128.

Tobin, M. J. (1994). *Principles and practice of mechanical ventilation.* New York: McGraw-Hill, Inc.

Tobin, M. J. et al. (1986). The pattern of breathing during successful and unsuccessful trials of weaning from mechanical ventilation. *Am Rev Respir Dis, 134,* 1111–1118.

CHAPTER TWELVE

MANAGEMENT OF MECHANICAL VENTILATION

David W. Chang

--- OUTLINE ---

KEY TERMS

- **alarm**

- **anion gap**

- **auto-PEEP**

- **culture and sensitivity**

- **extracellular fluid (ECF)**

- **Gram stain**

- **intracellular fluid (ICF)**

- **mechanical deadspace**

- **optimal PEEP**

- **oxygenation**

- **permissive hypercapnia**

- **refractory hypoxemia**

- **spontaneous ventilation**

INTRODUCTION

The primary function of mechanical ventilation is to support the ventilatory and oxygenation requirement of a patient until such time that the patient becomes self-sufficient. During mechanical ventilation, it is essential to maintain a patient's acid-base balance, nutritional and resting needs, and fluid and electrolyte balance because these factors can affect management strategies of mechanical ventilation and patient outcome.

This chapter discusses strategies to provide optimal ventilation and oxygenation during mechanical ventilation, as well as other methods to maintain essential physiologic functions through nutritional, fluid, and electrolyte support.

STRATEGIES TO IMPROVE VENTILATION

☑ $PaCO_2 > 45$ mm Hg is indicative of hypoventilation (the normal $PaCO_2$ for COPD patients is about 50 mm Hg).

Hypoventilation causes respiratory acidosis (ventilatory failure), and hypoxemia if supplemental oxygen is not provided to the patient. The best measure of a patient's ventilatory status is the $PaCO_2$ level. The normal $PaCO_2$ is 35 to 45 mm Hg; $PaCO_2$ greater than 45 mm Hg is indicative of hypoventilation. For COPD patients, however, the acceptable $PaCO_2$ should be the patient's normal value upon last hospital discharge and generally it is about 50 mm Hg. When the $PaCO_2$ level goes above this value, significant hypoventilation may be present.

Strategies for improving a patient's ventilation are summarized in Table 12-1.

auto-PEEP: *Uninten-tional PEEP associ-ated with pressure support ventilation, rapid respiratory rates, slow inspira-tory flow and air trapping.*

mechanical dead-space: *Volume of gas contained in the equipment and sup-plies (e.g., endotra-cheal tube, ventilator circuit) that does not take part in gas exchange.*

INCREASE MECHANICAL RATE

The most common approach to improve minute ventilation is to increase the respiratory rate (RR) of the ventilator. This may be the control rate in assist/control, the mandatory rate in intermittent mandatory ventilation, or other modes of ventilation that regulate the rate of the ventilator. However, the respiratory rate should not exceed 20/min. as **auto-PEEP** may occur at or above this rate, especially during pressure support ventilation (MacIntyre, 1986; Shapiro, 1994). The following equations show that an increase in respiratory rate causes a higher minute ventilation.

$\uparrow$ Minute Ventilation = (Ventilator $V_T \times \uparrow$ Ventilator RR) + (Spontaneous $V_T \times$ Spontaneous RR)

It is generally not desirable to increase the ventilator tidal volume beyond a level that is appropriate to the patient's body weight, generally 10 to 15 ml/kg (Burton et al., 1997). In volume-limited ventilators, a larger tidal volume requires a higher peak inspiratory pressure.

TABLE 12-1 Strategies to Improve Ventilation

PRIORITY	METHODS

1	Increase mechanical rate
	    Control rate in assist/control mode
	    Intermittent mandatory ventilation (IMV) rate
	    Synchronized IMV rate

2	Increase spontaneous tidal volume
	    Nutritional support and reconditioning of respiratory muscles
	    Administer bronchodilators
	    Initiate pressure support ventilation (PSV)
	    Use largest endotracheal tube possible

3	Increase mechanical tidal volume Tidal volume (V_T)

4	Reduce **mechanical deadspace**
	    Use low-compliance ventilator circuit
	    Cut endotracheal tube to appropriate length
	    Perform tracheotomy

5	Consider high frequency jet or oscillatory ventilation

☑ The most common approach to improve minute ventilation is to increase the respiratory rate of the ventilator.

☑ See Appendix 1 for example.

This high pressure condition increases the incidence of ventilator-related lung injuries such as cardiovascular impairment and barotrauma.

To estimate the mechanical rate needed to achieve a certain $PaCO_2$, the following formula may be used, assuming the ventilator tidal volume and deadspace volume stay the same (Barnes et al., 1993; Burton et al., 1997).

$$\text{New rate} = (\text{Rate} \times PaCO_2)/\text{Desired } PaCO_2$$

New rate : Ventilator rate needed for a desired $PaCO_2$
Rate : Original ventilator rate
$PaCO_2$: Original arterial carbon dioxide tension
Desired $PaCO_2$: Desired arterial carbon dioxide tension

INCREASE SPONTANEOUS TIDAL VOLUME OR RATE

☑ It is more advantageous for a patient to increase the spontaneous tidal volume since increasing the respiratory rate at low tidal volume promotes deadspace ventilation.

In most modes of mechanical ventilation, minute ventilation is the sum of the volume delivered by the ventilator and the volume achieved by a spontaneously breathing patient. For this reason, the patient can contribute to the minute ventilation by increasing either the spontaneous tidal volume or spontaneous rate.

$$\uparrow \text{Minute Ventilation} = (\text{Ventilator } V_T \times \text{Ventilator RR}) + (\uparrow \text{Spontaneous } V_T \times \uparrow \text{Spontaneous RR})$$

It is more advantageous for a patient to increase the spontaneous tidal volume since increasing the respiratory rate at low tidal volume promotes deadspace ventilation. A larger deadspace to tidal volume (VD/V_T) ratio results because of the constant anatomic deadspace volume at a reduced tidal volume.

spontaneous ventilation: Volume of gas inspired by a patient. It is directly related to the patient's spontaneous tidal volume and respiratory rate.

In some patients, the respiratory muscles are not sufficient to maintain prolonged **spontaneous ventilation** or to overcome air flow resistance imposed by the ventilator circuit and endotracheal tube. This condition may be compensated by using pressure support ventilation. The level of pressure support is usually started at 10 to 15 cm H_2O (Shapiro, 1994) and titrated until a desired spontaneous tidal volume and respiratory rate are obtained. The increase in spontaneous tidal volume improves the minute ventilation.

Low levels of pressure support ventilation (<10 cm H_2O) are titrated and used to overcome the air flow resistance of the ventilator circuit and endotracheal tube. At high levels of pressure support ventilation (>20 cm H_2O), the breathing pattern resembles pressure-limited assisted ventilation (Burton et al., 1997; Nathan et al., 1993). Pressure support ventilation increases spontaneous tidal volume, and therefore the minute ventilation.

☑ Pressure support ventilation increases spontaneous tidal volume, and therefore the minute ventilation.

$$\uparrow \text{Minute Ventilation} = (\text{Ventilator } V_T \times \text{Ventilator RR}) + (\uparrow \text{Spontaneous } V_T \times \text{Spontaneous RR})$$

INCREASE MECHANICAL TIDAL VOLUME

The ventilator tidal volume is usually set according to the patient's body weight and its range available for adjustments is rather narrow. Excessive ventilator tidal volume may increase the likelihood of ventilator-related lung injuries. On the other hand, inadequate ventilator tidal volume may induce atelectasis.

Before a decision is made to increase the ventilator tidal volume, one must first consider the detrimental side effects of excessive volume and pressure. It should be implemented only when the ventilator rate is too fast and exceeds the patient's ideal breathing pattern and inspiratory-expiratory relationship.

OTHER STRATEGIES TO IMPROVE VENTILATION

Other strategies to improve the minute ventilation may involve use of ventilator circuits with low compressible volume. This helps to reduce the mechanical deadspace and volume loss due to the tubing compression factor.

The endotracheal tube is sometimes cut shorter to facilitate tube management, to clear secretions, and to reduce tubing deadspace. Tracheostomy also improves ventilation by enhancing tube management and secretion removal. In addition, it provides easier access for oral care and lower tubing deadspace than an oral endotracheal tube.

High frequency jet ventilation has been used extensively only in the infant population. It is effective to improve ventilation in infants but its use in adult patients shows mixed results.

PERMISSIVE HYPERCAPNIA

In mechanical ventilation, peak airway pressure is used to create the pressure gradient and to deliver a predetermined tidal volume. Occasionally the peak airway pressure can be very high in the presence of high airway resistance and low compliance. This high level of pressure in the lungs may lead to ventilator-related lung injuries.

Permissive hypercapnia is a strategy to minimize the occurrence of ventilator-related lung injuries caused by positive pressure ventilation. This is done by ventilating the patient with a small tidal volume in a range of 4 to 7 ml/kg (normally 10 to 15 ml/kg) (Feihl et al., 1994), thus making it possible to ventilate the patient with a lower peak airway pressure, and to minimize potential pressure- or volume-related complications. Since the plateau pressure (i.e., end-inspiratory occlusion pressure) is the best estimate of the average peak alveolar pressure, it is often used as the target pressure when trying to avoid alveolar overdistention (Slutsky, 1994). Permissive hypercapnia using a low tidal volume (4 to 7 ml/kg) strategy is more likely to keep the plateau pressure lower than 35 cm H_2O.

Small tidal volume may cause hypoventilation, CO_2 retention, and acidosis. Acidosis causes the development of central nervous dysfunction, intracranial hypertension, neuromuscular weakness, cardiovascular impairment, and increased pulmonary vascular resistance.

permissive hypercapnia: Intentional hypoventilation of a patient by reducing the mechanical tidal volume to a range of 4 to 7 ml/kg (normally 10 to 15 ml/kg). It is used to lower the pulmonary pressures and to minimize the risk of ventilator-related lung injuries. The patient's $PaCO_2$ is significantly elevated but the acidotic pH may be neutralized by a bicarbonate IV drip.

☑ Permissive hypercapnia is a strategy to minimize the occurrence of ventilator-related lung injuries caused by positive pressure ventilation by using a *small* ventilator tidal volume (4 to 7 ml/kg).

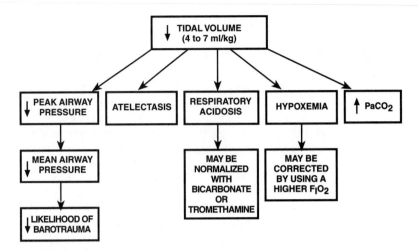

Figure 12-1 Mechanism and physiological changes of permissive hypercapnia.

☑ The plateau pressure should be kept below 35 cm H_2O to avoid alveolar overdistention or barotrauma.

These potential complications may be alleviated by keeping the pH within its normal range, between 7.35 to 7.45, either by renal compensation over time or by neutralizing the acid with bicarbonate or tromethamine (Marini, 1993).

By normalizing the pH, it appears that permissive hypercapnia may be a safe and beneficial strategy in the management of patients with status asthmaticus (Cox et al., 1991; Darioli et al., 1984), and adult respiratory distress syndrome (ARDS) (Feihl et al., 1994; Hickling et al., 1990; Lewandowski et al., 1992). The mechanism and physiological changes of permissive hypercapnia are outlined in Figure 12-1.

STRATEGIES TO IMPROVE OXYGENATION

oxygenation:
Amount of oxygen available for metabolic functions.

Oxygenation is dependent on adequate and well-balanced ventilation, diffusion, and perfusion. The strategies to improve oxygenation are therefore structured to improve the normal physiologic functions or to compensate for the abnormal functions. The prioritized methods to improve oxygenation, from simple to complex, are outlined in Table 12-2.

INCREASE INSPIRED OXYGEN FRACTION (F_IO_2)
Supplemental oxygen is most frequently used to manage hypoxemia because a high F_IO_2 increases the alveolar-capillary oxygen pressure gradient, thus enhancing diffusion of oxygen from the lungs to the pulmonary circulation. Oxygen readily corrects hypoxemia that is due to uncomplicated V/Q abnormalities.

☑ Oxygen readily corrects hypoxemia that is due to uncomplicated V/Q abnormalities.

TABLE 12-2 Strategies to Improve Oxygenation

PRIORITY	METHODS
1	Increase inspired oxygen fraction (F_IO_2)
2	Improve ventilation and reduce mechanical deadspace
3	Improve circulation 　　Fluid replacement if patient is hypovolemic 　　Vasopressors if patient is in shock 　　Cardiac drugs if patient is in congestive heart failure
4	Maintain normal hemoglobin level
5	Initiate continuous positive airway pressure (CPAP) only with *adequate* spontaneous ventilation
6	Initiate positive end-expiratory pressure (PEEP) 　　Titrate optimum PEEP
7	Consider inverse ratio ventilation
8	Consider extracorporeal membrane oxygenation (ECMO), high frequency ventilation, hyperbaric oxygenation, or intravascular oxygenation (IVOX) device

The following two-step procedure may be used to estimate the needed F_IO_2 for a desired PaO_2 assuming that there is no severe deadspace or shunt abnormalities (Burton et al., 1997; Krider et al., 1986).

$$\text{Step 1: } PAO_2 \text{ needed} = \frac{PaO_2 \text{ desired}}{(a/A \text{ ratio})}$$

$$\text{Step 2: } F_IO_2 = \frac{(PAO_2 \text{ needed} + 50)}{713}$$

PAO_2 needed : Alveolar oxygen tension needed for a desired PaO_2
PaO_2 desired : Arterial oxygen tension desired
a/A ratio : Arterial/alveolar oxygen tension ratio;
　　　　　　(PaO_2/PAO_2 before changes)
F_IO_2 : Inspired oxygen concentration needed to get
　　　　a desired PaO_2
50 : normal $PaCO_2$ / Respiratory Quotient =
　　(40 / 0.8) mm Hg
713 : $P_B - PH_2O = (760 - 47)$ mm Hg

✔ Hypoxemia related to hypoventilation may be partially corrected by improving ventilation. But in most cases, supplemental oxygen is also needed to treat hypoxemia.

Oxygen and Ventilation. Most patients with respiratory acidosis or ventilatory failure are also hypoxemic. Hypoxemia related to hypoventilation may be partially corrected by improving ventilation. But in most cases supplemental oxygen is also needed to treat hypoxemia. In a clinical setting, an elevated $PaCO_2$ along with hypoxemia should be treated with ventilation and oxygen.

*refractory hypox-
emia: Hypoxemia
that is commonly
caused by intrapul-
monary shunting
and does not re-
spond to high F_IO_2.*

✓ Refractory
hypoxemia re-
sponds well to sup-
plemental oxygen
when used with
CPAP or PEEP.

✓ Alveolar ventila-
tion may be
improved by ↑ me-
chanical rate or V_T or
↑ spontaneous rate
or V_T.

✓ Alveolar ventila-
tion may be im-
proved by ↓ the
anatomic, mechani-
cal, or alveolar
deadspace.

✓ Hypoperfusion
due to conges-
tive heart failure
may be corrected
by improving myo-
cardial function.

Oxygen and PEEP. Oxygen therapy alone may not be sufficient if the hypoxemia is caused by intrapulmonary shunting. This type of **refractory hypoxemia** requires oxygen and continuous positive airway pressure (CPAP) or positive end-expiratory pressure (PEEP).

Oxygen Toxicity. Sufficient oxygen should be given to the patient to maintain a PaO_2 of around 80 mm Hg (lower for COPD patients). Excessive oxygen is to be avoided because of the increased likelihood of developing oxygen toxicity, ciliary impairment, lung damage, respiratory distress syndrome, and pulmonary fibrosis (Otto, 1986). Since these complications may occur within 12 to 24 hours of exposure to 100% oxygen, the general guideline is to use an F_IO_2 lower than 60% and use high F_IO_2's for less than 24 hours, when possible (Winter et al., 1972).

IMPROVE VENTILATION AND REDUCE MECHANICAL DEADSPACE

Adequate ventilation is a prerequisite to oxygenation. Hypoxemia caused by hypoventilation is usually supported by supplemental oxygen during mechanical ventilation, but it must be corrected by improving alveolar ventilation. Arterial $PaCO_2$ is the best measure of a patient's ventilatory status. When $PaCO_2$ is elevated in conjunction with hypoxemia, improvement in the patient's oxygenation status may be possible by ventilation alone. The level of ventilation can be improved by increasing the mechanical rate or tidal volume; or the patient's spontaneous tidal volume or rate.

Alveolar ventilation may also be improved by reducing the deadspace volume. Endotracheal intubation and tracheostomy are both effective in reducing the anatomic deadspace. Mechanical deadspace of an endotracheal tube may be decreased by cutting it shorter than the original length. If a high V/Q mismatch (ventilation in excess of perfusion) exists, alveolar deadspace may be reduced by improving pulmonary perfusion.

IMPROVE CIRCULATION

Adequate pulmonary blood flow is necessary for proper gas exchange. If perfusion is too low relative to ventilation, deadspace ventilation (high V/Q) results. If perfusion is too high, pulmonary hypertension becomes the potential problem. In order to maintain a normal ventilation-perfusion relationship, the hemodynamic values should be monitored regularly, including systemic arterial pressure, central venous pressure, pulmonary artery pressure, and pulmonary capillary wedge pressure.

When hypovolemia occurs due to volume loss, fluid replacement is necessary. If the cause of hypovolemia is shock (relative hypovolemia; loss of venous tone), fluid replacement should be done with extreme caution because of the potential for fluid overload when

✓ In relative hypo-
volemia (loss
of venous tone),
fluid replacement
should be done with
extreme caution be-
cause of the poten-
tial for fluid overload
when vascular tone
returns to normal.

vascular tone returns to normal. Vasopressors are very useful to provide quick relief of hypovolemia due to shock but the condition should
be corrected by treating the cause of shock.

MAINTAIN NORMAL HEMOGLOBIN LEVEL

Monitoring of the PaO_2 alone for assessment of oxygenation status
may be inadequate when a patient's hemoglobin level is below normal. This is because PaO_2 measures the amount of oxygen dissolved
in the plasma whereas a vast majority (98%) of the oxygen in the blood
is combined with and carried by the hemoglobins. When anemic hypoxia is suspected, the hemoglobin level should be checked for the
presence of anemia (hemoglobin less than 10 gm/100 ml of blood).

Treatment of anemia must be specific to the cause. For example,
anemia due to excessive blood loss should be treated by stopping the
blood loss and replacing the blood volume. Anemia caused by insufficient hemoglobin should be treated by replacing the red blood cells.
Once the hemoglobin level is restored, the oxygen carrying capacity
and oxygen content should return to normal.

INITIATE CONTINUOUS POSITIVE AIRWAY PRESSURE (CPAP)

✓ CPAP is only
suitable for
patients who have
adequate respiratory
mechanics and can
sustain prolonged
spontaneous
breathing.

Continuous positive airway pressure (CPAP) provides positive airway
pressure throughout the respiratory cycle. It increases the functional
residual capacity and is therefore very useful to correct hypoxemia due
to intrapulmonary shunting. Since CPAP does not provide mechanical
ventilation, it is only suitable for patients who have adequate respiratory mechanics and can sustain prolonged spontaneous breathing.
Adequacy of spontaneous ventilation can be documented by trending
a patient's $PaCO_2$. An increasing $PaCO_2$ over time indicates that the
patient is tiring and continuation of CPAP must be reevaluated.

INITIATE POSITIVE END-EXPIRATORY PRESSURE (PEEP)

✓ Like CPAP, PEEP
increases the
functional residual
capacity and is
therefore very useful
to correct hypox-
emia due to intrapul-
monary shunting.

Positive end-expiratory pressure (PEEP) provides positive airway
pressure at the end of the expiratory phase. It is similar to CPAP with
the exception that PEEP is used in conjunction with mechanical ventilation. Spontaneous breathing is not required when PEEP is used as
the patient relies on the ventilator for ventilatory support. Like CPAP,
PEEP increases the functional residual capacity and is therefore very
useful to correct hypoxemia due to intrapulmonary shunting.

*optimal PEEP: The
lowest PEEP level
leading to the best
oxygenation (or
compliance) status
without causing car-
diopulmonary side
effects.*

In order to minimize the cardiovascular complications and barotrauma associated with excessive pulmonary pressures, the **optimal
PEEP** should be used. Optimal PEEP may be determined by measuring many different parameters, among them the PaO_2, PvO_2, compliance, and O_2 saturation. Table 12-3 shows that 10 cm H_2O is the
optimal PEEP since the next level of PEEP (12 cm H_2O) causes a
decrease of PaO_2 and compliance.

TABLE 12-3 Titration of Optimal PEEP Using PaO$_2$ and Compliance As Indicators

PEEP (cm H$_2$O)	PaO$_2$ (mm Hg)	COMPLIANCE (ml/cm H$_2$O)
0	43	26
5	67	33
8	77	37
10*	83	43
12	79	41

*10 cm H$_2$O is the optimal PEEP since the PaO$_2$ and compliance show a continuing upward trend with the increasing PEEP level from 0 to 10 cm H$_2$O. Beyond the optimal PEEP, the next PEEP setting (12 cm H$_2$O) causes the PaO$_2$ to drop from 83 to 79 mm Hg and the compliance to fall from 43 to 41 ml/cm H$_2$O. It is not necessary to use more than one indicator to titrate the optimal PEEP. As shown above, the PaO$_2$ indicator is more time-consuming and invasive than the compliance indicator.

TABLE 12-4 Weaning from PEEP and High F$_I$O$_2$

1. Maintain PEEP and decrease F$_I$O$_2$ to 40% or 50%	Keep PaO$_2$ > 60 mm Hg or SaO$_2$ > 90%. Monitor vital signs for acute changes.
2. Maintain F$_I$O$_2$ and decrease PEEP to about 3 cm H$_2$O (at 2 to 3 cm H$_2$O increments)	Keep PaO$_2$ > 60 mm Hg or SaO$_2$ > 90%. Monitor vital signs for acute changes.
3. Discontinue PEEP	Monitor vital signs for hypoxia and increased work of breathing.

☑ If the patient is hemodynamically stable and the risk of barotrauma or other PEEP complications appear minimal, it is advisable to decrease the F$_I$O$_2$ to 0.40 prior to decreasing the PEEP.

Weaning From PEEP. Since PEEP is used to treat refractory hypoxemia, a patient will typically be receiving high levels of oxygen. The first criterion is to reduce the F$_I$O$_2$ to nontoxic levels as quickly as the patient's condition allows. If the patient is hemodynamically stable and the risk of barotrauma or other PEEP complications appear minimal, it is advisable to decrease the F$_I$O$_2$ to 0.40 prior to decreasing the PEEP. PEEP should always be decreased in small increments while the patient's oxygen saturation is closely monitored. If at all possible, the patient's saturation should not be allowed to fall below 90%. The proper sequence of weaning PEEP is outlined in Table 12-4.

INVERSE RATIO VENTILATION (IRV)

Inverse ratio ventilation (IRV) is a technique used in mechanical ventilation in which the inspiratory time is longer than the expiratory time. The inspiratory time is prolonged by decreasing the inspiratory flow rate or by increasing the inflation hold time. IRV is also observed during airway pressure release ventilation where the pressure release rate is less than 20 per minute (or greater than six seconds per cycle). IRV has been used to treat ARDS patients with refractory hypoxemia not

☑ IRV helps to improve oxygenation by (1) overcoming non-compliant lung tissue, (2) recruiting collapsed alveoli, and (3) increasing the time for gas diffusion.

responsive to conventional mechanical ventilation and PEEP (Gurevitch et al., 1986).

The prolonged inspiratory time in IRV helps to improve oxygenation by (1) overcoming noncompliant lung tissues, (2) recruiting collapsed alveoli, and (3) increasing the time for gas diffusion. Since inspiratory time is a function of mean airway pressure, a prolonged inspiratory time can increase mean airway pressure and diminish the cardiovascular functions of a critically ill patient.

IRV can be effective in improving oxygenation in patients with ARDS. However, it should be tried on an individual basis and used as an alternative after other conventional mechanical ventilation strategies have failed to improve oxygenation.

EXTRACORPOREAL MEMBRANE OXYGENATION (ECMO)

The first use of the extracorporeal membrane oxygenator (ECMO) on an infant was done and described in 1971 (Zwischenberger et al., 1986). Since then, ECMO has been used with considerable success as an oxygenation strategy for infants with extreme hypoxemia. In adult patients, however, it has not been shown to provide better oxygenation over conventional mechanical ventilation with PEEP (Zapol et al., 1979).

ACID-BASE BALANCE

When interpreted correctly, blood gas studies are very useful in the evaluation of a patient's acid-base, ventilatory, and oxygenation status. Blood gas interpretation is most accurate when it is done in conjunction with the patient's medical history and diagnosis. This section covers two pairs of blood gas abnomalities that look very similar without a closeup examination: (1) respiratory acidosis and compensated metabolic alkalosis; and (2) respiratory alkalosis and compensated metabolic acidosis.

RESPIRATORY ACIDOSIS AND COMPENSATED METABOLIC ALKALOSIS

Respiratory acidosis (ventilatory failure) is caused by hypoventilation. The strategy to correct this abnormality is to improve ventilation. For specific procedures to improve ventilation, refer to the section on "Strategies to Improve Ventilation" at the beginning of this chapter.

☑ If hypoventilation occurs due to metabolic alkalosis, increasing mechanical ventilation may further reduce spontaneous ventilation.

The strategies to improve ventilation are useful only when respiratory acidosis is induced by hypoventilation. They should not be used when hypoventilation occurs as a compensatory mechanism for metabolic alkalosis. Compensated metabolic alkalosis has an elevated $PaCO_2$, thus mimicking the elevated $PaCO_2$ seen in primary or compensated respiratory acidosis.

Table 12-5 compares the typical blood gases of compensated respiratory acidosis and compensated metabolic alkalosis (both show high $PaCO_2$ and high HCO_3^-). Note that in primary respiratory acidosis, the HCO_3^- is within its normal range (i.e., no renal compensation). In compensated respiratory acidosis, the pH (7.37) is on the acidotic side of its normal range (7.35 to 7.45). In compensated metabolic alkalosis, the pH (7.42) is on the alkalotic side of its normal range (7.35 to 7.45). As with other blood gas abnormalities, the patient's medical history should be used to differentiate whether the condition is a respiratory or metabolic problem.

RESPIRATORY ALKALOSIS AND COMPENSATED METABOLIC ACIDOSIS

☑ If hyperventilation occurs due to acute hypoxia, weaning or use of mechanical deadspace should not be implemented.

Respiratory alkalosis is caused by alveolar hyperventilation. In general, this condition does not require mechanical ventilation intervention and it usually allows gradual weaning of the mechanical rate. However, if the hyperventilation is induced by acute hypoxia, the cause of hypoxia must be identified and treated. Otherwise, weaning the ventilator rate will cause further patient hyperventilation due to uncorrected and persistent hypoxia.

Additional deadspace tubing between the endotracheal tube and ventilator "Y" adaptor is sometimes used to partially correct persistent respiratory alkalosis. This may be necessary when the mechanical volume and rate cannot be reduced due to the patient's tidal volume and oxygenation requirements.

It is also important to note whether the respiratory alkalosis is a compensatory mechanism for metabolic acidosis. Compensated metabolic acidosis has a decreased $PaCO_2$, thus mimicking the reduced $PaCO_2$ seen in primary or compensated respiratory alkalosis.

Table 12-6 compares the typical blood gases of compensated respiratory alkalosis and compensated metabolic acidosis (both show low $PaCO_2$ and low HCO_3^-). Note that in primary respiratory alkalosis, the HCO_3^- is within its normal range (no renal compensation). In compensated respiratory alkalosis, the pH (7.42) is on the alkalotic side of its normal range (7.35 to 7.45). In compensated metabolic acidosis, the pH (7.37) is on the acidotic side of its normal range (7.35 to 7.45). As with

TABLE 12-5 Differentiation of Respiratory Acidosis and Compensated Metabolic Alkalosis

BLOOD GAS CONDITION	pH	PaCO$_2$ (mm Hg)	HCO$_3^-$ (mEq/L)
Primary respiratory acidosis	7.30	53	26
Compensated respiratory acidosis	7.37	52	30
Compensated metabolic alkalosis	7.42	50	32

TABLE 12-6 **Differentiation of Respiratory Alkalosis and Compensated Metabolic Acidosis**

BLOOD GAS CONDITION	pH	PaCO$_2$ (mm Hg)	HCO$_3^-$ (mEq/L)
Primary respiratory alkalosis	7.50	30	23
Compensated respiratory alkalosis	7.42	28	17
Compensated metabolic acidosis	7.37	29	15

other blood gas abnormalities, the patient's medical history should be used to differentiate a respiratory or metabolic problem.

METABOLIC ACID-BASE ABNORMALITIES

Metabolic acid-base abnormalities should be corrected by treating their respective causes. Three major causes of metabolic acidosis are renal failure, diabetic ketoacidosis, and lactic acidosis. One of the major causes of metabolic alkalosis is hypokalemia (Shapiro et al., 1994). Ventilatory (respiratory) interventions by mechanical ventilation should not be done to compensate or correct primary metabolic problems. One should refer to a blood gas textbook for further information on the diagnosis and treatment of metabolic abnormalities.

TROUBLESHOOTING OF COMMON VENTILATOR ALARMS AND EVENTS

alarm: An absolute value of a parameter on the ventilator beyond which an alert is invoked to warn that the safety limit has been breached.

The type of ventilator **alarm** is easy to spot since most ventilators provide an indicator (light or sound) for each event that triggers the alarm. Once the type of alarm is identified, steps can be taken to alleviate the problem by process of elimination. This section provides the common causes for each alarm.

LOW PRESSURE ALARM

The low pressure limit is set to ensure that a minimum pressure is present in the ventilator circuit during each inspiratory cycle.

☑ The low pressure alarm may be triggered in: (1) loss of circuit pressure (a common event), (2) loss of system pressure (an uncommon occurrence), (3) conditions leading to premature termination of inspiratory phase, and (4) inappropriate ventilator settings.

Low pressure alarms are triggered when the circuit pressure drops below the preset low pressure limit. If the preset low pressure limit is set at 40 cm H$_2$O, and the circuit pressure drops below 40 cm H$_2$O, the low pressure alarm will then be triggered. In all likelihood, the low volume alarm will also be triggered since pressure and volume are affected simultaneously by similar clinical conditions.

Conditions that may trigger the low pressure alarm may be grouped into four areas: (1) loss of circuit pressure (a common event), (2) loss of system pressure (an uncommon occurrence), (3) conditions leading to premature termination of inspiratory phase, and (4) inappropriate ventilator settings. These conditions and selected examples are listed in Table 12-7.

LOW EXPIRED VOLUME ALARM

☑ The low volume alarm is usually triggered along with the low pressure alarm because loss of airway pressure usually results in loss of volume delivered.

The low volume limit is set to ensure that the patient receives (and exhales) a minimum volume.

The low expired volume alarm is triggered when the expired volume drops below the preset low volume limit. If the preset low expired volume limit is set at 400 mL and the expired volume drops below 400 mL, the low volume alarm will be triggered.

As mentioned before, the low volume alarm is usually triggered along with the low pressure alarm because loss of airway pressure usually results in loss of volume delivered, thus the expired volume. See Table 12-7 for examples of conditions that may trigger low volume alarm.

HIGH PRESSURE ALARM

☑ The high pressure alarm may be triggered in the following conditions: (1) increase in air flow resistance, (2) decrease in lung or chest wall compliance.

The high pressure limit is set to control the maximum ventilator circuit pressure during a complete breathing cycle, usually during the inspiratory phase.

The high pressure alarm is triggered when the circuit pressure reaches or exceeds the preset high pressure limit. If the high pressure limit is set at 60 cm H_2O, and the circuit pressure reaches or exceeds 60 cm H_2O, the high pressure alarm will be triggered.

TABLE 12-7 Conditions That Trigger the Low Pressure/Low Volume Alarms

CONDITION	EXAMPLES
Loss of circuit pressure	Circuit disconnection Exhalation valve drive line disconnection Insufficient endotracheal tube cuff volume Loose circuit connection Loose humidifier connection
Loss of system pressure	Power failure Source gas failure or disconnection Air compressor failure
Premature termination of inspiratory phase	Excessive peak flow Insufficient inspiratory time (I time) Excessive expiratory time (E time) Inappropriate sensitivity setting (too sensitive)
Inappropriate ventilator settings	Excessive rate with insufficient peak flow Low pressure limit set too high Low tidal volume limit set too high

Conditions that trigger the high pressure alarm may be: (1) increase in air flow resistance, and (2) decrease in lung or chest wall compliance. These conditions and selected examples are shown in Table 12-8.

HIGH RESPIRATORY RATE ALARM

The high respiratory rate limit is set to alert the practitioner that the patient has experienced tachypnea.

✓ The high rate alarm may be triggered due to: (1) patient's need to increase ventilation, (2) excessive sensitivity setting.

This alarm is triggered when the total rate exceeds the high rate limit. This condition is most likely caused by a distressed patient when the need to increase ventilation (i.e., respiratory rate) becomes necessary. When the patient consistently sets off the high respiratory rate alarm, the practitioner may need to increase the level of ventilatory support to ease the patient's work of breathing.

Another cause of the high rate alarm is inappropriate sensitivity setting. When this control is set excessively sensitive to the patient's inspiratory effort, minimum inspiratory efforts or movements would cause the ventilator to initiate unwanted breaths and increase the total respiratory rate.

APNEA/LOW RESPIRATORY RATE ALARM

The apnea/low respiratory rate limit is set to ensure that a minimum number of breaths is delivered to the patient.

TABLE 12-8   Conditions That Trigger the High Pressure Alarm

CONDITION	EXAMPLES

Increase in air flow resistance	Mechanical Factors
	   Kinking of circuit
	   Kinking of ET tube
	   Blocked exhalation manifold
	   Water in circuit
	   Herniated ET tube cuff
	   Main-stem bronchial intubation
	   High pressure limit set too low
	
	Patient Factors
	   Bronchospasm
	   Coughing
	   Breathing pattern out of synchronization
	     with ventilator
	   Secretions in ET tube
	   Mucus plug

Decrease in lung or chest wall compliance	Tension pneumothorax Atelectasis ARDS Pneumonia

☑ Disconnection of
the ventilator
circuit from the pa-
tient's endotracheal
tube is the most fre-
quent trigger of the
apnea alarm.

The apnea or low respiratory rate alarm is triggered when the total rate drops below the low rate limit. Disconnection of the ventilator circuit from the patient's endotracheal tube is the most frequent trigger of the apnea alarm, since the ventilator cannot sense any air movement (respiratory effort) from a disconnected circuit. Other triggers of the apnea/low rate alarm include patient under respiratory depressants or muscle-paralyzing agents, conditions of respiratory center dysfunction, and respiratory muscle fatigue.

Some ventilators merely alert the practitioner that the patient is having periods of apnea; the practitioner must increase ventilation to alleviate the situation. Other ventilators (e.g., Puritan-Bennett 7200) switch to a backup ventilation mode to ventilate the patient until the problem is corrected.

HIGH PEEP ALARM

The high PEEP limit is set to prevent excessive PEEP being delivered to the patient. The alarm is triggered when the actual PEEP exceeds the preset PEEP limit. Inadvertent PEEP may occur in conditions of air trapping, insufficient inspiratory flow rate (long I time), or insufficient expiratory time (short E time).

Air trapping may be reduced by using bronchodilators in patients with reversible airway obstruction. Increasing the inspiratory peak flow provides a longer E time and this may also help to reduce air trapping.

LOW PEEP ALARM

The low PEEP limit is set to ensure that the preselected PEEP is delivered to the patient. The alarm is triggered when the actual PEEP drops below the preset low PEEP limit. Failure of the ventilator circuit to hold the PEEP is usually due to leakage in the circuit or endotracheal tube cuff.

AUTO-PEEP

Auto-PEEP (intrinsic PEEP, inadvertent PEEP, occult PEEP) is the unintentional PEEP during mechanical ventilation that is associated with pressure support ventilation, significant airway obstruction, rapid respiratory rates (>20/min), insufficient inspiratory flow rates, and relatively equal (about 1:1) I:E ratio. It is also more likely to occur when the patient has a history of air trapping (MacIntyre, 1986; Schuster, 1990). With auto-PEEP, the distal airway pressures in the lungs can be as high as 15 cm H_2O, while the ventilator's proximal airway pressure manometer shows zero pressure (or PEEP if PEEP is used). Auto-PEEP can be measured by occluding the expiratory port just before the next inspiration (Marini, 1988). To measure it accurately, the patient should be sedated or paralyzed.

☑ Auto-PEEP is
associated
with pressure
support ventilation,
significant airway
obstruction, rapid
respiratory rates
(>20/min), insuffi-
cient inspiratory
flow rates, relatively
equal (about 1:1) I:E
ratio, and history
of air trapping.

Auto-PEEP Increases Work of Breathing (See Figure 12-2A.)   Under normal conditions, a mechanical breath is initiated when the inspiratory

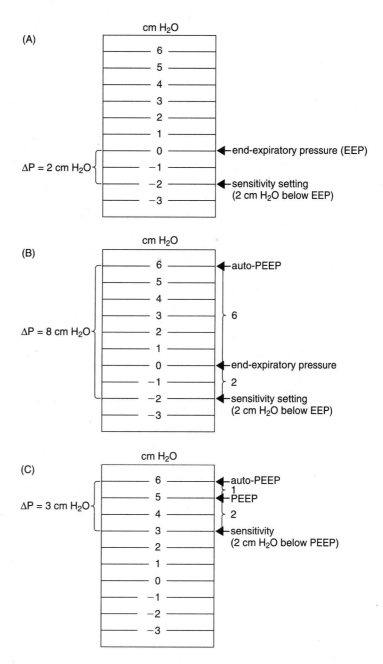

Figure 12-2 (A) Without auto-PEEP, the pressure gradient from end-expiratory pressure to sensitivity setting is 2 cm H_2O. (B) With auto-PEEP of 6 cm H_2O, the pressure gradient from auto-PEEP to sensitivity setting is 8 cm H_2O. (C) With auto-PEEP of 6 cm H_2O and PEEP setting of 5 cm H_2O, the pressure gradient from auto-PEEP to sensitivity setting is 3 cm H_2O.

negative pressure reaches the sensitivity setting of the ventilator. For example, when the normal end-expiratory pressure is 0 cm H_2O and the sensitivity is set at –2 cm H_2O, the pressure gradient (ΔP) or work of breathing to trigger a mechanical breath is 2 cm H_2O (from 0 cm H_2O to 2 cm H_2O).

If auto-PEEP is present, the work of breathing is increased because the level of auto-PEEP in the lungs at end-expiratory phase must first be overcome before additional inspiratory negative pressure can be used to reach the sensitivity setting. For example, when the auto-PEEP level is 6 cm H_2O and the sensitivity is set at –2 cm H_2O, the pressure gradient (ΔP) to trigger a mechanical breath becomes 8 cm H_2O. Figure 12-2B shows the distribution of 8 cm H_2O of pressure (6 cm H_2O to bring auto-PEEP from 5 to 0 cm H_2O plus 2 cm H_2O to reach the preset sensitivity level).

> ✓ Auto-PEEP may be reduced or eliminated by: (1) improving ventilation and reducing air trapping by bronchodilators, (2) prolonging the expiratory time by increasing the flow rate or reducing the tidal volume.

Strategies to Reduce Auto-Peep.   To reduce the likelihood of auto-PEEP, the respiratory rate during pressure support ventilation should be kept less than 20 breaths/min. if possible. Auto-PEEP may also be minimized or eliminated by improving ventilation or providing a longer expiratory time. Two methods may be useful to reduce or eliminate the auto-PEEP and they are: (1) improving ventilation and reducing air trapping by bronchodilators, (2) prolonging the expiratory time by increasing the flow rate or reducing the tidal volume.

Using PEEP to Reduce Effects of Auto-PEEP.   PEEP can be used to reduce the effects of auto-PEEP. The level of PEEP used to counter the effects of auto-PEEP should be kept below 85% of the measured auto-PEEP level (Scanlan et al., 1999). For example, PEEP level of up to 5 cm H_2O may be used when auto-PEEP of 6 cm H_2O is measured during mechanical ventilation. Figure 12-2C shows that the pressure gradient (ΔP) to trigger a mechanical breath drops to 3 cm H_2O (1 cm H_2O to bring auto-PEEP from 6 cm H_2O to 5 cm H_2O plus 2 cm H_2O to reach the preset sensitivity level).

CARE OF THE VENTILATOR CIRCUIT

The ventilator circuit serves as an important interface between the ventilator and the patient. Circuit compliance, circuit patency, humidity, and temperature are four essential factors to consider in the management of mechanical ventilation.

CIRCUIT COMPLIANCE

The compliance of ventilator circuits should be as low as possible. High circuit compliance leads to a higher compressible volume in the circuit during inspiration and this condition reduces the effective tidal volume delivered to the patient. For example, at a peak airway pressure of 40 cm H_2O, ventilator circuit with a compliance of 5 ml/cm H_2O would expand and hold 200 ml (40 cm $H_2O \times$ 5 ml/cm H_2O) of the mechanical tidal volume. At the same peak airway pressure, ventilator circuit with a compliance of 3 ml/cm H_2O would have a compressible volume of only 120 ml (40 cm $H_2O \times$ 3 ml/cm H_2O). Unless tidal volume adjustment is made to account for the circuit compliance factor, the effective tidal volume to the patient would be reduced substantially when high compliance circuits are used (Burton, 1997).

CIRCUIT PATENCY

Condensation imposes the most common threat to the patency of ventilator circuit. Gas temperature drops as it travels from the heated humidifier to the patient. As the temperature drops along the circuit, water vapor condenses and water collects in the tubing. This condition leads to significant airflow obstruction. Heated-wire circuit (Figure 12-3) and inline water trap (Figure 12-4) have been used successfully to reduce condensation and the amount of water in the circuit.

Heat and Moisture Exchanger (HME).   (Figure 12-5) is a device that may be used to replace the traditional heated humidifier. It is placed between the patient's artificial airway and the ventilator circuit. During exhalation, moisture and heat from the patient is absorbed into the

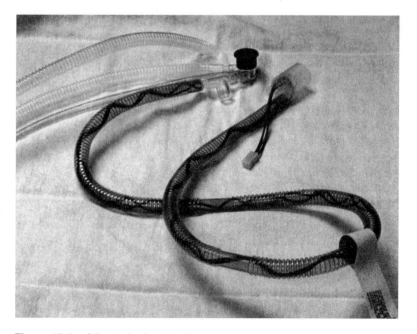

Figure 12-3   A heated-wire circuit.

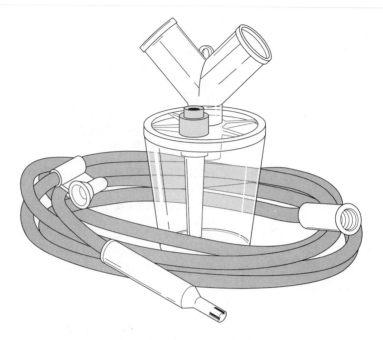

Figure 12-4 Inline water trap.

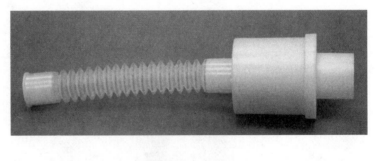

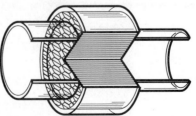

Figure 12-5 A photograph and a functional diagram of a heat and moisture exchanger (HME).

honeycomb structure of the exchanger. The moisture and heat is transferred back to the patient during the next inhalation. The efficiency of HME units ranges from 70% to 90% relative humidity and 30 to 31 degrees Celsius (White, 1999). Compared to the heated humidifier, ventilator circuits with a bacterial-viral filtering HME cost less to maintain and are less likely to colonize bacteria (Boots, Howe, George et al., 1997; Kirton, DeHaven, Morgan et al., 1997).

HME may not be suitable for certain patients due to problems associated with adequacy of airflow, humidity, and temperature. Contraindications for HME include a thick and large amount of secretions, minute volume exceeding 10 LPM, body temperature less than 32 degrees Celsius, and need for aerosolized medications (Scanlan et al., 1999).

HUMIDITY AND TEMPERATURE

Since the upper airway is bypassed during mechanical ventilation, the inspired gas temperature should be kept close to the body temperature. The temperature probe for the heated humidifier should be placed inside the inspiratory limb of the ventilator circuit as close to the patient as possible. Since water vapor saturation depends on the water content as well as the temperature, the temperature setting should be adjusted for a distal temperature reading of 37°C. This ensures proper temperature and humidification to the patient (Burton, 1997).

FREQUENCY OF CIRCUIT CHANGE

It has been well established that the optimal interval for ventilator circuit change is once per week (Fink, Krause & Barrett, 1998; Kotilainen & Keroack, 1997; Long, Wickstrom & Grimes et al., 1996; Stamm, 1998). When compared to more frequent circuit changes, weekly circuit change does not increase the incidence of nosocomial infection, including ventilator-associated pneumonia. Weekly change also saves manpower and reduces the direct replacement cost for new ventilator circuits. In one study, a cost savings of $26.46 was realized per circuit change (Kotilainen & Keroack, 1997).

CARE OF THE ARTIFICIAL AIRWAY

✓ Patency of the ET tube can only be ensured with adequate humidification and prompt removal of retained secretions.

Supplemental humidity must be provided during mechanical ventilation since the endotracheal (ET) tube does not receive humidification normally provided by the upper airway. In addition, secretions must be removed by suctioning if necessary because the ET tube and the ventilator circuit are a closed system. If not removed, any secretions coughed up by the patient are likely to stay in the ET tube. Patency of the ET tube can only be ensured with adequate humidification and prompt removal of retained secretions.

PATENCY OF THE ENDOTRACHEAL TUBE

In mechanical ventilation, the primary purpose of an ET tube is to conduct air flow between the ventilator and the lungs. Since air flow resistance is inversely related to the diameter of the tube, small tubes cause a tremendous increase in the work of breathing. In order to enhance air flow, the largest size ET tube that is appropriate to the patient should be used. Mucus in the ET tube should also be removed frequently in order to minimize air flow obstruction created by retained secretions.

Poiseuille's Law shows that when the radius of an airway is reduced by half, the driving pressure (work of breathing) must be increased 16 times in order to maintain the same flow rate. An obstructed airway hinders not only mechanical ventilation, but spontaneous ventilation as well. Airway management should always be an integral part of mechancial ventilation.

$$\text{Pressure change} = \frac{\text{Flow}}{r^4}$$

Other conditions that can affect the patency of the ET tube include: (1) kinking or bending of the tube due to poor positioning of the patient and placement of the ventilator circuit; (2) patient biting on the ET tube due to physical or psychological discomfort; and (3) malfunction of the ET tube cuff causing partial or complete blockage.

Frequent endotracheal suctioning is sometimes necessary to maintain the patency of the endotracheal tube. One of the problems with endotracheal suctioning is hypoxia. Suction-induced hypoxia may be minimized by preoxygenating the patient with oxygen prior to suction, limiting the total suction time to no more than 10 seconds, and using a closed tracheal suction system (Scanlan et al., 1999). Since one can perform suctioning without disconnecting the ventilator circuit, FIO_2 and PEEP levels may be maintained. Figure 12-6 shows a closed tracheal suction system.

HUMIDIFICATION AND REMOVAL OF SECRETIONS

Proper function of the ciliary blanket of the airway is dependent on adequate humidity. In mechanical ventilation, humidification of the airways and lungs is commonly provided by a heated cascade, heated wick humidifier, or heat and membrane exchanger (HME, or artificial nose). Occasionally, humidification and removal of the secretions are supplemented by use of a saline solution via a small volume nebulizer or direct endotracheal instillation.

Saline solution used in a small volume nebulizer is delivered in an aerosol form, and is thus capable of carrying pathogens into the lower airways. Instillation of saline solution directly into the trachea to facilitate endotracheal suctioning has also been implicated in the

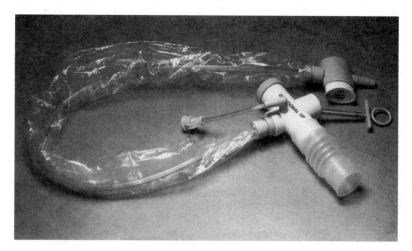

Figure 12-6 An example of a Closed Suction System manufactured by Ballard Medical, Inc.

contamination of the lower airways with pathogens (Hagler et al., 1994). For these reasons, aseptic techniques for equipment handling and sterile techniques for endotracheal suctioning must be followed in order to minimize the occurrence of pulmonary contamination and infection.

INFECTION CONTROL

Patients who are intubated and on mechanical ventilation are more prone to develop nosocomial pneumonia than nonintubated patients (Craven et al., 1989). The estimated incidence of ventilator-associated pneumonia ranges from 10% to 65%, with fatality rates of 13% to 55% (Kollef et al., 1994). The presence of an artificial airway bypasses the natural defense mechanism of the airway, causes local trauma and inflammation, and increases the risk of aspiration of pathogens from the oropharynx.

In one study, 45% of the patients developed pneumonia within three days of intubation (Lowy et al., 1987). This condition may be caused by microbes acquired from the patient's oropharynx, respiratory instruments, health care providers (Hu, 1991), endotracheal and nasogastric tubes (Joshi et al., 1993), and manual ventilation bags (Weber et al., 1990). Table 12-9 outlines the potential sources of ventilator-associated pneumonia. Strategies to decrease ventilator-associated pneumonias include proper handwashing techniques, closed suction systems (Figure 12-6), continuous feed humidification systems, and less frequent ventilator circuit changes.

Sputum Culture. Sputum cultures should be obtained if infection of the lungs is suspected. Since the patient is intubated, the sputum

Gram stain: A method for staining bacteria. Gram-positive bacteria (e.g., Staphlococcus) retain the gentian violet (purple) color and Gram-negative bacteria (e.g., Pseu-domonas) take the red counterstain.

culture and sensitivity: A laboratory procedure that grows the microbes in an agar plate and tests their sensitivity or resistance to different antimicrobial drugs.

✓ Gram stain is done for rapid selection of antibiotics.

✓ Acid-fast sputum analysis is for pulmonary tuberculosis. Silver stain is for *Pneumocystis carinii* pneumonia.

✓ Culture and sensitivity (c & s) is done to identify the microbes and effective antimicrobial agents.

TABLE 12-9 Potential Sources of Ventilator-Associated Pneumonia

POTENTIAL SOURCE	LOCATIONS
Patient	Oropharynx
Health care provider	Hands
Equipment and supplies	Respiratory instruments Aerosol nebulizers and humidifiers Endotracheal tube Nasogastric tube Manual ventilation bag

sample may be obtained via an endotracheal suction setup and a sputum trap (Figure 12-7). Sputum analyses are commonly done by the **Gram stain**, and the **culture and sensitivity** methods.

The Gram stain technique is done to quickly establish the general category (Gram-positive or Gram-negative) of the suspected microbes so that appropriate broad-spectrum antibiotics may be administered without delay. Acid-fast sputum analysis is for pulmonary tuberculosis and silver stain is for *Pneumocystis carinii* pneumonia. Culture and sensitivity is more time-consuming but it can identify the microbes in the sputum and the most suitable antibiotics for the infection.

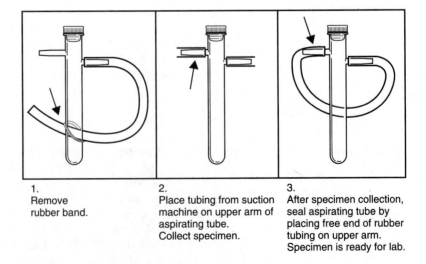

1.
Remove rubber band.

2.
Place tubing from suction machine on upper arm of aspirating tube. Collect specimen.

3.
After specimen collection, seal aspirating tube by placing free end of rubber tubing on upper arm. Specimen is ready for lab.

Figure 12-7 Sputum collecting tube used with a suction system. The upper outlet goes to the vacuum source and the lower outlet is connected to the suction catheter.

FLUID BALANCE

Fluid balance in the body is mainly affected by: (1) the blood and fluid volume in the blood vessels and cells, (2) the pressure gradient between the blood vessels and the tissues around them, and (3) electrolyte concentrations.

DISTRIBUTION OF BODY WATER

extracellular fluid (ECF): Fluid in the plasma and interstitial space. It accounts for 20% of total body water and is mainly affected by the sodium concentration in the plasma.

Water makes up about 60% of the body weight. The distribution of this volume is 20% in the plasma and interstitial fluid (**extracellular fluid, ECF**) and 40% within the cells (**intracellular fluid, ICF**). Table 12-10 shows the distribution of body water.

Changes in Extracellular Fluid Distribution. The distribution of body water in the ECF and ICF compartments is not a static measurement. Depending on the physiologic needs, fluid can move into and out of any compartment along with certain electrolytes. When an excessive volume of fluid moves out of the extracellular compartment, ECF deficit occurs.

intracellular fluid (ICF): Fluid within the cells. It accounts for 40% of total body water.

Fluid deficiency in the extracellular compartment (space) may be caused by one or a combination of these reasons: (1) inadequate intake (e.g., dehydration); (2) excessive loss (e.g., diarrhea); and (3) shifting of fluid along with the electrolytes into cells and tissues (e.g., swelling of tissues in burns).

CLINICAL SIGNS OF EXTRACELLULAR FLUID DEFICIT OR EXCESS

☑ When urine output drops below 20 ml/hr, it is indicative of fluid inadequacy.

Urine output is the most common method used to assess ECF abnormalities. When urine output drops below 20 ml/hr (or 400 ml in a 24-hour period, or 160 ml in 8 hours), it is called oliguria and is indicative of fluid inadequacy (Kraus et al., 1993). Excessive urine output is one of the signs of excessive ECF or excessive diuresis. Other clinical signs of ECF abnormalities include those involved with the central nervous system and the cardiovascular system. They are listed in Table 12-11.

TABLE 12-10   **Distribution of Body Water**

COMPARTMENT	SUBDIVISION	PERCENT OF WATER BY BODY WEIGHT
Extracellular	Plasma	5%
	Interstitial fluid	15%
Intracellular	Intracellular fluid	40%
Total		60% of body weight

TABLE 12-11   Signs of Extracellular Fluid (ECF) Deficit or Excess

SYSTEM	ECF DEFICIT	ECF EXCESS
CNS	Diminished sensorium Coma	None
Cardiovascular	Tachycardia Hypotension Cold extremities Poor peripheral pulse	Increased P_2 heart sound Increased cardiac output Bounding pulse Pulmonary edema
Renal	Oliguria Anuria (no urine)	Increased urine output

TREATMENT OF EXTRACELLULAR FLUID ABNORMALITIES

Treatment of ECF deficit is by fluid replacement with Ringer's lactate solution since it is similar to ECF in composition. Physiologic (0.9%) saline solution is an acceptable alternative. Success of fluid replacement therapy can be determined by reversal of those signs of ECF deficit in Table 12-11. For example, decrease in heart rate, increase in blood pressure, and urine output are signs of improvement in ECF deficit after fluid replacement.

Excessive fluid in the extracellular space is uncommon in a clinical setting. When it occurs, pulmonary edema is a common manifestation. The treatment for excessive ECF is to withhold fluid or to give a diuretic such as furosemide (Lasix). Mannitol should not be given for diuresis as it can increase plasma volume before inducing diuresis (Eggleston, 1985).

Use of diuretics will further increase the urine output. For this reason, reversal of the cardiovascular signs of ECF excess in Table 12-11 should be used to determine the success of treatment. For example, disappearance of the P_2 heart sound, reduction in pulse intensity, and clearing of pulmonary edema are signs of improvement in ECF excess due to fluid restriction or diuresis. Since diuresis can affect the electrolyte composition, monitoring of electrolyte balance is essential when diuretics are used to manage ECF excess.

☑ Decrease in heart rate, increase in blood pressure and urine output are signs of improvement in ECF deficit after fluid replacement.

☑ Disappearance of P_2 heart sound, reduction in pulse intensity, and clearing of pulmonary edema are signs of improvement in ECF excess.

ELECTROLYTE BALANCE

Electrolyte balance is the difference between the cations (positively charged ions) and the anions (negatively charged ions) in the plasma. Serum cations and anions are used to calculate the anion gap and assess a patient's electrolyte balance.

TABLE 12-12 **Normal Serum Electrolytes**

CATION	CONCENTRATION (mEq/L)	ANION	CONCENTRATION (mEq/L)
Na^+	140 (138 to 142)	Cl^-	103 (101 to 105)
K^+	4 (3 to 5)	HCO_3^-	25 (23 to 27)
Ca^{++}	5 (4.5 to 5.5)	Protein	16 (14 to 18)
Mg^{++}	2 (1.5 to 2.5)	HPO_4^{--}, $H_2PO_4^-$	2 (1.5 to 2.5)
		SO_4^{--}	1 (0.8 to 1.2)
		Organic acids	4 (3.5 to 4.5)
Total cations	151	Total Anions	151

NORMAL ELECTROLYTE BALANCE

Table 12-12 shows the normal values for serum electrolytes. Sodium is the major cation in the extracellular fluid compartment and it is directly related to the fluid level in the body. Potassium is the major cation in the intracellular fluid compartment and it is not related to the amount of fluid in the body.

Sodium and potassium are the two major electrolytes that must be monitored. In general, once the sodium and potassium concentrations are properly managed and returned to normal, the chloride concentration will be corrected as well without further intervention. The following sections cover sodium and potassium abnormalities.

Anion Gap.   Anion gap is the relationship of the cations [sodium (Na^+) and potassium (K^+)] to the anions [chloride (Cl^-) and bicarbonate (HCO_3^-)]. The normal range is 15 to 20 mEq/L when K^+ is included in the calculation (10 to 14 MEq/L when K^+ is excluded). When the anion gap is outside this range, electrolyte replacement may be necessary. See Chapter 9 for a discussion on the interpretation of anion gap in metabolic acidosis.

The anion gap is calculated as follows:

$$\text{Anion gap} = Na^+ + K^+ - Cl^- - HCO_3^-$$
or
$$\text{Anion gap} = Na^+ - Cl^- - HCO_3^-$$

anion gap: *The difference between cations (positive ions) and anions (negative ions) in the plasma. The normal range is 15 to 20 mEq/L when K^+ is included in the calculation (10 to 14 mEq/L when K^+ is excluded).*

✓ See Appendix 1 for example.

SODIUM ABNORMALITIES

Sodium is the major cation in the extracellular fluid (ECF) and it directly influences the ECF volume. The sodium concentration in the ECF may be higher than normal (hypernatremia) or lower than normal (hyponatremia). The clinical signs of sodium abnormalities are highlighted in Table 12-13.

TABLE 12-13   Clinical Signs of Sodium Abnormality

SYSTEM	HYPONATREMIA	HYPERNATREMIA
Central nervous system	Muscle twitching Loss of reflexes Increased intracranial pressure	Restlessness Weakness Delirium
Cardiovascular	Blood pressure change secondary to increased intracranial pressure	Tachycardia Hypotension (if severe)
Gastrointestinal	Watery diarrhea	None
Renal	Oliguria to anuria	Oliguria

☑ Hyponatremia is commonly related to ECF deficits (hypovolemia). The usual treatment is replenishment of sodium with saline solution.

☑ Hypernatremia is an uncommon problem and it is usually related to water deficit as a result of prolonged intravenous fluid administration with sufficient sodium but no dextrose.

☑ Potassium deficiency may be caused by excessive K⁺ loss (trauma, severe infection, vomiting, use of diuretics) or inadequate K⁺ intake (massive or prolonged intravenous fluid infusion without supplemental potassium).

Hyponatremia.   Hyponatremia is a more common form of sodium abnormality than hypernatremia. It is commonly related to ECF deficit (hypovolemia). The usual treatment is replenishment of sodium with saline solution (100 to 300 ml of 2.5% or 3% saline). It is not safe to administer fluids that have no sodium as "water intoxication" may occur. Rapid movement of sodium-free fluid into the brain cells and kidney cells by the action of osmosis may cause edema and shutdown of these organs (Eggleston, 1985).

Hypernatremia.   Hypernatremia is an uncommon problem in the clinical setting. When hypernatremia occurs, it is usually related to water deficit as a result of prolonged intravenous fluid administration with sufficient sodium but no dextrose. This condition is readily reversible by a water solution supplemented with dextrose (Eggleston, 1985).

POTASSIUM ABNORMALITIES

Potassium is the major cation in the intracellular fluid (ICF), therefore it has a narrow normal range (3 to 5 mEq/L) outside the cells. The potassium concentration in the ECF may be higher than normal (hyperkalemia) or lower than normal (hypokalemia). The clinical signs of potassium abnormality are outlined in Table 12-14.

Hypokalemia.   Hypokalemia is a more common form of potassium (K⁺) abnormality than hyperkalemia. Potassium deficiency may be caused by excessive K⁺ loss (e.g., trauma, severe infection, vomiting, use of diuretics) or inadequate K⁺ intake (e.g., massive or prolonged intravenous fluid infusion without supplemental potassium). Normal breakdown of body tissue produces some potassium as a by-product, but hypokalemia may still occur if excretion exceeds production.

Deficiency of serum potassium may be corrected by oral intake or slow intravenous infusion of potassium chloride. Potassium chloride is used because hypochloremia (low chloride) usually coexists with hypokalemia and the chloride ions must be replaced at the same time.

TABLE 12-14   Clinical Signs of Potassium Abnormality

SYSTEM	HYPOKALEMIA	HYPERKALEMIA
Neuromuscular	Decreased muscle functions	Increased neuromuscular conduction
Cardiac	Flattened T wave and depressed ST segment on ECG	Elevated T wave and depressed ST segment on ECG (mild)
	Arrhythmias	Cardiac arrest (severe)
Gastrointestinal	Decreased bowel activity	Increased bowel activity
	Diminished or absent bowel sounds	Diarrhea

☑ Oral intake of potassium replacement is safer. If intravenous route is used, precautions must be followed to ensure patient safety.

Oral intake of potassium replacement is safer. If intravenous route is used, there are four precautions that must be followed to ensure patient safety (Eggleston, 1985): (1) Consider replacement only if the urine output is at least 40 to 50 mL/hr; (2) Never use KCl undiluted as it can cause arrhythmias and cardiac arrest; (3) Do not give more than 40 mEq of potassium in any one hour or more than 200 mEq in 24 hours; and (4) Concentration of potassium in the intravenous drip should not be higher than 40 mEq/L.

☑ Hyperkalemia may be caused by renal failure.

Hyperkalemia.   Hyperkalemia is an uncommon condition in the clinical setting, but when hyperkalemia occurs it is usually caused by renal failure. Decrease in urine output (less than 200 to 300 ml per day) secondary to renal failure leads to retention of potassium ions. Therefore, the primary treatment for this form of hyperkalemia is to improve kidney function.

If hyperkalemia occurs in the presence of normal kidney function, it may be treated rapidly by using 80 mEq of sodium lactate, 100 ml of calcium gluconate, 100 ml of 50% dextrose in water, or 25 units of insulin (Eggleston, 1985).

NUTRITION

Nutritional intake should be adjusted according to a patient's requirements so inadequate intake may lead to impaired respiratory function due to reduction in the efficiency of respiratory muscles. Excessive intake may increase the patient's work of breathing due to the increased metabolic rate and carbon dioxide production.

UNDERNUTRITION

☑ Inadequate nutritional support can lead to fatigue of respiratory muscles.

Proper nutritional support is a therapeutic necessity for patients on a mechanical ventilator. Poor nutritional status may lead to rapid depletion of cellular stores of glycogen and protein in the diaphragm (Mlynarek et al., 1987). It also leads to fatigue of the major respiratory muscles in patients with or without lung diseases and contributes to impaired pulmonary function, hypercapnia, and inability to wean (Fiaccadori & Borghetti, 1991). Risk of infection becomes more likely when a patient is undernourished because of resultant decreased cell-mediated immunity. Interstitial and pulmonary edema may develop because of severe hypoalbuminemia in which the osmotic pressure is decreased and the fluid is shifted into the interstitial space (interstitial edema), and eventually into the alveoli (pulmonary edema). Other complications of undernutrition include poor wound healing and decreased surfactant production (Table 12-15) (Ideno et al., 1995).

OVERFEEDING

While undernutrition is undesirable for critically ill patients, overfeeding should be avoided. Excessive nutrition may significantly increase the work of breathing because of lipogenesis and increased carbon dioxide production. It may also lead to diminished surfactant production and fatty degeneration of the liver (Table 12-16) (Ideno et al., 1995).

High caloric enteric nutrition can cause a significant increase in oxygen consumption, carbon dioxide production, and respiratory quotient.

☑ High caloric enteric nutrition can cause a significant increase in oxygen consumption and carbon dioxide production. In turn, this can induce respiratory distress during weaning for patients with limited pulmonary reserve.

TABLE 12-15 Effects of Undernutrition

1. Depletion of cellular stores of glycogen and protein
2. Fatigue of respiratory muscles
3. Impaired pulmonary function
4. Decreased cell-mediated immunity
5. Interstitial or pulmonary edema
6. Poor wound healing
7. Decreased surfactant production

TABLE 12-16 Effects of Overfeeding

1. Increased oxygen consumption
2. Increased carbon dioxide production
3. Increased work of breathing
4. Decreased surfactant production
5. Interstitial or pulmonary edema
6. Fatty degeneration of liver

In turn, this can induce respiratory distress during weaning for patients with a limited pulmonary reserve.

Problems with overfeeding may also be found in total parenteral nutrition (TPN) provided via the intravenous route. Respiratory acidosis during mechanical ventilation has been reported within hours after initiation of TPN (van der Berg et al., 1988).

LOW-CARBOHYDRATE, HIGH-FAT DIET

✓ A low carbohydrate high-fat diet may maximize energy intake and minimize oxygen utilization and carbon dioxide production.

Each gram of hydrous dextrose (a form of glucose) produces 3.4 kilocalories. For the same amount of fat emulsion, it generates 9.1 kilocalories. The concentrated source of energy in fat emulsion is preferred for fluid-restricted patients. A fat-based diet also reduces carbon dioxide production and ventilatory requirements (Mlynarek et al., 1987).

For this reason, an increase in fat kilocalories with a concurrent decrease in carbohydrate (dextrose) intake has been done to maximize energy intake and to minimize oxygen utilization and carbon dioxide production. The fat-based diet should contain at least 40% total fat kilocalories and it should be based on the patient's clinical status since a metabolically stressed patient may become immunosuppressed because of insufficient fat in the diet (Ideno et al., 1995).

In one study, a high-calorie diet consisting of 28% carbohydrate, 55% fat, and balanced protein resulted in significantly lower CO_2 production and arterial PCO_2 in COPD patients with hypercapnia. Furthermore, two important lung function measurements (forced vital capacity and forced expiratory volume in 1 second) improved by 22% over baseline values with this low-carbohydrate, high-fat diet (Angelillo et al., 1985).

TOTAL CALORIC REQUIREMENTS

Energy requirements for the critically ill patient are commonly done by using the Harris-Benedict equation (Roza et al., 1984). This equation can be used to estimate a patient's resting energy expenditure (REE) and total energy expenditure (TEE).

✓ Hypophosphatemia (serum phosphate level < 1 mg/dL), in severe form, may cause the patient to experience confusion, muscle weakness, congestive heart failure, and respiratory failure.

REE is the minimum energy requirement for basic metabolic needs. TEE is the energy requirement based on a patient's disease state in which the metabolic rate is higher than normal. TEE is the product of REE and the activity/stress factors (TEE = REE × Activity × Stress Factors). These factors are used to make allowances for hypermetabolic or hypercatabolic conditions such as activity, trauma, infection, and burns. For ventilator-dependent patients, the TEE is calculated by multiplying the REE by factors ranging from 1.2 to 2.1 as shown in Table 12-17 (Askanazi et al., 1982; Roza et al., 1984).

PHOSPHATE SUPPLEMENT

In addition to the total caloric requirement, a patient's nutritional program should maintain a balanced serum phosphate level. Insufficient phosphate in a patient's diet may cause hypophosphatemia,

TABLE 12-17 Calculation of Daily REE and TEE in kcal

REE for men in kcal/day = 66 + 13.7 W + 5 H − 6.8 A
REE for women in kcal/day = 655 + 9.6 W + 1.85 H − 4.7 A
W = weight in kg; H = height in cm; A = age in yr

TEE for men in kcal/day = REE × activity factor × stress factor
TEE for women in kcal/day = REE × activity factor × stress factor
W = weight in kg; H = height in cm; A = age in yr

Activity factor
  Confined to bed   ×1.2
  Out of bed   ×1.3

Stress factor
  Minor operation   ×1.20
  Skeletal trauma   ×1.35
  Major sepsis   ×1.60
  Severe thermal burn ×2.10

a condition where the serum phosphate level is less than 1 mg/dL. Hypophosphatemia decreases tissue ATP (adenosine triphosphate) level, and in severe form it may cause the patient to experience confusion, muscle weakness, congestive heart failure, and respiratory failure (Mlynarek, 1987).

SUMMARY

This chapter outlines the essential strategies that are useful in the management of patients receiving mechanical ventilation. These strategies are straightforward and can be followed by using a logical deduction process. Careful observation of the patient and ventilator must be done in order to identify the problem at hand. Once the problem has been identified, appropriate steps may be taken. It is vital to remember that no changes to ventilator settings should be made unless the reasons for doing so are safe and justifiable.

Self-Assessment Questions

1. Strategies that are useful to improve ventilation include all of the following *except*:

A. increase mechanical deadspace.
B. increase tidal volume.
C. increase respiratory rate.
D. increase minute ventilation.

2. An endotracheal tube is sometimes cut shorter because a shorter ET tube:

A. increases the F_IO_2.

B. increases the mechanical deadspace volume.

C. facilitates airway management and secretions removal.

D. reduces the arterial pH.

3. The primary purpose of permissive hypercapnia is to reduce the patient's _____ during mechanical ventilation.

A. tidal volume

B. pH

C. pulmonary pressures

D. respiratory rate

4. Permissive hypercapnia is a technique in which the mechanical _____ is reduced. This leads to an increase of the patient's _____.

A. peak airway pressure, pH

B. peak airway pressure, PaO_2

C. tidal volume, pH

D. tidal volume, $PaCO_2$

5. CPAP and PEEP may be used to correct refractory hypoxemia caused by:

A. deadspace ventilation.

B. V/Q mismatch.

C. intrapulmonary shunting.

D. diffusion defect.

6. The PaO_2 of an ARDS patient has been deteriorating while on 50% oxygen. The physician asks you to suggest the best solution for this problem. You would recommend trying the following procedures in the order provided:

A. CPAP, mechanical ventilation with PEEP, inverse ratio ventilation.

B. mechanical ventilation, CPAP, inverse ratio ventilation with PEEP.

C. inverse ratio ventilation, mechanical ventilation, PEEP.

D. mechanical ventilation, inverse ratio ventilation, PEEP.

7. Compensated respiratory acidosis and compensated metabolic alkalosis have similar blood gas characteristics: normal pH, high $PaCO_2$, and high HCO_3^-. One useful clue to differentiate these two conditions is that in compensated:

A. respiratory acidosis, the pH is on the acidotic side of normal range.

B. metabolic alkalosis, the pH is on the acidotic side of normal range.

C. respiratory and metabolic acidosis, both pH are on the alkalotic side of normal range.

D. respiratory and metabolic alkalosis, both pH are on the acidotic side of normal range.

8. A patient's low pressure alarm is triggered while you are performing ventilator care. The likely causes of this condition include all of the following *except*:

   A. disconnection of ventilator circuit.   C. power failure.
   B. kinking of endotracheal tube.   D. leakage of endotracheal tube cuff.

9. While you are looking for the cause of low pressure alarm on a ventilator, the high pressure alarm is also triggered. This condition is likely caused by:

   A. disconnection of ventilator circuit.   C. loose ventilator humidifier fitting.
   B. low pressure limit set too high.   D. patient coughing.

10. Analysis of sputum samples by the culture and sensitivity method is _____. It provides information on the type of _____ that the microbes are sensitive to.

   A. quick, sterilizing agents   C. time-consuming, sterilizing agents
   B. quick, antibiotics   D. time-consuming, antibiotics

11. The average urine output of a patient is 15 ml/hr. This output is _____ than normal and it implies that there is too _____ fluid in the extracellular fluid compartment.

   A. higher, much   C. lower, much
   B. higher, little   D. lower, little

12. The following electrolyte values are collected from a patient with severe sepsis who has been on a mechanical ventilator for two weeks. Which of the following electrolytes is out of its normal range?

Electrolyte	Value (mEq/L)
A. Na^+	138
B. K^+	1.5
C. Cl^-	105
D. HCO_3^-	25

13. In replacing fluids to a volume-depleted patient, it is not safe to administer fluids that have no sodium because _____ movement of sodium-free fluid into the brain and kidney cells may cause _____ of these organs.

   A. rapid, swelling   C. slow, swelling
   B. rapid, dehydration   D. slow, dehydration

14. Decreased muscle function, flattened T wave and depressed ST segment on the electro-cardiogram, and diminished bowel sounds are some signs of:

    A. hyperkalemia.   C. hypernatremia.
    B. hypokalemia.   D. hyponatremia.

15. Proper nutrition is essential to patients receiving mechanical ventilation because under-nutrition can cause:

    A. increased surfactant production.   C. increased metabolic rate.
    B. improved pulmonary function.   D. fatigue of respiratory muscles.

16. A diet consisting of low carbohydrate and high fat is more suitable for ventilator patients because _____ generates more calories per gram and produces less _____.

    A. fat, CO_2 C. carbohydrate, CO_2
    B. fat, O_2 D. carbohydrate, O_2

17. The total energy expenditure (TEE) is _____ than the resting energy expenditure (REE) because TEE _____ accounts for patient factors such as activity, trauma, and infection.

    A. higher, does   C. lower, does
    B. higher, does not   D. lower, does not

References

Angelillo, V. A. et al. (1985). Effects of low and high carbohydrate feedings in ambulatory patients with chronic obstructive pulmonary disease and chronic hypercapnia. *Ann Intern Med, 103*(6, Pt. 1), 883–885.

Askanazi, J. et al. (1982). Nutrition and the respiratory system. *Crit Care Med, 10,* 163–172.

Barnes, T. A. et al. (1993). *Core textbook of respiratory care practice.* St. Louis: Mosby-Year Book.

Boots, R. J., Howe, S., & George, N. et al. (1997). Clinical utility of hygroscopic heat and moisture exchangers in intensive care patients. *Crit Care Med, 25*(10), 1707–1712.

Burton, G. G. et al. (1997). *Respiratory care: A guide to clinical practice* (4th ed.). Philadelphia: J.B. Lippincott.

Cox, R. G. et al. (1991). Efficacy, results, and complications of mechanical ventilation in children with status asthmaticus. *Pediatr Pulmonol, 11*(2), 120–126.

Craven, D. E. et al. (1989). Nosocomial pneumonia in the intubated patient. New concepts on pathogenesis and prevention. *Infect Dis Clin North Am, 3*(4), 843–866.

Darioli, R. et al. (1984). Mechanical controlled hypertension in status asthmaticus. *Am Rev Respir Dis, 129,* 385–387.

Eggleston, F. C. (1985). Simplified management of fluid and electrolyte problems. Normal balance, abnormalities and practical management. *Tropical Doctor, 15*(2), 55–64.

Feihl, F. et al. (1994). Permissive hypercapnia: How permissive should we be? *Am J Respir Crit Care Med, 150*(6, Pt. 1), 1722–1737.

Fiaccadori, E., & Borghetti, A. (1991). Pathophysiology of respiratory muscles in course of undernutrition. *Ann Ital Med Int (AUZ), 6*(4), 402–407.

Gurevitch, M. J. et al. (1986). Improved oxygenation and lower peak airway pressure in severe adult respiratory distress syndrome: Treatment with inverse ratio ventilation. *Chest, 89,* 211.

Fink, J. B., Krause, S. A., & Barrett, L. (1998). Extending ventilator circuit change interval beyond 2 days reduces the likelihood of ventilator-associated pneumonia. *Chest, 113*(2), 405–411.

Hagler, D. A. et al. (1994). Endotracheal saline and suction catheters: Sources of lower airway contamination. *Am J Crit Care, 3*(6), 444–447.

Hickling, K. G. et al. (1990). Low mortality associated with permissive hypercapnia in severe adult respiratory distress syndrome. *Intensive Care Med, 16,* 372–377.

Hu, B. (1991). Lower respiratory tract flora in intubated patients. *Chung Hua I Hsueh Tsa Chih (Chinese), 71*(5), 243–245.

Ideno, K. T. et al. (1995, April/May). Managing respiratory patients' nutritional outcomes. *Journal for Respiratory Care Practitioners*, 111–118.

Joshi, N. et al. (1993). A predictive risk index for nosocomial pneumonia in the intensive care unit. *Am J Med, 93*(2), 135–142.

Kirton, O. C., DeHaven, B., & Morgan, J. et al. (1997). A prospective, randomized comparison of an in-line heat moisture exchange filter and heated wire humidifiers: Rates of ventilator-associated early-onset (community-acquired) or late-onset (hospital-acquired) pneumonia and incidence of endotracheal tube occlusion. *Chest, 112*(4), 1055–1059.

Kollef, M. H. et al. (1994). Ventilator-associated pneumonia: Clinical considerations. *Am J Roentgen, 163,* 1031–1035.

Kotilainen, H. R., & Keroack, M. A. (1997). Cost analysis and clinical impact of weekly ventilator circuit changes in patients in intensive care unit. *Am J Infect Control, 25*(2), 117–120.

Kraus, P. A. et al. (1993). Acute lung injury at Baragwanath ICU—An eight-month audit and call for consensus for other organ failure in the adult respiratory distress syndrome. *Chest, 103*(6), 1832–1836.

Krider, T. M. et al. (1986). *Master guide for passing the Respiratory Care Credentialing Exam.* Claremont, CA: Education Resource Consortium.

Lewandowski, K. et al. (1992). Approaches to improve survival in severe ARDS. In J. L. Vincent (Ed.), *Update in intensive care and emergency medicine* (pp. 372–377). Berlin: Springer-Verlag.

Long, M. N., Wickstrom, G., & Grimes, A. et al. (1996). Prospective, randomized study of ventilator-associated pneumonia in patients with one versus three ventilator circuit changes per week. *Infect Control Hosp Epidemiol, 17*(1):14–19.

Lowy, F. D. et al. (1987). The incidence of nosocomial pneumonia following urgent endotracheal intubation. *Infect Control, 8*(6), 245–248.

MacIntyre, N. R. (1986). Pressure support ventilation. *Respir Care, 31,* 189–190.

Marini, J. J. (1988). Monitoring during mechanical ventilation. *Clin Chest Med, 9,* 73–100.

Marini, J. J. (1993). New options for the ventilatory management of acute lung injury. *New Horiz, 1*(4), 489–503.

Mlynarek, M. et al. (1987). Individualizing nutrition in patients with acute respiratory failure requiring mechanical ventilation. *Drug intelligence and clinical pharmacy, 21,* 865–869.

Nathan, S. D. et al. (1993). Prediction of minimal pressure support during weaning from mechanical ventilation. *Chest, 103,* 1215–1219.

Otto, C. W. (1986). Ventilatory management in the critically ill. *Emerg Med Clin North Am, 4*(4), 635–654.

Roza, A. M. et al. (1984). The Harris-Benedict equation reevaluated: Resting energy requirements and the body cell mass. *Am J Clin Nutr, 40,* 168–182.

Scanlan, C. L. et al. (1999). *Egan's fundamentals of respiratory care* (7th ed.) St. Louis, MO: Mosby-Year Book.

Schuster, D. P. (1990). A physiologic approach to initiating, maintaining, and withdrawing mechanical ventilatory support during acute respiratory failure. *Am J Med, 88,* 268–278.

Shapiro, B. A. (1994). A historical perspective on ventilator management. *New Horiz, 2*(1), 8–18.

Shapiro, B. A. et al. (1994). *Clinical application of blood gases* (5th ed.). St. Louis: Mosby-Year Book.

Slutsky, A. S. (1994). Consensus conference on mechanical ventilation—January 28–30, 1993 at Northbrook, IL, USA, Part I. *Int Care Med, 20,* 64–79.

Stamm, A. M. (1998). Ventilator-associated pneumonia and frequency of circuit changes. *Am J Infect Control, 26*(1):71–73.

van der Berg, B. et al. (1988). Metabolic and respiratory effects of enteral nutrition in patients during mechanical ventilation. *Int Care Med, 14,* 206–211.

Weber, D. J. et al. (1990). Manual ventilation bags as a source for bacterial colonization of intubated patients. *Am Rev Respir Dis, 142*(4), 892–894.

White, G. C. (1999). *Equipment theory for respiratory care* (3rd ed.). Albany, NY: Delmar Publishers.

Winter, P. M. et al. (1972). The toxicity of oxygen. *Anesthesiology, 37,* 210.

Zapol, W. M. et al. (1979). Extracorporeal membrane oxygenation in severe acute respiratory failure. *JAMA, 242,* 2193–2196.

Zwischenberger, J. B. et al. (1986). The role of extracorporeal membrane oxygenation in the management of respiratory failure in the newborn. *Resp Care, 31*(6).

CHAPTER THIRTEEN

PHARMACOTHERAPY FOR MECHANICAL VENTILATION

Sandra Gaviola
Luis S. Gonzalez

OUTLINE

KEY TERMS

- acetylcholine
- antiemetic
- anxiolysis
- barbiturates
- benzodiazepines
- cathartic agents
- chronotropic
- corticosteroids
- depolarizing agents

- GABA (gamma-aminobutyric acid)
- inotropic
- narcotic analgesics
- nondepolarizing agents
- parasympatholytic bronchodilators
- Ramsay Scale
- sympathomimetic bronchodilators
- xanthine bronchodilators

INTRODUCTION

Two primary purposes of drug therapy for patients using mechanical ventilation are that they: (1) provide patient comfort, and (2) facilitate airway management and mechanical ventilation. For example, some drugs are used to facilitate intubation (neuromuscular blockers and sedatives) and reduce air flow resistance (bronchodilators), while others are necessary to manage pain (narcotics) and induce sedation (sedatives). Proper use of drug therapy is necessary to achieve desired outcomes. A clear understanding of these drugs is also essential to avoid misuse, complications, and prolonged mechanical ventilation.

DRUGS FOR IMPROVING VENTILATION

Airway narrowing is a common complication in patients receiving mechanical ventilation. Increasing peak airway pressure, wheezing, hypoxemia, and agitation are some clinical signs that indicate the presence of airway distress.

For the ventilator patient, airway distress may be caused by: (1) preexisting airway disease (chronic bronchitis, asthma), (2) drug-induced bronchospasm, (3) accumulated secretions, and (4) mechanical irritation. Whatever the cause, the distress must be recognized and corrected quickly to prevent hypoxemia and further deterioration.

Along with regular endotracheal suctioning, bronchodilators and corticosteroids play a critical role in achieving optimal airway patency and constitute the majority of nebulized drugs used in respiratory care.

THE AUTONOMIC NERVOUS SYSTEM

The smooth muscles of the airway are under autonomic (involuntary) nervous control. For this reason, the patient has no control over the patency of the affected airways. When airways constrict, bronchodilators are necessary to provide airway dilation and relief.

Sympathetic and Parasympathetic Branches. The autonomic nervous system (ANS) is comprised of motor neurons that innervate tissues under involuntary control. Among important functions regulated by the ANS are respiration, heart rate, blood pressure, perspiration and glandular secretions. The sympathetic and parasympathetic fibers are the basic subdivisions of the ANS and, for the most part, elicit responses in an opposing manner (at the effector sites). For example, stimulation of the sympathetic branch results in bronchodilation whereas stimulation of the parasympathetic branch causes bronchoconstriction (Tortora et al., 1987).

Adrenergic and Cholinergic Responses. The neurotransmitter substance released at the sympathetic terminal axon is epinephrine (adrenaline) and it elicits an adrenergic response.

The neurotransmitter substance released at the terminal axon of the parasympathetic fiber is acetylcholine (ACh) and it elicits a cholinergic response.

Bronchodilation can be achieved by eliciting an adrenergic response (sympathomimetic action) or by interfering with the cholinergic response (parasympatholytic action). Many bronchodilators use the sympathomimetic action (**sympathomimetic bronchodilators**) while other bronchodilators take advantage of the parasympatholytic action (**parasympatholytic bronchodilators**). Table 13-1 shows these two pathways to achieve bronchodilation.

sympathomimetic bronchodilators:
Adrenergic agonists. Drugs that dilate the airways by stimulating the Beta 2 receptors of the sympathetic nervous system. Examples are epinephrine (Adrenaline) and albuterol (Ventolin, Proventil).

parasympatholytic bronchodilators:
Anticholinergic bronchodilators. Drugs that dilate the airways by inhibiting the parasympathetic branch of the autonomic nervous system. Examples are atropine, and ipratropium bromide (Atrovent).

TABLE 13-1 Two Autonomic Nervous System (ANS) Pathways for Bronchodilation

SYMPATHETIC PATHWAY	PARASYMPATHETIC PATHWAY
Stimulation of adrenergic response	Interference of cholinergic response
↓	↓
↑ Sympathomimetic activity (Stimulation of sympathetic activity)	↑ Parasympatholytic activity (Inhibition of parasympathetic activity)
↓	↓
Bronchodilation	Relative increase of sympathetic activity
	↓
	Bronchodilation

ADRENERGIC BRONCHODILATORS (SYMPATHOMIMETICS)

Adrenergic bronchodilators are agents that stimulate the adrenergic receptors via the sympathetic nerve fibers of the autonomic nervous system.

Mechanism of Action. Sympathetic adrenergic receptors are distributed throughout the body. They are identified and classified according to their response to specific neurotransmitter substances. Alpha 1, alpha 2, beta 1, and beta 2 are the types that have been identified. Some important effects associated with these receptors are shown in Table 13-2.

In the lungs, β-2 receptors are found in the smaller airways, alveolar walls, and submucosal glands. The primary goal of beta-2 adrenergic drugs is to combine with these receptors to initiate bronchodilation.

Adrenergic bronchodilators are classified as catecholamines or catecholamine derivatives.

Catecholamines. Catecholamines such as norepinephrine, epinephrine, isoproterenol, and isoetharine share the following characteristics: (1) rapid onset, (2) rapid degradation by catechol-O-methyltransferase (COMT) in the liver, kidney, and throughout the body and the intraneuronal enzyme monoamine oxidase (MAO), (3) ineffective when taken enterally, and (4) nonspecific receptor binding.

inotropic: affecting the contraction.

Catecholamine derivatives. Catecholamine derivatives such as metaproterenol, terbutaline, albuterol, and pirbuterol have a more complex chemical structure than catecholamines. The modification in the chemical structure results in more specific beta-2 receptor binding and delayed degradation by COMT and MAO. As a result, catecholamine derivatives (noncatecholamines) offer less cardiac adverse effects and prolonged bronchodilation than the catecholamines. Additionally, resistance to COMT degradation makes these agents suitable

chronotropic: affecting the rate.

TABLE 13-2 **Major Effects of Alpha and Beta Receptors**

RECEPTOR	MAJOR EFFECTS
Alpha-1 (α-1)	Vasoconstriction Constriction of pupils
Alpha-2 (α-2)	Decreased gastrointestinal activity
Beta-1 (β-1)	Positive **inotropic** effect ($\uparrow$ muscular contractility) Positive **chronotropic** effect ($\uparrow$ heart rate)
Beta-2 (β-2)	Bronchodilation Peripheral vasodilation Decreased gastrointestinal activity

for enteral administration—although, beta-2 specificity may be lost via this route (Rau, 1998).

Table 13-3 shows the relative receptor actions, dosage, and frequency of use of some common sympathomimetics.

Adverse Effects.   The adverse effects of adrenergic bronchodilators include tachycardia, palpitations, skeletal muscle tremors and nervousness. The degree of adverse effects depends on the mode of administration, dosage, frequency of administration, presence of preexisting cardiac disease, and the specific adrenergic agent used. In most cases the benefits of bronchodilation will outweigh the potential adverse effects.

TABLE 13-3   Adrenergic Bronchodilators

CATECHOLAMINES	ACTION RECEPTOR	INHALATION	DOSAGE	FREQUENCY
Epinephrine (adrenaline)	a > β-1 > β-2	Neb (1%)	0.25 to 0.5 ml	QID
Racemic Epinephrine (MicroNefrin, Vaponefrin, Asmanefrin)	a > β-1 > β-2	Neb (2.25%)	0.25 to 0.5 ml	QID
Isoetharine (Bronkosol, Bronkometer)	β-1 = β-2	Neb (1%) MDI	0.25 to 0.5 ml 1 to 2 puffs	QID QID
Isoproterenol (Isuprel)	β-1 < β-2	Neb (0.5%)	0.25 to 0.5 ml	QID
CATECHOLAMINE DERIVATIVES				
Bitolterol (prodrug) (Tornalate)	β-1 < β-2	MDI	2 puffs	Q 4 to 6°
Metaproterenol (Alupent, Metaprel)	β-1 < β-2	Neb MDI	(5%) 0.3 ml 2 to 3 puffs	TID/QID Q 4°
Albuterol (Proventil, Ventolin)	β-1 < β-2	Neb (0.5%) MDI	0.5 ml 2 puffs	TID/QID TID/QID
Terbutaline (Brethaire, Brethine, Bricanyl)	β-1 < β-2 DPI	MDI 1 puff	2 puffs QID	QID
Pirbuterol (Maxair)	β-1 < β-2	MDI	1 to 2 puffs	Q 4 to 6°
Salmeterol Xinafoate (Serevent)	β-1 < β-2	MDI	2 puffs	BID

Special Considerations. The primary purpose of beta agonists is bronchodilation. For patients with inflammatory airway disease (i.e., asthma and chronic bronchitis) intermittent use of beta agonists may not be sufficient. Deaths have been reported in asthmatics following regular and prolonged use of these agents. Uncontrolled inflammation and mucosal edema are likely the cause of this adverse outcome (Witek, 1994).

Desensitization of receptor sites has been documented with regular use of beta agonists. Two mechanisms appear to be responsible: (1) the loss of receptor from the surface of cells, and (2) the failure of the cell to function (Cottrell et al., 1995). The practitioner may wish to combine beta agonists with other categories of drugs to achieve bronchodilation. For example, a combination of corticosteroid and beta agonist may potentiate their individual effects and produce bronchodilation.

However, paradoxical bronchospasm may occur with combined use of adrenergic agonist and corticosteroid. Its occurrence is rare, but the onset can be sudden. For this reason, practitioners should be aware of the hazard.

ANTICHOLINERGIC BRONCHODILATORS (PARASYMPATHOLYTICS)

Anticholinergic bronchodilators are agents that impede the impulses of the cholinergic, especially the parasympathetic nerve fibers of the autonomic nervous system.

acetylcholine: An ester that plays a role in the transmission of nerve impulses at synapses and neuromuscular junctions. It is metabolized by an enzyme, cholinesterase. Too much or too little of acetylcholine at the motor endplates may lead to muscle blockade.

Mechanism of Action. Parasympathetic receptors (muscarinic and nicotinic) are found throughout the body. They are classified according to whether they respond to muscarine or nicotine. In the lungs, muscarinic receptors are found in submucosal glands, mast cells and smooth muscles of the larger airways.

The combination of **acetylcholine** with muscarinic receptors results in increased bronchial tone and increased secretion from mucosal glands. Anticholinergic agents (atropine and atropine derivatives) block these physiologic responses and they may be useful for the reversal of vagally mediated bronchospasm. Table 13-4 shows the usage of three common anticholinergic bronchodilators.

TABLE 13-4 Anticholinergic Bronchodilators

DRUG	INHALATION DOSAGE		FREQUENCY
Atropine	Neb	0.3 to 0.5 ml	Up to 4 times/day
Ipratropium bromide (Atrovent)	MDI Neb (0.025%)	1 to 2 puffs 1 to 2 ml	QID Q 4 to 6°
Glycopyrrolate (Robinul)	Neb (0.02%)	5.0 ml	Q 4 to 6°

✓ Atropine is an anticholinergic agent used as a secondary bronchodilator. It is also used for symptomatic bradycardia and prophylactic drying of secretions before surgery.

Adverse Effects.   When inhaled, atropine is readily distributed throughout the body and may cause systemic effects such as tachycardia, nervousness, headache, and dried secretions. Atropine easily penetrates the blood brain barrier and at higher levels may cause hallucination or mental confusion. Patients with atropine-induced hallucinations have been erroneously diagnosed with psychiatric disorders.

Other anticholinergic agents such as ipratropium bromide (Atrovent) and glycopyrrolate (Robinul, an atropine derivative) are not well absorbed systemically and when inhaled, produce fewer adverse effects than those produced by atropine. Drying of secretions is an adverse effect of Atrovent, but it can be prevented by proper humidification or systemic hydration.

Clinical Considerations.   Ipratropium bromide is not indicated for the initial treatment of acute episodes of bronchospasm where immediate response is required. These agents are commonly used in addition to the rapid-acting beta agonists.

XANTHINE BRONCHODILATORS

xanthine bronchodilators: Drugs that produce bronchodilation by inhibiting phosphodiesterase, an enzyme that inactivates cyclic 3, 5-AMP (a substance that promotes bronchodilation). Examples are oral theophylline (Theo-Dur, Slo-bid), and aminophylline, a water-soluble theophylline (Aminophyllin, Somophyllin).

The third class of bronchodilators, the **xanthines,** include the drugs theophylline and its salt form aminophylline. Theophylline is a stimulant found in tea leaves and is chemically related to other stimulants found in coffee and colas. To the consumers of caffeine, the effects of tachycardia, central nervous stimulation (wakefulness) and diuresis may be well known.

Xanthines are used for their relaxing effects on smooth muscles and ability to inhibit inflammation. Clinically, the xanthines are considered to be less effective in acute broncospasm than the beta agonists and are more useful in the management of inflammation associated with asthma and COPD. For individuals with carbon dioxide retention, xanthines improve ventilation by heightening carbon dioxide sensitivity in the central nervous system and enhancing diaphragmatic contractility. Water-soluble aminophylline is suitable for intravenous administration and is indicated for acute bronchospasm or periods of apnea associated with narcotic overdose, head trauma, and congestive heart failure (Cottrell et al., 1995). Table 13-5 lists the oral and intravenous xanthine bronchodilators.

Mechanism of Action.   Multiple theories on the mechanism of theophylline have been described. Although one generally accepted mechanism is that theophylline produces bronchodilation by inhibiting phosphodiesterase (PDE). Recall that PDE rapidly inactivates cyclic 3'5' AMP, the substance that relaxes the airway smooth muscles and inhibits mast cell histamine release. By inhibiting PDE, xanthine indirectly increases cyclic 3'5' AMP levels. A second theory describes theophylline as an adenosine antagonist. Normally, the stimulation

TABLE 13-5 **Xanthine Bronchodilators**

GENERIC NAME	TRADE NAMES	ADMINISTRATION
Theophylline (100% anhydrous)	(Aerolate, Constant-T, Respbid, Slo-bid, Theo-Dur, Uniphyl)	Oral
Aminophylline (78-86% theophylline, water soluble)	(Aminophyllin, Somophyllin)	Intravenous

☑ Inhibition of phosphodi-esterase, acting as an adenosine antagonist, and increased catecholamine release are three proposed mechanisms of action of theophylline.

of adenosine receptors results in histamine release, thus a blocking effect provides anti-inflammatory benefits. And finally, theophylline has been shown to increase catecholamine release in some studies. The enhanced sympathomimeticlike adverse effects experienced with a nonautonomic drug such as theophylline seems to support this finding (Rau, 1998).

Adverse Effects. Unlike the adrenergic and anticholinergic bronchodilators, xanthines are not useful via inhalation due to their lack of ability to penetrate the mucosal lining of the airways. Xanthines are available for systemic administration via the intravenous and oral routes and, thus, produce widespread effects.

Some of the adverse effects (tachycardia and skeletal muscle and CNS stimulation) can occur even at therapeutic serum theophylline ranges of 10 to 20 µg/mL. Routine monitoring of serum theophylline levels is one way to prevent these effects from intensifying to the degree of toxicity. However, the practitioner should be able to recognize the early warning signs of theophylline toxicity since a narrow margin between therapeutic and toxic levels exists. Patients with mild to moderate toxicity (20 to 30 µg/mL) may experience tachypnea, palpitations, nausea, vomiting, headache, and agitation. Severe toxicity (>40 µg/mL) is marked by gastric bleeding, arrhythmias and seizures (Scanlan et al., 1999; Witek, 1994).

☑ Nausea, vomiting, abdominal pain, diarrhea, and nervousness are some initial signs of theophylline toxicity.

Clinical Considerations. Nausea, vomiting, abdominal pain, diarrhea, and nervousness are some initial signs of theophylline toxicity. These signs may not be apparent in or communicated by the sedated or paralyzed patient. If xanthines are used in a paralyzed patient, the serum theophylline level should be monitored closely to prevent inadvertent overdose. Toxic adverse effects can be minimized when the serum theophylline level is within its therapeutic range (10 to 20 µg/mL) (Witek, 1994).

☑ Theophylline toxicity may be avoided by keeping its serum level within therapeutic range (10 to 20 µg/mL).

Most of the theophylline is metabolized by the liver and excreted in the urine. Patients at risk for theophylline toxicity are those with heart failure or liver disease. Diminished liver perfusion (due to heart failure) or impaired liver function can reduce the metabolism and clearance rate of theophylline. The end result is excessive theophylline accumulation and toxicity.

On the other hand, patients at risk for inadequate theophylline are those who smoke. Smoking increases the level of hepatic enzyme and theophylline clearance. The end result for these individuals is higher maintenance theophylline dosages to maintain bronchodilation (Cottrell et al., 1995).

ANTI-INFLAMMATORY AGENTS (CORTICOSTEROIDS)

Corticosteroids are powerful, naturally occurring hormones that are released from the adrenal cortex. Their anti-inflammatory effects make them first-line drugs in the management of chronic asthma and other long-term airway inflammatory conditions. In the intensive care setting, they have been used with favorable results in status asthmaticus, acute exacerbation of COPD, inhalation airway injury, drug-induced pneumonitis, septic shock, ARDS, and spinal cord injury.

Corticosteroids have no bronchodilator effect and should not be given alone during an acute asthma attack. The effects of corticosteroids require an onset time of about 2 to 24 hours, further demonstrating their inappropriateness in acute situations.

Mechanism of Action.   The general functions of corticosteroids include: (1) carbohydrate metabolism, (2) immunosuppression, and (3) reduced inflammation. Their specific mechanism in reducing inflammation is complex, involving genetic changes to target cells of inflammation. The combination of the steroid with its receptor site (nucleus of target cell) results in altered cellular function.

Normally, an inflammatory response results in the release of histamine and bradykinin (among other mediators) from the mast cell causing bronchoconstriction and increased capillary permeability. This leads to early-phase bronchoconstriction and late-phase submucosal edema and hyperactivity (Rau, 1998). With altered cellular function, these and other mediators are blocked and inflammation is reduced.

Adverse Effects.   Corticosteroids are available for oral, intravenous, and inhalation administration (Tables 13-6 and 13-7), and as with most agents, the inhalation route is favored for its convenience, smaller dosage, and fewer adverse effects.

The most frequent adverse effects reported with metered-dose inhaler (MDI) use are hoarseness and oral fungal infections (e.g., candidiasis). To prevent fungal superinfections, patients should be instructed to rinse and gargle the mouth after each treatment. MDI corticosteroids are rarely used in the ventilator patient.

There are many serious adverse effects associated with systemic corticosteroid therapy. Abrupt withdrawal following long-term systemic therapy may cause serious complications from adrenal insufficiency.

corticosteroids:
Hormones that are released from the cortex of the adrenal gland. Their potent anti-inflammatory effects make corticosteroids useful in the treatment of asthma and chronic bronchitis. Corticosteroids are available for intravenous administration as well as inhalation. Examples of inhaled steroids are dexamethasone (Decadron, Respihaler), beclomethasone (Beclovent, Vanceril), flunisolide (AeroBid), and triamcinolone (Azmacort).

☑ Corticosteroids may be used when other traditional bronchodilators have failed to relieve bronchospasm.

☑ Corticosteroids return constricted airways to normal by blocking the inflammatory mediators.

TABLE 13-6 Corticosteroids for Metered-Dose Inhaler (MDI) Use

DRUG	MDI DOSAGE	FREQUENCY
Dexamethasone (Decadron, Respihaler)	2 to 3 puffs	3 to 4 times/day
Beclomethasone (Beclovent, Vanceril)	2 puffs	3 to 4 times/day
Flunisolide (AeroBid)	2 puffs	2 times/day
Triamcinolone (Azmacort)	2 puffs	3 to 4 times/day

TABLE 13-7 Corticosteroids for Systemic Use

DRUG	ROUTE OF ADMINISTRATION
Hydrocortisone Cortisone Prednisolone Dexamethasone	Oral Parenteral (intravenous, intramuscular, subcutaneous, or mucosal)
Prednisone	Oral

Recovery time varies depending on the dosage and duration of therapy. Another serious effect is an increased susceptibility to opportunistic infections.

Clinical Considerations.   Corticosteroids are not bronchodilators. Their use in the treatment of bronchospasm is limited to situations where patients have lost beta agonist responsiveness or when other bronchodilators have failed. Their primary role is in the management of long-term airway inflammation. Systemic corticosteroids should be used cautiously with patients receiving steroidal based neuromuscular blocking agents (vecuronium bromide and pancuronium bromide) because of the potential of prolonged blockade (Kupfer et al., 1987).

DELIVERY OF MDI MEDICATIONS

Many bronchodilators and steroids come in a metered-dose inhaler (MDI). With proper adapter or fittings, MDI medications may be administered via the ventilator circuit without interruption to mechanical ventilation or airway pressure. MDI may be given with a right-angle adapter or with a spacer. Studies have shown that an MDI with spacer is a more efficient method for delivering inhaled medications to the

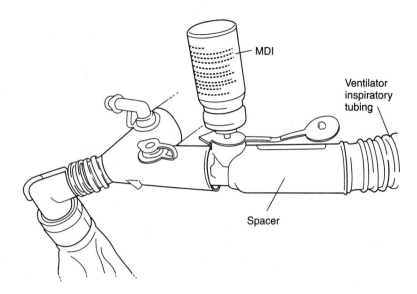

Figure 13-1 An MDI with spacer on a ventilator circuit.

lungs than the right-angle MDI port (Marik, Hogan & Krikorian, 1999; Mouloudi, Katsanoulas & Anastasaki et al., 1998). In addition, the efficacy of MDI medications does not improve with end-inspiratory pause during delivery (Mouloudi, Katsanoulas & Anastasaki et al., 1998). Figure 13-1 shows a typical setup of an MDI on the ventilator circuit.

NEUROMUSCULAR BLOCKING AGENTS

Neuromuscular blocking agents are administered when temporary paralysis of skeletal muscles is desired. Pharmacological paralysis is most commonly induced to (1) ease endotracheal intubation, (2) relieve laryngeal spasm, (3) provide muscle relaxation during surgery, or (4) maintain mechanical ventilation.

Paralyzing agents are used on ventilator patients in difficult situations due to underlying pathology, unnatural modes of ventilation, or psychological unacceptance. If any of these conditions prevent adequate ventilation, oxygenation or patient comfort, a paralyzing agent should be considered. The benefits of paralysis during controlled ventilation are given in Table 13-8.

Since serious adverse effects can occur with the use of these agents, they should not be given routinely or before alternative management is considered. If paralysis is indicated, a sedative drug, such as the

TABLE 13-8   Benefits of Paralysis during Controlled Ventilation

1. Reduced combativeness and agitation
2. Relaxation of respiratory muscles
3. Increased chest wall compliance
4. Synchronization during unnatural modes of ventilation (e.g., inverse I:E)
5. Prevention of hypoxemia associated with increased work of breathing
6. Decreased intracranial pressures caused by excessive movement

benzodiazepines along with a narcotic analgesic should be provided for patient comfort. This is necessary because perception and pain threshold of a patient still exist with use of neuromuscular blocking drugs.

The following testimonies affirm the need for adequate sedation and analgesia during paralysis. One patient who was pharmacologically paralyzed and not sedated described his experience as "a feeling of being buried alive." Another patient thought that she had died (Halloran, 1991). A trauma survivor recalls the sensation of endotracheal tube suctioning being like that of a red-hot burning iron passed into the trachea (Hansen-Flaschen et al., 1993).

MECHANISM OF ACTION

During normal neuromuscular transmission, the nerve axon reaches the muscle fibers and it branches out to form many fine nerve terminals. These nerve terminals are rich in mitochondria, cytoplasmic enzymes, and vesicles. Acetylcholine (ACh), the major chemical in the transmission of nerve impulses, is stored in these vesicles.

When the nerve terminal is stimulated by nerve impulses, acetylcholine is released into the synaptic cleft. From there, some of the acetylcholine is broken down by acetylcholinesterase (AChe) and other ACh diffuses to the muscle end plate producing depolarization and muscle contraction. Figure 13-2 is the functional illustration of neuromuscular transmission.

The sequence of events at the neuromuscular junction is as follows. A repeating sequence of depolarization and repolarization is required for continued and coordinated muscular movement. Interruption at any point of the sequence causes muscle relaxation or paralysis, depending on the effective dosage.

Neuromuscular blocking drugs are typically divided into two groups depending on the modes of action at the neuromuscular junction.

depolarizing agents:
Drugs that prolong the depolarization phase of muscle contraction, thus rendering the repolarization/depolarization sequence (normal mechanism for muscle movement) impossible and causing muscle blockade. An example is succinylcholine (Anectine, Quelicin).

Depolarizing Agents.   The first group of neuromuscular blockers is classified as **depolarizing agents**. This type of agent (e.g., succinylcholine) binds with the receptor site, producing quick onset and

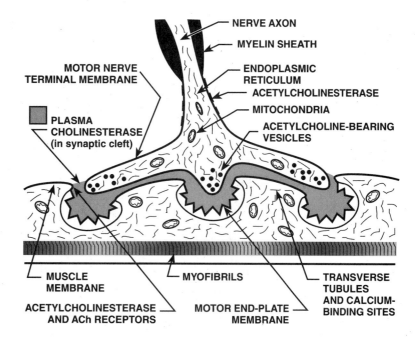

Figure 13-2 Functional illustration of neuromuscular transmission.

sustaining depolarization. Uncoordinated muscle contraction called fasciculation marks the onset. Subsequent neuromuscular transmission is inhibited during the time that adequate concentration of succinylcholine is bound to the receptor site (Ebadi, 1993).

There is no antidote for depolarizing agents. Succinylcholine is however, rapidly hydrolyzed by plasma pseudocholinesterase (PCHE). A small percentage of the population has an abnormal plasma cholinesterase that does not hydrolyze succinylcholine within minutes, as expected. Plasma PCHE level may also be decreased in patients with insecticide poisoning, liver disorders (hepatitis, cirrhosis, obstructive jaundice), malnutrition, acute infections, and anemias (Kee, 1995). These individuals may require ventilatory support for hours because of insufficient plasma PCHE.

Nondepolarizing Agents.   The second group of neuromuscular blockers is classified as **nondepolarizing agents**. These agents (e.g., tubocurarine) compete with acetylcholine for the receptor sites at the motor endplates, thus blocking the normal action of acetylcholine. Since the nondepolarizing agents compete for the receptor sites, they are also called competitive agents. They are antagonized by anticholinesterase agents such as endrophonium, pyridostigmine, and neostigmine. Anticholinesterase agents allow ACh levels to rise.

nondepolarizing agents: *Drugs that compete with acetylcholine for the receptor sites at the motor endplates, thus blocking the normal action of acetylcholine and causing muscle blockade. Examples are tubocurarine chloride (Tubarine), and pancuronium bromide (Pavulon).*

CHARACTERISTICS OF NEUROMUSCULAR BLOCKING AGENTS

Pharmacologically induced blockade progresses in the following sequence: rapidly contracting muscles (eyes and digits) followed by larger and slower contracting muscles (extremities, trunk and diaphragm) (Halloran, 1991). Depolarizing agents (e.g., succinylcholine) have a quick onset but are short-lasting, making them the drugs of choice for emergency intubation. Nondepolarizing agents have longer onsets ranging from 3 to 10 minutes, but are longer lasting. These drugs are more appropriate for controlled ventilation in the intensive care unit. Table 13-9 shows the characteristics of selected depolarizing and nondepolarizing neuromuscular blocking agents.

FACTORS AFFECTING NEUROMUSCULAR BLOCKADE

Several factors can alter neuromuscular transmission and blockade. They include organ failure, drug interaction, electrolyte imbalance, and acid-base status.

☑ Organ failure may decrease drug clearance, increase drug accumulation and prolonged neuromuscular blockade.

Organ Failure. Patients with altered renal or hepatic function have an increased risk of prolonged blockade. These patients can remain profoundly weak long after the drug is discontinued. Both pancuronium bromide and vecuronium bromide have been implicated in drug accumulation in patients with renal insufficiency. Vecuronium is also poorly eliminated in patients with hepatic failure. Atracurium is preferred in the presence of organ failure because it is self destroying and does not rely on organ metabolism and excretion (Halloran, 1991).

☑ Beta blockers, procainamide, quinidine, calcium channel blockers and nitroglycerine may potentiate the effects of nondepolarizing agents.

Drug Interaction. Some cardiovascular and antiarrhythmic agents may interact and potentiate the effects of nondepolarizing agents. They include beta blockers, procainamide, quinidine, calcium channel blockers and nitroglycerine. High concentrations of antibiotics may also potentiate the effects of competitive agents by decreasing the release of ACh. These antibiotics include the aminoglycosides and polymyxins as well as tetracycline, erythromycin, and vancomycin (Halloran, 1991).

Steroidal based vecuronium bromide and pancuronium bromide may be particularly dangerous if administered along with systemic corticosteroids (Watling et al., 1994). A significant number of asthmatics receiving these neuromuscular blocking agents in combination with steroid therapy have experienced prolonged blockade for several days following discontinuation of the paralyzing agent (Kupfer et al., 1987). This prolonged blockade is possibly related to the comparable chemical structure of steroid and steroidal based agents. Figure 13-3 shows the basic steroid structure and pipecuronium, a steroidal based paralyzing agent. Until studies become conclusive, use of corticosteroids should

TABLE 13-9 Depolarizing and Nondepolarizing Agents

AGENTS	INITIAL DOSE (mg/kg)	ONSET (min)	DURATION	DRUG CLEARANCE
Depolarizing				
Succinylcholine (Anectine, Quelicin, Sux-Cert, Sucostrin)	0.3 to 1.1	1	Short	Metabolized by plasma cholinesterase
Nondepolarizing				
Tubocurarine chloride (Tubarine)	0.5	5	Long	Excreted unchanged in urine
Pancuronium bromide (Pavulon)	0.07	5 to 7	Long	Metabolized by liver, excreted in urine
Metocurine iodide (Metubine)	0.2 to 0.4	4	Long	Excreted unchanged in urine
Atracurium (Tracrium)	0.4 to 0.5	4 to 5	Intermediate	Self-destroying
Vecuronium bromide (Norcuron)	0.05	4 to 6	Intermediate	Metabolized by liver, excreted in urine
Pipecuronium bromide (Arduan)	0.05 to 0.06	4 to 6	Long	Renal
Doxacurium chloride (Neuromax)	0.03	8 to 12	Long	Renal
Mivacurium chloride (Mivacron)	0.01	3 to 6	Short	Metabolized by plasma cholinesterase
Rocuronium (Zemuron)	0.3	3 to 4	Short	Metabolized by liver

☑ ↑ Ca^{++} may lead to ↑ release of Ach and ↑ muscular contraction.

☑ ↑ Mg^{++} may lead to ↓ release of Ach and ↓ muscular contraction.

be avoided during prolonged muscle blockade with steroidal based blocking agents (pancuronium bromide and vecuronium bromide) (Hansen-Flaschen et al., 1993).

Electrolyte Imbalance.   The normal physiology of muscle contraction depends on the regulation of electrolytes. Abnormal levels of calcium and magnesium affect the quality of contraction, while imbalances in potassium and sodium levels alter the excitability at the motor endplate. For example, the release of ACh depends on extracellular calcium and magnesium concentrations. Calcium functions

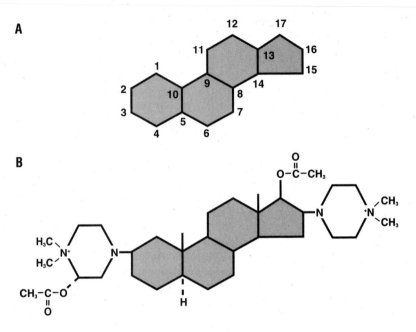

Figure 13-3 (A) Basic steroid structure; (B) A steroidal based neuromuscular blocking agent, pipecuronium.

✓ ↓ Ca++ or ↑ Mg++ enhances neuromuscular blockade with *nondepolarizing* agents.

✓ ↑ Mg++ enhances neuromuscular blockade with *depolarizing* agents.

✓ Diuretic-induced hypokalemia causes ↑ blockade with nondepolarizing agents and ↓ blockade with depolarizing agents.

to release ACh from the vesicles and expose myosin-binding sites on actin. Myosin-binding site exposure is a structural change that is necessary for the sliding of thin myofilaments past thick myofilaments. The sliding of these filaments results in muscular contraction (Tortora et al., 1987). Magnesium works in opposition to calcium. It decreases the release of ACh as well as the membrane's sensitivity, thus inhibiting muscle contraction (Ebadi, 1993).

Consequently, low calcium and high magnesium levels can enhance the effects of nondepolarizing agents. Increased magnesium levels can magnify the effects of depolarizing agents.

Sodium and potassium function in the process of depolarization. When a muscle cell is at rest, or not depolarized, there is a considerable difference between the concentration of sodium and potassium outside and inside the plasma membrane. At rest, there is an increased concentration of sodium extracellularly and an increased concentration of potassium intracellularly. The difference in charge on either side of the membrane of the resting cell is known as the resting potential and is said to be polarized or charged (Tortora et al., 1987).

An acute decrease in extracellular potassium will result in hyperpolarization and an increased resistance to depolarization. Hence, hypokalemia augments nondepolarizing agents and antagonizes depolarizing agents (Ebadi, 1993). Diuretic-induced hypokalemia should be corrected to prevent altered effects (potentiation of blockade with non-depolarizing agents; hinderance of blockade with depolarizing agents) (Halloran, 1991).

Acid-Base Status.   Acidemia intensifies neuromuscular blockade requiring a lower dosage of paralyzing agent or a higher dosage of reversal agent such as neostigmine (Kupfer et al., 1987). On the other hand, alkalemia necessitates a higher dosage of paralyzing agent to maintain neuromuscular blockade. These alterations are likely the result of potassium shift (extracellularly) associated with acidemia, H^+ moves into cells to be buffered, and K^+ moves out to maintain ionic neutrality. One might find these effects to be significant when intracranial pressure is being reduced via hyperventilation (respiratory alkalosis).

Although the preceding factors can alter the action of neuromuscular blocking agents, the net effects following the initial dosage can be titrated based on the results of patient monitoring. Since there is no standard level of paralysis to be achieved, the desired depth of blockade will depend on the clinical objectives of the physician.

ADVERSE EFFECTS

Apnea is the most immediate and life-threatening adverse effect associated with both depolarizing and nondepolarizing agents. For this reason, practitioners experienced in airway management must be present when these drugs are administered. For a patient who is already intubated and committed to a mechanical ventilator, the following alarms should be employed.

- Apnea alarm
- Low pressure/disconnect
- Low exhaled tidal volume
- Low exhaled minute volume
- Low SaO_2 or SpO_2 (pulse oximetry)

Deaths due to apnea have been reported in cases where alarms were inappropriately set or inactivated. It is possible that the incidence of fatal outcome is underreported (Halloran, 1991).

Other undesirable effects of neuromuscular blocking agents include loss of cough mechanism, blunted neurological assessment, emotional trauma due to inadequate sedation, disuse muscle atrophy, pressure sores, and increased iatrogenic morbidity and mortality associated with extended ICU exposure.

Histamine release is a property shared by most nondepolarizing agents. The presence of histamine may be manifested clinically as vasodilation, flushing, and bronchospasm. The degree of histamine release differs among the drugs. Succinylcholine, tubocurarine, metocurine, and atracurium have been known to provoke broncho-

---

☑️ Acidemia intensifies the effects of neuromuscular blockade.

☑️ Alkalemia diminishes the effects of neuromuscular blockade.

☑️ Succinylcholine, tubocurarine, metocurine, and atracurium may provoke bronchospasm and hypotension due to histamine release.

spasm and hypotension related to moderate histamine release, whereas pancuronium elicits only minimal release. Histamine release is not likely with the use of vecuronium (Ebadi, 1993).

Cardiovascular effects range from minimal to moderate, including bradycardia, tachycardia, arrhythmias, and circulatory collapse. Sudden changes in drug levels associated with intermittent administration (versus continuous infusion) seem to be responsible for these adverse effects (Watling et al., 1994). Table 13-10 summarizes the bronchopulmonary and cardiovascular adverse effects of neuromuscular blocking agents.

TABLE 13-10 Adverse Effects of Neuromuscular Blocking Agents

AGENTS	HISTAMINE RELEASE	CARDIOVASCULAR IMPAIRMENT	CLINICAL CONSIDERATIONS
Depolarizing			
Succinylcholine (Anectine, Quelicin, Sux-Cert, Sucostrin)	Moderate	Moderate	Caution with plasma cholinesterase disorder
Nondepolarizing			
Tubocurarine chloride (Tubarine)	Moderate	Moderate	
Pancuronium bromide (Pavulon)	Minimal	Moderate	Steroidal based Use corticosteroids with caution
Metocurine iodide (Metubine)	Moderate	Moderate	Appropriate dosage highly variable About 3 times as potent as tubocurarine, but shorter acting
Atracurium (Tracrium)	Moderate	Minimal	Not affected by organ dysfunction
Vecuronium bromide (Norcuron)	Not likely	Minimal	Steroidal based Use corticosteroids with caution
Pipecuronium bromide (Arduan)	Minimal	Minimal	
Doxacurium chloride (Neuromax)	Minimal	Minimal	Caution with plasma cholinesterase disorder
Mivacurium chloride (Mivacron)	Moderate	Minimal	Steroidal based
Rocuronium (Zemuron)	Minimal	Minimal	Use corticosteroids with caution

EVALUATION OF NEUROMUSCULAR BLOCKADE

To prevent unintentional overdosing, clinicians must establish an objective method of monitoring the depth of paralysis. This is especially meaningful in the management of patients with potential for drug accumulation secondary to renal or hepatic dysfunction.

The Train-of-Four, a peripheral nerve stimulator, is a valuable tool used in the evaluation of patients who are pharmacologically paralyzed. It determines the degree of blockade by measuring the muscle twitches in response to a controlled stimulus. Two electrodes are placed along a nerve path where an electrical stimulus is delivered four times in 0.5 second intervals. As the degree of blockade increases, the number of elicited responses decreases. The ulnar, facial, and posterior tibial nerves are commonly used because they are superficial and easy to locate. Figure 13-4 shows the electrode placement along the ulnar nerve.

A clinically useful but less objective method of measuring the depth of blockade is by assessing the patient's spontaneous muscle effort. Recovery of muscle blockade occurs in a reverse sequence. The ability to open one's eyes widely, sustain head lift, and protrude the tongue for more than five seconds confirms adequate reversal.

☑ The ability to open eyes widely, sustain head lift, and protrude the tongue for more than five seconds confirms adequate reversal of neuromuscular blockade.

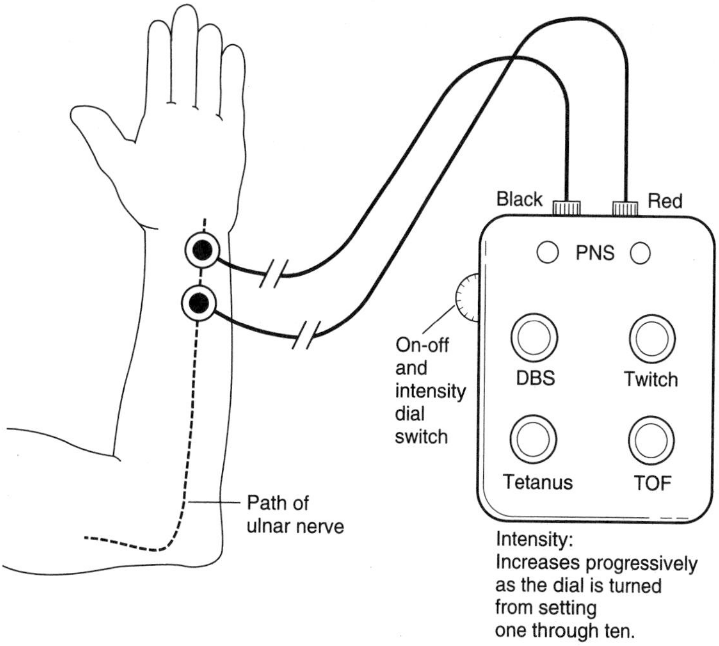

Figure 13-4 Placement of the Train-of-Four electrodes along the ulnar nerve. (Courtesy of Organon, Inc., West Orange, N.J.)

TABLE 13-11   Assessment of Neuromuscular Blockade Reversal

1. Head lift five seconds
2. Tongue protrusion five seconds
3. Hand grip
4. Arterial blood gases with PaO_2 > 80 mm Hg and $PaCO_2$ < 45 mm Hg*
5. Maximal inspiratory pressure (MIP) at least –25 cm H_2O
6. Vital capacity greater than 900 mL

* Slightly higher $PaCO_2$ is acceptable for patients with chronic CO_2 retention.

☑ Return of diaphragm function is assessed by acceptable blood gases, MIP > –25 cm H_2O, VC > 900 mL.

Ventilator support, however, should not be discontinued until the diaphragm is able to provide adequate ventilation. Arterial blood gases and spontaneous maneuvers [e.g., maximal inspiratory pressure [MIP] and vital capacity [VC]) can provide evidence of partial or full diaphragm recovery (Halloran, 1991). Table 13-11 outlines the method for assessment of neuromuscular blockade reversal.

SEDATIVES AND ANTIANXIETY AGENTS (BENZODIAZEPINES)

benzodiazepines: A group of drugs with strong hypnotic and sedative actions; used mainly to reduce anxiety and to induce sleep.

Benzodiazepines are given to patients to reduce anxiety, provide amnesia, and improve tolerance of mechanical ventilation. In addition, they facilitate invasive procedures (e.g., bronchoscopy, intravenous access, suctioning), decrease oxygen consumption, and protect the patient from self-injury.

MECHANISM OF ACTION

GABA (gamma-aminobutyric acid): A major central nervous system inhibitory transmitter that regulates the chloride ion channel and hyperpolarizes the neurons. Once the neurons are hyperpolarized and become resistant to repeated depolarization, sedation results.

Binding receptors for benzodiazepines have been identified in the limbic, thalamic, and hypothalamic levels of the central nervous system (Mohler et al., 1977). These receptor sites appear to be involved in a large molecular complex that includes **gamma-aminobutyric acid (GABA)** receptors and GABA-regulated chloride ion channels (Figure 13-5).

GABA Mechanism.   GABA is a major central nervous system inhibitory transmitter that opens chloride ion channels. Once hyperpolarized by the GABA action, the neurons become more resistant to repeated depolarization and sedation results (Mohler et al., 1988). Benzodiazepines facilitate the action of GABA, thus producing clinical sedation, **anxiolysis**, anticonvulsant effects, amnesia, slowing of reaction time, visual accommodation difficulties, and ataxia.

anxiolysis: Diminishing anxiety.

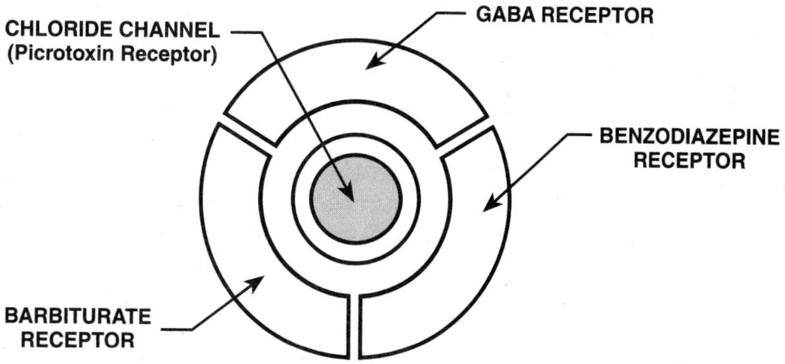

Figure 13-5 GABA (gamma-aminobutyric acid) receptor complex. GABA is the most common inhibitory neurotransmitter in the central nervous system (CNS). Activation of the postsynaptic GABA receptor increases chloride conductance through the ion channel thus hyperpolarizing it and inhibiting the postsynaptic neuron. Once the postsynaptic neurons are inhibited, depression of the CNS and neuromuscular blockade result.

> ☑ With benzodi-
> azepines, the in-
> travenous route of
> administration is
> preferred.

Absorption. Benzodiazepines are normally well absorbed in the gastrointestinal (GI) tract. In unstable patients, GI tract absorption may be unreliable and parenteral administration is preferred. Lorazepam and midazolam are rapidly and completely absorbed intramuscularly, whereas the absorption of chlordiazepoxide and diazepam is slow and erratic (McEvoy, 1995). Because of the slower onset of action and pain associated with intramuscular administration, the intravenous route is preferred in the critically ill. The lipid solubility of the drugs allows rapid distribution across the blood-brain barrier with midazolam being the most lipophilic, followed by diazepam and chlordiazepoxide, and then lorazepam (McEvoy, 1995).

Excretion. Benzodiazepines are metabolized in the liver to active and inactive metabolites that are excreted mainly in the urine. Although the pharmacokinetics of drugs are often used to explain correlations between plasma concentrations and effect, benzodiazepines do not exhibit this relationship. Furthermore, carefully controlled clinical trials have not shown the superiority of one agent over another for various ICU indications (Dasta et al., 1994). Therefore, the choice of benzodiazepine is often based on cost.

ADVERSE EFFECTS

> ☑ Dose-dependent
> adverse CNS
> effects include con-
> fusion, weakness,
> dizziness, drowsi-
> ness, ataxia, syn-
> cope, vertigo, and
> amnesia.

Dose-dependent adverse central nervous system effects are very common with benzodiazepines. They are an extension of the pharmacologic actions of the drugs and include confusion, weakness, dizziness, drowsiness, ataxia, syncope, vertigo, and amnesia (McEvoy, 1995). Central nervous system stimulation occurs occasionally in patients

☑ **Withdrawal syndrome** (anxiety, tachycardia, diaphoresis, hypertension, and occasionally, seizures) may occur if benzodiazepines are abruptly discontinued.

☑ **Benzodiazepines may decrease** the mean arterial pressure, stroke volume, cardiac output, and systemic vascular resistance.

☑ **Ramsay Scale is used to assess** a patient's sedation state.

☑ **Ramsay Scale is not suitable for** paralyzed patients since they cannot perform those required commands.

Ramsay Scale: *The scoring system with a scale ranging from level I to level VI; used to assess the degree of sedation.*

with underlying psychiatric disorders. These patients present with restlessness, mania, euphoria, acute rage reactions, and sleep disorders (McCartney et al., 1993). A withdrawal syndrome may occur if these drugs are abruptly discontinued in patients on prolonged therapy or high doses. This may be manifested by severe anxiety, tachycardia, diaphoresis, hypertension, and, occasionally, seizures (McCartney et al., 1994).

Parenteral administration of benzodiazepines may result in a dose-dependent respiratory depression (Forster et al., 1980) which is additive to that produced by narcotics. Elderly and COPD patients are at the greatest risk (Levine, 1994). Although depression of the respiratory drive is not usually as great with benzodiazepines as with other sedative agents, apnea may occur. Careful dosing of these agents is also necessary to avoid prolonged mechanical ventilation.

Benzodiazepines may also have direct effects on cardiovascular hemodynamics. They have been shown to decrease mean arterial pressure, stroke volume, cardiac output, and systemic vascular resistance (Reves et al., 1990). Additive decreases in blood pressure may occur when narcotics are administered concurrently. Table 13-12 outlines the cardiovascular effects of benzodiazepines.

ASSESSMENT OF SEDATION

The indication for benzodiazepines and the estimated duration of therapy may be helpful in deciding whether to administer these drugs intermittently or continuously. If a short period of sedation is needed, intermittent intravenous bolus dosing may prevent oversedation. If prolonged periods of sedation are required, a bolus followed by a continuous infusion may provide optimal patient comfort. If the indication is to facilitate an uncomfortable procedure, an intravenous bolus dose should be given.

Since individual patient response to benzodiazepines is highly variable, monitoring is essential to ensure correct dosing and reduce costs. Assessment of a patient's sedation state may be done with the **Ramsay Scale** for Assessment of Sedation as outlined in Table 13-13 (Ramsay et al., 1974). Using the Ramsay Scale and the appropriate types and dosages of benzodiazepines (Table 13-14), a desired level of sedation may be determined.

TABLE 13-12   Cardiovascular Effects of Benzodiazepines

1. ↓ Mean arterial pressure
2. ↓ Stroke volume
3. ↓ Cardiac output
4. ↓ Systemic vascular resistance
5. ↓ Blood pressure

TABLE 13-13   Ramsay Scale for Assessment of Sedation

LEVEL/SCORE	CLINICAL DESCRIPTION
I	Anxious and agitated
II	Cooperative, oriented, tranquil
III	Responds only to verbal commands
IV	Asleep with brisk response to light stimulation
V	Asleep with sluggish response to stimulation
VI	Asleep without response to stimulation

TABLE 13-14   Common Benzodiazepines Used in Mechanical Ventilation

DRUG	INITIAL DOSE	ONSET	DURATION
Diazepam (Valium)	2.5 to 10 mg IV	Fast	Short initially; multiple doses result in prolonged effect
Lorazepam (Ativan)	0.5 to 2 mg IV	Intermediate	Intermediate
Midazolam (Versed)	1 to 5 mg IV	Fast	Short, but may be prolonged if not carefully dosed

☑ Autonomic signs (tachycardia, diaphoresis, hypertension, and lacrimation) may suggest inadequate sedation or pain control.

It is important to note that the Ramsay Scale is not suitable for paralyzed patients. Since they cannot perform those required commands for the Ramsay Scale, autonomic signs such as tachycardia, diaphoresis, hypertension, and lacrimation may suggest inadequate sedation or pain control (Shelly et al., 1986).

NARCOTIC ANALGESICS

Patients on mechanical ventilation may have a variety of medical or surgical problems that necessitate attention to pain control. In these patients, however, pain is difficult to assess because of their inability to speak. Hemodynamic and respiratory instability, and immediate life-threatening concerns also overshadow the presence of pain. Subsequently, pain control for these patients is often inadequate (Wheeler, 1993).

narcotic analgesics:
Drugs that are used to control pain via the central nervous system. Examples are morphine, codeine, and meperidine (Demerol, a synthetic compound).

Pain can cause anxiety, discomfort, and delirium in patients on mechanical ventilation. Interference with sleep also compounds the level of anxiety thus further elevating the perception of pain. Pain is also associated with many adverse outcomes in the intensive care unit (Table 13-15). **Narcotic analgesics** are commonly used to control pain to allow earlier patient mobilization and to decrease hospital stay.

TABLE 13-15 Adverse Patient Outcomes Associated with Pain

REACTION INDUCED BY PAIN	ADVERSE OUTCOMES
Tissue initiated stress hormone response	Breakdown of body tissue Increased blood clotting Increased metabolic rate Increased water retention Decreased immune function
Activation of autonomic functions	Increased blood pressure Increased heart rate
Muscle splinting	Decreased tidal volume Decreased respiratory rate Decreased minute ventilation
Immobility	Formation of deep vein thrombosis and pulmonary embolism
Diminished gastrointestinal function	Delay of bowel and gastric function

MECHANISM OF ACTION

Narcotic analgesics produce analgesia by binding to opioid receptors in and outside the central nervous system. Several subtypes of opiate receptors have been identified. The mu, kappa, and sigma receptors are known to have important nociceptive (neural receptors for painful stimulus) properties in humans. Binding and activating these receptors also helps to explain the adverse pharmacologic profile of these drugs (Table 13-16) (Teeple, 1990).

Opiates may be further classified depending on whether they are agonists, agonist-antagonists, or pure antagonists at these receptors

TABLE 13-16 Narcotic Receptor Classifications

PHYSICAL PARAMETER	mu	kappa	sigma
Pain sensation	−	−	0
Body temperature	−	0	+
Pulse rate	−	0	+
Pupils	−	−	+
Respiratory rate	−	−	+
CNS effect	Sedation	Hypnosis	Delirium

+ increased effect
− reduced effect
0 no effect

TABLE 13-17 Opioid Drug Classifications

DRUGS [SELECTED EXAMPLES]	mu	kappa	sigma
1. Agonist [morphine, meperidine, fentanyl]	+	+	0
2. Agonist-antagonist [pentazocine, butorphanol]	–	+	+
3. Antagonist [naloxone (Narcan)]	–	–	–

+ *agonist*
– *antagonist*
0 *no effect*

✓ Full agonists produce a maximal response within cells to which they bind.

✓ Agonist-antagonists activate one type of opiate receptor while blocking another.

✓ Antagonists block opiate receptors.

✓ Sedation, respiratory depression, and shallow breathing are the primary adverse effects of narcotic analgesics on the CNS.

✓ Myoclonus (twitching or spasm of muscles), convulsions, and chest wall rigidity are the primary adverse effects of narcotic analgesics on the muscle group.

(Table 13-17). Full agonists produce a maximal response within cells to which they bind; agonist-antagonists activate one type of opiate receptor while blocking another; and antagonists only block opiate receptors (Teeple, 1990).

Table 13-17 contains only representative samples from each class. It is not a complete listing of all opioids.

Most agonist-antagonist drugs are agonists at the sigma receptor. As the dose of these drugs is increased for deeper analgesia, the more likely they may cause significant psychological effects such as delirium. This class of drugs is not routinely used in ventilator patients and will not be discussed further.

Antagonist drugs such as naloxone (Narcan) are primarily used to reverse overdose of narcotics. Special care must be exercised with the use of naloxone in a patient being treated for severe pain. It may reverse an untoward adverse effect such as respiratory depression while causing the return of severe pain (Levine, 1994).

ADVERSE EFFECTS

Narcotic analgesics produce many adverse effects. Table 13-18 outlines the adverse effects that may occur to various systems or body locations of the patient.

Central Nervous System. Opiates cause sedation, respiratory depression, and myoclonus (twitching or spasm of muscles) and their effects are dose-dependent (Levine, 1994). Clinically significant respiratory depression is more likely to occur with a large initial dose or in patients with underlying pulmonary disease. Respiratory depression (decreased tidal volume and respiratory rate) is mediated by opioid agonist activity at the mu receptors of the brain stem (Teeple, 1990). Since opiates suppress deep breathing, they may induce atelectasis, which can be prevented by activating the automatic sigh mode on the ventilator.

Muscle Groups. Myoclonus (twitching or spasm of muscles) and other neuroexcitatory phenomena have been reported with opioid analgesics. Myoclonus may be prevented by switching to another

TABLE 13-18   Adverse Effects of Narcotic Analgesics

LOCATION	ADVERSE EFFECTS
Central nervous system	Sedation Respiratory depression Shallow breathing (and atelectasis)
Muscle groups	Myoclonus (twitching or spasm of muscles) Convulsions Chest wall rigidity
Cardiovascular	Direct vasodilation Vagally mediated bradycardia Hypotension
Gastrointestinal	Delayed gastric emptying Constipation Nausea
Others	Miosis (contraction of pupils) Altered levels of stress hormones Uncommon allergic reactions

opioid, lowering the dosage, or using a benzodiazepine (Valium), an antianxiety and hypnotic agent. Convulsions have been reported with high doses of any opioid in an intolerant patient, but are most common with normeperidine—a liver metabolite of meperidine (Demerol) (Brucera et al., 1992). Naloxone (Narcan) may be used to reverse convulsions caused by opiates with the exception of those caused by use of meperidine.

Chest wall rigidity is a complication that may develop after administration of any opiate, but it is most commonly reported with fentanyl (Sublimaze). This adverse effect is most often seen at the time of anesthesia induction or after surgery. It may be so severe that the patient may require intubation, mechanical ventilation, and chemical paralysis. Patients at risk for this untoward effect appear to be the elderly, patient's with renal failure, and those receiving large doses of opioids (Wheeler, 1993).

✓ Direct vasodilation, vagally mediated bradycardia, and hypotension are the primary adverse effects of narcotic analgesics on the cardiovascular system.

Cardiovascular Effects.   Opioids can affect a patient's hemodynamic status. Hypotension may develop as a result of direct vasodilation, histamine release, and vagally mediated bradycardia (Levine, 1994). These complications may be prevented by using the lowest effective dose, providing an adequate intravascular volume, or decreasing the rate of administration. (Note: Meperidine's [Demerol's] structure resembles that of atropine; thus it may cause tachycardia rather than bradycardia.)

Although opioids may produce a dose-dependent clinical spectrum ranging from pain relief to sedation, deep coma, and anesthesia, low-dose opiates are often combined with low-dose sedatives (benzodiazepines) to minimize the adverse effects of these two agents.

☑ Delayed gastric emptying, constipation, nausea are the primary adverse effects of narcotic analgesics on the GI system.

cathartic agents:
Active purgatives used to produce bowel movements.

Gastrointestinal Effects.   The gastrointestinal effects of opioids include delayed gastric emptying, constipation, and nausea (Levine, 1994). Since tolerance to constipation does not occur, or occurs very slowly during opiate administration, **cathartic agents** should be given on a regular basis to activate bowel movements.

Nausea and vomiting during opiate administration may be due to three different mechanisms. Opiates may reduce gastric motility that results in nausea after eating. Secondly, opioids seem to cause nausea that is due to sensitization of the vestibular apparatus. This type of nausea is brought on by changes in position or head movement. Third, these drugs may directly stimulate the medullary chemoreceptor trigger zone. Nausea from this mechanism is usually present continuously (Jacox et al., 1994).

Other adverse effects related to opioid use include miosis (contraction of pupils), altered levels of stress hormones, and uncommon allergic reactions.

CLINICAL CONSIDERATIONS

Opioid tolerance, physical dependence, and psychological dependence are important concepts to understand when considering analgesic therapy. Misuse of these terms has led to ineffective practices in prescribing, administering, and treatment of patients in pain.

Tolerance.   Tolerance is defined as the need to increase dosage requirements to maintain effective pain relief. In addition, tolerance may occur to some adverse opioid effects such as respiratory depression, miosis, sedation, and nausea (Foley, 1993).

Physical Dependence.   Physical dependence is defined as the precipitation of a withdrawal syndrome upon abrupt termination of the drug or after administration of a narcotic antagonist (naloxone). Clinically, the withdrawal symptoms include irritability, joint pain, chills and hot flashes, anxiety, nausea, vomiting, lacrimation, rhinorrhea, diaphoresis, abdominal cramps, and diarrhea. Withdrawal symptoms may be avoided in physically dependent patients by gradual dosage reduction of the opiate (Hammack et al., 1994).

Psychological Dependence.   Psychological dependence is an additive behavior characterized by drug seeking, preoccupation with obtaining and using the drug, and drug use for other than analgesic purposes (euphoria).

☑ Since ventilator patients cannot communicate effectively, these clinical signs may be used to reflect inadequate pain control.

TABLE 13-19 Clinical Signs of Inadequate Pain Control

Tachycardia in the absence of hypoxemia

Blood pressure changes

Dilated pupils

Diaphoresis

Grimacing

Restlessness

Guarding

ASSESSMENT OF ADEQUATE PAIN CONTROL

Pain assessment is important in ensuring adequate pain relief and enhancing patient recovery. Cooperative, awake, and alert patients may be assessed with pain intensity and pain distress scales. Unfortunately, ventilator patients are frequently unable to participate in their pain management plan. In this case, clinical signs such as tachycardia, blood pressure changes, dilated pupils, diaphoresis, grimacing, restlessness, and guarding may be signs that indicate inadequate analgesia (Table 13-19).

barbiturates: A group of drugs that depresses the central nervous system. Adverse effects are many, including alteration of the respiration, heart rate, blood pressure, and temperature. It is used in seizure disorders, control of elevated intracranial pressure, and intubation enhancement.

AGENTS FOR SEIZURES AND ELEVATED INTRACRANIAL PRESSURE (BARBITURATES)

Barbiturates, once widely used in the critically ill for sedation and anxiolysis, have limited applications in patients on mechanical ventilation because of respiratory and cardiovascular depression. For sedative action, they have been replaced by safer drugs such as benzodiazepines. Barbiturates may be preferred in certain situations, such as seizure disorders, control of elevated intracranial pressure, and "rapid sequence intubation."

Table 13-20 lists the selected barbiturates that are used in different situations because of the wide range of duration of action, ranging from ultra short-acting (0.2 hour) to long-lasting (4 to 12 hours).

☑ Barbiturates may be preferred in seizure disorders, control of elevated intracranial pressure, and "rapid sequence intubation."

MECHANISM OF ACTION

Barbiturates are capable of producing all levels of CNS depression, ranging from mild sedation to hypnosis to deep coma to death. As previously discussed in the benzodiazepine section, GABA is the most common CNS inhibitory neurotransmitter. The GABA receptor exists as a complex involving the benzodiazepine receptor, the barbiturate

TABLE 13-20 **Selected Barbiturates**

NAMES	DURATION OF ACTION	DURATION OF HYPNOTIC* EFFECT
Thiopental Methohexital	Ultra short-acting	0.2 hr
Pentobarbital	Short-acting	1 to 4 hrs
Amobarbital	Intermediate-acting	2 to 8 hrs
Phenobarbital	Long-acting	4 to 12 hrs

*The anesthetic dose is about three times the hypnotic dose; the lethal dose is about six times the hypnotic dose (Cottrell et al., 1995; Ziment, 1978).

☑ GABA-mediated hyperpolarization of the neuron makes the neuron more resistant to depolarization causing depression of CNS function.

receptor, and the GABA receptor and its associated chloride ion channel (Figure 13-5) (Olson, 1988). Drug binding to this receptor complex facilitates GABA-mediated hyperpolarization of the neuron via an increase in chloride ion entry into the cell. This hyperpolarization makes the neuron more resistant to depolarization causing depression of CNS function. The importance of this cellular mechanism in producing the clinical effects of barbiturates is unclear.

Higher doses of barbiturates may directly activate the chloride ion channel independent of the barbiturate-GABA receptor complex (Levine, 1994). This results in a progressive depression of central nervous system function ranging from deep sedation to coma. When coma is induced, these agents are capable of decreasing cerebral metabolic oxygen consumption. Through autoregulation, the brain decreases cerebral blood flow thereby lowering intracranial pressure.

ADVERSE EFFECTS

☑ Venodilation with peripheral pooling of blood, tachycardia, and depressed myocardial contractility may result in hypotension in patients with poor cardiac function.

These once widely used agents now have limited applications in critically ill patients because of dose-dependent cardiovascular and respiratory depression (Price-Roberts, 1984). Venodilation with peripheral pooling of blood, tachycardia, and depressed myocardial contractility may result in hypotension especially in elderly patients with poor cardiac function.

Respiratory adverse effects to barbiturates include blunted ventilatory response to hypoxia and hypercapnia, reduced tidal volume and respiratory rate. Other adverse effects attributed to barbiturates include rashes and gastrointestinal upset.

DRUG INTERACTIONS

☑ Barbiturates increase the clearance of those drugs that are metabolized by the liver.

Barbiturates may induce tolerance as well as physical and psychological dependence. These concepts have been discussed at length in the section on narcotic therapy. Another problem complicating barbiturate therapy is the potential for numerous drug interactions. When barbiturates are in use, liver metabolism of other drugs may be enhanced thus decreasing their effects. Caution should be exercised when adding to

✔ Barbiturates do not relieve pain and may paradoxically heighten the sensation of pain.

or deleting a drug from a therapeutic regimen containing a barbiturate, giving consideration to the possible need for dosage adjustment.

Barbiturates do not relieve pain and may paradoxically heighten pain intensity (Dundee et al., 1988). Therefore it is necessary to reassess analgesic efficacy when these drugs are used in patients requiring analgesia.

OTHER AGENTS USED IN MECHANICAL VENTILATION

Other agents used in mechanical ventilation include propofol (for sedation and maintenance of anesthesia), haloperidol (for sedation and reduction of anxiety), and nitric oxide (for dilation of pulmonary vessels).

PROPOFOL

✔ Depending on the dosage, propofol provides a spectrum of CNS depression ranging from light sedation to deep general anesthesia.

Propofol (Diprivan) is an intravenous (IV) drug administered together with other anesthetics to produce and maintain anesthesia. A hypnotic effect is produced within 40 seconds after a rapid IV bolus administration (1 to 2.5 mg/kg). The maintenance dose is 0.05 to 0.2 mg/kg/min by IV infusion (Reiss et al., 1993). Propofol is used to provide sedation in ventilator patients and induction and maintenance of anesthesia.

Mechanism of Action. Propofol appears to enhance GABA-activated chloride ion channel function (for a complete discussion, see Sedatives and Antianxiety Agents [Benzodiazepines] in this chapter) (Fragen et al., 1992). The mechanism of action may involve a separate receptor recognition site or may involve a different mechanism from that previously discussed for barbiturates and benzodiazepines.

✔ Propofol is formulated in an oil-in-water vehicle and it could contribute a significant amount of calories from fat.

✔ Since fat emulsion provides an excellent medium for microbial growth, strict aseptic techniques are essential.

Adverse Effects. Adverse reactions reported with propofol use include apnea, bradycardia, laryngospasm, bronchospasm, coughing, dyspnea, hypotension, and burning or pain at the site of infusion. Discoloration of the urine to green or red-brown may occur due to liver metabolites of propofol (Mirenda et al., 1995; Reiss et al., 1993).

Propofol is highly fat soluble and is formulated in an oil-in-water vehicle. The soybean oil in this vehicle could contribute a significant amount of calories from fat. Therefore, other sources of dietary intake must be adjusted to compensate for the amount of fat infused. In addition, patients receiving propofol should be monitored for elevations in serum triglycerides. Because fat emulsion provides an excellent medium for microbial growth, and propofol contains no preservatives, strict aseptic administration techniques are important to prevent iatrogenic sepsis.

✓ Propofol has no analgesic properties. Additional analgesics are needed for pain control.

Clinical Considerations. Propofol has no analgesic properties, therefore attention must be paid to providing adequate analgesia in patients requiring pain relief. When opioid analgesics are used in combination with a propofol additive, hypotension may occur.

Since propofol does not promote salivation or vomiting, its use can be an advantage for intubated patients (Reiss et al., 1993). The rapid onset and offset of sedation may be a disadvantage if patients are allowed to awaken abruptly in pain or to great environmental disorientation (Levine, 1994). This problem can be avoided by decreasing the infusion rate so the patient awakens slowly.

As discussed previously in the benzodiazepine section, monitoring the level of sedation is important to avoid over- or undersedation. The Ramsay scale (refer to Sedatives and Antianxiety Agents [Benzodiazepines] in this chapter for a discussion) or computer-assisted cerebral function monitoring can be used to determine the patient's level of sedation. The latter notes changes in brain function on a real-time basis and with adequate training, the changes may be interpreted by caregivers.

HALOPERIDOL

✓ Haloperidol (Haldol) may be effective in sedating patients who have concurrent agitation and delirium caused by use of sedatives.

Pharmacotherapy for sedation and anxiolysis may in some patients paradoxically cause agitation and delirium. Haloperidol (Haldol) may be effective in these situations. Delirium may be defined as a reversible global impairment of cognitive processes manifested chiefly by disorientation, impaired short-term memory, arousal, attention, illusions, and hallucinations (McCartney et al., 1993). The initial approach to a ventilator patient presenting with delirium should be a search for reversible causes. See Table 13-21 for examples of reversible causes of delirium.

TABLE 13-21 Reversible Causes of Delirium

WITHDRAWAL OF MEDICATIONS	IMPROVEMENT OF CLINICAL CONDITIONS
Alcohol	Fever
Analgesics	Head injury
Anticholinergics	Hepatic failure
Anticonvulsants	Hyperparathyroidism and hypoparathyroidism
Antihistamines	Hyperthyroidism and hypothyroidism
Antihypertensives	Renal failure
Antiparkinsonian agents	
Cardiac drugs	
Corticosteroids	
Psychiatric agents	

Nonpharmacologic approaches such as repeated reorientation and explanation (explain treatment plans to the patient), minimize environmental stress, and enhance communication (written or hand signals in intubated patients may also be helpful). Drug therapy should be added to nonpharmacologic approaches if the latter are ineffective and a reversible cause is not found.

Indications. Haloperidol is primarily used in the critically ill ventilator patient for the control of agitation and delirium. The intravenous route of administration is preferred in the intensive care setting although the drug may be given intramuscularly or orally.

Mechanism of Action. An increase in dopamine release and metabolism have been postulated as one of the central nervous system derangements manifesting as agitation and delirium. Haloperidol blocks dopamine receptors in the central nervous system (limbic, basal ganglia, and brain stem) producing a calming effect (McEvoy, 1995). In addition, haloperidol blocks dopamine receptors in the chemoreceptor trigger zone that may be responsible for its **antiemetic** activity.

antiemetic: Preventing nausea and vomiting.

Adverse Effects. Blockade of dopamine receptors in the central nervous system may interfere with normal motor function. These adverse effects are called extrapyramidal reactions (EPS) and may include unilateral cervical muscle contraction with neck twisting (torticollis), swollen tongue (laryngeal dystonia), jaw muscle spasm (trismus), and flexion of head and feet backward (opisthotonus) (McEvoy, 1995). EPS occurs much less frequently with IV haloperidol than that observed with intramuscular or oral therapy. The reason for this is currently unknown (Fish, 1991).

Neuroleptic malignant syndrome is a rare, idiosyncratic, life-threatening reaction that may occur after a single dose of haloperidol. Hyperthermia, altered consciousness, labile blood pressure, diaphoresis, and tachyarrhythmias are suggestive of this condition (Simon, 1993).

Haloperidol may also prolong the electrocardiographic QT interval that on rare occasions can produce a polymorphic form of ventricular tachycardia known as torsade de pointes (Fish, 1991).

☑ Neck twisting, swollen tongue, jaw muscle spasm, and flexion of head and feet backward are some adverse effects of haloperidol.

Clinical Considerations. Combination therapy including a benzodiazepine, opioid, and haloperidol is often necessary for control of extremely agitated, delirious patients requiring critical care. The critical care team must be diligent in the search for reversible causes of agitation and delirium and if found, correct them whenever possible.

☑ Combined use of benzodiazepine, opioid, and haloperidol is often necessary for control of extremely agitated, delirious patients.

NITRIC OXIDE

Nitric oxide is endogenously synthesized in vascular endothelium from the amino acid L-arginine (Palmer et al., 1987). After being released from the endothelium, nitric oxide diffuses into vascular smooth muscle cells where it stimulates production of 3' 5'-cyclic guanosine monophosphate (cGMP). cGMP decreases the concentration of calcium in the muscle resulting in vasodilatation. Because nitric oxide is extremely labile (rapidly inactivated by hemoglobin) it causes only local regulation of endothelial tone without systemic hypotensive effects.

Indications.   Inhaled nitric oxide (NO) therapy has been used as a treatment or supportive modality for a variety of clinical conditions. Some of these conditions include persistent pulmonary hypertension and hypoxemic respiratory failure of the newborn (Abman & Kinsella, 1999), respiratory distress syndrome and hypoxemic respiratory failure of older infants and children (Dobyns, Cornfield & Anas et al., 1999), and adult respiratory distress syndrome (Burke-Martindale, 1998). In addition, NO therapy has been effective in increasing pulmonary blood flow and oxygenation and improving systemic cardiopulmonary hemo-dynamics in infants (Ochikubo, Waffarn & Turbow et al., 1997).

> ✓ Inhaled nitric oxide produces local vasodilation of vascular smooth muscles.

Mechanism of Action.   Inhaled nitric oxide produces local vaso-dilation of vascular smooth muscles. Because the gas is delivered to alveolar units still presumably participating in gas exchange, these alveolar capillary units are preferentially vasodilated, diverting blood from hypoxic capillary beds with high vascular resistance (Stamler et al., 1992). The net physiologic results are reduction of pulmonary vascular resistance, reversal of hypoxic pulmonary vasoconstriction in unobstructed airway (improvement of V/Q matching), and im-provement of oxygenation (Figure 13-6).

> ✓ Pulmonary vaso-dilation may reduce pulmonary vascular resistance, correct V/Q mis-match, and improve oxygenation.

> ✓ Nitric and nitrous acid are lung inflammatory by-products of nitric oxide therapy.

Adverse Effects.   Adverse effects of NO therapy are dependent on the dosage and concentration of inhaled NO. When combined with oxygen, NO is converted to nitrogen dioxide (NO_2). NO_2 levels of higher than 10 ppm can cause cell damage, hemorrhage, pulmonary edema, and death. However, at therapeutic dosages (less than 2 ppm), adverse effects and toxicity caused by inhalation of NO are rare (Linberg & Rydgren, 1999; Scanlan et al., 1999).

NO and NO_2 may be converted to nitric acid (HNO_3) and nitrous acid (HNO_2), respectively, both of which may cause lung inflammation (interstitial pneumonitis). Toxicology information on these compounds is primarily available from administration of various concentrations of NO and NO_2 to healthy animals or volunteers with normal lungs (Lunn, 1995). Further research is necessary to determine the adverse effects of prolonged exposure of NO and NO_2 in patients with lung diseases.

NO is inactivated by combining with hemoglobin to form methe-moglobin (hemoglobin in blood oxidized to ferric form that is incapable of transporting oxygen). The amount formed during therapy depends on the amount of NO administered and the amount of methemoglobin elim-inated by an enzyme (methemoglobin reductase). Partial or complete

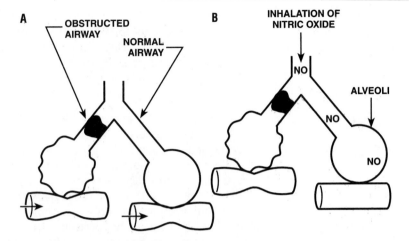

Figure 13-6 (A) Ventilation/perfusion (V/Q) relationship of an obstructed airway and a normal airway. The perfusion to both is decreased because of hypoxic vasoconstriction. In the obstructed airway, V/Q is absent. In the unobstructed airway, a high V/Q (deadspace ventilation) is seen. (B) Inhalation of nitric oxide (NO) selectively dilates the pulmonary vessels of the ventilated alveoli, thus improving perfusion and restoring normal V/Q in unobstructed airway.

deficiencies of this enzyme may exist in some patients, predisposing them to methemoglobinemia.

Other potential adverse effects of NO are inhibition of platelet aggregation and possible negative inotropic effect.

Clinical Considerations.   Most of the patients who receive NO therapy are on mechanical ventilation. Two components are necessary for the delivery of NO to these patients: in-line monitoring of NO and NO_2, and a delivery source of NO gas (Wessel et al., 1994).

At this time, NO is regulated by the Food and Drug Administration and is available as an investigational agent. It is supplied as cylinders containing either 800 parts per million (ppm) or 2,200 ppm with nitrogen as the inert balance gas.

SUMMARY

In mechanical ventilation, different drugs are used to (1) provide bronchodilation, (2) facilitate intubation, (3) relieve pain and anxiety, and (4) treat seizures or elevated intracranial pressure. These drugs can be very useful when they are used as directed. At the same time, they must be used with care, since adverse effects can be dangerous or even life-threatening. For this reason, practitioners are expected to have a thorough knowledge of the indications, contraindications, and adverse effects of the drugs that are administered to patients on mechanical ventilation.

Self-Assessment Questions

1. Bronchodilation may be induced by all of the following mechanisms *except*:

   A. stimulating the sympathetic branch of the autonomic nervous system.
   B. stimulating the parasympathetic branch of the autonomic nervous system.
   C. inhibiting the enzyme phosphodiesterase.
   D. inhibiting the parasympathetic branch of the autonomic nervous system.

2. A patient who has been using Theo-Dur at home states that she experiences palpitations, nausea, vomiting, headache, and agitation each time after taking the medication. The proper management technique for this patient includes monitoring of the _____ level and titrating the dosage to a therapeutic range of _____.

   A. serum theophylline, 10 to 20 µg/ml
   B. corticosteroid, 10 to 20 µg/ml
   C. serum theophylline, 40 to 60 µg/ml
   D. corticosteroid, 40 to 60 µg/ml

3. An asthmatic patient who has been using Ventolin for several months complains of shortness of breath and states that "the Ventolin is not working any more." The physician asks for your suggestion. You would recommend a trial use of:

   A. Proventil.
   B. Alupent.
   C. Brethine.
   D. Vanceril.

4. Which of the following is *not* an indication for using a neuromuscular blocking agent?

   A. relieve laryngeal spasm
   B. maintain mechanical ventilation
   C. facilitate endotracheal suctioning
   D. enhance endotracheal intubation

5. Succinylcholine (Anectine, Quelicin) is a _____ neuromuscular blocking agent. It induces muscle blockade by _____.

   A. depolarizing, binding to the receptor sites and causing sustained depolarization
   B. nondepolarizing, binding to the receptor sites and causing sustained depolarization
   C. depolarizing, competing for the receptor sites and blocking the action of acetylcholine
   D. nondepolarizing, competing for the receptor sites and blocking the action of acetylcholine

6. All of the following are potential complications of a neuromuscular blocking agent *except*:

   A. oversedation.
   B. prolonged muscle blockade.
   C. apnea.
   D. bronchospasm.

7. A patient who has been given Norcuron one hour ago is recovering in the surgical intensive care unit. The physician wants to know whether neuromuscular blockade reversal has occurred. You would check all of the following *except*:

 A. tongue protusion.
 B. serum Anectine level.

 C. hand grip.
 D. head lift.

8. A ventilator patient has been receiving diazepam (Valium) for better tolerance of mechanical ventilation and related procedures. The cardiovascular adverse effects for his patient may include:

 A. decreased cardiac output.
 B. increased stroke volume.

 C. increased mean arterial pressure.
 D. increased systemic vascular resistance.

9. The Ramsay Scale is commonly used to assess the degree of:

 A. ventilation.
 B. pain.

 C. bronchodilation.
 D. sedation.

10. Inadequate pain control may lead to all of the following complications *except*:

 A. increased blood pressure.
 B. increased immune function.

 C. decreased lung function.
 D. decreased patient mobility.

11. A patient is given naloxone upon returning from surgery. You may conclude that the patient has received too much _____ during surgery.

 A. narcotic analgesic
 B. neuromuscular blocking agent

 C. benzodiazepine
 D. nitric oxide

12. For seizure disorders and control of elevated intracranial pressure, _____ may be useful.

 A. neuromuscular blocking agent
 B. nitric oxide

 C. barbiturate
 D. corticosteroid

13. Haloperidol (Haldol) should be considered for controlling agitation and delirium:

 A. as soon as a patient is placed on mechanical ventilator.
 B. when narcotic analgesic is given to a patient.

 C. when a patient experiences pain.
 D. after reversible causes of delirium have been ruled out.

References

Abman, S. H. & Kinsella, J. P. (1998). Inhaled nitric oxide therapy for pulmonary disease in pediatrics. *Curr Opin Pediatr, 10*(3), 236–242.

Brucera, E. et al. (1992). Organic hallucinosis in patients receiving high doses of opiates for cancer pain. *Pain, 48,* 397–399.

Burke-Martindale, C. H. (1998). Inhaled nitric oxide therapy for adult respiratory distress syndrome. *Crit Care Nurse, 18*(6), 21–27.

Cottrell, G. et al. (1995). *Pharmacology for respiratory care practitioners.* Philadelphia: F.A. Davis Co.

Dasta, J. F. et al. (1994). Pattern of prescribing and administering drugs for agitation and pain in patients in surgical intensive care unit. *Crit Care Med, 22,* 974–980.

Dobyns, E. L., Cornfield, D. N. & Anas, N. G. et al. (1999). Multicenter randomized controlled trial of the effects of inhaled nitric oxide therapy on gas exchange in children with acute hypoxemic respiratory failure. *J Pediatr, 134*(4), 406–412.

Dundee, J. W. et al. (1988). *Intravenous anaesthesia* (2nd ed.). New York: Churchill Livingstone.

Ebadi, M. (1993). *Pharmacology* (2nd ed.). Boston: Little, Brown and Co.

Fish, D. N. (1991). Treatment of delirium in the critically ill patient. *Clin Pharmacy, 10,* 456–466.

Foley, K. M. (1993). Changing concepts of tolerance to opioids: What the cancer patient has taught us. In C. R. Chapman, & K. M. Foley (Eds.), *Current and emerging issues in cancer pain: Research and practice* (pp. 331–350). New York: Raven Press, Ltd.

Forster, A. et al. (1980). Respiratory depression by midazolam and diazepam. *Anesthesiology, 53,* 494–497.

Fragen, R. J. et al. (1992). Nonopioid intravenous anesthetics. In P. G. Barash, B. F. Cullen, & R. K. Stoetling (Eds.), *Clinical Anesthesia* (pp. 385–412). Philadelphia: J.B. Lippincott.

Halloran, T. (1991). Use of sedation and neuromuscular paralysis during mechanical ventilation. *Crit Care Nur Clin of North Am, 3*(4), 651–657.

Hammack, J. E. et al. (1994). Use of orally administered opioids for cancer-related pain. *Mayo Clinic Proc, 69,* 384–390.

Hansen-Flaschen, J. et al. (1993). Neuromuscular blockade in the intensive care unit: More than we bargain for. *Am Rev of Respir Dis, 147*(1), 234–236.

Jacox, A. et al. (1994, March). Management of cancer pain. *Clinical Practice Guideline No. 9* AHCPR Publication No. 94-0592. Rockville, MD. Agency for Health Care Policy and Research, U. S. Department of Health and Human Services, Public Health Service.

Kee, J. L. (1995). *Laboratory and diagnostic tests with nursing implications* (4th ed.). Norwalk, CT: Appleton & Lange.

Kinsella, J. P. & Abman, S. H. (1999). Recent developments in inhaled nitric oxide therapy of the newborn. *Curr Opin Pediatr, 11*(2), 121–125.

Kupfer, Y. et al. (1987). Disuse atrophy in a ventilated patient with status asthmaticus receiving neuromuscular blockade. *Crit Care Med, 15*(8), 795–799.

Levine, R. L. (1994). Pharmacology of intravenous sedatives and opioids in critically ill patients. *Crit Care Clin, 10,* 709–731.

Lindberg, L. & Rydgren, G. (1999). Production of nitrogen dioxide during nitric oxide therapy using the Servo Ventilator 300 during volume-controlled ventilation. *Acta Anaesthesiol Scand, 43*(3), 289–294.

Lunn, R. J. (1995). Inhaled nitric oxide therapy. *Mayo Clin Proc, 70*(3), 247–255.

Marik, P., Hogan, J. & Krikorian, J. (1999). A comparison of bronchodilator therapy delivered by nebulization and meter-dose inhaler in mechanically ventilated patients. *Chest, 115*(6), 1653–1657.

McCartney, J. R. et al. (1993). Understanding and managing behavioral disturbances in the ICU. *J Crit Illness,* 87–97.

McCartney, J. R. et al. (1994). Anxiety and delirium in the intensive care unit. *Crit Care Clin, 10,* 673–680.

McEvoy, G. K. (Ed.). (1995). *AHFS drug information.* Bethesda: American Society of Health System Pharmacists.

Mirenda, J. et al. (1995). Propofol as used for sedation in the ICU. *Chest, 108,* 539–548.

Mohler, H. et al. (1977). Demonstration of benzodiazepine receptors in the central nervous system. *Science, 198,* 849–851.

Mohler, H. et al. (1988). The benzodiazepine receptor: A pharmacological control element of brain function. *Eur J Anaesthesiology,* (Suppl. 2), 15–24.

Mouloudi, E., Katsanoulas, K. & Anastasaki, M. et al. (1998). Bronchodilator delivery by metered-dose inhaler in mechanically ventilated COPD patients: Influence of end-inspiratory pause. *Eur Respir J, 12*(1), 165–169.

Ochikubo, C. G., Waffarn, F. & Turbow, R. et al. (1997). Echocardiographic evidence of improved hemodynamics during inhaled nitric oxide therapy for persistent pulmonary hypertension of the newborn. *Pediatr Cardiol, 18*(4), 282–287.

Olson, R. W. (1988). Barbiturates. *Int Anesthesiol Clin, 26,* 254.

Palmer, R. M. et al. (1987). Nitric oxide release accounts for the biological activity of endothelium-derived relaxing factor. *Nature, 327,* 425–526.

Price-Roberts, C. (1984). Cardiovascular and ventilatory effects of intrevenous anaesthetics. *Clin Anaesth 2,* 203.

Ramsay, M. A. E. et al. (1974). Controlled sedation with alphaloxone-alphadone. *Br Med J, 2,* 656–659.

Rau, J. L. (1998). *Respiratory care pharmacology (*4th ed.). Philadelphia: Mosby.

Reiss, B. S. et al. (1993). *Pharmacological aspects of nursing care* (4th ed.). Albany, NY: Delmar Publishers, Inc.

Reves, J. G. et al. (1990). Nonbarbiturate intravenous anesthetics. Chapter 9. In R. D. Miller (Ed.), *Anesthesia* (3rd ed.). New York: Churchill Livingstone.

Scanlan, C. L. et al. (1999). Egan's fundamentals of respiratory care. St. Louis: Mosby-Year Book.

Shelly, M. P. et al. (1986). Assessing sedation. *Crit Care Clin, 3,* 170–178.

Simon, H. B. (1993). Hyperthermia. *New Eng Journal of Medicine, 329,* 483–486.

Stamler, J. S. et al. (1992). Biochemistry of nitric oxide and its redox-activated forms. *Science, 258,* 1899–1902.

Teeple, J. R. E. (1990). Pharmacology and physiology of narcotics. *Crit Care Clin, 6,* 255–282.

Tortora, G. et al. (1999). *Principles of anatomy and physiology* (9th ed.). New York: John Wiley & Sons.

Watling, S. M. et al. (1994). Prolonged paralysis in an intensive care unit patient after the use of a neuromuscular blockade. *Crit Care Nur, 22*(5), 884–891.

Wessel, D. L. et al. (1994). Delivery and monitoring of inhaled nitric oxide in patients with pulmonary hypertension. *Crit Care Med, 22,* 930–938.

Wheeler, A. P. (1993). Sedation, analgesia and paralysis in the intensive care unit. *Chest, 104,* 566–576.

Witek, T. J. (1994). *Pharmacology and therapeutics in respiratory care.* Philadelphia: W.B. Saunders Co.

Ziment, I. (1978). *Respiratory pharmacology and therapeutics.* Philadelphia: W.B. Saunders Co.

Suggested Reading

Acute Pain Management Guideline Panel. (1992, February). Acute pain management: Operative or medical procedures and trauma. *Clinical Practice Guideline.* AHCPR Pub. No. 92-0032. Rockville, MD: Agency for Health Care Policy and Research, U.S. Department of Health and Human Services, Public Health Service.

Johnson, J. (1990). Delirium in the elderly. *Emerg Med Clin N Amer, 8,* 255–265.

Kehlet, H. (1989). Surgical stress: The role of pain and analgesia. *British Journal of Anaesthesia, 63,* 189–195.

Murray, M. J. (1990). Pain problems in the ICU. *Crit Care Clin, 6,* 235–253.

Reves, J. G. et al. (1990). Nonbarbiturate intravenous anesthetics. Chapter 9. In R. D. Miller (Ed.), *Anesthesia* (3rd ed.). New York: Churchill Livingstone.

Simon, H. B. (1993). Hyperthermia. *New Eng Journal of Medicine, 329,* 483–486.

Wattwil, M. (1989). Postoperative pain relief and gastrointestinal motility. *Acta Churgica Scandinavia, 550* (Suppl.), 140–145.

Westreich, L. et al. (1992). Delirium and acute psychosis. *Postgrad Med, 92,* 319–332.

CHAPTER FOURTEEN

WEANING FROM MECHANICAL VENTILATION

David W. Chang
James H. Hiers

OUTLINE

KEY TERMS

- compliance rate oxygenation and pressure (CROP) index
- pressure support ventilation (PSV)
- respiratory frequency to tidal volume (f/V_T) ratio
- simplified weaning index (SWI)
- SIMV (synchronized intermittent mandatory ventilation)
- T-tube weaning
- weaning procedure

INTRODUCTION

Weaning is the process of withdrawing mechanical ventilatory support and transferring the work of breathing from the ventilator to the patient. Weaning may be accomplished abruptly with the patient being directly transitioned from full ventilatory support to unassisted spontaneous breathing. This weaning approach is sometimes referred to as "taking the patient off the ventilator" or simply "discontinuing the ventilator."

Some patients can tolerate an abrupt termination of ventilatory support; this would include those who have been on the ventilator for a relatively short time (usually no more than one to two days) and who have also regained normal cardiopulmonary function. Examples include patients recovering from postanesthesia, drug overdose, and status asthmaticus.

For other patients, successful weaning requires a more gradual withdrawal of mechanical ventilatory support. Generally, the longer the patient has been on mechanical ventilation, the more gradual the weaning process should be. The process of gradually reducing mechanical ventilatory support must be individualized for each patient and the weaning process may take from days to weeks or even months. Indeed, some patients become ventilator dependent and may not be able to maintain adequate ventilation without mechanical assistance. Examples of these patients include high cervical spine (C-2) injury and some neuromuscular diseases.

DEFINITION OF WEANING SUCCESS AND FAILURE

✓ The process of gradually reducing mechanical ventilatory support must be individualized for each patient.

The ability to breathe spontaneously is the criterion to gauge the success or failure of weaning attempts. Weaning success means that a patient is able to maintain spontaneous breathing for a prescribed period of time. This usually leads to termination of mechanical ventilation. Weaning failure generally means that a patient is returned to mechanical ventilation after a period of unsustained spontaneous breathing.

WEANING SUCCESS

Weaning success is defined as effective spontaneous breathing without any mechanical assistance for 24 hours or more (Fiastro et al., 1988; Morganroth et al., 1984). While the spontaneous breaths are unassisted by mechanical means, supplemental oxygen, bronchodilators, pressure support, or continuous positive airway pressure are often used to support and maintain adequate spontaneous ventilation and oxygenation.

Success Rate.   Not all patients can be weaned from mechanical ventilation successfully on first attempt. In one study, the first weaning trial was successful in only 52% of 110 patients requiring mechanical ventilation (Pardee et al., 1984). The duration needed to wean a patient from mechanical ventilation may also vary greatly. Nett et al. (1984) reported that 15% of ventilator patients required more than 7 days to be weaned successfully.

The success rate of weaning attempts is partly dependent on the patient population. It is generally more difficult to predict the weaning outcome of medical patients. Since medical patients often have coexisting problems, they usually take more time to complete the weaning process than surgical patients (Yang et al., 1991).

WEANING FAILURE

Weaning failure is harder to define than weaning success. This is because whenever a patient is placed back on the ventilator, weaning attempt has failed in one form or another. However, most studies have defined weaning failure on the basis of abnormal blood gases at the end of weaning trial or clinical deterioration to an unacceptable critical threshold (Sahn et al, 1973; Tobin et al., 1986). Signs of worsening clinical condition include diaphoresis, evidence of increasing respiratory effort, tachycardia, arrhythmias, and hypotension (Yang et al., 1991).

Determining the threshold of abnormal blood gases and clinical condition can be a rather subjective process, depending on the background and experience of the physician. Also, the aggressiveness of one's weaning approach may also differ as to at what point the weaning trial has failed.

Since there are no simple objective measures for the assessment of weaning failure, it is defined here that weaning failure has occurred when the patient is returned to mechanical ventilation after any length of weaning trial.

Impact of Weaning Failure.   It is obvious that patients who require prolonged ventilator support have a severe impact on the use of health care resources, including financial, physical, and human resources. In addition, the longer a patient stays on the ventilator, emotional and psychological pains also take a toll. For these reasons, different strategies have been devised to enhance the weaning process. These strategies are

---

☑ Weaning success is defined as effective spontaneous breathing without any mechanical assistance for 24 hours or more.

☑ Since medical patients often have coexisting problems, they usually take more time to complete the weaning process than surgical patients.

☑ Signs of weaning failure include: abnormal blood gases, diaphoresis, increasing respiratory effort, tachycardia, arrhythmias, and hypotension.

TABLE 14-1   Conditions That May Hinder a Successful Weaning Outcome

CONDITIONS	EXAMPLES
Patient/pathophysiologic	Fever Infection Renal failure Sepsis Sleep deprivation
Cardiac/circulatory	Arrhythmias Blood pressure (high or low) Cardiac output (high or low) Fluid imbalance
Dietary/acid-base/electrolytes	Acid-base imbalance Electrolytes disturbance Anemia/dysfunctional hemoglobins

designed to minimize the use of our limited resources, and to keep the patients from the uncomfortable and sometimes painful diagnostic and therapeutic procedures associated with mechanical ventilation.

PATIENT CONDITION PRIOR TO WEANING

☑ Before weaning is attempted, the patient should be fully recovered and be able to assume spontaneous breathing.

Perhaps the first criterion to consider before any weaning attempt is to assess the patient's overall clinical condition. Two important questions pertaining to the patient's clinical condition are: (1) Has the patient significantly recovered from the disease or injury that prompted the need for mechanical ventilation? and, (2) Are there other clinical conditions that may interfere with the patient's ability to maintain the work of spontaneous breathing?

Assessment of the patient's overall clinical condition should include an evaluation of the clinical conditions in Table 14-1. Depending on the severity of these clinical conditions, they should be corrected or normalized prior to a weaning attempt.

WEANING CRITERIA

Weaning criteria are used to evaluate the readiness of a patient for weaning trial and the likelihood of weaning success. Weaning is more likely to succeed if a patient meets most of the criteria. On the other

TABLE 14-2 **Common Weaning Criteria**

CATEGORY	EXAMPLES	VALUES
Ventilatory criteria	$PaCO_2$	< 50 mm Hg with normal pH
	Vital capacity	> 10 to 15 ml/kg
	Spontaneous V_T	> 5 to 8 ml/kg
	Spontaneous RR (f)	< 30/min
	Minute ventilation	< 10 L
Oxygenation criteria	PaO_2 without PEEP	> 60 mm Hg @ F_IO_2 up to 0.4
	PaO_2 with PEEP	> 100 mm Hg @ F_IO_2 up to 0.4
	SaO_2	> 90% @ F_IO_2 up to 0.4
	Q_S/Q_T	< 20%
	$P(A-a)O_2$	< 350 mm Hg @ F_IO_2 of 1.0
	PaO_2/F_IO_2	> 200 mm Hg
Pulmonary reserve	Max. Voluntary Vent.	2x min vent @ F_IO_2 up to 0.4
	Max. Insp. Pressure	> −20 to −30 cm H_2O in 20 sec
Pulmonary measurements	Static compliance	> 30 ml/cm H_2O
	Airway Resistance	Observe trend
	V_D/V_T	< 60%

(Data from Burton et al., 1997; Caruso et al., 1999; Girault et al., 1994; Tobin et al., 1990; Yang et al., 1991.)

hand, if a patient can only meet one or two of the weaning criteria, the success rate is likely to be low.

Both subjective and objective measurements have been developed to determine a patient's readiness for weaning. The common weaning criteria are summarized in Table 14-2.

VENTILATORY CRITERIA

The ventilatory status of a patient may be used to evaluate the readiness and outcome of weaning attempts. Weaning success will be more likely if the patient can sustain an adequate ventilation. The generally acccepted ventilatory weaning criteria include a $PaCO_2$ of less than 50 mm Hg with normal pH, a vital capacity of greater than 10 to 15 ml/kg, a spontaneous V_T of greater than 5 to 8 ml/kg, a spontaneous respiratory rate of less than 30/min, and a minute ventilation of less than 10 L with satisfactory blood gases.

$PaCO_2$. The partial pressure of carbon dioxide in the arterial blood ($PaCO_2$) is the most reliable indicator of the patient's ventilatory status. Weaning from mechanical ventilation should be attempted only when the $PaCO_2$ is less than 50 mm Hg with a compensated pH (in the non-COPD patient).

In patients with normal lung functions, the $PaCO_2$ should be within the normal range of 35 to 45 mm Hg and the pH should be between

☑ The $PaCO_2$ should be between 35 and 45 mm Hg and the pH between 7.35 and 7.45 (COPD patients, the $PaCO_2$ may be around 50 mm Hg with a pH near 7.35).

7.35 to 7.45. However, in COPD patients, the acceptable $PaCO_2$ may be slightly higher and the pH slightly lower, depending on the patient's normal values prior to mechanical ventilation (Millbern et al., 1978).

Vital Capacity and Spontaneous Tidal Volume. The mechanical condition of the lungs may be evaluated by measuring the vital capacity and spontaneous tidal volume. It is generally accepted that the minimal vital capacity and spontaneous tidal volume consistent with successful weaning are 10 to 15 ml/kg, and 5 to 8 ml/kg, respectively (Pierson, 1982; Pierson, 1983; Tahvanainen et al., 1983). The results of 11 studies indicate that spontaneous tidal volume averaged 368 ml in weaned patients but only averaged 277 ml in nonweaned patients (Jabour et al., 1991).

✓ The minimal vital capacity and spontaneous tidal volume consistent with successful weaning are 10 to 15 ml/kg, and 5 to 8 ml/kg, respectively.

If the patient has been receiving full ventilatory support, it is advisable to allow the patient to breathe spontaneously for three minutes under close observation prior to measuring the vital capacity and spontaneous tidal volume. An equilibration period is needed to obtain the spontaneous effort based on the patient's actual respiratory requirement.

Unlike spontaneous tidal volume, vital capacity requires active patient effort and cooperation. Vital capacity measures the maximal amount of volume that the patient can expire following a maximal inspiration. For this reason, its validity is effort-dependent, and proper teaching and coaching are required for accurate measurements. Poor effort or inability to follow commands may result in lower than actual vital capacity measurement.

✓ The vital capacity maneuver is effort-dependent. Proper teaching and coaching are required for accurate and valid measurements.

Spontaneous Respiratory Rate. For a successful weaning outcome, the spontaneous respiratory rate should be less than 30 to 35 breaths per minute while the corresponding $PaCO_2$ should be less than 50 mm Hg (Pierson, 1983; Tahvanainen et al., 1983). A rate of greater than 35 breaths per minute is associated with an increased work of breathing that probably cannot be sustained by the patient. Increases in spontaneous respiratory rate after discontinuation of mechanical ventilation are strongly associated with weaning failure (Jabour et al., 1991).

✓ For a successful weaning outcome, the spontaneous respiratory rate should be less than 30 to 35 breaths per minute, while the corresponding $PaCO_2$ should be less than 50 mm Hg.

As with the spontaneous tidal volume measurement, if the patient has been receiving full ventilatory support, the patient should be allowed to breathe spontaneously for three minutes off the ventilator prior to measuring the spontaneous respiratory rate. This method allows the patient ample time to normalize the breathing pattern, thus more reflective of the patient's response to the respiratory requirements.

✓ The patient's minute volume should be *less* than 10 liters per minute for a successful weaning outcome.

Minute Ventilation. The patient's minute volume (either spontaneous or assisted) should be *less* than 10 liters per minute for a successful weaning outcome (assuming the corresponding $PaCO_2$ is normal). A high minute ventilation requirement (>10 L) needed to normalize the $PaCO_2$ implies that the work of spontaneous breathing will be excessive. The patient is unlikely to be able to sustain the increased work of breathing once the ventilator rate begins to reduce.

An excessive minute volume requirement may result from increased carbon dioxide production secondary to an increased metabolic rate, an increase in alveolar deadspace, or metabolic acidosis. Causes for increased carbon dioxide production include extensive burn injuries, an elevated body temperature, and sometimes overfeeding, especially with carbohydrate supplements. Alveolar deadspace will be increased if the alveolar ventilation exceeds the alveolar perfusion ($V/Q > 0.8$). This condition may occur when: (1) the alveoli are overventilated as in hyperinflation of the lungs (e.g., emphysema); and (2) the pulmonary circulation is underperfused (e.g., pulmonary embolism, decreased cardiac output).

OXYGENATION CRITERIA

The oxygenation status of a patient may be used to evaluate the readiness and outcome of weaning attempts. Weaning success will be more likely if the patient is adequately oxygenated. The generally accepted oxygenation weaning criteria include a PaO_2 of greater than 60 mm Hg (or $SaO_2 > 90\%$) on an F_IO_2 of 0.40 or less (Barnes, 1994), an intrapulmonary shunt of less than 20%, an alveolar-arterial oxygen tension gradient [$P(A\text{-}a)O_2$] gradient less than 350 mm Hg, and a PaO_2/F_IO_2 ratio greater than 200 mm Hg (Feeley et al., 1975; Girault et al., 1994).

☑ For a successful weaning outcome, the PaO_2 should be > 60 mm Hg on F_IO_2 ≤ 40%.

PaO_2 and SaO_2. A PaO_2 of 60 mm Hg corresponds to an SaO_2 of about 90%. It is essential to note that in patients with anemia or increased level of dysfunctional hemoglobins (carboxyhemoglobin), the PaO_2 and SaO_2 do not reflect the true oxygenation status of the patient. In those instances, the arterial oxygen content (CaO_2) should be measured and used.

If pulse oximetry is used to monitor a patient's oxygenation status, the pulse oximetry O_2 saturation (SpO_2) should be kept in the mid-90s for allowance of machine inaccuracies because SpO_2 readings in critical care are accurate to within 2 to 4% of the SaO_2 (Malley, 1990).

Q_S/Q_T. The physiologic shunt to total perfusion (Q_S/Q_T) ratio is used to estimate how much pulmonary perfusion is wasted. Shunted pulmonary perfusion cannot take part in gas exchange due to lack of ventilation (e.g., atelectasis). The Q_S/Q_T ratio can be calculated as follows using the classic physiologic shunt equation:

☑ See Appendix 1 for example.

$Q_S/Q_T = (CcO_2 - CaO_2) / (CcO_2 - CvO_2)$
Q_S/Q_T: Shunt percent in %
CcO_2: End-capillary oxygen content in vol%
CaO_2: Arterial oxygen content in vol%
CvO_2: Mixed venous oxygen content in vol%

☑ For a successful weaning outcome, the Q_S/Q_T should be < 20%.

In clinical settings, a calculated physiologic shunt of 10% or less is considered normal. Shunt of 10 to 20% indicates mild physiologic shunt, and shunt of 20 to 30% shows significant physiologic shunt. Greater than 30% shunt reflects critical and severe shunt (Malley, 1990; Shapiro et al., 1993).

Since physiologic shunt in mechanical ventilation is usually intrapulmonary in origin (inadequate ventilation in relation to pulmonary perfusion), weaning failure becomes very likely when spontaneous ventilation cannot keep up with the pulmonary perfusion. For this reason, significant and severe intrapulmonary shunt ($Q_S/Q_T > 20\%$) should be corrected in order to enhance the weaning process and secure a successful weaning outcome.

P(A-a)O_2. The alveolar-arterial oxygen tension gradient [$P(A-a)O_2$] is used to estimate the degree of hypoxemia and the degree of physiologic shunt. The $P(A-a)O_2$ gradient may be obtained by subtracting the measured PaO_2 from the calculated PAO_2 value. This gradient is directly related to the degree of hypoxemia or shunt (a larger gradient reflects more severe hypoxemia or shunt).

The alveolar-arterial oxygen tension gradient [$P(A-a)O_2$] can be calculated as follows:

$$P(A-a)O_2 = PAO_2 - PaO_2$$
$P(A-a)O_2$: Alveolar-arterial oxygen tension gradient in mm Hg
PAO_2: Alveolar oxygen tension in mm Hg
PaO_2: Arterial oxygen tension in mm Hg

☑ On 100% oxygen, every 50 mm Hg difference in $P(A-a)O_2$ approximates 2% physiologic shunt.

On room air, the $P(A-a)O_2$ should be less than 4 mm Hg for every 10 years in age. For example, the $P(A-a)O_2$ should be less than 24 for a 60-year-old patient. On 100% oxygen, every 50 mm Hg difference in $P(A-a)O_2$ approximates 2% physiologic shunt (Barnes, 1994; Burton et al., 1997; Shapiro et al., 1993).

☑ For a successful weaning outcome, the $P(A-a)O_2$ should be < 350 mm Hg while on 100% O_2.

In mechanical ventilation, $P(A-a)O_2$ of less than 350 mm Hg while on 100% oxygen suggests a strong likelihood of weaning success. $P(A-a)O_2$ of 350 mm Hg while on 100% oxygen approximates 14% shunt and values of greater than 350 mm Hg may hinder the weaning process. Any large $P(A-a)O_2$ gradient (> 350 mm Hg) should be corrected prior to the weaning trial.

☑ For a successful weaning outcome, the PaO_2/F_IO_2 index should be ≥ 200 mm Hg.

PaO_2/F_IO_2. The arterial oxygen tension to inspired oxygen concentration (PaO_2/F_IO_2) index is a simplified method for estimating the degree of intrapulmonary shunt. A PaO_2/F_IO_2 index of 200 mm Hg or higher is indicative of normal physiologic shunt and compatible to successful weaning trial (Girault et al., 1994).

PULMONARY RESERVE

A patient's pulmonary reserve may be assessed by measuring the vital capacity (VC) and maximum inspiratory pressure (MIP). The VC and MIP maneuvers require active patient cooperation and therefore these two measurements are effort dependent. Proper explanation, vigorous coaching, and allowance of an equilibration period to stimulate active respiratory drive are the prerequisites for valid and meaningful measurements.

☑ For a successful weaning outcome, the patient should have a VC > 10 to 15 ml/kg.

Vital Capacity (VC). The vital capacity (VC) reflects a patient's pulmonary reserve as it includes three lung volumes: inspiratory reserve volume, tidal volume, and expiratory reserve volume. VC measures the maximum amount of lung volume that the patient can exhale following maximal inspiration. Typically the patient is instructed to breathe in as deep as possible and exhale all the air into a spirometer. Unlike the forced vital capacity obtained in the pulmonary function lab, this VC maneuver does not require forceful exhalation. For successful weaning, the patient should have a VC of greater than 10 to 15 ml/kg (Pierson, 1982; Pierson, 1983; Tahvanainen et al., 1983).

☑ For a successful weaning outcome, the patient should be able to generate an MIP of > –30 cm H_2O.

Maximum Inspiratory Pressure (MIP). The maximum inspiratory pressure (also called negative inspiratory force) is the amount of negative pressure that the patient can generate in 20 seconds when inspiring against an occluded measuring device (negative pressure manometer) (Marini et al., 1986). If the patient is alert, explain the procedure and encourage the patient to attempt to inspire as forcibly as possible. The MIP is considered a measure of ventilatory muscle strength and weaning will likely be successful if the patient can generate an MIP of at least –30 cm H_2O. The results of 11 studies indicate that the MIP averaged –37 cm H_2O for weaned patients versus only –30 cm H_2O for nonweaned patients (Jabour et al., 1991).

PULMONARY MEASUREMENTS

Static compliance, airway resistance, and deadspace to tidal volume (V_D/V_T) ratio are three measurements that are not dependent on a patient's cooperation or effort. They are used to indicate the amount of pulmonary workload that is needed to support spontaneous ventilation. In general, low compliance, high airway resistance, and high V_D/V_T ratio all contribute to an increased workload. When these undesirable conditions reach the patient's threshold, they may hinder the weaning process and outcome.

☑ For a successful weaning outcome, the compliance should be ≥ 30 ml/cm H_2O.

Static Compliance. The static lung compliance is measured by dividing the patient's tidal volume (measured at the airway opening) by the difference in the plateau pressure and the PEEP. The lower the compliance, the greater the work of breathing will be. The minimal compliance value consistent with successful weaning is 30 ml/cm H_2O or greater (Hess et al., 1991).

The static lung compliance may be calculated as follows:

☑ See Appendix 1 for example.

$Cst = \Delta V / \Delta P$
Cst: Static lung compliance in mL/cm H_2O
ΔV: Corrected tidal volume in mL
ΔP: Pressure change (Plateau–PEEP) in cm H_2O

pressure support ventilation (PSV): *PSV is a mode in which the patient's spontaneous tidal volume is augmented by the application of a preset pressure plateau to the patient's airway for the duration of a spontaneous breath. It is used to reduce the work of breathing imposed by the endotracheal tube and ventilator circuit.*

Airway Resistance. The airway resistance can be calculated by dividing the difference in the peak inspiratory pressure and the plateau pressure by *constant* inspiratory flow rate. The normal range for airway resistance is 0.6 to 2.4 cm H_2O/L/sec (Burton et al., 1991) and higher for ventilator patients because of the associated pathological conditions (e.g., bronchospasm) and tubing resistance (e.g., endotracheal tube, ventilator circuit).

Although no critical weaning value for airway resistance has been established in the literature, the higher the airway resistance, the greater the work of breathing will be. The endotracheal (ET) tube contributes significantly to the airway resistance. The effect of resistance through the tube can be minimized by insuring that the ET tube is not kinked or the suction catheter of a continuous suction system (Ballard suction system) is not protruding into the tube. Since retained secretions and bronchospasm contribute to the airway resistance, the patient's airways and lungs should be suctioned as needed. Use of bronchodilators also may be helpful to reduce or reverse bronchospasm.

Pressure support ventilation (PSV) has been used successfully in reducing the circuit and airway resistance during spontaneous breathing. This strategy may be used in conjunction with the **SIMV** mode or other modes that include spontaneous ventilation.

SIMV (synchronized intermittent mandatory ventilation): *A mode of ventilation that permits spontaneous breaths between preset (mandatory) ventilator breaths. The ventilator breaths are synchronized (mandatory breaths that may come slightly sooner or later) to coincide with the patient's next inspiratory effort.*

Deadspace/Tidal Volume (V_D/V_T) Ratio. The deadspace to tidal volume (V_D/V_T) ratio indicates the amount of each breath that is "wasted" or not being perfused by pulmonary circulation. The higher the V_D/V_T ratio, the greater the minute volume demand will be. The V_D/V_T ratio can be calculated as the partial pressure of arterial carbon dioxide minus the mean partial pressure of the carbon dioxide in the exhaled air divided by the arterial blood carbon dioxide tension. For a successful weaning outcome, the V_D/V_T ratio should be 60% or less (Fitzgerald et al., 1976).

The deadspace to tidal volume (V_D/V_T) ratio can be calculated as follows:

☑ For a successful weaning outcome, the V_D/V_T ratio should be ≤ 60%.

☑ See Appendix 1 for example.

$V_D/V_T = (PaCO_2 - P\bar{E}CO_2) / PaCO_2$
V_D/V_T: Deadspace to tidal volume ratio in %
$PaCO_2$: Arterial carbon dioxide tension in mm Hg
$P\bar{E}CO_2$: Mixed expired carbon dioxide tension in mm Hg

COMBINED WEANING INDICES

In the early 1990s, some of the independent weaning criteria were combined to make up a cumulative index of weaning. Among the indices developed, three are simple to use and highly accurate in predicting weaning success. They are (1) Respiratory Frequency to Tidal Volume (f/V_T) Ratio, (2) Simplified Weaning Index (SWI), and (3) Compliance Rate Oxygenation and Pressure (CROP) Index. These combined weaning indices and the threshold values for successful weaning are listed in Table 14-3.

RESPIRATORY FREQUENCY TO TIDAL VOLUME RATIO (f/V_T)

Failure of weaning may be related to the development of a spontaneous breathing pattern that is rapid (high respiratory rate), and shallow (low tidal volume). The ratio of spontaneous respiratory rate divided by the spontaneous tidal volume (in liters) has been used to evaluate the presence and severity of this breathing pattern (Jacob et al., 1997; Tobin et al., 1986; Vassilakopoulos et al., 1998; Yang et al., 1991).

Rapid shallow breathing is quantified as the f (number of breaths per minute) divided by the V_T in liters and this breathing pattern induces inefficient, deadspace ventilation. When the f/V_T ratio becomes greater than 100 cycles/L, it suggests potential weaning failure. On the other hand, absence of rapid shallow breathing, as defined by an f/V_T ratio of less than 100 cycles/L, is a very accurate predictor of weaning success (Yang et al., 1991).

To measure the f/V_T ratio, the patient is taken off the ventilator and allowed to breathe spontaneously for three minutes or until a stable breathing pattern has been established. The minute expired volume (V_E) and respiratory frequency (f) are measured. The V_T is calculated by dividing the V_E by f. The procedure for measuring and calculating the f/V_T is outlined in Table 14-4.

respiratory frequency to tidal volume (f/V_T) ratio: The f/V_T ratio quantifies rapid shallow spontaneous breathing as the f (rate of spontaneous breathing) is divided by the V_T (depth of spontaneous breathing) in liters. Absence of rapid shallow breathing, as defined by an f/V_T ratio of less than 100 cycles/liter, is a very accurate predictor of weaning success.

☑ Rapid shallow breathing induces inefficient, deadspace ventilation.

☑ For a successful weaning outcome, the f/V_T ratio should be < 100 cycles/L.

TABLE 14-3 Combined Weaning Indices

TERM	NORMAL THRESHOLD FOR SUCCESSFUL WEANING
Respiratory Frequency to Tidal Volume Ratio (f/V_T)	< 100 breaths/min/L
Simplified Weaning Index (SWI)	< 9/min
Compliance Rate Oxygenation and Pressure (CROP) Index	≥ 13 ml/cycles/min

TABLE 14-4 Procedures to Obtain the f/V_T Ratio

PROCEDURE

1. Allow the patient to stabilize spontaneous breathing pattern
2. Use respirometer to measure expired volume and respiratory frequency for one minute
3. Divide minute volume by frequency (f) to obtain an average tidal volume (V_T)
4. Divide f by V_T to obtain f/V_T ratio

NOTE: See Appendix 1 for example.

SIMPLIFIED WEANING INDEX (SWI)

Calculation of the Simplified Weaning Index (SWI) is based on the following parameters: Ventilator respiratory rate (f_{mv}), peak inspiratory pressure (PIP), PEEP, spontaneous maximum inspiratory pressure (MIP), and $PaCO_2$ while receiving full ventilatory support ($PaCO_{2\ mv}$). The SWI can be calculated as follows:

☑ See Appendix 1 for example.

simplified weaning index (SWI): SWI evaluates a patient's ventilatory endurance and the efficiency of gas exchange. An SWI of less than 9/minute is highly predictive (93%) of weaning success.

$$SWI = \frac{f_{mv}\,(PIP - PEEP)}{MIP} \times \frac{PaCO_{2\ mv}}{40}$$

SWI: Simplified Weaning Index / min
f_{mv}: Ventilator frequency
PIP: Peak inspiratory pressure
PEEP: Positive end-expiratory pressure
MIP: Maximal inspiratory pressure
$PaCO_{2\ mv}$: Arterial CO_2 tension while on ventilator

When the SWI is less than 9/min, it is highly predictive (93%) of weaning success and when the SWI is greater than 11/min, there is a 95% probability of weaning failure (Jabour et al., 1991). SWI evaluates a patient's ventilatory endurance and the efficiency of gas exchange. Even though SWI is a simplified version of the original weaning index, its simplicity and exclusive use of common parameters make this index a practical method of assessment during routine ventilator care.

☑ When the SWI is less than 9/min, it is highly predictive (93%) of weaning success.

COMPLIANCE RATE OXYGENATION AND PRESSURE (CROP) INDEX

The Compliance Rate Oxygenation and Pressure (CROP) Index evaluates a patient's pulmonary gas exchange and the balance between respiratory demands and respiratory neuromuscular reserve. A CROP index of 13 ml/breaths/min. or higher is predictive of weaning success (Yang et al., 1991). The CROP index is calculated as follows:

$$CROP = \frac{\left[C_{DYN} \times MIP \times \dfrac{PaO_2}{PAO_2} \right]}{f}$$

compliance rate oxy-genation and pres-sure (CROP) index:
The CROP index evaluates a patient's pulmonary gas exchange and the balance between respiratory demands and respiratory neu-romuscular reserve. A CROP index of 13 ml/breaths/min or higher is predictive of weaning success.

weaning procedure:
A systemic approach to wean a patient off mechanical ventila-tion by using a set of clinical measure-ments as a guide.

T-tube weaning: A technique of wean-ing by alternating the patient between spontaneous aerosol T-tube breathing (5 minutes) and full ventilatory support (30 to 180 minutes). The duration of T-tube use is gradu-ally increased as tolerated by the patient.

CROP: Compliance Rate Oxygenation and Pressure Index
C_{DYN} (dynamic compliance): Volume delivered/(peak airway pressure – PEEP)
MIP (maximum inspiratory pressure): Most negative pressure recorded during 20 seconds of airway occlusion
PaO_2: Arterial oxygen tension
PAO_2: Alveolar oxygen tension
f (frequency): Spontaneous respiratory rate per minute

WEANING PROCEDURE

The **weaning procedure** may be carried out by one or more of the following procedures: **T-tube weaning**, synchronized intermittent mandatory ventilation (SIMV), and pressure support ventilation (PSV). Selection of the weaning procedure is dependent on the pa-tient's ability to breathe spontaneously and the level of muscular strength to overcome the airway resistance. The suggested steps for each procedure are outlined in Table 14-5.

T-TUBE WEANING

Once a decision is made to proceed with weaning, the patient may be discontinued from full ventilator support and placed on an aerosol T-tube or weaned more gradually by progressively decreasing the level of ventilatory support (Dries, 1997; Vallverdu et al., 1998). The T-tube weaning method may be useful for patients with normal car-diopulmonary status who require only brief mechanical ventilation. Abrupt termination of ventilatory support is usually reserved for patients who have been on the ventilator for a relatively short time (usually for no more than two to three days), and who appear to have substantially recovered from the need for mechanical ventilation. Generally speaking, the longer a patient has been on the ventilator, the longer the weaning process.

If a patient is to be weaned gradually, there are basically three approaches that may be used. Prior to the introduction of IMV/SIMV, the only available method of "gradually" weaning a patient was the technique of alternating the patient between spontaneous aerosol T-tube breathing and full ventilatory support (Nett et al., 1984). Initially, the patient is placed on a T-tube for 5 minutes and returned to full support for approximately 30 to 180 minutes. The process is repeated with progressively more time on the T-tube and less time on full support until either the patient is weaned or it appears that the patient is not ready to be weaned.

SIMV

SIMV weaning alleviates the need to alternate the patient on T-tube and ventilatory support. Since most current generation ventilators

TABLE 14-5   **Common Weaning Procedures**

PROCEDURE	STEPS
T-Tube weaning	(1) May use new aerosol setup or existing ventilator circuit; (2) Let patient breathe spontaneously for up to 5 min every 30 to 180 min; (3) Return patient to mechanical ventilation to rest; (4) Increase duration of spontaneous breathing gradually for up to 2 hours each time; (5) If patient tolerates step (4), consider extubation when blood gases and vital signs are satisfactory.
SIMV	(1) Reduce SIMV (ventilator) rate by 1 to 3 breaths per min; (2) Obtain blood gases after 30 min; (3) Reduce SIMV rate further until a rate of close to 0 is reached. This may take only hours for patients with normal cardiopulmonary functions but days for those with abnormal functions; (4) If patient tolerates step (3), consider extubation when blood gases and vital signs are satisfactory.
PSV	(1) PSV may be used in conjunction with spontaneous breathing or SIMV mode; (2) Start PSV at a level of 5 to 15 cm H_2O (up to 40 cm H_2O) to augment spontaneous V_T until a desired (high) V_T or (low) spontaneous RR is obtained; (3) Decrease pressure support (PS) level by 3 to 6 cm H_2O intervals until a level of close to 0 is reached; (4) If patient tolerates step (3), consider extubation when blood gases and vital signs are satisfactory.

(Data from Downs et al., 1974; Girault et al., 1999; MacIntyre, 1986; Milbern et al., 1978; Nett et al., 1984; Tobin et al., 1990.)

have an SIMV mode, weaning with the SIMV mode is probably the most simple and common weaning approach. Weaning with SIMV is accomplished by progressive decreases in the mandatory SIMV respiratory rate (usually 1 to 3 breaths per minute at each step). Arterial blood gases are measured after 30 minutes or more at that setting (Tobin et al., 1990). If the pH remains above 7.30 or 7.35 (Downs et al., 1974; Milbern et al., 1978), the SIMV rate is further reduced in further steps until a rate of close to zero is reached. The pace of SIMV weaning is dictated by the patient's tolerance. Some patients may be weaned using SIMV in a few hours while other patients may take much longer.

☑ The pace of SIMV weaning is dictated by the patient's tolerance.

PRESSURE SUPPORT VENTILATION

Pressure support ventilation (PSV) is also commonly applied during SIMV weaning. PSV helps to reduce the airway resistance imposed on the patient by the endotracheal tube and ventilator circuit. Some clinicians advocate weaning with pressure support as a stand alone mode.

✓ Weaning with PSV is done by starting the pressure support level at 5 to 15 cm H$_2$O and adjusting it gradually (up to 40 cm H$_2$O) until a desired spontaneous V$_T$ or spontaneous rate (<25/min) is obtained.

Regardless of the weaning approach used, it is advisable to provide full ventilatory support at night to allow the patient to rest (Barnes, 1994).

Weaning with PSV is done by starting the pressure support level at 5 to 15 cm H$_2$O and adjusting it gradually (up to 40 cm H$_2$O) until a desired V$_T$ is obtained (MacIntyre, 1986). Some practitioners titrate the pressure support level until a desired spontaneous rate is reached, typically 25 BPM or less. This approach is clinically relevant since an increased spontaneous tidal volume corresponds with a decreased spontaneous rate. If the patient tolerates the weaning process well, the pressure support level is gradually decreased by 3 to 6 cm H$_2$O increments until a level of close to 0 cm H$_2$O is reached. Extubation may be considered when the patient's blood gases and vital signs remain satisfactory (Tobin et al., 1990).

SIGNS OF WEANING FAILURE

Once the weaning process has been started, the previously described weaning criteria should be monitored closely to insure that the patient is tolerating the weaning attempt. When the mechanical ventilatory support is decreased, part of the work of breathing is shifted to the patient. The goal for the patient is to maintain the work of spontaneous breathing and adequate oxygenation. If the patient tolerates the increased work of breathing and the weaning criteria remain within acceptable limits, then the amount of ventilatory support (e.g., SIMV rate, pressure support level) should again be decreased. This process is repeated if the patient tolerates the decrease of ventilatory support. The weaning process should be stopped if the patient shows signs of muscle fatigue or ventilatory failure.

✓ Early signs of weaning failure include: tachypnea, use of accessory muscles and paradoxical abdominal movements, dyspnea, chest pain, chest-abdomen asynchrony, and diaphoresis.

Early signs of weaning failure include tachypnea, use of accessory muscles, and paradoxical abdominal movements (Cohen et al., 1982). Other indications that the patient cannot maintain the work of breathing may include dyspnea, chest pain, chest-abdomen asynchrony, and diaphoresis (Jabour et al., 1991). Some specific indicators of weaning failure are listed in Table 14-6.

If the patient does not tolerate the weaning procedure, the patient should be returned to full ventilatory support and be allowed to rest. The patient should then be reassessed in order to determine the cause of weaning failure. Appropriate therapies may then be applied before attempting the weaning process again.

CAUSES OF WEANING FAILURE

Aside from the pathological conditions that lead to the need for mechanical ventilation, weaning failure may occur when the work

TABLE 14-6   Indicators of Weaning Failure

INDICATORS	EXAMPLES
Blood Gases	Increasing $PaCO_2$ (> 50 mm Hg) Decreasing pH (< 7.30) Decreasing PaO_2 (< 60 mm Hg) Decreasing SpO_2 (< 90%)
Vital Signs	Changing blood pressures (20 mm Hg systolic or 10 mm Hg diastolic) Increasing heart rate (by 20/min, or > 110/min) Abnormal ECG (presence of arrhythmias)
Respiratory Parameters	Decreasing V_T (< 250 ml) Increasing RR (f) (> 30/min) Increasing RR/V_T (f/V_T) ratio (> 100 cycles/L) Decreasing MIP (< −20 cm H_2O) Decreasing static compliance (< 30 mL/cm H_2O) Increasing V_D/V_T (> 60%)

(Data from Burton et al., 1997; Girault et al., 1994; Jabour et al., 1991; Jubran & Tobin, 1997; Tobin et al., 1990; Yang et al., 1991.)

☑ Weaning failure is generally related to (1) increase of air flow resistance, (2) decrease of compliance, or (3) respiratory muscle fatigue.

of spontaneous breathing becomes too great for the patient to sustain. Weaning failure is generally related to (1) increase of air flow resistance, (2) decrease of compliance, or (3) respiratory muscle fatigue.

INCREASE OF AIR FLOW RESISTANCE

Normal subjects using an endotracheal (ET) tube have an increase of 54% to 240% in the work of breathing depending on the size of the ET tube and ventilator flow rate (Fiastro et al., 1988). An 8-mm ET tube has a cross-sectional area of 50 mm², which is slightly smaller than the average cross-sectional area of the adult glottis (66 mm²), the narrowest part of the airway (Kaplan et al., 1991). To minimize the effects of artificial airway on air flow resistance, ET tubes of size 8 or larger should be used when it is appropriate to the patient's size. In addition, the ET tube may be cut to about an inch from the patient's lips so as to minimize the air flow resistance contributed by the length of the ET tube. The cut section of the ET tube should be displayed prominently so others would not presume that the ET tube had been moved deep into the brochus.

☑ ET tubes of size 8 or larger should be used to reduce the air flow resistance.

Other strategies for decreasing airway resistance can easily be done by periodic monitoring of the ET tube for kinking or obstructions by secretions, or other devices attached to the ET tube such as a continuous suction catheter, heat and moisture exchanger (HME, "artificial nose") or end-tidal CO_2 monitor probe. Frequent suctioning to remove retained secretions and use of bronchodilators to relieve bronchospasm have also been used successfully to reduce the air flow resistance.

Other causes for an increased work of breathing include abdominal distention or an increased carbon dioxide production. Abdominal distention may contribute to an increased work of breathing if it interferes with diaphragmatic movement. An increased metabolic rate will result in an increased carbon dioxide production which in turn will require an increased minute volume to "blow off" the CO_2. An increased metabolic rate may be due to disease or injury or it may result from excessive nutritional support, especially if carbohydrate substrates are being administered.

Tracheal obstruction may cause weaning failure in patients requiring long-term mechanical ventilation (Rumbak et al., 1999). The ventilator may also contribute to an increased work of breathing. A low demand valve sensitivity, a relatively long demand valve response time, or an inadequate inspiratory flow delivered by the ventilator are conditions that increase the patient's work of breathing.

DECREASE OF COMPLIANCE

☑ Low lung or thoracic compliance makes lung expansion difficult and it is a major contributing factor to respiratory muscle fatigue and weaning failure.

Abnormally low lung or thoracic compliance impairs the patient's ability to maintain efficient gas exchange. Low compliance makes lung expansion difficult and it is a major contributing factor to respiratory muscle fatigue and weaning failure.

In situations where the compliance gradually decreases (ARDS), the resultant refractory hypoxemia and increased work of breathing may lead to muscle fatigue and ventilatory failure. When this occurs to a patient undergoing a weaning trial, return to the mechanical ventilator is almost inevitable. Table 14-7 shows some examples that lead to a decreased compliance measurement.

RESPIRATORY MUSCLE FATIGUE

Respiratory work is a product of transpulmonary pressure and tidal volume. Studies have been done to evaluate the relationship between the work of breathing and a patient's ability to sustain adequate spontaneous ventilation.

TABLE 14-7 Clinical Conditions that Decrease the Compliance

TYPE OF COMPLIANCE	CLINICAL CONDITIONS
Static compliance	Atelectasis
	ARDS
	Tension pneumothorax
	Obesity
	Retained secretions
Dynamic compliance	Bronchospasm
	Kinking of ET tube
	Airway obstruction

Work of Breathing = P_{TP} (transpulmonary pressure) $\times$ V_T (tidal volume)

The transpulmonary pressure is increased in conditions of low compliance or high airway resistance. Normally a threshold work value of 1.6 kg.m/min or less is needed before ventilator-dependent patients can be weaned and assume adequate spontaneous breathing. Conditions leading to an increased work load such as low compliance and high air flow resistance may lead to respiratory muscle fatigue and eventual ventilatory failure. A threshold work value of 1.7 kg.m/min or higher is associated with failure to wean from mechancial ventilation (Tobin et al., 1990; Vassilakopoulos et al., 1996).

Another condition that may cause respiratory muscle dysfunction is due to muscular atrophy secondary to prolonged full ventilatory support and muscle disuse. Other factors that may contribute to muscle weakness include a low oxygen delivery (low O_2 content or cardiac output), insufficient nutrition or electrolyte imbalance, especially hypokalemia, hypophosphatemia, hypocalcemia, and hypomagnesemia (Knochel, 1982).

Retraining of atrophied muscles may be accomplished by short T-tube trials that improve strength. Pressure support ventilation may also be tried as it increases diaphragmatic endurance (Hess et al., 1991).

TERMINAL WEANING

☑ Terminal weaning is defined as withdrawal of mechanical ventilation that results in the death of a patient.

Terminal weaning is defined as withdrawal of mechanical ventilation that results in the death of a patient. This differs from withholding of mechanical ventilation in which the patient is not placed on any mechanical ventilatory support.

Decisions to withdraw life-support measures (e.g., mechanical ventilation, nutritional support) have become more common. This trend is partly due to the public's awareness of the quality of life issue, and their knowledge that death is an inevitable process in spite of medical advances, state-of-the-art medical equipment, and pulmonary rehabilitation strategies (Jacavone & Young, 1998). It is also partly due to the availability of living wills, and the choices available to the patient and family members.

When terminal weaning is considered, three concerns must be evaluated and discussed: (1) patient's informed request, (2) medical futility, and (3) reduction of pain and suffering (Campbell et al., 1992).

☑ Discussions on a patient's informed consent should be done over a period of time so that emotion, pain, and other intangible factors do not interfere with an informed and valid decision.

Patients' informed consent means that patients agree to have the life-sustaining devices removed, and that they understand the potential consequences (including death). No matter who initiates the discussion, the talk with patients must be open and honest. These discussions should also be done over a period of time so that emotion, pain, and other intangible factors do not interfere with an informed and valid decision.

☑ **Terminal weaning may be justified if medical intervention is futile or hopeless.**

Terminal weaning may be justified if medical intervention is futile or hopeless. The interpretation of futility (hopelessness) is based on the past experience of the primary physician or specialist. Schneiderman et al. (1990) suggested that medical treatments may be futile if physicians have concluded that in the last 100 similar cases the treatments were useless. This type of objective assessment may be helpful to the patients or family members who have reservations about terminal weaning and uncertainties about the chances of recovery.

☑ **Another reason for terminal weaning is to stop pain and suffering.**

Another reason for terminal weaning is to stop pain and suffering associated with the disease process (e.g., cancer), medical treatments (e.g., radiation therapy), medical procedures (e.g., arterial puncture, incisional wounds), and psychological trauma (e.g., being totally dependent on others in an unfamiliar surrounding, unable to care for self, to eat, or talk).

Terminal weaning carries many ethical and legal implications. Each health care facility should have resource persons and standard protocol on terminal weaning available to the patients and family members, preferably before the needs arise. It is beyond the scope of this section to cover the ethical implications of terminal weaning in detail. The readers are encouraged to seek other available medical ethics books to learn more about this topic.

SUMMARY

Weaning from mechanical ventilation is not always easy because there are no absolute criteria that can guarantee successful weaning every time. The criteria for weaning provided in this chapter are based on results of research studies and experience of clinical trials from many sources. While these criteria cannot be expected to be accurate at all times, they are nevertheless very useful as a guide and a starting point for weaning trials.

From the review of available literature, it is reasonable to conclude that the more weaning criteria that are met by a patient, the more likely the weaning process will be successful. In addition to using as many clinical parameters as feasible, the patient's progress should also be monitored on a continuing basis. From these data and trends, changes and adjustments on the ventilator and treatment plan may then be made to enhance the weaning outcome.

Self-Assessment Questions

1. Which of the following patient conditions is the *least important* consideration prior to weaning a patient off mechanical ventilation?

   A. frequent arrhythmias

   B. ventilatory failure

   C. severe acidosis

   D. use of positive end-expiratory pressure (PEEP)

2. The physician asks you to evaluate the following ventilatory parameters for possible weaning attempt on a 40-year-old patient. You would report to the physician that the only parameter that suggests successful weaning is:

A. spontaneous RR (f) = 40/min.

C. minute ventilation = 12 L.

B. spontaneous V_T = 7 ml/kg.

D. $PaCO_2$ = 55 mm Hg.

3. The oxygenation status of a 30-year-old postoperative patient shows: PaO_2 = 65 mm Hg, SaO_2 = 85%, Q_S/Q_T = 25%, PaO_2/F_IO_2 = 118 mm Hg, F_IO_2 = 55%. Based on these measurements, you would recommend to the physician that weaning _____ begin because _____ of the measurements presented above are within the normal limits for a weaning attempt.

A. should, 50%

C. should not, none

B. should, all

D. should not, 50%

4. All of the following pulmonary measurements suggest readiness for weaning attempt *except*:

A. maximal inspiratory pressure = −18 cm H_2O.

C. static compliance = 32 ml/cm H_2O.

B. V_D/V_T = 50%.

D. maximum voluntary ventilation = 3 times the minute ventilation.

5. A ventilator patient has the following oxygen content measurements: CcO_2 = 21.1 vol %, CaO_2 = 18.8 vol %. CvO_2 = 14.4 vol %. The calculated shunt is about _____ and it can be interpreted as _____ shunt.

A. 3.4%, mild

C. 34%, severe

B. 17%, significant

D. 66%, severe

6. The PaO_2 of a ventilator patient is 250 mm Hg on 100% oxygen. If the PAO_2 is 680 mm Hg, what is the alveolar-arterial oxygen tension gradient? What is the estimated shunt if every 50% mm Hg difference approximates 2% shunt?

A. 430 mm Hg, 8%

C. 940 mm Hg, 17%

B. 430 mm Hg, 17%

D. 940 mm Hg, 34%

7. Ms. Warren, a ventilator patient recovering from drug overdose, has a PaO_2 of 76 mm Hg on 30% (0.30) oxygen. What is the PaO_2/F_IO_2 ratio? Is it normal based on the oxygenation criteria for weaning?

A. 25.3, normal

C. 253, normal

B. 25.3, abnormal

D. 253, abnormal

8. A patient has the following measurements while receiving mechanical ventilation: corrected tidal volume = 480 ml, peak airway pressure = 45 cm H_2O, plateau pressure = 30 cm

H_2O, PEEP = 8 cm H_2O. What is the calculated static compliance? Is it normal based on the pulmonary measurement criteria for weaning?

A. 11 ml/cm H_2O, normal

B. 11 ml/cm H_2O, abnormal

C. 22 ml/cm H_2O, normal

D. 22 ml/cm H_2O, abnormal

9 to 11. Match the combined weaning indices with the normal threshold for a successful weaning attempt.

Combined Weaning Index	Normal Threshold
9. Respiratory Frequency to Tidal Volume Ratio (f/V_T)	A. < 9/min
10. Simplified Weaning Index (SWI)	B. $\geq$ 13 ml/cycles/min
11. Compliance Rate Oxygenation and Pressure (CROP) Index	C. < 100 breaths/min/L

12. _____ weaning is done by reducing the ventilator respiratory rate gradually.

A. T-tube

B. Synchronized intermittent mandatory ventilation (SIMV)

C. Positive end-expiratory pressure (PEEP)

D. Pressure support ventilation (PSV)

13. All of the following trends may be used as indicators of weaning failure with the *exception* of:

A. decreasing PaO_2.

B. increasing $PaCO_2$.

C. increasing V_T.

D. decreasing static compliance.

14. Terminal weaning is defined as _____ of mechanical ventilation that results in the _____ of a patient.

A. withholding, vegetative state

B. withholding, death

C. withdrawal, vegetative state

D. withdrawal, death

References

Barnes, T. A. (1994). *Core textbook of respiratory care practice* (2nd ed.). St. Louis: Mosby-Year Book.

Baumeister, B. L. et al. (1997). Evaluation of predictors of weaning from mechanical ventilation in pediatric patients. *Pediatr Pulmonol, 24*(5), 344–352.

Burton, G. G. et al. (1997). *Respiratory care: A guide to clinical practice* (4th ed.). Philadelphia: J.B. Lippincott.

Campbell, M. L. et al. (1992). Terminal weaning from mechanical ventilation: Ethical and practical considerations for patient management. *Am J Crit Care, 3,* 52–56.

Caruso, P. et al. (1999). The unidirectional valve is the best method to determine maximal inspiratory pressure during weaning. *Chest, 115*(4), 1096–1101.

Cohen, C. A. et al. (1982). Clinical manifestations of inspiratory muscle fatigue. *Am J Med, 73,* 308–316.

Downs, J. B. et al. (1974). Intermittent mandatory ventilation: An evaluation. *Arch Surg, 109,* 519–523.

Dries, D. J. (1997). Weaning from mechanical ventilation. *J Trauma, 43*(2), 372–384.

Feeley, T. W. et al. (1975). Weaning from controlled ventilation and supplemental oxygen weaning from intermittent positive pressure ventilation. *N Engl J Med, 292,* 903–906.

Fiastro, J. F. et al. (1988). Comparison of standard parameters and the mechanical work of breathing in mechanically ventilated patients. *Chest, 94,* 232–238.

Fiastro, J. F. et al. (1988). Pressure support compensation for inspiratory work due to endotracheal tubes and demand continuous positive airway pressure. *Chest, 93,* 499–505.

Fitzgerald, L. M. et al. (1976). Weaning the patient from mechanical ventilation. *Heart Lung, 5,* 228–234.

Girault, C. et al. (1994). Weaning criteria from mechanical ventilation. *Monaldi Arch Chest Dis, 49*(2), 118–124.

Girault, C. et al. (1999). Noninvasive ventilation as a systematic extubation and weaning in acute-on-chronic respiratory failure: A prospective, randomized controlled study. *Am J Respir Crit Care Med, 160*(10), 86–92.

Hess, D. et al. (1991). Mechanical ventilation: Initiation, management and weaning. In G. G. Burton, J. E. Hodgkin, J. J. Ward (Eds.), *Respiratory care: A guide to clinical practice* (3rd ed.). Philadelphia: J.B. Lippincott.

Jabour, E. R. et al. (1991). Evaluation of a new weaning index based on ventilatory endurance and the efficiency of gas exchange. *Am Rev Respir Dis, 144,* 531–537.

Jacavone, J. & Young, J. (1998). Use of pulmonary rehabilitation strategies to wean a difficult-to-wean patient: Case study. *Crit Care Nurse, 18*(6), 29–37.

Jacob, B. et al. (1997). The unassisted respiratory rate/tidal volume ratio accurately predicts weaning outcome in postoperative patients. *Crit Care Med, 25*(2), 253–257.

Jubran, A. & Tobin, M. J. (1997). Pathophysiologic basis of acute respiratory distress in patients who fail a trial of weaning from mechanical ventilation. *Am J Respir Crit Care Med, 155*(3), 906–915.

Kaplan, J. D. et al. (1991). Physiologic consequence of tracheal intubation. *Clin Chest Med, 12,* 425–432.

Knochel, J. P. (1982). Neuromuscular manifestations of electrolyte disorders. *Am J Med, 72,* 521–533.

MacIntyre, N. R. (1986). Respiratory function during pressure support ventilation. *Chest, 89,* 677–683.

Malley, W. J. (1990). *Clinical blood gases—Application and noninvasive alternatives.* Philadelphia: W.B. Saunders Co.

Marini, J. J. et al. (1986). Estimation of inspiratory muscle strength in mechanically ventilated patients: The measurement of maximal inspiratory pressure. *J Crit Care, 1,* 32–38.

Millbern, S. M. et al. (1978). Evaluation of criteria for discontinuing mechanical ventilatory support. *Arch Surg, 113,* 1441–1443.

Morganroth, M. L. et al. (1984). Criteria for weaning from prolonged mechanical ventilation. *Arch Intern Med, 144,* 1012–1016.

Nett, L. M. et al. (1984). Weaning from mechanical ventilation: A prospective and review of techniques. In R. C. Bone (Ed.), *Critical care: A comprehensive approach.* Park Ridge, IL: American College of Chest Physicians.

Pardee, N. E. et al. (1984). Bedside evaluation of respiratory distress. *Chest, 85,* 203–206.

Pierson, D. J. (1982). Acute respiratory failure. In S. A. Sahn (Ed.), *Pulmonary emergencies.* New York: Churchill Livingstone.

Pierson, D. J. (1983). Weaning from mechanical ventilation in acute respiratory failure: Concepts, indications and techniques. *Respir Care, 28,* 646–662.

Rumbak, M. J. et al. (1999). Significant tracheal obstruction causing failure to wean in patients requiring prolonged mechanical ventilation: A forgotten complication of long-term mechanical ventilation. *Chest, 115*(4), 1092–1095.

Sahn, S. A. et al. (1973). Bedside criteria for discontinuation of mechanical ventilation. *Chest, 63,* 1002–1005.

Schneiderman, L. J. et al. (1990). Medical futility: Its meaning and ethical implications. *Ann Intern Med, 112,* 949–954.

Shapiro, B. A. et al. (1993). *Clinical application of blood gases* (5th ed.). St. Louis: Mosby-Year Book.

Tahvanainen, J. et al. (1983). Extubation criteria after weaning from intermittent mandatory ventilation and continuous positive airway pressure. *Crit Care Med, 11,* 702–707.

Tobin, M. J. et al. (1986). The pattern of breathing during successful and unsuccessful trials of weaning from mechanical ventilation. *Am Rev Respir Dis, 134,* 1111–1118.

Tobin, M. J. et al. (1990). Weaning from mechanical ventilation. *Crit Care Med, 6*(3), 725–747.

Vallverdú, I. et al. (1998). Clinical characteristics, respiratory functional parameters, and outcome of a two-hour T-piece trial in patients weaning from mechanical ventilation. *Am J Respir Crit Care Med, 158*(6), 1855–1862.

Vassilakopoulos, T. et al. (1996). Respiratory muscles and weaning failure. *Eur Respir J, 9*(11), 2383–2400.

Vassilakopoulos, T. et al. (1998). The tension-time index and the frequency/tidal volume ratio are the major pathophysiologic determinants of weaning failure and success. *Am J Respir Crit Care Med, 158*(2), 378–385.

Yang, K. L. et al. (1991). A prospective study of indexes predicting the outcome of trials of weaning from mechanical ventilation. *N Engl J Med, 324,* 1445–1450.

Suggested Reading

Terminal Weaning

American Thoracic Society Medical Section of the American Lung Association. (1991). Withholding and withdrawal of life-sustaining therapy. *Am Rev Respir Dis. 144,* 726–731.

Bone, R. C. et al. (1990). ACCP/SCCM consensus panel: Ethical and moral guidelines for the initiation, continuation and withdrawal of intensive care. *Chest, 97,* 949–958.

Campbell, M. L. et al. (1999). Patient responses during rapid terminal weaning from mechanical ventilation: A prospective study. *Crit Care Med, 27*(1), 73–77.

The Ethics Committee of the Society of Critical Care Medicine. (1997). Consensus statement of the Society of Critical Care Medicine's Ethics Committee regarding futile and other possibly inadvisable treatments. *Crit Care Med, 25,* 887–891.

Fair allocation of intensive care unit resources. (1997). Official Statement of the American Thoracic Society. *Am J Respir Crit Care Med 156,* 1282–1301.

Gilligan, T. & Raffin, T. A. (1996). Withdrawing life support: Extubation and prolonged terminal weans are inappropriate. *Crit Care Med, 24*(2), 352–353.

Robb, Y. A. (1997). Ethical considerations relating to terminal weaning in intensive care. *Intensive Crit Care Nurs, 13*(3), 156–162.

Tasota, F. J. & Hoffman, L. A. (1996). Terminal weaning from mechanical ventilation: Planning and process. *Crit Care Nurs Q, 19*(3), 36–51.

Therapist-driven Protocol

Ely, E. W. et al. (1999). Large scale implementation of a respiratory therapist-driven protocol for ventilator weaning. *Am J Respir Crit Care Med, 159*(2), 439–446.

Weaning

Chao, D. C. & Scheinhorn, D. J. (1998). Weaning from mechanical ventilation. *Crit Care Clin, 14*(4), 799–817, viii.

Leitch, E. A. et al. (1996). Weaning and extubation in the intensive care unit. Clinical or index-driven approach? *Intensive Care Med, 22*(8), 752–759.

Vassilakopoulos, T. et al. (1999). Weaning from mechanical ventilation. *J Crit Care, 14*(1), 39–62.

Weaning of Infant/Pediatric Patients

Baumeister, B. L. et al. (1997). Evaluation of predictors of weaning from mechanical ventilation in pediatric patients. *Pediatr Pulmonol 24*(5), 344–352.

Khan, N. et al. (1996). Predictors of extubation success and failure in mechanically ventilated infants and children. *Crit Care Med 24*(9), 1568–1579.

CHAPTER FIFTEEN

NEONATAL MECHANICAL VENTILATION

Kent B. Whitaker

——— OUTLINE ———

KEY TERMS

- **compression factor**
- **extracorporeal membrane oxygenation (ECMO)**
- **high frequency ventilation (HFV)**
- **inspiratory time (I Time)**
- **mean airway pressure (MAWP)**

- **peak inspiratory pressure**
- **pressure-limited ventilator**
- **surfactant**
- **surfactant replacement**

INTRODUCTION

Neonatal mechanical ventilation provides a different kind of challenge to many respiratory care practitioners because neonates have different requirements (normal and abnormal physiologic and laboratory values) from those of adults. Also, caring for neonates often requires very different respiratory care equipment, supplies, and techniques. Above all, keen senses and the ability to observe and evaluate a neonate in distress is the most critical element because they cannot talk.

This chapter provides a working outline of respiratory care procedures in caring for a neonate in distress. These procedures focus on neonatal care and range from intubation and surfactant instillation immediately after birth to different types of neonatal mechanical ventilation.

INTUBATION

In most instances, intubation of the trachea is a necessary part of mechanical ventilation of the neonate. An exception is the use of external negative thoracic pressure. It is beyond the scope of this chapter to cover in detail the procedure for neonatal intubation. Those interested in studying the procedure are referred to any of the several excellent neonatal/pediatric respiratory texts for that information. Here, the indications, equipment, and general considerations of neonatal mechanical ventilation are covered.

☑ Indications for intubation include an Apgar score of 0 to 3, difficult to ventilate, thick meconium stain, and diaphragmatic hernia.

INDICATIONS

The most common situation requiring intubation is during resuscitative efforts following delivery. Intubation is indicated during a resuscitation if: 1) the patient has an Apgar score of 0 to 3, indicating secondary apnea (please note that this is based on an immediate evaluation of the newborn, not at 3 minutes); 2) bag and mask ventilation is difficult or ineffective; 3) thick meconium is present in the amniotic fluid; or 4) the neonate is suspected of having a diaphragmatic hernia. Intubation is additionally indicated in the presence of obstructive lesions such as Pierre-Robin syndrome, tracheomalacia, tracheal web, tracheal stenosis, laryngeal paralysis, and extrinsic masses. Other indications include assisting in removal of pulmonary secretions, maintaining the airway during surgery, and obtaining tracheal cultures.

Table 15-1 shows a method of assessing the neonate using the Apgar score. Parameters listed are assigned points based on findings shown in the table. The scores range from 0 to 10. It is done immediately after birth (usually called 1-minute Apgar) and after 3 or 5 minutes.

EQUIPMENT

The first piece of equipment needed for an intubation is a laryngo-scope and blade with a functioning light. A Miller blade, size 0 is used for most newborns and all preemies. Some newborns and older infants (generally > 5 kg) require a Miller size 1. Next, an appropriately sized endotracheal tube (ETT) is obtained. While the ultimate decision of ETT size is based on the experience of the intubator and possibly the guidelines of the specific hospital, Table 15-2 outlines a general guide for determining ETT size.

Equipment to suction the airway, adhesive tape or other securing device for the ETT, a resuscitation bag and mask with a 100% oxygen

✓ Use laryngo-scope blade size 0 for most newborns and all preemies; size 1 for older infants (> 5 kg).

TABLE 15-1 Apgar Score

	0	1	2
Heart rate	None	Slow (<100) Irregular	Over 100
Respiratory effort	Apnea	Irregular, shallow Gasping	Good, crying
Muscle tone	Flaccid	Some flexion of extremities	Well flexed
Reflex	No response to stimulus	Grimace	Cough or sneeze
Color	Pale blue	Blue extremities, pink body	Pink all over

TABLE 15-2 Appropriate-Sized Neonatal Endotracheal Tubes

TUBE SIZE (ID MM)	WEIGHT	GESTATIONAL AGE
2.5	Below 1,000 gm	Below 28 weeks
3.0	1,000 to 2,000 gm	28 to 34 weeks
3.5	2,000 to 3,000 gm	34 to 38 weeks
4.0	Above 3,000 gm	Above 38 weeks

source, and an assistant are also needed. The assistant helps by handing equipment to the intubator, monitoring the patient during the attempt, and helping secure the tube. The patient should be continuously monitored during the attempt with an ECG and pulse oximeter. Intubation attempts should be limited to 30 seconds to minimize hypoxia. Between attempts, the neonate is manually ventilated with 1.0 F_IO_2 to help stabilize the PaO_2.

SURFACTANT REPLACEMENT THERAPY

It has long been understood that the primary dysfunction in respiratory distress syndrome (RDS) is abnormally high alveolar surface tension resulting from a lack of pulmonary **surfactant.** Thus it became an item of major interest in the scientific community to develop a surfactant that can be administered to an infant to replace that which is lacking (Robertson & Halliday, 1998).

Naturally occurring surfactant is composed of several phospholipids and lipids, and four or more specific apoproteins. Each component appears to have its own distinct characteristics with regard to production, secretion, and removal (Jobe & Ilkegami, 1993). These factors have made it difficult to produce an ideal replacement surfactant.

Approximately 90% of surfactant is phospholipid, with phosphatidylcholine (PC) comprising 85% of the total amount. Roughly 60% of the PC is dipalmitoyl phosphatidylcholine (DPPC). It is the DPPC that allows surfactant to lower the surface tension of alveoli (Holm & Waring, 1993). The remaining phospholipids are phosphatidylglycerol (PG) and phosphatidylinositol (PI). Cholesterol is the predominant neutral lipid in surfactant. The four proteins found in surfactant, given the names of surfactant proteins A, B, C, and D (SP-A, etc.), make up 5% to 10% of the total. While small in quantity, their presence is essential for proper activity of pulmonary surfactant (Holm & Waring, 1993).

HISTORY

Early studies were discouraging as researchers could not find the right combination of components that formed an effective surfactant. Effective dosages and ideal method of delivery were two other questions that hindered the development of **surfactant replacement** therapy.

Early surfactants were made with DPPC and were nebulized into the trachea. This type of surfactant alone and method of delivery did not produce the desired results. Continued research and later studies of surfactant and its biochemical and biophysical properties illustrated the important role of the other proteins and lipids. New surfactants were developed that included the additional lipids and proteins.

Delivery was changed from nebulization to direct instillation of surfactant into the trachea at higher dosages than had previously been used. These discoveries had dramatic effects on the surfactant-deficient premature lung, with rapid weaning of pressures and F_IO_2 levels.

INDICATIONS

There are currently two protocols for the administration of surfactant. Prophylactic administration of surfactant is indicated for those infants who are at a high risk of developing RDS. Included are those infants born before 32 weeks, with weight less than 1,300 grams, and those with a lecithin to sphingomyelin (L/S) ratio less than 2:1, or the absence of phosphatidylglycerol (PG) in the amniotic fluid. Under this protocol, the infant receives the surfactant as quickly following delivery as possible (Table 15-3).

Therapeutic ("rescue") administration is not given until the patient develops signs of RDS. Indications include those infants who require ventilatory assistance due to increased work of breathing (grunting, nasal flaring, retractions), those with increasing oxygen requirements (shunting), and those who have chest radiographic evidence of RDS (ground glass appearance).

TYPES OF SURFACTANT AND DOSAGES

Currently used surfactants fall into one of two categories: those obtained from mammalian lungs and those that are synthetically produced. Typically, the mammalian preparations contain all surfactant proteins, whereas the synthetics are protein-free. There are currently two surfactants that are FDA-approved. Survanta®, which is produced by mincing bovine (cow) lung tissue and Exosurf Neonatal®, which is synthetic. A randomized trial comparing the two surfactants failed to find any advantage in using one over the other (Horbar et al., 1993). Both surfactants have been found to be effective for the treatment of RDS (Modanlou et al., 1997).

☑ Prophylactic use of surfactant is indicated for infants at risk of RDS, less than 32-week gestation, less than 1,300 grams, L/S ratio less than 2:1, or absence of PG in the amniotic fluid.

☑ Therapeutic (rescue) use of surfactant is indicated in RDS (grunting, nasal flaring, retractions), increasing oxygen requirements and positive chest radiograph.

☑ Survanta® is produced by mincing cow lung tissue. Exosurf Neonatal® is a synthetic preparation.

TABLE 15-3   Indications of Surfactant Replacement

APPLICATION	CRITERIA
Prophylactic use	Gestational age < 32 weeks Body weight < 1,300 gm L/S ratio < 2:1 Absence of PG in amniotic fluid

Therapeutic (rescue) use	Signs of RDS
	    (grunting, nasal flaring, retractions, cyanosis)
	Increasing oxygen requirement
	Positive chest radiograph for RDS
	    (ground glass appearance)

In prophylatic therapy Exosurf Neonatal® (colfosceril palmitate) is administered as soon as possible after birth in a dosage of 5 ml/kg birth weight. (Each ml of Exosurf contains 13.5 mg of active ingredient.) If necessary, second and third doses may be given 12 and 24 hours following the initial dose. For rescue therapy, 5 ml/kg is given, and it is followed by another dose 12 hours later (Witek & Schachter, 1994).

The recommended dosage for prophylatic or rescue use of Survanta (beractant) is 4 ml/kg or 100 mg/kg birth weight. (Each ml of Survanta contains 25 mg of active ingredient.) Repeat doses of the same amount may be given at least 6 hours following the preceding dose (Witek & Schachter, 1994; Robertson & Halliday, 1998).

OUTCOMES

✓ Surfactant replacement therapy reduces the severity of RDS and the incidence of some related cardiopulmonary complications.

On the positive side, surfactant replacement therapy appears to reduce the severity of RDS, pulmonary interstitial emphysema (PIE), and epithelial necrosis (Pinar et al., 1994), reduces pulmonary vascular resistance (Kaapa et al., 1993), improves lung function (Yuksel et al., 1993), and has beneficial long-term effects on airway resistance (Abbasi et al., 1993). Additionally, synthetic surfactants may reduce the incidence of bronchopulmonary dysplasia (BPD) and intraventricular hemorrhage (IVH) (Long, 1993).

Another study found that surfactant replacement therapy may actually predispose an infant to intraventricular hemorrhage (IVH) (Gunkel & Banks, 1993). Surfactant replacement does not work on all patients. It is not known why some patients have a transient response and others have no response. Perhaps as knowledge and understanding continue to advance in this area, we will discover those unknown factors that prevent successful use of surfactant replacement therapy in all neonates.

Since coming of age, surfactant replacement therapy has dramatically decreased the mortality rate from RDS in neonates. It should now be considered the standard of care for those neonates with RDS who require mechanical ventilation (Parmigiani et al., 1997; Wiswell & Mendiola, 1993).

BASIC PRINCIPLES OF NEONATAL VENTILATION

Essentially all mechanical ventilators used in the neonatal population are classified as pressure-limited ventilators. They generate a sufficient flow and deliver variable tidal volumes by a preset pressure limit. Recently, mechanical ventilation by monitoring and adjusting the volume setting has gained some popularity.

pressure-limited ventilator: A ventilator that ends the inspiratory phase once the preset pressure limit is reached. The volume delivered by a pressure-limited ventilator is directly related to the preset pressure and is variable dependent on the compliance and airway resistance of a patient.

PRESSURE-LIMITED, TIME-CYCLED VENTILATION

Most neonatal ventilators are classified as continuous flow, pressure-limited, and time-cycled. In contrast to a volume-cycled ventilator, a **pressure-limited ventilator** delivers variable tidal volumes depending on the patient's compliance and airway resistance.

In general, a decreasing compliance or an increasing airway resistance requires a higher pressure limit to maintain the same tidal volume. As the patient's condition improves (increased compliance or decreased airway resistance), the pressure limit may be decreased to avoid excessive ventilation and possible barotrauma.

Basic Design. Figure 15-1 shows the basic design of neonatal pressure-limited ventilators. Compressed air and oxygen are connected to an oxygen blender, either within the ventilator or attached to the exterior.

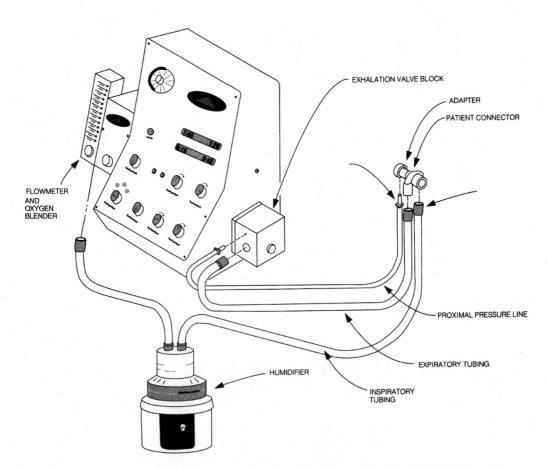

Figure 15-1 Basic design of a neonatal pressure-limited ventilator (Sechrist IV–100B) showing the flowmeter and oxygen blender, patient circuit, and humidifier.

☑ Pressure-limited ventilators deliver a variable tidal volume depending on the patient's compliance and airway resistance. Conditions accompanied by low compliance or high airway resistance require a higher pressure limit on the ventilator.

A flowmeter is placed on the outflow of the blender and delivers a steady flow of mixed gas into the patient circuit. The gas is then warmed and humidified and is carried along the inspiratory line to the patient connection.

During the expiratory phase, the gas continues past the patient connection into the expiratory tubing. The expiratory tubing connects to the expiratory valve, which uses a rubber diaphragm or a balloon to seal off the expiratory line during inspiration.

Altering Frequency. Neonatal ventilators use either a rate knob or an expiratory timer to determine frequency of ventilation. When the determined time for exhalation has ended, the timing mechanism of the rate knob or the expiratory timer signals the closure of the expiratory valve. This occurs mechanically with a solenoid valve or a flow of gas that pushes against a rubber diaphragm and seals off the expiratory line. Other ventilators inflate a small rubber balloon in the expiratory valve that occludes the expiratory line. With the occlusion of the expiratory line, the continuous flow of gas builds up pressure within the circuit, and flow is diverted into the endotracheal tube and the patient's lungs.

Older neonatal ventilators offer the choice of intermittent mandatory ventilation (IMV) and CPAP. Newer generation ventilators now offer synchronized IMV (SIMV) and Assist Mode, in addition to IMV and CPAP.

peak inspiratory pressure: The maximum pressure reached by a ventilator during the inspiratory phase.

Determining Peak Inspiratory Pressure. The level to which the pressure builds up in the circuit is preset by the operator. The **peak inspiratory pressure** is limited by a pop-off valve, or by limiting the pressure applied to the expiratory valve, allowing excess pressure in the circuit to slowly escape the valve. This pressure limit does not stop inspiration, but merely limits the inspiratory pressure.

Once the inspiratory pressure limit is reached, flow is diverted out of the pop-off valve or out the expiratory valve and flow to the patient virtually ceases. The result is an inspiratory hold, where the volume in the lungs remains static until expiration occurs.

inspiratory time (I time): The time required to complete the inspiratory phase. I time (sec) multiplied by the flow rate (ml/sec) approximates the tidal volume (ml).

Setting Inspiratory Time. The duration of inspiration, or **inspiratory time (I time),** is determined by an inspiratory timer control and is set by the operator. The inspiratory timer begins timing the breath at the instant the expiratory timer signals the closure of the valve. When the predetermined time has been reached, the inspiratory timer opens the valve and exhalation occurs passively from the lungs.

VENTILATOR CIRCUITS AND HUMIDIFIERS

During mechanical ventilation, some of the ventilator volume is "lost" within the circuit and humidifier and is not delivered to the patient. This wasted volume is called the compressible volume, and it is partly *compression factor: The amount of expansion of the ventilator circuit or humidifier during the inspiratory phase measured in ml/cm H_2O. This volume is considered "lost" and unavailable to the patient.*

✓ To minimize volume loss the circuit and humidifier used in a neonatal ventilator should have small compressible volume.

✓ Heated wire inside the inspiratory tubing reduces condensation.

caused by the positive pressure applied to these devices. Higher inspiratory pressures would cause the circuit and humidifier to expand more than those under low pressures. This compressible volume is also dependent on the characteristics of the circuit and humidifier. More compliant circuits and humidifiers would expand more under positive pressure than those with low compliance.

Circuit Compression Factor. Neonatal ventilator circuits should have a very low **compression factor**, that is, they should have minimal expansion when pressure is applied. A highly compliant circuit would expand under pressure and absorb a large portion of the volume of gas that should be delivered to the patient.

Humidifiers. Humidifiers that are used in a neonatal circuit should possess a small compressible volume. The larger the compressible volume, the more expansion occurs under pressure. A humidifier with a large compressible volume may hold more volume than the patient's lungs and thus greatly reduce patient ventilation.

The ideal humidifiers for neonatal ventilation are types that incorporate a wick-type system, as they provide excellent warming and humidifying properties and maintain a low compressible volume.

Ideally, the temperature of the gas at the trachea should be 32 to 34°C (Chatburn, 1991). When inspired gas temperature is measured at the patient connection, the humidifier must heat the gas 3 or 4 degrees above the desired temperature to overcome the loss of heat after the gas exits the humidifier. One problem that occurs in this type of ventilator circuit is condensation or "rain-out" inside the tubing.

"Rain-out" occurs when the warmed and humidified gas exits the humidifier and makes contact with the cooler walls of the tubing. This causes the gas temperature to decrease and condensation to occur on the tubing wall. The water accumulated in the ventilator tubing may result in increased airway resistance, a higher risk of contamination, and the potential of accidentally draining the water into the patient's lungs. A water trap placed in-line with the ventilator circuit helps to prevent these hazards.

Heated Wire Circuits. To counter this problem, many ventilator circuits have a heated wire inside the inspiratory tubing that runs from the humidifier to the patient connection, shown in Figure 15-2. The heated wire is attached to a servo-controller before its entry into the circuit. The temperature of the gas is measured as it exits the canister and is controlled by the humidifier. The temperature is again measured at the patient connection by the servo-controller.

The servo heats the gas flow in the inspiratory tubing by heating the wire, which then heats the inspired gas. Both the humidifier and servo work from a negative feedback mechanism. The desired temperature becomes the set point and as the actual temperature drops

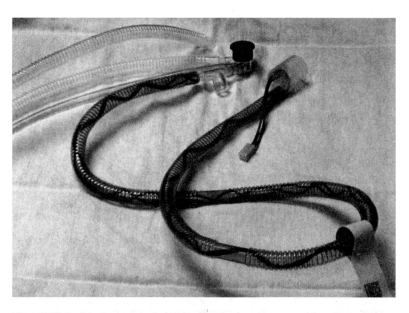

Figure 15-2   Heated wire circuit inside the inspiratory tubing that runs from the humidifier to the patient connection. The heated wire is attached to a servo-controller for temperature regulation.

below the set point, power is increased until the temperature returns to the desired level. Newer circuits heat the expiratory gas in addition to the inspiratory flow, thus minimizing condensation in the expiratory line.

One potential problem with this system is found when the distal temperature probe is placed at the patient connection inside a heated incubator that is set at a higher temperature than the humidifier. As the inspiratory tubing enters the incubator, the gas is heated to the set temperature of the incubator environment. This causes the temperature probe to sense the higher temperature and shut down the heater wires. The result is a buildup of condensation in the inspiratory tubing.

The solution to this problem is to place the distal temperature probe just outside the inlet to the incubator. This allows the probe to measure the actual gas temperature and properly regulate the heater wires (Chatburn, 1991).

☑ To prevent premature shutdown (power off) of the heated wire, the temperature probe should be placed just outside the inlet to the incubator.

INITIATION OF NEONATAL VENTILATOR SUPPORT

Indications for neonatal ventilatory support are based on three general guidelines: apnea, hypercapnia, and hypoxemia. These guidelines are similar to those used for adult patients. Unlike adult ventilators that use a tidal volume control to adjust the tidal volume, neonatal ventilators use a peak inspiratory pressure control to deliver an approximate tidal volume. Another unique feature of most neonatal ventilators includes the use of the flow rate and inspiratory time (I time) to fine tune the tidal volume. The suggested initial ventilatory parameters for neonatal mechanical ventilation are discussed below.

INDICATIONS FOR MECHANICAL VENTILATION

Mechanical ventilation provides two important physiologic functions. First, it maintains elastic properties and lung volumes by preventing or correcting atelectasis. By maintaining an appropriate FRC, lung compliance is maintained at an optimal level. Mechanical ventilation supplies the work of breathing when the patient is unable to maintain these properties. Second, mechanical ventilation provides the appropriate removal of CO_2 and the addition of inspired oxygen to meet the needs of the patient who cannot maintain arterial PO_2 or PCO_2 at normal levels.

☑ Mechanical ventilation is indicated when the patient is unable to maintain adequate blood gas values through spontaneous breathing.

Mechanical ventilation is therefore indicated when any condition causes a decrease in lung function and an increase in work of breathing that the patient is unable to overcome and when the patient is unable to maintain normal blood gas values through spontaneous breathing. The exact criteria used to determine the need for mechanical ventilation are difficult to define. Each institution establishes its own criteria for initiation of mechanical ventilation. Table 15-4 lists general guidelines used to indicate the need for mechanical ventilation.

INITIAL VENTILATOR PARAMETERS

The initial ventilator parameters depend on several factors, including the gestational age and weight of the neonate, the disease state present, and the type of ventilator being used. In general, the smaller the neonate, the higher the incidence of barotrauma. Therefore, it is desirable to initiate these patients at lower pressures when possible. Disease states in which lung compliance is reduced will require higher initial pressures than normal or high compliance states. The presence of air leaks requires low pressures and high rates. Finally, some ventilators may require a tidal volume to be set by the operator.

☑ The initial pressure setting is higher for neonates with low compliance; lower for air leaks.

TABLE 15-4 General Indications for Initiating Neonatal Mechanical Ventilation

1. Apnea
   a. due to prematurity
   b. secondary to intraventricular hemorrhage
   c. due to drug depression
2. $PaCO_2$ acutely rising with concurrent decrease in pH
3. PaO_2 acutely below 50 mm Hg with supplemental oxygen

With respect to the above factors, Table 15-5 lists suggested starting ventilator parameters.

Since the tidal volume (V_T) control is not available on a pressure-limited ventilator, an estimated V_T can be calculated by multiplying the inspiratory time (I time) and flow rate, as follows:

Example: On a pressure-limited ventilator, the I time and flow rate are set at 0.5 sec and 6 LPM, respectively. What is the calculated V_T?

$$V_T = \text{I time (second)} \times \text{flow rate (liters per minute)}$$
$$= 0.5 \text{ sec} \times 6 \text{ l/m}$$
$$= 0.5 \text{ sec} \times 6000 \text{ ml}/60 \text{ sec}$$
$$= 0.5 \text{ sec} \times 100 \text{ ml/sec}$$
$$= 50 \text{ ml}$$

Once mechanical ventilation is initiated, the ventilator settings are fine tuned until appropriate arterial blood gases are achieved. Blood gas measurement can be achieved by obtaining arterial blood from a peripheral or umbilical artery catheter (UAC), peripheral artery puncture, or capillary blood from a finger or heel stick. Under most circumstances, a $PaO_2 > 50$ mm Hg, a $PaCO_2$ 35 to 45 mm Hg, and a pH between 7.3 to 7.45, are acceptable for a UAC sample. An appropriately done capillary sample will roughly correlate with arterial PCO_2, pH and HCO_3^-, and thus share the same acceptable values. A capillary PO_2 is usually not acceptable as a determinant of oxygenation status and requires the use of a pulse oximeter or transcutaneous PO_2 monitor.

☑ The normal arterial blood gases for neonates are: $PO_2 > 50$ mm Hg, a $PaCO_2$ 35 to 45 mm Hg, and a pH between 7.3 to 7.45. For capillary samples, a lower PO_2 is acceptable.

TABLE 15-5 **Initial Neonatal Mechanical Ventilation Parameters**

PARAMETER	NORMAL COMPLIANCE	LOW COMPLIANCE
PIP	15 to 20 cm H_2O	20 to 40 cm H_2O
PEEP	3 to 5 cm H_2O	up to 8 cm H_2O
V_T*	10 to 12 ml/kg	10 to 12 ml/kg
Rate	40/min	Up to 150/min (esp. with air leak)
Flow Rate	6 to 8 LPM	6 to 8 LPM
I Time	0.5 sec	Change according to rate to maintain an I:E ratio of 1:1
I:E Ratio	1:1.5 to 1:2	At least 1:1
F_IO_2	Set to keep patient pink using SpO_2 or transcutaneous pO_2 readings	Set to keep patient pink using SpO_2 or transcutaneous pO_2 readings Use with appropriate PEEP level

*On ventilators that are capable of providing a preset tidal volume (volume-controlled ventilation).
(Data from Bandy et al., 1992; Goldsmith et al., 1993.)

Common exceptions to these values are in the case of chronic lung disease patients such as pulmonary interstitial emphysema in which higher $PaCO_2$'s are acceptable, and patients treated for pulmonary hypertension, where high PO_2's, low PCO_2's and high pH's are used.

HIGH FREQUENCY VENTILATION (HFV)

high frequency ventilation (HFV): *A type of ventilation that uses very high frequencies. It is subdivided into three categories: high frequency positive pressure ventilation (60 to 150 cycles/minute); high frequency jet ventilation (240 to 660 cycles/minute); and high frequency oscillatory ventilation (480 to 1,800 cycles/minute).*

Since the explosion of research in neonatal medicine started some 20 years ago, there is an ongoing search for a better method of ventilation to maintain adequate blood gas levels without inflicting damage on the premature lung. Several exciting methods have evolved to address these concerns.

The normally held understanding of ventilation is that the tidal volume must exceed the amount of physiologic deadspace for alveolar ventilation to occur. Conventional ventilation utilizes this principle by inflating the patient's lungs with a tidal volume that exceeds deadspace and inflates the alveoli. Expiration then occurs by the passive recoil of the thorax and lung.

High frequency ventilation (HFV) is a ventilation technique that delivers small tidal volumes at very high frequencies. Early studies involving HFV showed that adequate ventilation occurred even when tidal volumes far below deadspace were used (Carlo & Chatburn, 1988).

☑ HFV is a technique of ventilation that delivers small tidal volumes at very high frequencies.

The major advantage of delivering small tidal volumes is that it can be done at relatively low pressures, greatly reducing the risk of barotrauma. Despite the fact that HFV offers the advantage of oxygenation and ventilation at a lower risk of barotrauma, it has not been shown to be superior to conventional ventilation and its use is often limited to those situations in which conventional ventilation has failed. It appears to be most useful in treating RDS and pneumonia (Clark, 1994).

☑ HFV uses low pressures to deliver small tidal volumes. This reduces the risk of barotrauma.

HFV is delivered at rates between 150 and 3,000 cycles/minute (breaths/minute). The major types of HFV are categorized by the frequency of ventilation and the method with which the tidal volume is delivered. The three categories examined here are high frequency positive pressure ventilation, high frequency jet ventilation, and high frequency oscillation (Table 15-6).

HIGH FREQUENCY POSITIVE PRESSURE VENTILATION (HFPPV)

HFPPV is simply conventional ventilatory breaths delivered at rates between 60 and 150 breaths/minute (1 to 2.5 Hz). The delivery of tidal volume during HFPPV appears to occur via convective air movement, in which tidal volume exceeds deadspace (Boynton, 1986). Modern neonatal ventilators can deliver HFPPV at rates up to 150/minute.

TABLE 15-6 Classification of High Frequency Ventilation

TYPE OF HIGH FREQUENCY VENTILATOR	FREQUENCY (HERTZ)*	FREQUENCY (CYCLES/MIN)
High Frequency Positive Pressure Ventilation (HFPPV)	1 to 2.5 Hz	60 to 150
High Frequency Jet Ventilation (HFJV)	4 to 11 Hz	240 to 660
High Frequency Oscillatory Ventilation (HFOV or HFO)	8 to 30 Hz	480 to 1800

*1 Hertz (Hz) = 1 cycle/sec or 60 cycles/min

✔ HFPPV is indicated on those patients who are hypoxemic or hypercapnic despite adequate and appropriate conventional ventilation.

Indications. HFPPV is indicated on those patients who are hypoxemic or hypercapnic despite adequate and appropriate conventional ventilation. Studies have shown a reduction in $PaCO_2$ and in F_IO_2 when HFPPV was used on these patients. These studies additionally showed a lower incidence of pneumothoraces in the neonates ventilated with HFPPV when compared to those receiving conventional ventilation (Boynton, 1986). There are also studies that have shown that fighting the ventilator by the neonate may be eliminated at ventilatory rates of 100 to 120 breaths/minute (Milner & Hoskins, 1989).

mean airway pressure (MAWP): The average airway pressure during a complete respiratory cycle. It is directly affected by the respiratory rate, inspiratory time, peak inspiratory pressure, and positive end-expiratory pressure.

Clinical Use. In the presence of severely noncompliant lungs, increases in peak inspiratory pressure may reach dangerous levels before an adequate tidal volume is achieved. In these cases, the rate is increased to increase minute ventilation, allowing the peak pressure to remain lower. As rates increase, the inspiratory time is decreased to allow adequate exhalation of the tidal volume. This requires that time constants be low to allow exhalation and prevent air trapping. Continuous monitoring of $PaCO_2$ and PaO_2 will help the practitioner achieve the rate needed to attain the desired minute ventilation.

✔ HFPPV increases the risk of barotrauma and cardiac compromise.

Hazards. As the rate of positive pressure breaths increases, the **mean airway pressure (MAWP)** increases concurrently. The increasing MAWP greatly heightens the risk for barotrauma and cardiac compromise. The neonate is also at a higher risk of developing intracranial bleeding with increasing MAWP. The ability to suction the airway is diminished, as even short-term removal from the ventilator may result in severe hypoxemia and hypercapnia.

✔ See Appendix 1 for example.

$$MAWP = \left[\left(\frac{RR \times I\ time}{60}\right) \times (PIP - PEEP)\right] - PEEP$$

MAWP: Mean airway pressure
RR: Respiratory rate
I time: Inspiratory time
PIP: Peak inspiratory pressure
PEEP: Positive end-expiratory pressure

HIGH FREQUENCY JET VENTILATION (HFJV)

High frequency jet ventilators generally operate at rates between 240 to 660 per minute (4 to 11 Hz). The high frequency jet ventilator delivers a high pressure pulse of gas to the patient's airway. This is done through a special adaptor attached to the endotracheal tube, or through a specially designed endotracheal tube that allows the pulsed gas to exit inside the endotracheal tube, depicted in Figure 15-3.

☑ The indications for using HFJV include severe pulmonary disease that is complicated by air leaks and other pulmonary problems.

Indications.   The indications for using HFJV include severe pulmonary disease that is complicated by air leaks, pulmonary hypoplasia, restrictive lung disease, and persistent pulmonary hypertension (Gordin, 1989).

Clinical Use.   HFJV is used in tandem with conventional ventilators. The purpose of the conventional ventilator is threefold. First, it provides occasional sighs that help stimulate the production of surfactant and prevent microatelectasis. Second, the conventional ventilator provides PEEP to the patient's airway. Third, it makes a continuous flow of gas available at the endotracheal tube for entrainment by the jet ventilation (Gordin, 1989).

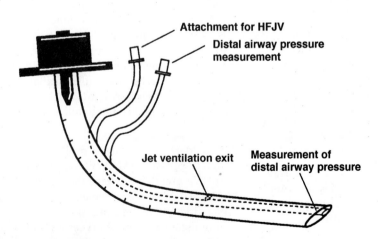

Attachment for HFJV
Distal airway pressure measurement
Jet ventilation exit
Measurement of distal airway pressure

Figure 15-3   The high frequency jet ventilator (HFJV) delivers a high pressure pulse of gas to the patient's airway through a specially designed endotracheal tube that allows the pulsed gas to exit inside the endotracheal tube.

✓ The principle hazard of HFJV is damage to the trachea and large airways leading to necrotizing tracheo-bronchitis.

✓ To minimize tracheal damage, the high pressure pulse of gas exits inside the endotracheal tube via a special tube.

✓ Transillumination of the infant chest can be used to detect tension pneumothorax.

Hazards. The principle hazard of HFJV is damage to the trachea and large airways leading to necrotizing tracheobronchitis. Originally thought to be caused by poor humidification, it is now believed to be caused by the impact of the high pressure gas "bullets" on the wall of these airways (Milner & Hoskins, 1989).

To offset damage, HFJV should only be delivered through a special catheter that exits internally to the endotracheal tube or via a special triple-lumen endotracheal tube, previously mentioned. The triple-lumen tube incorporates the jet injector and a pressure monitoring port in the lumen of standard-sized endotracheal tubes.

Other hazards include gas trapping, hyperinflation, obstruction of the airway with secretions, hypotension, and inflammatory injury to the trachea (Gordin, 1989; Richardson, 1988).

Of concern with the use of HFJV is the difficulty encountered in assessing the patient. Auscultation of breath sounds and heart sounds is difficult due to the constant vibration and noise produced by the ventilator. Assessment of these patients is based on the observation of other clinical signs. Decreased lung compliance and pneumothoraces are observed by a decrease in chest wall vibration, increased $PaCO_2$, and a decreased PaO_2. A decrease in chest wall vibration and an increase in $PaCO_2$, without a drop in PaO_2, indicate an obstruction or malposition of the endotracheal tube. Microatelectasis and hyperinflation may be seen clinically as a decrease in the PaO_2. Neonates on HFJV should also be closely monitored for fluid, electrolyte, and neurological status (Gordin, 1989).

HIGH FREQUENCY OSCILLATORY VENTILATION (HFOV OR HFO)

High frequency oscillatory ventilation (HFOV) utilizes the highest of rates, usually in the range of 480 to 1,800 per minute (8 to 30 Hz). The oscillatory waves that deliver the gas to the lungs, are produced by either a piston pump or by the use of a loudspeaker.

Concept of Operation. A unique feature of HFOV is that it produces a positive as well as a negative stroke, which assists both inspiration and expiration (Figure 15-4). The HFOV device is placed inline with the endotracheal tube and a gas source is passed perpendicularly into the tube, as illustrated in Figure 15-5.

As the fresh gas enters the endotracheal tube, it is driven to the patient by the waves coming from the oscillator. Expiration occurs opposite to where the gas enters the endotracheal tube through an expiratory limb that has a high impedance to oscillations, but low impedance when there is a steady flow of gas. Modern HFOV devices use traditional endotracheal tubes and are not used in tandem with conventional ventilators (Meredith, 1995).

Theories of Gas Exchange. As with all theories of gas exchange during HFV, it may be easiest to just say "We don't know why, it just

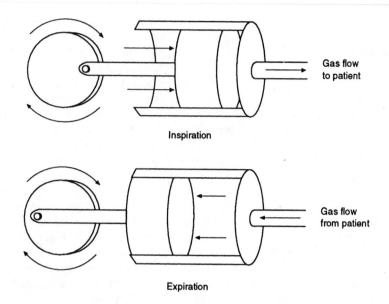

Figure 15-4 In high frequency oscillatory ventilation (HFOV), positive and negative strokes are provided to assist both inspiration and expiration.

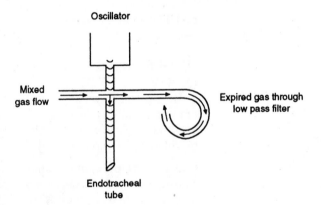

Figure 15-5 The oscillator or high frequency oscillatory ventilation (HFOV) device is placed inline with the endotracheal tube and a gas source is passed perpendicularly into the tube.

works." Even those who experiment, compute, and mathematically examine these theories, conclude that what happens in simulations may not be what is happening in real lungs (Pedley et al., 1994).

Indications. HFOV is indicated for use on neonates with severe RDS complicated with pulmonary hypertension and hypercapnia

☑ HFOV is indicated for use on neonates with severe RDS complicated with pulmonary hypertension and hypercapnia.

(Vierzig et al., 1994). It is effectively used to stabilize newborns with congenital diaphragmatic hernia (Miguet et al., 1994) and to treat pediatric patients with respiratory failure (Grenier & Thompson, 1996). HFOV is a safe and effective rescue technique in treating patients in whom conventional ventilation has failed (Clark et al., 1994). It is of interest to note that the presence of airleaks and failure to show early improvement indicate a poor prognosis (Chan et al., 1994).

Benefits. Three benefits of HFOV have been demonstrated. First it appears as though HFOV prevents the release of inflammatory chemical mediators in the lung, resulting in less lung injury than is seen with conventional ventilation (Imai et al., 1994). When used in conjunction with surfactant replacement therapy during the first hours of life, the incidence and severity of BPD may be reduced (Jackson et al., 1994). The third benefit of HFOV is that when applied early to maintain ventilation with optimal lung volume, oxygenation is increased in acute stage of RDS. This improvement in oxygenation reduces the need for surfactant administration (Plavka et al., 1999).

Complications. The ability of HFOV to oxygenate the blood is not as good as with other methods. This often requires the use of high levels of PEEP, often in excess of 15 cm H_2O (Milner & Hoskins, 1989). Combined with evidence that HFOV causes hyperinflation of the alveoli, high levels of PEEP may compromise cardiac output and lead to a higher risk of developing barotrauma (Milner & Hoskins, 1989).

There are several technical problems encountered in the use of HFOV. One problem is in the measurement of pressure at the distal end of the endotracheal tube. It is likely that alveolar pressures are quite different from those measured at the carina. An additional problem is a general lack of HFOV devices and training for its use in level I and level II nurseries.

☑ During HFJV and HFOV, cardiopulmonary assessment of the patient is difficult. Signs of pallor, cyanosis, bradycardia, hypotension, and increased respiratory effort indicate a worsening of status.

As with HFJV, cardiopulmonary assessment of the patient is difficult when HFOV is being used. The infant must be frequently assessed for signs of pallor, cyanosis, bradycardia, hypotension, and increased respiratory effort, all of which indicate a worsening of status.

OTHER METHODS OF VENTILATION

In addition to research into new ventilatory techniques, several advances have been made in the use of conventional ventilation. Much of the focus is on synchronizing the ventilator with the neonate's own spontaneous breathing to lessen the effect of fighting the ventilator and to improve flow dynamics into the airways. One new mode is flow-synchronization, in which the patient triggers the ventilator, with flow changing to meet the patient's inspiratory needs. This method of ventilation has been shown to allow weaning and extubation more rapidly when compared to conventional ventilation (Donn, 1990).

Other approaches include synchronized assisted ventilation (Blocker et al., 1994; Visveshwara et al., 1991), negative pressure ventilation, pressure support ventilation, and pressure-controlled inverse ratio ventilation. Some of these methods of mechanical ventilation are discussed elsewhere in this book.

LIQUID VENTILATION

An exciting technology in the area of neonatal ventilation is liquid ventilation. Although not a new concept, the ability to successfully utilize this technology has only recently been developed. The concept behind liquid ventilation is to obliterate the air/liquid interface in the alveoli with resultant lowering of surface tension. Mechanical inflation could then occur at pressures low enough to prevent damage to lung tissues.

Perfluorocarbon (PFC) liquids are the first substances that have been shown to support respiration while remaining relatively nontoxic to the lungs.

Liquid ventilation has potential applications for use in several diseases that traditionally have been difficult to treat. Included are RDS, aspiration syndromes, persistent pulmonary hypertension of the newborn, and pneumonia (Greenspan, 1993). While the potential of a favorable impact on the treatment of neonates is nearer, much research is still necessary before liquid ventilation takes its place among current treatment modalities.

EXTRACORPOREAL MEMBRANE OXYGENATION (ECMO)

With patients for whom it is difficult or near impossible to maintain adequate oxygenation by conventional means (oxygen therapy, CPAP, PEEP), it may become necessary to oxygenate the blood outside the body. One method used with moderate success is the procedure of **extracorporeal membrane oxygenation (ECMO)**.

extracorporeal membrane oxygenation (ECMO): Oxygenation of blood outside the body through a membrane oxygenator.

HISTORY

Oxygenation of blood outside the body, through a membrane oxygenator, was first developed for use in open heart surgery in the 1950s. The technology continued to improve and modifications allowed long-term use of the technique in the 1960s (Carlo & Chatburn, 1988).

The first use of the extracorporeal membrane oxygenator on an infant was done and described in 1971 (Zwischenberger et al., 1986). This paved the way for perfection and refinement of the technique. Today ECMO is used in many institutions across the country.

☑ ECMO is not recommended for infants of less than 34 weeks gestational age, weighing less than 2,000 grams, having evidence of intracranial hemorrhage (ICH).

PATIENT SELECTION

Because of the potential risks associated with ECMO, the clinical criteria used selects only those infants who are at an 80% or greater risk of mortality if conventional methods are used.

Several limitations have been established that help to define the ECMO population. Those infants at a gestational age less than 34 weeks or weighing less than 2,000 grams are excluded from consideration. This is due to the significant mortality associated with intracranial hemorrhage (ICH) (Revenis et al., 1992). Any patient with an existing ICH is not a candidate for ECMO. This is because of the need for systemic heparinization during the procedure, which could worsen an intracranial bleed. This also requires that any coagulopathy be corrected before initiating ECMO.

ECMO is contraindicated when mechanical ventilation has been used for more than two weeks prior to the initiation of ECMO. This is because of the likelihood of the development of chronic lung disease, which ECMO cannot reverse (Short, 1994). Additionally, candidates must have a reversible lung disease and should be free of significant cardiac disease.

☑ ECMO candidates should have less than two weeks of ventilator assistance, and have reversible lung disease.

☑ The mortality rate of infants under conventional ventilator care strategies can be predicted by three methods: P(A–a)O$_2$, oxygen index, PaO$_2$ or pH measurements.

ECMO CRITERIA

Since ECMO therapy is reserved for candidates with an extremely high mortality rate (80% or greater) under conventional ventilator care strategies, there are three ways to predict the occurrence of this mortality rate: (1) Alveolar-arterial oxygen pressure gradient [P(A–a)O$_2$ or A–aDO$_2$], (2) oxygen index, and (3) PaO$_2$ or pH measurements.

Using the P(A–a)O$_2$.   The P(A–a)O$_2$ is measured and calculated with the patient on 100% oxygen:

$$P(A–a)O_2 = \text{barometric pressure} – 47 – PaCO_2 – PaO_2$$

P(A–a)O$_2$ of 605 to 620 mm Hg (at 100% F$_I$O$_2$) for 4 to 12 hours indicates a need for ECMO therapy.

Using the Oxygen Index.   The OI is determined as follows:

$$OI = \frac{(\text{Mean Airway Pressure} \times F_I O_2)}{PaO_2}$$

An oxygen index of 0.35 to 0.6 for 0.5 to 6 hours is inclusive for ECMO therapy.

A study by Durand and associates (1990), described the use of the OI in addition to MAWP to identify a select group of meconium aspiration patients for ECMO. Their conclusions were that an OI greater than 0.4 in association with a MAWP of 20 cm H$_2$O or greater, may be helpful in identifying those patients who could benefit from ECMO.

☑ In the venoarte-
    rial route, blood
    goes from the
right atrium (via the
internal jugular vein)
to the aortic arch (via
the right common
carotid artery). This
route oxygenates the
blood and supports
the patient's cardiac
function.

☑ In the venove-
    nous route,
    blood goes from
the right atrium
(via the right internal
jugular vein) and
returns to the right
atrium (via the
femoral vein). This
route oxygenates
the blood only and
does not support
the patient's cardiac
function.

Using the PaO₂ or pH.   A third criteria used is the presence of a PaO_2 of 35 to 50 mm Hg for 2 to 12 hours or a pH of < 7.25 for 2 hours with hypotension (Short, 1994). Table 15-7 summarizes the parameters and critical values that may be used to determine the need for ECMO therapy.

MECHANISMS OF BYPASS

Two types of ECMO can be done: venoarterial and venovenous.

Venoarterial.   In the venoarterial route, blood is drawn from the right atrium via the internal jugular vein. The oxygenated blood is returned to the aortic arch via the right common carotid artery, as shown in Figure 15-6. Venoarterial ECMO not only oxygenates the blood, but also supports the cardiac function of the patient, because the blood return to the aortic arch is supported by the ECMO machine. For this reason, the venoarterial route is most commonly used for the ECMO procedure (Donn, 1990).

Venovenous.   In the venovenous route, blood is removed from the right atrium via a catheter inserted in the right internal jugular vein. The oxygenated blood is returned to the right atrium through a catheter inserted via the femoral vein. This method oxygenates the blood and does not support cardiac output.

In the venovenous method, blood flow from right to left heart remains the sole function of the heart.

ECMO Circuit.   The ECMO circuit uses a modified heart-lung bypass machine consisting of a venous-blood drainage reservoir, a blood pump, the membrane oxygenator where the exchange of O_2 and CO_2 takes place, and a heat exchanger to maintain temperature. Figure 15-7 depicts a typical ECMO circuit.

COMPLICATIONS

Complications of ECMO are both mechanical and physiologic. Common physiologic complications of ECMO are those related to bleeding,

TABLE 15-7   Criteria for ECMO Therapy

PARAMETER	CRITICAL VALUE
Alveolar-arterial oxygen tension gradient (A-aDO₂) on 100% F₁O₂	605 to 620 mm Hg for 4 to 12 hrs
Oxygen index (OI)	0.35 to 0.6 for 0.5 to 6 hrs
PaO₂	35 to 50 mm Hg for 2 to 12 hrs
pH	< 7.25 for 2 hrs with hypotension

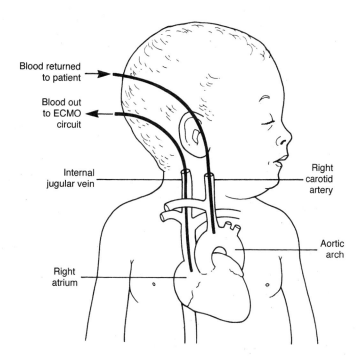

Figure 15-6 Venoarterial route of ECMO setup. Blood is drawn from the right atrium via the internal jugular vein. The oxygenated blood is returned to the aortic arch via the right carotid artery.

☑ Bleeding, ICH, pulmonary edema, and hemorrage are some potential complications of ECMO therapy.

secondary to the high level of heparin required for anticoagulation. Intracranial hemorrhage (ICH) has been reported to affect 14% of ECMO patients in one study (Donn, 1990). The incidence of ICH may be decreased if cephalic jugular venous drainage is used in conjunction with ECMO (O'Connor, 1993).

There is also a high incidence of seizures in ECMO patients. It is unknown whether the seizures are caused by the therapy, the disease, or both (Donn, 1990). Pulmonary edema, the release of vasoactive substances secondary to platelet-membrane interaction, and pulmonary hemorrhage are potential pulmonary complications.

Cardiovascular complications arise from hypo- and hypervolemia leading to hypo- and hypertension in the infant. Hypertension is seen in about 7% of ECMO patients (Donn, 1990). Alteration of the renin-angiotensin-aldosterone cycle, secondary to the nonpulsatile perfusion, may lead to renal complications.

Anemia, leukopenia and thrombocytopenia are all possible hematologic complications caused by the consumption of blood components by the membrane oxygenator (Carlo & Chatburn, 1988). Due to the invasive nature of ECMO, there is an increased risk of infection. Roughly 6% of patients on ECMO have positive blood cultures (Donn, 1990).

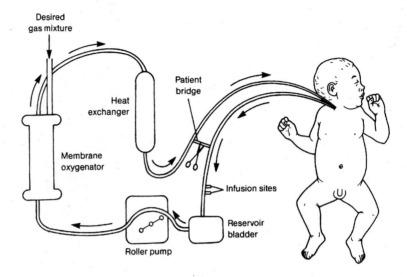

Figure 15-7 A typical ECMO circuit.

Mechanical complications arise in approximately 10% of ECMO cases and include failure of the pump, rupture of the tubing, failure of the membrane, and difficulties with the cannulas (Donn, 1990).

Implications. The initial hope that ECMO could provide a safe means of ventilating the sick neonate has not been realized. It became apparent early on that there are many hazards and complications that make the procedure suitable in only a few selected clinical conditions. The long-term complications of ECMO are still unknown. It is necessary to permanently ligate the carotid artery used to cannulate the patient, and the effects of having a single carotid artery as the patient grows older have yet to be determined.

The ECMO procedure is expensive and requires around-the-clock monitoring by specially trained personnel, which increases the cost tremendously. The high cost is often offset however, by a decreased number of days spent in the hospital. Patients receiving ECMO averaged 25 days in the hospital, compared to 76 days for those treated conventionally (Wagner, 1989).

SUMMARY

Neonatal mechanical ventilation is an area that requires additional training and clinical experience beyond the basics of respiratory care. Neonates are not just smaller adults because the ventilator settings, normal values, and treatment plans are all unique and sometimes wearisome to manage. This is particularly true for respiratory care practitioners who "wear more than one hat" and work in both the adult and neonatal intensive care units.

Since the materials presented in this chapter are relevant to actual clinical practice, they should be very useful to respiratory care students as they get ready to practice in the neonatal intensive care units. For seasoned practitioners, the reference sources should provide additional information on the topics presented in this chapter.

Self-Assessment Questions

1. Intubation of neonates following delivery is indicated under all of the following conditions *except*:

   A. meconium staining of amniotic fluid.
   B. difficulty ventilating by bag and mask.
   C. Apgar score greater than 8.
   D. presence of diaphragmatic hernia.

2. For neonates below 1,000 gm body weight, the proper size of laryngoscope blade should be size _____ and endotracheal tube size _____ (internal diameter, mm):

   A. 0, 1.5
   B. 0, 2.5
   C. 1, 1.5
   D. 1, 2.5

3. The most common cause of respiratory distress syndrome in newborns is:

   A. surfactant deficiency.
   B. oxygen toxicity.
   C. congenital heart disease.
   D. low body weight.

4. A preterm infant has a diagnosis of respiratory distress syndrome. You would expect to read in the chart that, immediately after delivery, the neonate showed all of the following signs *except*:

   A. expiratory grunting.
   B. nasal flaring.
   C. apnea.
   D. chest retraction.

5. Which of the following statements is *true* regarding to surfactant replacement therapy?

   A. Survanta® is a synthetic preparation.
   B. Exosurf Neonatal® is a preparation from cow lung tissue.
   C. Surfactant replacement works on all preterm infants.
   D. Surfactant replacement reduces the severity of RDS.

6. The major difference between adult and neonatal ventilators is that neonatal ventilators are mostly _____-limited and they deliver a variable _____ depending on a patient's lung compliance or airway resistance.

   A. pressure, volume
   B. pressure, pressure
   C. volume, pressure
   D. volume, volume

7. Keeping the same preset pressure on a pressure-limited ventilator, a lower tidal volume would result when the patient's compliance is _____ or airway resistance is _____.

    A. increased, increased

    B. increased, decreased

    C. decreased, increased

    D. decreased, decreased

8. A blood gas report done on a neonate shows a $PaCO_2$ of 58 mm Hg. The physician asks you to increase the tidal volume to be delivered by the pressure-limited ventilator. You would increase the _____ setting on the ventilator.

    A. tidal volume

    B. inspiratory pressure

    C. expiratory time

    D. positive end-expiratory pressure

9. During mechanical ventilation, the volume loss in the circuit and humidifier may be minimized by using a circuit and humidifier with:

    A. large mechanical deadspace volume.

    B. heated wire.

    C. low compression factor.

    D. high compression factor.

10. A heated wire is sometimes placed on the inspiratory side of the circuit to reduce _____ in the ventilator circuit.

    A. airway resistance

    B. condensation

    C. contamination

    D. circuit temperature

11. The general indications for mechanical ventilation include all of the following *except*:

    A. acute alveolar hyperventilation.

    B. apnea.

    C. acute respiratory acidosis.

    D. acute hypoxemia (PaO_2 < 50 mm Hg with supplemental oxygen).

12. When using a pressure-limited ventilator, the tidal volume delivered by the ventilator may be estimated by:

    A. I time + Flow rate.

    B. I time × Flow rate.

    C. I time + E time.

    D. Flow rate / I time.

13. The normal blood gas values of an umbilical artery sample include all of the following *except*:

    A. pH from 7.3 to 7.45.

    B. PCO_2 from 35 to 45 mm Hg.

    C. PO_2 greater than 50 mm Hg.

    D. SaO_2 from 60% to 90%.

14. High frequency ventilation has the advantages of delivering _____ and reducing the incidence of _____.

A. small tidal volume, barotrauma

B. large tidal volume, barotrauma

C. large mean airway pressure, necrotizing trachbronchitis

D. low peak inspiratory pressure, air trapping

15 to 17. Match the type of high frequency ventilator with the respective frequency (cycles/minute). Use each answer once.

Type of High Frequency Ventilator	Frequency (Cycles/min)
15. High Frequency Jet Ventilation (HFJV)	A. 60 to 150
16. High Frequency Oscillatory Ventilation (HFOV or HFO)	B. 240 to 660
17. High Frequency Positive Pressure Ventilation (HFPPV)	C. 480 to 1800

18. To minimize tracheal damage caused by high pressure gas jets in high frequency jet ventilation (HFJV), a specially-designed tube allows pulsed gas to exit _____ the endotracheal tube.

A. at the distal end of
B. at the proximal end of

C. at the middle and inside of
D. at the middle and outside of

19. During high frequency jet ventilation (HFJV) or high frequency oscillatory ventilation (HFOV), assessment of a patient's cardiopulmonary status is difficult. Signs of deterioration may include all of the following *except*:

A. respiratory distress.
B. tachycardia.

C. hypotension.
D. pallor.

20. A neonate who is diagnosed with severe RDS has been deteriorating over the past 12 hours. The physician asks you to evaluate this neonate for possible extracorporeal membrane oxygenation (ECMO) therapy. You would *recommend* the neonate for ECMO therapy if she:

A. has a gestational age of more than 34 weeks.
B. weighs less than 2,000 grams.

C. has evidence of intracranial hemorrhage (ICH).
D. has been mechanically ventilated for more than 2 weeks.

21. Extracorporeal membrane oxygenation (ECMO) therapy should be considered only when the patient has a(n) _____ percent mortality rate using the conventional ventilator management strategies.

    A. 20   C. 60
    B. 40   D. 80

22. All of the following may be used to predict an 80% mortality rate under conventional ventilator management strategies *except*:

    A. A-a gradient of 605 to 620 mm Hg for 4 to 12 hours.
    B. oxygen index of 0.35 to 0.6 for 30 minutes to 6 hours.
    C. PaO_2 of 35 to 50 for 2 to 12 hours.
    D. pH of less than 7.25 for 2 hours with hypertension.

23. Which of the following statements is *true* concerning the *venoarterial* route in ECMO therapy?

    A. Blood is removed from the right common carotid artery.
    B. Blood is removed from the brachial or femoral artery.
    C. Blood is returned to the aortic arch via the right common carotid artery.
    D. Blood is returned to the aortic arch via the internal jugular vein.

24. Which of the following statements is *true* concerning the *venovenous* route in ECMO therapy?

    A. Blood is removed from the right atrium via the right carotid artery.
    B. Blood is removed from the right atrium via the femoral vein.
    C. Blood is returned to the right atrium via the femoral vein.
    D. Blood is returned to the aortic arch via the internal jugular vein.

25. The _____ route in ECMO therapy supports cardiac function because the blood is returned to the _____.

    A. venoarterial, aortic arch via the common carotid artery
    B. venoarterial, right atrium via the femoral vein
    C. venovenous, aortic arch via the common carotid artery
    D. venovenous, right atrium via the femoral vein

References

Abbasi, S. et al. (1993). Long-term pulmonary consequences of respiratory distress syndrome in preterm infants treated with exogenous surfactant. *J Pediatr, 122*(3).

Bandy, K. P. et al. (1992, May/June). Volume-controlled ventilation for severe neonatal respiratory failure. *Neonatal Intensive Care,* 70–73.

Blocker, D. et al. (1994, November/December). Synchronized assisted ventilation of infants (SAVI) examined as part of a quality improvement study: West Paces Medical Center, Atlanta, Georgia. *Neonatal Intensive Care,* 32–35.

Boynton, B. R. (1986). High frequency ventilation in newborn infants. *Respiratory Care, 31*(6).

Carlo, W. A., & Chatburn, R. L. (1988). *Neonatal respiratory care* (2nd ed.). Chicago: Year Book Medical Publishers, Inc.

Chan, V. et al. (1994). High frequency oscillation for preterm infants with severe respiratory failure. *Arch Dis Child, 70*(Spec. No. 1).

Chatburn, R. L. (1991). Principles and practice of neonatal and pediatric mechanical ventilation. *Resp Care, 36*(6).

Clark, R. H. (1994). High frequency ventilation in acute pediatric respiratory failure. (Editorial). *Chest, 105*(3).

Clark, R. H. et al. (1994). Prospective, randomized comparison of high frequency oscillation and conventional ventilation in candidates for extracorporeal membrane oxygenation. *J Pediatr, 124*(3).

Donn, S. M. (1990). ECMO indications and complications. *Hosp Practice, 25*(6).

Durand, M. et al. (1990). Oxygenation index in patients with meconium aspiration: Conventional and extracorporeal membrane oxygenation therapy. *Crit Care Med, 18*(4).

Goldsmith, J. P. et al. (1993). Ventilatory management casebook. *J Perinatology, 8*(1).

Gordin, P. (1989). High frequency jet ventilation for severe respiratory failure. *Pediatr Nurs, 15*(6).

Greenspan, J. S. (1993). Liquid ventilation: A developing technology. *Neonatal Network, 12*(4).

Grenier, B. & Thompson, J. (1996). High-frequency oscillatory ventilation in pediatric patients. *Respir Care Clin N Am, 2*(4), 545–575.

Gunkel, J. H., & Banks, P. L. (1993). Surfactant therapy and intracranial hemorrhage: Review of the literature and results of new analyses. *Pediatrics, 92*(6).

Holm, B. A., & Waring, A. J. (1993). Designer surfactants: The next generation in surfactant replacement. *Clin Perinat, 20*(4).

Horbar, J. D. et al. (1993). A multicenter randomized trial comparing two surfactants for the treatment of neonatal respiratory distress syndrome. *J Pediatr, 123*(5).

Imai, Y. et al. (1994). Inflammatory chemical mediators during conventional ventilation and during high frequency oscillatory ventilation. *Am J Resp Crit Care Med, 150*(6, Pt. 1).

Jackson, J. C. et al. (1994). Reduction in lung injury after combined surfactant and high frequency ventilation. *Am J Resp Crit Care Med, 150*(2).

Jobe, A. H., & Ikegami, M. (1993). Surfactant metabolism. *Clin Perinat, 20*(4).

Kaapa, P. et al. (1993). Pulmonary hemodynamics after synthetic surfactant replacement in neonatal respiratory distress syndrome. *J Pediatr, 123*(1).

Long, W. (1993). Synthetic surfactant. *Semin Perinatol, 17*(4).

Meredith, K. S. (1995). High frequency ventilation. In S. L. Barnhart, & M. P. Czervinske, *Perinatal and pediatric respiratory care.* Philadelphia: W.B. Saunders Co.

Miguet, D. et al. (1994). Preoperative stabilization using high frequency oscillatory ventilation in the management of congenital diaphragmatic hernia. *Crit Care Med, 22*(Suppl. 9).

Milner, A. D., & Hoskins, E. W. (1989). High frequency positive pressure ventilation in neonates. *Arch Dis Child, 64*(1), [Fetal Neonatal ed.].

Modanlou, H. D. et al. (1997). Comparative efficacy of Exosurf® and Survanta® surfactants on early clinical course of respiratory distress syndrome and complications of prematurity. *J Perinatol, 17*(6), 455–460.

O'Connor, T. A. (1993). Decreased incidence of intracranial hemorrhage using cephalic jugular venous drainage during neonatal extracorporeal membrane oxygenation. *J Pediatr Surg, 28*(10).

Parmigiani, S. et al. (1997). Evolution of respiratory mechanics in preterm babies after surfactant administration in the neonatal period. *Acta Biomed Ateneo Parmense, 68*(Suppl. 1), 65–73.

Pedley, T. J. et al. (1994). Gas flow and mixing in the airways. *Crit Care Med, 22*(Suppl. 9).

Pinar, H. et al. (1994). Pathology of the lung in surfactant-treated neonates. *Pediatr Pathol, 14*(4).

Plavka, R. et al. (1999). A prospective randomized comparison of conventional mechanical ventilation and very early high frequency oscillatory ventilation in extremely premature newborns with respiratory distress syndrome. *Intensive Care Med, 25*(1), 68–75.

Revenis, M. E. et al. (1992). Mortality and morbidity among lower birth weight (2–2.5 kg) infants treated with extracorporeal membrane oxygenation (ECMO). *J Pediatr, 121*.

Richardson, C. (1988). Hyaline membrane disease: Future treatment modalities. *J Perinat Neonat Nurs, 2*(1).

Robertson, B. & Halliday, H. L. (1998). Principles of surfactant replacement. *Biochim Biophys Acta, 1408*(2–3), 346–361.

Short, B. L. (1994). Extracorporeal membrane oxygenation. In G. B. Avery et al. (Eds.), *Neonatology: pathophysiology and management of the newborn* (4th ed.). Philadelphia: J.B. Lippincott.

Vierzig, A. et al. (1994). Clinical experiences with high frequency oscillatory ventilation in newborns with severe respiratory distress syndrome. *Crit Care Med, 22*(Suppl. 9).

Visveshwara, N. et al. (1991). Patient-triggered synchronized assisted ventilation of newborns. Report of a preliminary study and three years' experience. *Journal of Perinatology, 11*(4), 347–354.

Wagner, M. (1989). New technology for critically ill newborns needs solid planning. *Modern Healthcare, 19*(29).

Wiswell, T. E., & Mendiola, J. (1993). Respiratory distress syndrome in the newborn: Innovative therapies. *Am Fam Phys, 47*(2).

Witek, T. J. & E. N. Schachter. (1994). *Pharmacology and therapeutics in respiratory care.* W. B. Saunders Company, Philadelphia.

Yuksel, B. et al. (1993). Respiratory function at follow-up after neonatal surfactant replacement therapy. *Respir Med, 87*(3).

Zwischenberger, J. B. et al. (1986). The role of extracorporeal membrane oxygenation in the management of respiratory failure in the newborn. *Resp Care, 31*(6).

Suggested Reading

Mechanical Ventilation and Monitoring

Bignall, S. et al. (1997). Monitoring interactions between spontaneous respiration and mechanical inflations in preterm neonates. *Crit Care Med, 25*(3), 545–553.

Despotova-Toleva, L. & Petrov, A. (1997). Feasibility for evaluation of the efficacy of conventional ventilatory support in very low birth weight infants. *Folia Med* (Plovdiv), *39*(4), 55–64.

Mammel, M. C. & Bing, D. R. (1996). Mechanical ventilation of the newborn. An overview. *Clin Chest Med, 17*(3), 603–613.

Sinha, S. K. et al. (1997). Randomized trial of volume controlled versus time cycled, pressure limited ventilation in preterm infants with respiratory distress syndrome. *Arch Dis Child Fetal Neonatal Ed, 77*(3), F202–205.

High-Frequency Ventilation

Hoehn, T. et al. (1998). High-frequency ventilation augments the effect of inhaled nitric oxide in persistent pulmonary hypertension of the newborn. *Eur Respir J, 11*(1), 234–238.

Jouvet, P. et al. (1997). Assessment of high-frequency neonatal ventilator performances. *Intensive Care Med, 23*(2), 208–213.

Kalenga, M. et al. (1998). High-frequency oscillatory ventilation in neonatal RDS: Initial volume optimization and respiratory mechanics. *J Appl Physiol, 84*(4), 1174–1177.

Extracorporeal Gas Exchange

Alpard, S. K. & Zwischenberger, J. B. (1998). Extracorporeal gas exchange. *Respir Care Clin N Am, 4*(4), 711–738, ix.

CHAPTER SIXTEEN

HOME MECHANICAL VENTILATION

David W. Chang

KEY TERMS

- acute care
- acute exacerbation
- desaturation
- home care

- learning objectives
- quality of life
- team approach

INTRODUCTION

Home mechanical ventilation made its first major appearance in the United States during the poliomyelitis epidemics of the mid-twentieth century. At that time, negative pressure ventilators (iron lungs) were used to sustain the lives of those who lost the ability to breathe. Today, health care reform and cost containment strategies are limiting the resources available for acute care in the hospitals. Since there are few nursing homes or extended care facilities that will accept the increasing number of ventilator patients, home care becomes an important and viable option for ventilator-dependent patients.

GOALS OF HOME MECHANICAL VENTILATION

acute care: Patient care provided in facilities where life-sustaining equipment and qualified personnel are always available.

quality of life: The most important, positive features of daily living for a patient based on his/her current physical and mental conditions. The quality varies among different individuals and its definition may change over time.

Mechanical ventilation provided in the home is drastically different from that delivered in an **acute care** setting. In an acute care setting such as the hospital, the patient is surrounded by an array of medical equipment and supplies. Specialized health care practitioners are available at all times to provide diagnostic and therapeutic procedures. In addition, the patient in an acute care setting gets little rest because of frequent vital sign assessments and routine laboratory tests. For patients who require long-term mechanical ventilation, it may not be logical or financially feasible to provide mechanical ventilation in an acute care setting.

An alternative to the acute care setting is to provide mechanical ventilation in a nonacute environment such as the patient's home. Three unique and beneficial goals of home ventilator care have been identified and they are: (1) extension of the patient's life and enhancement of the **quality of life**, (2) creation of an environment that will develop and strengthen the patient's physical and physiological functions, and (3) reduction of the cost for ventilator care (O'Donohue et al., 1986).

Extension of the patient's life is a primary goal of medical and health care procedures. Quality of life is an important issue since a life that has poor quality or little meaning may cause the patient a great deal of anxiety and unnecessary suffering. For this reason, the patient must be involved and be part of the decision-making process before changing the ventilator care plan from an acute care setting to the patient's home.

✓ To spend much of the day in a familiar home environment is one benefit that cannot be provided by the hospital.

To be able to spend much of the day in a familiar home environment is one benefit that cannot be provided by the hospital. At home, the patient is likely to become more active in the rehabilitation process. There is an incentive for the patient to try to get well and be weaned off the ventilator. Furthermore, interactions with family members and friends will enhance the patient's psychological well-being and quality of life.

✓ The cost savings of providing mechanical ventilation at home can be drastic but it should not be the *primary* consideration.

Reduction of the cost for patient care is another goal of home mechanical ventilation. The cost savings of providing mechanical ventilation at home can be drastic but should not be the primary consideration. It is vital to ensure that quality care is provided to the patient at or below the cost of patient care in an acute care setting.

team approach: A unified and supportive way of taking care of a patient by medical and nonmedical individuals who share a common goal.

As we see later in this chapter, the success of home ventilator care requires a team that consists of medical professionals (physicians, nurses, respiratory therapists, social workers) and nonmedical laypersons (relatives, friends, support group members). No matter what their background or training, a **team approach** dedicated and committed to quality care is vital to any successful home ventilator care program (Gower et al., 1985).

INDICATIONS

✓ A team approach dedicated and committed to quality care is vital to any successful home ventilator care program.

Before a decision is made to provide home ventilator care for a patient, four questions may help to assess the need for home ventilator care: (1) Does the patient have a disease state (high cervical spine injury, severe respiratory muscle paralysis) which may result in ventilatory failure and the need for long-term ventilator care? (2) Does the patient exhibit clinical characteristics (impending ventilatory failure, cerebral hypoxia) that require mechanical ventilation? (3) Is the patient clinically stable enough to be managed outside an acute care setting? and (4) Are there other noninvasive alternatives besides artificial airway and mechanical ventilation (diaphragm pacing, pneumobelt) suitable for the patient (O'Donohue et al., 1986)?

DISEASES THAT MAY JUSTIFY HOME MECHANICAL VENTILATION

Lung diseases that may justify ventilator care provided outside an acute care setting may be grouped into four categories. They are: (1) chronic obstructive lung diseases (COPD), (2) restrictive lung diseases, (3) ventilatory muscle dysfunction, and (4) central hypoventilation syndromes (Ferns, 1994; Goldstein et al., 1995; O'Donohue et al.,

1986). Since the severity and coexisting conditions of a disease vary greatly among patients with the same diagnosis, a thorough patient evaluation is a prerequisite for home ventilator care. The diseases that may benefit from home mechanical ventilation are summarized in Table 16-1.

COPD.   COPD is a group of lung impairments that includes chronic asthma, chronic bronchitis, emphysema, and bronchiectasis. Air flow obstruction is the primary clinical feature of these patients. Typically, stable COPD patients require only minimal care such as bronchodilators, flu vaccines, and bronchopulmonary hygiene. Only on rare occasions, do they require ventilatory assistance.

COPD patients who require mechanical ventilation are those who develop ventilatory failure or oxygenation failure, or both. On occasion, these patients may deteriorate to a point requiring mechanical ventilation as a result of pneumonia or major surgical procedure. When this occurs, blood gases usually reveal acute ventilatory failure (acute respiratory acidosis) superimposed on chronic ventilatory failure (compensated respiratory acidosis). This condition of acute hypercapnia in COPD is also called **acute exacerbation** of COPD (Malley, 1990). Table 16-2 shows the changes in blood gas reports when a stable COPD patient goes into ventilatory failure requiring mechanical ventilation.

Once placed on a ventilator, COPD patients may be difficult to wean off mechanical ventilation because of insufficient alveolar ventilation. This problem is due primarily to air flow obstruction, loss of elastic recoil, and air trapping. In addition, COPD patients usually have coexisting medical problems that are related to the primary lung disease. Some examples of these related medical problems are ventilation/perfusion mismatch, pulmonary hypertension, and cor pulmonale.

acute exacerbation: A sudden aggravation of symptoms or increase in the severity of a disease. This condition is often caused by a secondary medical problem such as a severe infection.

☑ COPD patients are difficult to wean because of insufficient alveolar ventilation caused by air flow obstruction, loss of elastic recoil, and air trapping.

TABLE 16-1   Diseases That May Justify Home Mechanical Ventilation

PULMONARY PROBLEM	CLINICAL COURSE
COPD	Air flow obstruction Excessively high compliance Air trapping Acute exacerbation (pneumonia)
Restrictive lung disease	Reduction of lung volumes and capacities Deadspace ventilation Muscle fatigue
Ventilatory muscle dysfunction	Inefficient ventilatory muscle Atelectasis and pneumonia
Central hypoventilation syndrome	Apnea Chronic hypoventilation Atelectasis and pneumonia

TABLE 16-2 Blood Gas Characteristics of Acute Exacerbation of COPD

CONDITION	TYPICAL BLOOD GASES
Chronic ventilatory failure in a stable COPD patient	pH = 7.36, $PaCO_2$ = 55 mm Hg, PaO_2 = 50 mm Hg, HCO_3^- = 30 mEq/L
Acute ventilatory failure in a normal patient due to pneumonia or major surgical procedure	pH = 7.30, $PaCO_2$ = 55 mm Hg, PaO_2 = 75 mm Hg, HCO_3^- = 26 mEq/L
Acute ventilatory failure superimposed on chronic ventilatory failure (e.g., COPD patient with pneumonia)	pH = 7.27, $PaCO_2$ = 74 mm Hg, PaO_2 = 43 mm Hg, HCO_3^- = 33 mEq/L

desaturation: A significant decrease in arterial oxygen saturation (SaO_2) or pulse oximetry saturation (SpO_2) from the normal baseline value.

☑ The amount of deadspace ventilation is increased in rapid shallow breathing.

COPD patients also require a high level of care in maintaining the airway. Because of copious amounts of pulmonary secretions and inability to clear secretions effectively, they often require suctioning of the airways and bronchopulmonary drainage. The oxygenation levels also fluctuate widely depending on unanticipated events such as bronchospasm and mucus plugging. Since the weaning process for COPD patients may take days or weeks, home ventilator care becomes a viable option once they are clinically stable and without significant oxygen **desaturation**. When significant oxygen desaturation (SaO_2 or SpO_2 < 90%) occurs, its cause must be identified and corrected before transferring the patient from hospital to home.

Restrictive Lung Diseases. Restrictive lung diseases such as pulmonary fibrosis and atelectasis limit the patient's ability to expand the lungs. As a result, lung volumes and capacities are reduced. Since minute ventilation requires an adequate tidal volume and respiratory rate, patients with restrictive lung disease assume a rapid breathing pattern because of the reduction of tidal volume.

The amount of deadspace ventilation is increased in rapid shallow breathing. Furthermore, the work of breathing in restrictive lung diseases is increased because of low lung compliance. High inflation pressures and respiratory rates are usually required to maintain adequate ventilation in these patients. Over time, these patients develop ventilatory failure secondary to excessive work of breathing and muscle fatigue. Home ventilator care should be considered for patients who have chronic restrictive lung disease and are clinically stable.

Ventilatory Muscle Dysfunction. Patients with ventilatory muscle dysfunction include those afflicted with spinal cord injury or polyneuropathy. Since the primary problem of ventilation is with the ventilatory muscles, they usually have healthy lungs and a good prognosis. Home ventilator care is usually carried out without any complications. Unless there is an infection, these patients generally maintain healthy lungs and normal lung functions. When lung infection occurs, it often leads to pneumonia and atelectasis.

Long-term mechanical ventilation is often necessary for these patients because of the chronic nature of the diseases affecting the respiratory system. These patients often recover and do not require prolonged mechanical ventilation except in cases of high spinal (cervical 1 and 2) injuries. Aggressive airway care and broncho-pulmonary hygiene should be done to avoid complications resulting from the use of mechanical ventilation and artificial airway.

Central Hypoventilation Syndrome.   Patients with central hypo-ventilation syndrome often exhibit apnea or variable periods of hypoventilation due to failure or dysfunction of the autonomic control of breathing. Because of the range of severity and complications in central hypoventilation syndrome, some patients may require mechanical ventilation only during sleep while others may need it continuously. In patients who have persistent hypoventilation, poor lung expansion may lead to lung infection, atelectasis, and pneumonia. Careful evaluation of these patients in the hospital can help to formulate a care plan for mechanical ventilation in the home.

PATIENT SELECTION

Not all patients receiving mechanical ventilation in an acute care setting are suitable candidates for home ventilator care. Typically, a patient who requires a good deal of monitoring and laboratory tests or one who is clinically unstable is ruled out for home ventilator care. Aside from the evaluations based on the medical perspective, four nonmedical factors are crucial in the patient selection process. They are: (1) desires of the patient, (2) desires of the family, (3) cost, and (4) available resources (Eigen et al., 1990; O'Donohue et al., 1986; Smith, 1994).

DESIRES OF THE PATIENT

Likely candidates for home ventilator care should be told about the potential advantages and disadvantages of leaving the hospital. The advantage of being at home is the opportunity for the patient to stay closer to family members and to live in a familiar environment. The disadvantage of leaving the hospital is the feeling of isolation from professional help and the assumption of medical care by self and family members. The discussion on the topic of home ventilator care should be done when the patient can comprehend the meaning and implications of leaving the acute care setting. It should not take place when the patient is hypoxic, confused, or under emotional distress.

✔ Discussions concerning home ventilator care should not take place when the patient is hypoxic, confused, or under emotional distress.

home care: Patient care provided in the home or other nonacute care settings (nursing homes, extended care facilities) where minimal medical equipment and personnel are available.

☑ Adaptation of home ventilator care depends on the level of communication within the family and the degree of commitment between all family members.

☑ The cost of home ventilator care varies greatly and depends primarily on the type of equipment and the extent of professional care required.

Finally, the decision to implement home ventilator care should not be rushed. Ample time should be provided to the patient so that the decision may reflect the patient's true desire. Hasty discussions and decisions often lead to inaccurate perceptions and poor transition from the hospital to the **home care** setting.

DESIRES OF THE FAMILY

The desires of family members must be considered because they will be the key persons taking care of the patient and ventilator at home. Depending on the level of ventilator care required by the patient, personal sacrifices must be made. These sacrifices may range from giving up some free time and leisure activities to terminating one's job or career (Smith, 1994). Successful home ventilator care requires a total commitment from family members. They must also be able and willing to assume this unfamiliar task of home ventilator care for the duration of time that the patient remains on the ventilator. In one study, the most important factor associated with adaptation of home ventilator care was the level of communication within the family and the degree of commitment between all family members (Glass, 1993).

COST

The cost of home ventilator care varies greatly and depends primarily on the type of equipment and the extent of professional care required. Ventilator, a back up ventilator, and oxygen supplies are some major equipment expenditures, either obtained by purchase or through a rental agreement. Use of home care professionals can also be costly. Depending on the patient's needs, nurses and respiratory therapists may be a costly expenditure (Murray, 1989; O'Donohue et al., 1986).

The complexity and available features of a ventilator can affect the equipment cost. As a rule, more complex equipment and supplies cost more. For patients who cannot breathe spontaneously and require continuous ventilatory support, a backup ventilator may also be necessary. Those patients who require around-the-clock care may also need medical professionals to make frequent home visits. Family members may also need to hire a home care aide to provide periodic relief for leisure time and other family or work obligations.

A study on the financial aspects of pediatric home ventilator care, it shows a significant reduction in the total cost (Hazlett, 1989). Of course, home ventilator care cannot be justified from a financial standpoint if its total cost is higher than the cost of comparable hospital care. Careful cost analysis should be done based on the patient's requirements. The resultant cost for the entire home ventilator care program may be part of the patient selection process.

AVAILABLE RESOURCES

The primary resources that are vital to the success of home ventilator care include physical environment, technical support, and emotional support. The physical environment for home ventilator care must provide adequate space for the ventilator, special bed, wheelchair, oxygen units, and supplies. Suitable and sufficient electrical outlets are also needed for the ventilator, alarms, and other related equipment. Technical support should include one or more home health agencies that have ample equipment and supplies, qualified medical professionals, and around-the-clock coverage. Emotional support may include psychosocial assistance provided to the patient and family members by community agencies, support groups, and friends.

EQUIPMENT SELECTION

Although positive pressure ventilation with an artifical airway is the most common modality in home ventilator care, there are several factors to consider before prescribing the equipment for the patient. The primary factor of equipment selection should result in a ventilator or device that suits the patient's immediate and long-term needs. The secondary factor should deal with the use and maintenance of the equipment.

TYPES OF VENTILATORY SUPPORT

If the patient does not have adequate spontaneous ventilation for an extended time, positive pressure or negative pressure ventilators are the equipment of choice. Positive pressure ventilation requires an artificial airway whereas negative pressure ventilation can be provided without an artificial airway. One exception to this practice is the presence of significant airway obstruction.

☑ A backup ventilator may be necessary if the patient is totally dependent on mechanical ventilation.

A backup ventilator may be necessary if the patient is totally dependent on mechanical ventilation. For patients who are using mechanical ventilation on a part-time basis (e.g., during sleep), a backup system may not be needed or financially justifiable.

Other modes of ventilatory support include the chest cuirass, raincoat or wrap, pneumobelt, rocking bed, and diaphragmatic pacing. A chest cuirass ventilator is a shell that fits over the patient's chest wall (Figure 16-1). The raincoat or wrap is an airtight jacket that seals at the arms, hips, and neck (Figure 16-2). It covers a larger area than the chest cuirass and does not impinge on the chest and abdomen. For this reason, it offers a larger inspiratory volume to the user. The raincoat or wrap is more difficult to get into and usually requires help from another person in the home. The pneumobelt is a corsetlike belt attached to a positive pressure generator. The positive pressure inflates the belt, squeezes the abdomen, and pushes the diaphragm upward. An alternating sequence of positive pressure and ambient pressure provided to the pneumobelt produces active ventilation. The rocking bed relies on motion to displace the abdominal contents

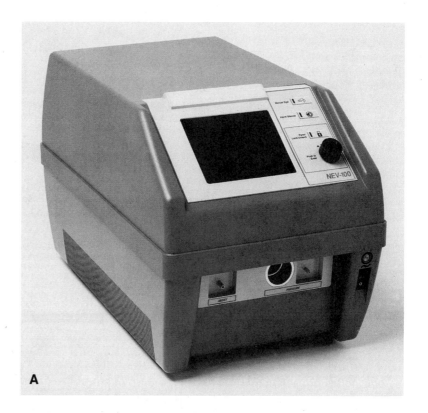

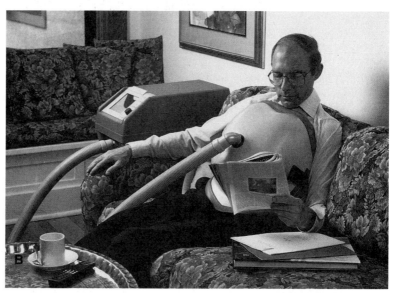

Figure 16-1 (A) LIFECARE's Noninvasive Extrathoracic Ventilator NEV-100;
(B) NEV-100 in use with a chest shell (cuirass).

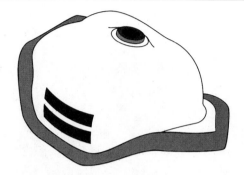

Figure 16-1 *(continued)* (C) LIFECARE Soft Seal Chest Shell. (Courtesy of LIFECARE, Westminster, Colo.)

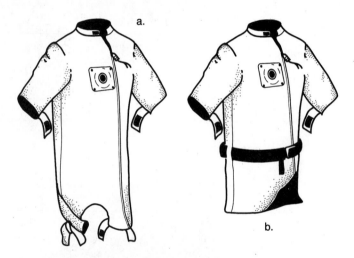

Figure 16-2 LIFECARE's Nu-Mo Suit (a) and Pulmo Wrap (b). (Courtesy of LIFECARE, Westminster, Colo.)

to facilitate diaphragmatic motion and ventilation (Hill, 1994; Votroubek, 1995).

Diaphragmatic Pacing. Diaphragmatic pacing or bilateral pacing of the phrenic nerves does not actually provide mechanical ventilation. Rather, it is used to augment spontaneous ventilation. Diaphragmatic pacing has been used in infants and children for more than a decade (Ilbawi et al., 1985). The pacing system includes an external transmitter and antenna placed on the skin over a receiver implanted subcutaneously. At a predetermined interval, the receiver sends electrical energy to an electrode placed near the thoracic phrenic nerves.

When the phrenic nerves are stimulated by electrical energy, the diaphragm contracts (Votroubek, 1995).

RELIABILITY AND SAFETY

The ventilator used at home should be highly dependable and require little or no maintenance by nonmedical personnel such as the patient, family members, and home care aides. Each ventilator should have safety features such as high pressure, low pressure, and ventilator failure alarms. These features must not be too complicated for those working with the patient and ventilator.

SIMPLICITY AND PORTABILITY

The operation and maintenance of home care ventilators should be direct and simple. Dials and alarms on the ventilator that are illogical and hard to understand are likely to confuse the users. The ventilator circuits should be easy to clean if they are reusable.

Ventilators that are small, compact, and portable will provide the most flexibility when the patient wants to move around the home. Ventilators with built-in rechargeable battery packs are also very versatile in the event of brief power failure. The patient may also take advantage of this feature to make physician office visits or brief shopping trips.

LEARNING OBJECTIVES FOR POSITIVE PRESSURE VENTILATION IN THE HOME

This section provides complete coverage of the essential and important aspects of providing positive pressure ventilation in the home. These topics are presented in the form of **learning objectives** and they should be a useful resource for respiratory care students, discharge planners, medical care providers, and family members. Family members, who work closely with the patient and ventilator are often the ones who receive the least training and instruction. Thus, they often have a great deal of apprehension about the equipment and procedures used in home mechanical ventilation (Smith, 1994).

By following the learning objectives, the team members may learn how to perform those essential procedures for successful mechanical ventilation in the home. The complete learning objectives are provided by the National Center for Home Mechanical Ventilation and National Jewish Center for Immunology and Respiratory Medicine (Glenn et al., 1993) and they are used with permission (Table 16-3).

Sidebar notes:

✓ A home care ventilator and its safety features must not be too complicated for those working with the patient and ventilator.

✓ Ventilators with built-in rechargeable battery packs are versatile in the event of brief power failure. The patient may also take advantage of this feature to make physician office visits or brief shopping trips.

learning objectives: A set of goals that outline the specific topics to be taught and learned.

✓ The learning objectives for positive pressure ventilation in the home can be a very useful resource for respiratory care students, discharge planners, medical care providers, and especially for family members.

TABLE 16-3   Learning Objectives for Positive Pressure Ventilation in the Home

INTRODUCTION

This is a comprehensive list of possible learning objectives for ventilator-assisted individuals in the home. The objectives are patient oriented but are also applicable to lay caregivers and health professionals. The National Center for Home Mechanical Ventilation (1400 Jackson Street, Denver, CO 80206) developed and originally published these objectives in July, 1993. These objectives are intended to facilitate development and implementation of home ventilator education plans that are specific to the needs of individual patients, families, and caregivers.

Not all of these objectives are appropriate for each patient and listing of an educational objective does not constitute endorsement of the objective by the National Center for Home Mechanical Ventilation. The health care professional(s) responsible for patient education should develop a list of Learning Objectives specific for each patient and caregiver based on the patient's diagnosis, age, ventilator, route of application, need for oxygen and other respiratory care, and precise prescription for ventilatory assistance. In some cases these objectives are general and might be made more specific for individual patients. For example, with the objective "Explain why secretion color is important," patients at risk for aspiration should be taught both about secretion color as an indication of infection as well as a sign of food material in secretions. It is suggested that the final objectives be given to each patient and used by health care professionals as a guide to education and training. Before the patient and caregivers use the ventilation system independently at home, they should be able to meet the appropriate Learning Objectives.

These objectives should be accompanied by written materials, diagrams, and simple step-by-step instructions whenever possible. Manufacturer-developed materials and instructions specific to the model, brand, and unit of ventilators and other equipment in use should always be incorporated into the educational process when they are available to maximize knowledge and familiarity with the equipment to be used.

SUGGESTIONS FOR USE OF THESE OBJECTIVES

The objectives are organized with the equipment or subject category at the top of each page. In the table that follows, the *Topic* column identifies specific issues that relate to the listed category, and the *Objective* column lists specific key points that may be addressed in the education of the patient and caregiver. The final two columns, *Presentation* and *Review/Demonstration,* are available to denote (a) when and by whom training has been performed, and (b) when the patient and caregiver have been tested and found to meet each objective.

It should be assumed that each objective is prefaced by the phrase "The patient and caregiver should be able to . . ."

(Table courtesy of National Center for Home Mechanical Ventilation and National Jewish Center for Immunology and Respiratory Medicine©. Used with permission.)

Note: Codes for Table 16-3: P = Presentation, R/D = Review/Demonstration

(continued)

Learning Objectives	GENERAL		
Topic	**Objective**	**P**	**R/D**
a. Need for ventilation	1. State respiratory diagnosis and all medical conditions. 2. Describe how the lungs work and why breathing is important. 3. Describe why the ventilator is needed. 4. Explain how it might feel and what might happen without the ventilator or if it is used less than prescribed.		
b. Ventilator schedule	1. Write the daily schedule for ventilator use. 2. Explain any changes that should be made to the ventilator settings for exertional activities or exercise. 3. Explain any changes that should be made to the ventilator settings for sleep. 4. Write the schedule for checking the ventilator. 5. Write the schedule for cleaning the ventilator.		
c. Supplies needed	1. List the supplies and amounts needed in the home. 2. List the equipment needed in the home. 3. Name the cleaning solution. 4. Explain how to mix the cleaning solution and when to change the solution. 5. Explain where and when to get the cleaning solution. 6. Make a list of places to get supplies not available from the respiratory home care company. Include vendor name, address, phone number, and manufacturer name of the supply and part number.		
d. Medical assistance information	1. List names and phone numbers of persons to contact for: • medical emergencies • equipment emergencies • power emergencies 2. Name the home respiratory care company that will assist with care and provide respiratory equipment and supplies. 3. Identify the agency or person responsible for the home: • nurse • health aide • attendants • social worker • physical therapy • respiratory therapy 4. List the name and phone number of the doctor.		

(continued)

Learning Objectives	**GENERAL** *(continued)*		
Topic	**Objective**	**P**	**R/D**
	5. Record the above contacts and numbers and describe how and where to keep them close to the ventilator.		
	6. Describe the situations when you should contact the: • doctor • home nurse • respiratory home care company • emergency service (such as an ambulance)		

Learning Objectives	**VENTILATOR**		
Topic	**Objective**	**P**	**R/D**
a. Principles of operation	1. Describe what a ventilator does. 2. Explain how the ventilator helps breathing. 3. Name the parts of the ventilation system (ventilator, tubing, humidifier, alarm, application device, oxygen, and others)		
b. Power	1. List each kind of power source available. 2. Describe the advantages and disadvantages of each kind of power source. 3. Demonstrate how to connect the ventilator to each power source. 4. List the number of hours of use to expect from: • the internal battery • the external battery • electrical outlet 5. Demonstrate how to check the external battery charge. 6. Demonstrate how to check the internal battery charge. 7. Describe when, how, and how long to charge (and discharge) the internal battery. 8. Describe when, how, and how long to charge the external battery.		
c. Settings	1. Explain each of the following elements of the ventilator settings: • ventilator mode • sensitivity • tidal volume • respiratory rate • peak pressure setting • pressure pop-off setting • inspiratory time • flow rate		

(continued)

Learning Objectives	VENTILATOR *(continued)*		
Topic	**Objective**	**P**	**R/D**

- percent inspiratory time
- inspiratory positive assist pressure (IPAP)
- expiratory positive assist pressure (EPAP)
- positive end-expiratory pressure (PEEP)

2. Locate the prescribed setting information on the ventilator information sheet:
   - ventilator mode
   - sensitivity
   - tidal volume
   - respiratory rate
   - peak pressure setting
   - pressure pop-off setting
   - inspiratory time
   - flow rate
   - percent inspiratory time
   - inspiratory positive airway pressure (IPAP)
   - expiratory positive airway pressure (EPAP)
   - positive end-expiratory pressure (PEEP)

3. Locate each of the following controls on the ventilator:
   - ventilator mode
   - sensitivity
   - tidal volume
   - respiratory rate
   - peak pressure setting
   - pressure pop-off setting
   - inspiratory time
   - flow rate
   - percent inspiratory time
   - inspiratory positive airway pressure (IPAP)
   - expiratory positive airway pressure (EPAP)

4. Demonstrate how to set each of the following controls:
   - ventilator mode
   - sensitivity
   - tidal volume
   - respiratory rate
   - peak pressure setting
   - pressure pop-off setting
   - inspiratory time
   - flow rate
   - percent inspiratory time
   - inspiratory positive airway pressure (IPAP)

(continued)

Learning Objectives	**VENTILATOR** *(continued)*		
Topic	**Objective**	**P**	**R/D**
	• expiratory positive airway pressure (EPAP) • positive end-expiratory pressure (PEEP) 5. Describe the situations when you should change any ventilator settings.		
d. Operational check	1. Explain why routine checks of the ventilation system are necessary. 2. Explain why water must be drained from tubings. 3. Demonstrate how to drain the water from the tubings. 4. Demonstrate how to check all ventilator settings. 5. Demonstrate how to check all ventilator alarms. 6. Demonstrate how to record each ventilator check. 7. Demonstrate how to secure the ventilator tubing to the mask/mouth piece/tracheostomy tube.		
e. Preventive maintenance	1. Explain why preventive maintenance is necessary. 2. Demonstrate where to find the hour meter on the ventilator. 3. Demonstrate where to find the preventive maintenance schedule for the ventilator. 4. Identify the company/person to contact to schedule preventive maintenance for the ventilator. 5. Explain what ventilator will be used while one ventilator is out of the home for preventive maintenance. 6. List the cleaning schedule for the ventilator filter(s). 7. Demonstrate how to change the ventilator filter. 8. Demonstrate how to clean the ventilator case. 9. Demonstrate how to charge the internal battery.		
f. Problems	1. Explain what to do if you suspect that the ventilator is not working right. 2. List and demonstrate what to do if the ventilator stops working. 3. List the steps to take if the ventilator begins alarming and you can't figure out why. 4. Explain what to do if there is a power failure when the ventilator is in use. 5. Explain what to do if the low internal battery alarm begins sounding.		

Learning Objectives	**ALARMS**		
Topic	**Objective**	**P**	**R/D**
a. Principles	1. Explain the purpose and function of each of the following alarms or warnings:		

(continued)

Learning Objectives	ALARMS *(continued)*		
Topic	**Objective**	**P**	**R/D**

<table>
<tr><td></td><td>

• low pressure alarm
• high pressure alarm
• remote alarm
• call system
• additional alarm
• power/battery alarm

2. Demonstrate where to find setting information on the ventilator information sheet for each of the following:
  • low pressure alarm
  • high pressure alarm
  • remote alarm
  • additional alarm

3. Identify the ordered setting for each of the following:
  • low pressure alarm
  • high pressure alarm
  • remote alarm
  • additional alarm

4. Locate each of the following controls on the ventilator:
  • low pressure alarm
  • high pressure alarm
  • remote alarm
  • call system
  • additional alarm

</td><td></td><td></td></tr>
<tr><td>

b. Settings

</td><td>

1. Demonstrate how to connect the following:
  • manual alarm or call system
  • additional alarm
  • remote alarm

2. Demonstrate how to set each of the following alarms or warnings:
  • low pressure alarm
  • high pressure alarm
  • remote alarm
  • call system

3. Demonstrate how to check the operation of each of the following:
  • low pressure alarm
  • high pressure alarm
  • remote alarm
  • call system
  • additional alarm
  • power/battery alarm

</td><td></td><td></td></tr>
</table>

(continued)

Learning Objectives	**ALARMS** *(continued)*		
Topic	**Objective**	**P**	**R/D**
c. Responses	1. List the first step to take whenever an alarm sounds.		
	2. List the reasons why the low pressure alarm may sound.		
	3. Demonstrate how to isolate and correct a low pressure alarm condition.		
	4. Explain situations when the low pressure alarm might not sound when the ventilator is disconnected.		
	5. List the reasons why the high pressure alarm may sound.		
	6. Demonstrate how to isolate and correct a high pressure alarm condition.		
	7. Explain situations when the high pressure alarm could unexpectedly sound.		
	8. Demonstrate how to respond to, evaluate, and correct a power/battery alarm condition.		
	9. Demonstrate how to respond to, evaluate, and correct a remote alarm condition.		
	10. List the reasons why the additional alarm may sound.		
	11. Demonstrate how to respond to, evaluate, and correct an additional alarm condition.		
	12. Explain situations when the additional alarm might sound incorrectly.		
	13. Demonstrate how to check and change batteries in remote alarms or call systems.		
d. Problems	1. Explain what to do if you suspect that an alarm has not sounded when it should.		
	2. Explain what to do if you cannot figure out why an alarm is sounding.		
	3. Explain what to do if an alarm sounds when you think it should not.		

Learning Objectives	**VENTILATOR TUBING**		
Topic	**Objective**	**P**	**R/D**
a. Application	1. Identify each of the following parts of the ventilator circuit: • large bore tubing • pressure line tubing • exhalation valve tubing • exhalation valve • bacteria filter		

(continued)

Learning Objectives	**VENTILATOR TUBING** (continued)		
Topic	**Objective**	**P**	**R/D**

<table>
<tr><td></td><td>

- water trap
- thermometer
- circuit one-way valve
- swivel connector
- "other" _____

2. Explain the purpose for each of the following parts of the ventilator circuit:
   - large bore tubing
   - pressure line tubing
   - exhalation valve
   - exhalation valve tubing
   - bacteria filter
   - water trap
   - circuit one-way valve
   - thermometer
   - swivel connector

3. Demonstrate how to empty water from each of the following parts of the ventilator circuit:
   - large bore tubing
   - pressure line tubing
   - exhalation valve
   - exhalation valve tubing
   - circuit one-way valve
   - bacteria filter
   - water trap

</td><td></td><td></td></tr>
<tr><td>

b. Changes

</td><td>

1. Demonstrate how to change all the tubing on the ventilator while:
   - the ventilator is not in use
   - the ventilator is in use

2. Demonstrate how to change and refill the humidifier when:
   - the ventilator is not in use
   - the ventilator is in use

</td><td></td><td></td></tr>
<tr><td>

c. Cleaning

</td><td>

1. List when to clean the tubing.
2. Demonstrate how to take the circuit tubing apart.
3. Demonstrate how to clean the tubing, including use of the disinfecting solution.
4. Demonstrate how to dry the tubing and exhalation valve.
5. Demonstrate how to put the ventilator circuit tubing back together.
6. Demonstrate how to replace the humidifier on the ventilator.

</td><td></td><td></td></tr>
</table>

(continued)

Learning Objectives	**VENTILATOR TUBING** *(continued)*		
Topic	**Objective**	**P**	**R/D**
	7. Demonstrate how to test the circuit for leaks.		
	8. Explain how to store the clean, dry tubings.		
	9. Demonstrate how and where to write down the circuit change and cleaning on the ventilator information sheet.		
d. Problems	1. Demonstrate how to find leaks in the ventilator circuit.		
	2. Describe how to fix leaks in the ventilator circuit.		
	3. Demonstrate how to empty water from each of the tubings.		

Learning Objectives	**EXHALATION VALVE**		
Topic	**Objective**	**P**	**R/D**
a. Application	1. Identify the exhalation valve.		
	2. Explain why the exhalation valve is necessary.		
	3. Explain how the exhalation valve works.		
b. Changes	1. Explain when to change the exhalation valve other than for regular cleaning.		
	2. Demonstrate how to change the exhalation valve while the ventilator is not in use.		
	3. Demonstrate how to change the exhalation valve while the ventilator is in use.		
c. Cleaning	1. List when to clean the exhalation valve.		
	2. Demonstrate how to take the exhalation valve apart.		
	3. Demonstrate how to clean the valve, including using the disinfecting solution.		
	4. Demonstrate how to dry the exhalation valve.		
	5. Demonstrate how to put the exhalation valve back together.		
	6. Demonstrate how to change the exhalation valve on the ventilator.		
	7. Demonstrate how to test the exhalation valve for leaks.		
	8. Explain how to store the clean, dry exhalation valve.		
d. Problems	1. Identify some signs that would lead you to check that the exhalation valve is working right.		
	2. Demonstrate how to find leaks in the exhalation valve.		
	3. Demonstrate how to empty water or mucus from the exhalation valve.		

(continued)

Learning Objectives	TRACHEOSTOMY		
Topic	**Objective**	**P**	**R/D**
a. Principles	1. Explain the purpose and function of a tracheostomy.		
	2. Explain why a tracheostomy tube is being used.		
	3. Explain how the tracheostomy tube changes the way air goes into the lungs and how this affects speaking.		
	4. List the brand, model, type, and size of the tracheostomy tube in use.		
	5. Identify the following parts of the tracheostomy tube: • cuff • pilot balloon, balloon valve, and tubing • obturator • inner cannula • flanges • fenestration • plug • ties or chain • stoma		
	6. Explain the purpose of each of the following parts of the tracheostomy tube: • cuff • pilot balloon, balloon valve, and tubing • obturator • inner cannula • flanges • fenestration • plug • ties or chain • stoma		
	7. List and explain the other equipment or supplies needed because air does not go in through the nose and mouth.		
	8. Explain why regular careful stoma inspection is important.		
	9. Explain how to speak with a tracheostomy tube.		
b. Stoma care	1. List the stoma care schedule.		
	2. List the supplies and equipment needed to clean the stoma.		
	3. Demonstrate stoma care.		
	4. Explain what to look for when you inspect the stoma.		

(continued)

Learning Objectives	TRACHEOSTOMY *(continued)*		
Topic	**Objective**	**P**	**R/D**
c. Cuff care	1. Explain why the pilot balloon and cuff are important. 2. Demonstrate how to inflate the cuff. 3. Demonstrate how to make sure there is the right amount of air in the cuff. 4. Demonstrate how to deflate the cuff. 5. Demonstrate how to speak/communicate with a cuffed tracheostomy tube. 6. Explain the hazards of excessive cuff inflation. 7. Indicate the volume of air used for cuff inflation and the cuff inflation-deflation schedule.		
d. Securing the tracheostomy tube	1. Explain why it is important to keep the tracheostomy tube fastened around the neck at all times. 2. Demonstrate how to fasten the tracheostomy tube with: • tracheostomy tape • a chain • a tracheostomy securing device 3. Explain why it is important to routinely look carefully at the neck underneath the tracheostomy ties. 4. Demonstrate how to attach the ventilator tubing to the tracheostomy tube.		
e. Tube care	1. List the tracheostomy tube cleaning schedule. 2. List the supplies and equipment needed to clean the tracheostomy tube. 3. Demonstrate tracheostomy tube cleaning with the tube in place. 4. Describe the equipment/supplies needed when breathing through the open tracheostomy tube, including use of: • oxygen • humidification		
f. Inner cannula	1. Explain when to have the inner cannula in/out. 2. List the cleaning/replacement schedule for the inner cannula. 3. Demonstrate changing the inner cannula. 4. Demonstrate cleaning the inner cannula.		
g. Tube changes	1. List the tracheostomy tube changing schedule. 2. Identify the people who should change the tracheostomy tube. 3. List the supplies and equipment needed to change the tracheostomy tube. 4. Demonstrate changing the tracheostomy tube.		

(continued)

Learning Objectives	TRACHEOSTOMY *(continued)*		
Topic	**Objective**	**P**	**R/D**
	5. Explain how to store the extra, clean tracheostomy tube.		
h. Using a tracheostomy plug	1. Explain why to use a tracheostomy tube plug.		
	2. Write the schedule for use of the tracheostomy tube plug.		
	3. Demonstrate the steps to follow to switch to the tracheostomy plug.		
	4. Demonstrate how to use extra oxygen with the plug in place.		
	5. Demonstrate how to clean and store the tracheostomy plug.		
i. Problems	1. List other situations or times beyond the regular schedule when a tracheostomy tube or inner cannula change might be necessary.		
	2. Describe how to recognize and respond to: • a cuff that has a leak • aspiration • bloody sputum • an air leak around the cuff • a leaky pilot balloon or valve • a blocked tracheostomy tube • accidental tracheostomy tube removal • bleeding from or around the tracheostomy tube • signs of infection around the tracheostomy tube		
	3. Explain what to do if different parts of the tracheostomy tube break or crack.		
	4. Explain what to do if the tracheostomy tube will not slip back into the neck.		
	5. Explain what to do if the tracheostomy tube will not slip out of the neck.		
	6. Explain what to do if the ventilator tubing will not disconnect from the tracheostomy tube.		

Learning Objectives	NASAL MASK		
Topic	**Objective**	**P**	**R/D**
a. Application	1. Explain why a nasal mask is needed.		
	2. Identify the parts of the nasal mask.		
	3. Demonstrate how to put on and adjust the mask.		
b. Cleaning	1. Describe when to clean the mask.		
	2. Demonstrate how to put the nasal mask together and take it apart.		
	3. Demonstrate how to clean and dry the nasal mask.		

(continued)

Learning Objectives	**NASAL MASK** *(continued)*		
Topic	**Objective**	**P**	**R/D**
	4. Demonstrate how to attach the mask to the ventilator tubing.		
c. Problems	1. Demonstrate what to do if air leaks around the mask.		
	2. List ways to relieve any sore spots, redness, or irritation on the face or around the mask.		
	3. Describe what to do if there is a lot of stomach bloating or burping.		

Learning Objectives	**MOUTHPIECE VENTILATION**		
Topic	**Objective**	**P**	**R/D**
a. Application	1. Explain why a mouthpiece is used.		
	2. Identify the mouthpiece and lip seal.		
	3. Demonstrate how to use the mouthpiece/lip seal and keep a seal.		
b. Cleaning	1. Describe when to clean the mouthpiece/lip seal.		
	2. Demonstrate how to clean and dry the mouthpiece/lip seal.		
c. Problems	1. Demonstrate what to do if air leaks around the mouth during sleep.		
	2. List different ways to relieve any sore spots, redness, or irritation around or in the mouth.		
	3. Describe what to do if there is a lot of stomach bloating or burping.		
	4. Describe what to do if any of the following occur: morning headaches, sudden waking up with shortness of breath, or a heart rate much faster than usual.		

Learning Objectives	**HUMIDIFICATION/HEAT AND MOISTURE EXCHANGER (HME)**		
Topic	**Objective**	**P**	**R/D**
a. Principles	1. Explain why a humidifier/HME is needed.		
	2. State the brand and type of humidifier/HME.		
b. Humidifier use on the ventilator	1. List the schedule for using the humidifier/HME.		
	2. State what kind of water to use in the humidifier.		
	3. Demonstrate how to connect the humidifier/HME to the ventilator tubing.		
	4. Demonstrate how to add water to the humidifier.		
	5. Explain why not to drain water from the tubings back into the humidifier.		
	6. State whether the humidifier needs electricity and where to plug it in.		

(continued)

Learning Objectives	**HUMIDIFICATION/HEAT AND**		
	MOISTURE EXCHANGER (HME) *(continued)*		
Topic	**Objective**	**P**	**R/D**
	7. Demonstrate how to set the temperature of the humidifier.		
	8. State the prescribed temperature range for the humidifier.		
	9. Explain when and how to check the humidifier temperature.		
	10. Explain any differences between the humidifier used with the primary ventilator and the humidifier used with the backup ventilator.		
c. Humidifier use off the ventilator	1. List the schedule for using the humidifier/ HME.		
	2. State what kind of water to use in the humidifier.		
	3. Demonstrate how to connect the humidifier/HME to the tubing.		
	4. Demonstrate how to add water to the humidifier.		
	5. Explain why not to empty water from the tubings back into the humidifier.		
	6. State whether the humidifier needs electricity and where to plug it in.		
	7. Demonstrate how to set the humidifier temperature.		
	8. State the prescribed temperature range for the humidifier.		
	9. Explain when and how to check the humidifier temperature.		
d. Cleaning	1. State when to clean the humidifier/HME.		
	2. Demonstrate how to put the humidifier together.		
	3. Demonstrate how to take the humidifier apart.		
	4. Demonstrate how to clean the HME.		
	5. Demonstrate how to clean and dry the humidifier.		
	6. Demonstrate how to change the humidifier/HME while the ventilator is in use.		
	7. Demonstrate how to change the humidifier/ HME while the ventilator is not in use.		
e. Changes	1. Explain why changing the humidifier/HME is important.		
	2. List when to change the humidifier/HME.		
f. Problems	1. Demonstrate how to find and correct a humidifier/HME air leak.		
	2. Demonstrate how to recognize and correct a blocked HME.		

(continued)

Learning Objectives	OXYGEN		
Topic	Objective	P	R/D

a. Prescription for use	1. Explain why extra oxygen is needed.
	2. State the amount of oxygen to use at these times:
	  • when the ventilator is in use
	  • when the ventilator is not in use
	  • with activity
	  • during sleep		

b. Application	1. Name the type of oxygen supply in use. 2. Demonstrate how to connect the oxygen to the ventilator tubing. 3. Demonstrate how to use extra oxygen when the ventilator is not in use. 4. Explain any differences between connecting oxygen to the usual ventilator and circuit and the circuit for the backup ventilator. 5. Demonstrate how to set or change the oxygen flow. 6. Demonstrate how to use oxygen when moving away from the main oxygen supply. 7. Demonstrate how to fill the portable oxygen system.		
c. Supply on hand	1. Demonstrate how to tell how much oxygen is left. 2. Estimate how long the oxygen supply will last. 3. Identify the oxygen supply level when you should call for replacement/refill of the oxygen supply. 4. Identify who to call for more oxygen.		
d. Safety	1. List the safety rules to follow with extra oxygen in the home. 2. List the safety rules to follow when transporting oxygen equipment. 3. List the safety rules to follow when storing oxygen.		

Learning Objectives	BACK-UP/SECONDARY VENTILATOR		
Topic	Objective	P	R/D
a. Purpose	1. Explain why a backup or second ventilator is important. 2. Describe the differences between the usual ventilator and the backup ventilator. 3. Explain any differences between the usual ventilator circuit and the circuit for the backup ventilator. 4. Explain when and how to use the backup or secondary ventilator.		

(continued)

Learning Objectives	BACK-UP/SECONDARY VENTILATOR *(continued)*		
Topic	**Objective**	**P**	**R/D**
	5. Explain when to change to the backup ventilator.		
b. Equipment	1. Demonstrate how to connect the circuit, humidifier, and alarms to the backup ventilator.		
	2. Demonstrate when and how to test the backup ventilator.		
	3. Demonstrate how to check the backup ventilator.		
	4. Explain why it is important to always keep the backup ventilator internal battery charged.		
	5. Explain how to keep a full charge on the backup ventilator internal battery.		
	6. Identify where to store the backup ventilator when not in use.		
	7. Demonstrate where to find the backup ventilator preventive maintenance schedule.		
c. Settings	1. Locate setting information for the backup/secondary ventilator.		
	2. Demonstrate how to set each of the following controls:		
	• ventilator mode		
	• sensitivity		
	• tidal volume		
	• respiratory rate		
	• peak pressure setting		
	• pressure pop-off setting		
	• inspiratory time		
	• flow rate		
	• percent inspiratory time		
	• inspiratory positive assist pressure (IPAP)		
	• expiratory positive assist pressure (EPAP)		
	3. List the power source(s) for the backup/secondary ventilator.		
	4. Demonstrate where to find setting information for the following alarms:		
	• low pressure alarm		
	• high pressure alarm		
	• additional alarm		
	5. Demonstrate how to set each of the following alarms or warnings:		
	• low pressure alarm		
	• high pressure alarm		
	• additional alarm		
	6. Demonstrate how to check the operation of each of the following:		

(continued)

Learning Objectives	BACK-UP/SECONDARY VENTILATOR *(continued)*		
Topic	**Objective**	**P**	**R/D**
	• low pressure alarm • high pressure alarm • additional alarm • power/battery alarm 7. Demonstrate how to perform and record a ventilator check on this machine.		
d. Problems	1. Explain what to do if you think there might be a problem with the backup ventilator. 2. Demonstrate what to do if the backup ventilator stops working. 3. List who to call if the backup ventilator stops working.		

Learning Objectives	TRACHEOSTOMY ONE-WAY VALVE		
Topic	**Objective**	**P**	**R/D**
a. Purpose	1. Identify the tracheostomy one-way valve, the brand name, type, and model. 2. Explain the purpose of the one-way valve and how it works. 3. Explain why a one-way valve is being used. 4. Explain the schedule to follow to use the one-way valve. 5. Explain the differences between how to breathe with and without the one-way valve. 6. Explain what times of day are best to use the one-way valve.		
b. Equipment	1. Demonstrate how to take out the inner cannula. 2. Demonstrate how to deflate the cuff. 3. Demonstrate how to put on the one-way valve. 4. Describe the differences that could be felt when using the one-way valve. 5. List signs to watch for that could mean its time to take the one-way valve off. 6. Demonstrate how to take off the one-way valve and resume using the ventilator. 7. Demonstrate how and where to write down the one-way valve use for the doctor and home care company. 8. Demonstrate cleaning and storage of the one-way valve.		
c. Problems	1. List signs indicating that fatigue is setting in during one-way valve use.		

(continued)

Learning Objectives	**TRACHEOSTOMY ONE-WAY VALVE** *(continued)*		
Topic	**Objective**	**P**	**R/D**
	2. Explain when to return to using the ventilator.		
	3. Explain what to do if shortness of breath continues after resuming ventilator use following one-way valve use.		

Learning Objectives	**OTHER EQUIPMENT**		
Topic	**Objective**	**P**	**R/D**
a. Manual resuscitator	1. Explain the purpose and function of a manual resuscitator.		
	2. Explain why a manual resuscitator is important.		
	3. Explain how the air goes through the manual resuscitator.		
	4. Demonstrate how to hook up extra oxygen to the manual resuscitator.		
	5. Identify ways a manual resuscitator can be harmful and how to prevent each one.		
	6. Demonstrate how to put the manual resuscitator together.		
	7. Demonstrate how to test the manual resuscitator.		
	8. Demonstrate how to find the cause of a leaky manual resuscitator and fix it.		
	9. Demonstrate how to use a manual resuscitator.		
	10. Demonstrate how to take the manual resuscitator apart.		
	11. Demonstrate how to clean the manual resuscitator.		
	12. Demonstrate how to dry and store the resuscitator.		
b. Suction	1. Identify the portable battery-powered suction machine.		
	2. Identify the battery for the portable suction machine and how to check the battery charge.		
	3. Demonstrate how to get the portable suction machine ready to use.		
	4. Demonstrate how to use the portable suction machine.		
	5. Demonstrate how and explain when to clean the suction machine.		
	6. List the causes of weak suction.		
	7. Explain how to correct each cause of weak suction.		
c. External battery	1. Identify the external battery.		
	2. List the safety rules to follow with the external battery.		
	3. Demonstrate how to hook the external battery to the ventilator.		

(continued)

Learning Objectives	OTHER EQUIPMENT *(continued)*		
Topic	**Objective**	**P**	**R/D**
	4. State how long to expect a fully charged external battery to power the ventilator.		
	5. Demonstrate how to check the charge in the external battery.		
	6. Demonstrate how and when to recharge the external battery and know how long it will take.		
d. Call unit	1. Identify the purpose of the call unit.		
	2. Demonstrate how to connect the call unit to the ventilator.		
	3. Demonstrate how to change the batteries in the call unit.		
	4. Demonstrate how and when to test the call unit.		
e. Extra alarm	1. State the purpose of the extra alarm.		
	2. Demonstrate how to connect the extra alarm to the ventilator.		
	3. Demonstrate how to change batteries in the extra alarm.		
	4. Explain when to use the extra alarm.		
	5. Demonstrate how to set the extra alarm.		
	6. Demonstrate how and when to test the extra alarm.		
	7. Identify times when the extra alarm can sound when it should not.		
	8. Identify times when the extra alarm might not sound when it should.		
f. Apnea monitor	1. Explain apnea.		
	2. Explain why an apnea alarm is being used.		
	3. Explain how the apnea alarm works.		
	4. Demonstrate how to connect this alarm to the individual and the power source.		
	5. Demonstrate how to change batteries in the apnea alarm.		
	6. Demonstrate how to set the apnea alarm.		
	7. Demonstrate how and when to test the apnea alarm.		
	8. Identify times when the apnea alarm can be misleading.		
	9. Demonstrate what to do if the apnea alarm sounds.		
g. Oxygen analyzer	1. Identify the oxygen analyzer.		
	2. Explain what an oxygen analyzer is.		
	3. Demonstrate how to check and change the batteries in the oxygen analyzer.		
	4. Demonstrate how to "zero" and calibrate the oxygen analyzer.		

(continued)

Learning Objectives	**OTHER EQUIPMENT** *(continued)*		
Topic	**Objective**	**P**	**R/D**

	5. Explain what to do if the analyzer will not "zero" or calibrate.		
	6. Demonstrate how and where to connect the analyzer to the ventilator tubing.		
	7. Demonstrate how and when to measure the amount of oxygen going through the tubing.		
	8. Demonstrate how to adjust the oxygen connected to the ventilator based on the oxygen analyzer reading.		
	9. Demonstrate how and where to write down the oxygen analyzer reading and oxygen flow.		
	10. Demonstrate how to remove the oxygen analyzer from the ventilator tubing.		
	11. Explain how to take care of the oxygen analyzer.		
	12. Explain how to store the oxygen analyzer.		
	13. Explain what to do if you think the analyzer is not accurate.		
h. Oximeter	1. Explain what the oximeter measures and why this is important.		
	2. Identify the oximeter and its parts including: • power cord • power switch • sensor • oxygen saturation display • heart rate display • alarm display • signal display • alarm controls		
	3. Demonstrate how to turn the oximeter on and make sure it is working right.		
	4. Explain when to use the oximeter.		
	5. Demonstrate how to attach the oximeter.		
	6. Demonstrate how to set the oximeter alarms.		
	7. State the expected oxygen saturation range.		
	8. Explain how to respond if the oxygen saturation is above the expected range.		
	9. Explain how to respond if the oxygen saturation is below the expected range.		
	10. Identify times when the oxygen saturation reading can be wrong.		
	11. Demonstrate how to respond to an alarming oximeter.		
i. Speaking	1. Explain why communicating can present special challenges.		

(continued)

Learning Objectives	**OTHER EQUIPMENT** *(continued)*		
Topic	**Objective**	**P**	**R/D**
	2. Discuss and demonstrate how to communicate using: • deflated cuff on the tracheostomy tube • Passy-Muir Valve • electronic larynx • talking tracheostomy tube • plugged tracheostomy tube • computer • communication board • lipreading		

Learning Objectives	**MONITORING**		
Topic	**Objective**	**P**	**R/D**
a. Ventilator	1. Explain why routine monitoring is important on and off the ventilator. 2. Identify the ventilator monitoring sheet. 3. List the parts of the ventilator system to check at regular times, and when to check them. 4. Explain peak inspiratory pressure. 5. State the normal peak inspiratory pressure range. 6. Demonstrate how and when to measure peak inspiratory pressure.		
b. Vital signs	1. State the normal range for each of the following vital signs: • heart rate • respiratory rate 2. Explain some normal activities during the day that could cause an increase or decrease in: • heart rate • respiratory rate 3. Demonstrate how and when to count and where to write down: • heart rate • respiratory rate 4. Identify one other place where heart rate can be counted. 5. Explain what to do if each of the following is above normal range: • heart rate • respiratory rate 6. Explain what to do if each of the following is below normal range: • heart rate		

(continued)

Learning Objectives　　　　　　　　**MONITORING** *(continued)*

Topic	Objective	P	R/D
	• respiratory rate		
c. Ease of breathing	1. List several things to notice if breathing is difficult: • when not using the ventilator • when using the ventilator 2. List the steps to take to make breathing easier. 3. List the steps to take to check the equipment.		
d. Skin & mucous membranes	1. List several parts of physical appearance that can show breathing is okay. 2. Explain why skin color is important. 3. Explain what to do if skin color is gray or blue. 4. Explain why skin and body temperature are important things to observe. 5. Explain what to do if there is a fever. 6. Explain what to do if the skin feels "cold and clammy."		
e. Secretions	1. Explain why each of the following mucous characteristics are important: • color • amount • thickness • odor 2. Explain what to do if a change is seen in any of these mucous characteristics: • color • amount • thickness • odor 3. Demonstrate where to write down notes about mucous.		
f. Signs of infection	1. Explain the signs of a lung infection. 2. List what to do if you think a lung infection may be starting. 3. Discuss how to prevent a lung infection.		
g. Routine medical follow-up	1. Explain why routine follow-up appointments with the doctor are important. 2. Explain the need for medical testing. 3. Explain the purpose of each of these tests the doctor may order: • blood gas (daytime and/or nighttime) • oximetry (daytime and/or nighttime) • sleep study • end tidal carbon dioxide measurement • complete blood count		

(continued)

Learning Objectives	MONITORING *(continued)*		
Topic	**Objective**	**P**	**R/D**
	• chest X-ray • sputum exam 4. Explain why routine home follow-up visits by the respiratory home care company representative are important.		

Learning Objectives	INHALED MEDICATIONS		
Topic	**Objective**	**P**	**R/D**
a. Purpose	1. Explain why aerosol/metered dose inhaled medication is needed. 2. Explain what each medication does.		
b. Prescription	1. State each medication name, schedule, and dosage. 2. Identify the container of each medication. 3. Identify how long to expect one container of each medication to last. 4. Identify how to store each medication. 5. Identify any normal side effects that could happen with each medication and what to do if they happen. 6. Identify possible serious side effects that might happen from each medication and what to do about them. 7. Identify how it might feel if a dose of each medication is missed. 8. Identify how it might feel if a dose of each medication is taken too soon. 9. List and explain which medications have any special instructions (tapering/discontinuing/increasing frequency).		

c. Aerosol equipment	1. Explain when to use the aerosol equipment.
	2. List the equipment and supplies needed for an aerosol treatment:
	  • when the ventilator is in use
	  • when the ventilator is not in use
	3. Demonstrate how to put the equipment together for an aerosol treatment.
	4. Demonstrate how to measure and mix the aerosol medication.
	5. Demonstrate an aerosol treatment:
	  • when the ventilator is in use
	  • when the ventilator is not in use
	6. Demonstrate how to monitor an aerosol treatment.		

(continued)

Learning Objectives	INHALED MEDICATIONS *(continued)*		
Topic	**Objective**	**P**	**R/D**
	7. Demonstrate how to write down an aerosol treatment on the ventilator sheet.		
d. Metered dose inhaler equipment	1. List the equipment and supplies needed for a metered dose inhaler treatment: • when the ventilator is in use • when the ventilator is not in use 2. Demonstrate a metered dose inhaler treatment: • when the ventilator is in use • when the ventilator is not in use 3. Explain what to observe before and after a metered dose inhaler treatment. 4. Demonstrate how to record a metered dose inhaler treatment. 5. Demonstrate how to clean the metered dose inhaler spacer and inspect it for excessive wear.		
e. Cleaning	1. List the cleaning schedule for the medication treatment equipment. 2. Demonstrate how to take the medication equipment apart. 3. Demonstrate how to clean and dry the medication equipment. 4. Demonstrate how to store the medication equipment.		

Learning Objectives	AIRWAY SECRETION CLEARANCE		
Topic	**Objective**	**P**	**R/D**
a. Principles	1. Explain the need for getting secretions out of the breathing passages. 2. Explain some ways to get the secretions out of the breathing passages when there is a tracheostomy tube. 3. Explain some ways to get secretions out of the breathing passages when a tracheostomy tube is not present.		
b. Assisted coughing	1. Demonstrate the use of manually assisted coughing while using tracheostomy ventilation. 2. Demonstrate the use of manually assisted coughing while using other kinds of ventilation or breathing without the ventilator.		
c. Suctioning	1. Explain tracheal suctioning. 2. Explain why suctioning is used. 3. Explain when tracheal suctioning should be done.		

(continued)

Learning Objectives	**AIRWAY SECRETION CLEARANCE** *(continued)*		
Topic	**Objective**	**P**	**R/D**
	4. Explain why it is important to look for changes in sputum color, thickness, quantity, or odor.		
	5. List the supplies needed to perform suctioning.		
	6. Explain how to observe tolerance for suctioning.		
d. Suctioning technique	1. Demonstrate how to set up all the supplies and equipment needed for suctioning.		
	2. Demonstrate safe suctioning using clean technique.		
e. Suction equipment cleaning	1. List the suction equipment cleaning schedule.		
	2. Demonstrate how to take the equipment apart.		
	3. Demonstrate how to clean and dry the equipment.		
	4. Demonstrate how to routinely inspect and store the equipment after cleaning.		
	5. Demonstrate proper disposal of used suction supplies.		
f. Problems	1. List the steps to take and demonstrate what to do for:		
	• unusual shortness of breath during suctioning		
	• difficulty removing the suction tube from the tracheostomy tube		
	• bright red blood coming out of the tracheostomy tube		
	• breathing that stops during suctioning		
	• unresponsiveness during suctioning		
	2. List the causes of weak suction machine.		
	3. Explain how to correct each cause of weak suction machine.		
	4. Explain what to do if food is suctioned from tracheostomy tube.		

Educational Objectives	**MOBILITY**		
Topic	**Objective**	**P**	**R/D**
a. Ventilator	1. Identify the changes to make to the ventilator and circuit to prepare to move around while the ventilator is in use.		
	2. List the positions in which the ventilator can be safely used.		
	3. Identify how access to the ventilator will be limited when it is secured for travel.		
	4. Explain the safety rules to follow with the external battery during mobile use.		

(continued)

Learning Objectives	**MOBILITY** *(continued)*		
Topic	**Objective**	**P**	**R/D**
	5. Demonstrate how to prepare the ventilator and accessory equipment such as humidifier and battery before moving around when the ventilator is in use.		
	6. Demonstrate how to secure the ventilator and battery on a wheelchair or cart to move around.		
	7. List what to do if there is a ventilator problem when away from home.		
b. Oxygen	1. Explain the precautions to take when traveling with the oxygen system.		
	2. Demonstrate how to check the amount of oxygen left in the portable supply.		
	3. Estimate how long the remaining oxygen supply will last.		
	4. List what to do if oxygen runs out or there is a problem with the supply.		
	5. Explain what to do if you think the oxygen flow is not right.		
c. Suction	1. Demonstrate how to use the battery-powered suction machine.		
	2. Demonstrate how to check and change the power for the portable suction machine.		
	3. Demonstrate how to use a delee suction catheter.		
	4. Explain how to dispose of used suction supplies when away from home.		
d. Supplies	1. List the supplies to have at all times, including when moving around the home.		
	2. List the equipment to have along whenever away from home.		

Learning Objectives	**THERAPIES AND DAILY ACTIVITIES**		
Topic	**Objective**	**P**	**R/D**
a. Positioning and transfers	1. Explain why regular repositioning is important.		
	2. List ventilator-related items to check before repositioning or moving from a bed to a chair.		
	3. Demonstrate how to move from a bed to a chair.		
b. Assisted cough	1. Explain the purpose and function of an assisted cough.		
	2. Explain how assisted coughing can be helpful.		
	3. Demonstrate an assisted cough.		
c. Postural drainage and percussion	1. Explain percussion and postural drainage.		
	2. List precautions to take before doing percussion or postural drainage.		

(continued)

Learning Objectives THERAPIES AND DAILY ACTIVITIES *(continued)*

Topic	Objective	P	R/D
	3. Explain why percussion and postural drainage are important.		
	4. Identify what part of the chest to emphasize.		
	5. Demonstrate percussion and postural drainage including proper positioning as prescribed.		
d. Range of motion	1. Explain why maintaining range of motion is important.		
	2. List the times and exercises that need to be done.		
	3. Demonstrate the upper body range-of-motion exercises.		
	4. Demonstrate the lower body range-of-motion exercises.		
e. Relaxation and pacing techniques	1. Explain why stress or anxiety changes respiratory needs.		
	2. Explain why relaxation techniques are important.		
	3. Demonstrate relaxation techniques.		
	4. Explain why energy conservation and pacing are important.		
	5. List energy conservation techniques.		
	6. Demonstrate energy conservation techniques for usual daily activities such as face washing.		
f. Exercise program	1. Explain why maintaining upper and lower body strength is important.		
	2. List the times and exercises that should be done.		
	3. Demonstrate upper body strengthening exercises.		
	4. Demonstrate lower body strengthening exercises.		
g. Maintaining proper fluid intake	1. Explain why the right amount of fluids is important.		
	2. List signs that might occur when fluid intake is too low.		
	3. List signs that might occur when fluid intake is too high.		
	4. Identify what to do if fluid intake might be too high or too low.		
h. Diet instruction	1. List special diet needs.		
	2. Explain why timing of meals is important.		
	3. List the ideal timing of meals.		
i. Tube feedings	1. Identify the gastrostomy tube.		
	2. Explain why tube feedings are necessary.		
	3. Demonstrate a tube feeding.		
	4. List precautions to take with a tube feeding.		
	5. Explain how to know if the gastrostomy tube is blocked.		

(continued)

Learning Objectives   **THERAPIES AND DAILY ACTIVITIES** *(continued)*

Topic	Objective	P	R/D
	6. Explain what to do if the gastrostomy tube comes out.		
	7. Explain why routine inspection of the tube and skin around it is important.		
	8. Explain when to clean the gastrostomy tube and surrounding skin.		
	9. Demonstrate cleaning of the gastrostomy tube and the skin around it.		
	10. Demonstrate how to change the dressing around the gastrostomy tube.		
	11. List signs of possible problems to look for around the gastrostomy tube.		
j. Assistance with other daily activities	1. Explain why proper skin care is important.		
	2. List signs to watch for when doing skin care and bathing.		
	3. Demonstrate skin care and bathing.		
	4. Explain the bowel or bladder routine (intermittent catheterization if necessary).		
	5. List the precautions to take with bowel and bladder care.		
	6. Demonstrate bowel and bladder care.		

Learning Objectives   **TIME WITHOUT THE VENTILATOR**

Topic	Objective	P	R/D
a. Purpose	1. Explain why spending time without the ventilator is important.		
	2. Explain the schedule for time without the ventilator.		
	3. Explain what times of day are better for breathing independently.		
b. Equipment	1. Demonstrate how to set up the equipment that will be used during time without the ventilator.		
	2. Demonstrate how to test the equipment used during times without the ventilator.		
	3. Demonstrate how to connect to and use the breathing equipment during times without the ventilator.		
	4. Demonstrate how to record time spent without the ventilator for the doctor and home care company.		
c. Problems	1. List several signs of tiring to watch for during times without the ventilator.		
	2. Explain when ventilator use should be resumed.		
	3. Explain what to do if shortness of breath continues after resuming ventilator use.		

(continued)

Learning Objectives	**EMERGENCIES**		
Topic	**Objective**	**P**	**R/D**
a. Equipment and information	1. Make a list of emergency phone numbers and explain when to call: • the home care company • the doctor • the hospital • the power company • rescue/ambulance • fire department 2. List the equipment to have available at all times. 3. List the supplies to have available at all times.		
b. Manual resuscitator	1. Demonstrate how to hook up oxygen to the manual resuscitator. 2. Demonstrate how to use the manual resuscitator. 3. Demonstrate how to find and fix the cause of a leaky manual resuscitator.		
c. Dyspnea	1. List things to notice if breathing is difficult when not using the ventilator. 2. List things to notice if breathing is difficult during ventilator use. 3. List the steps to make breathing easier when the ventilator is in use. 4. List the steps to make breathing easier when the ventilator is not in use. 5. List the steps to check the equipment.		
d. Ventilator problems	1. Explain what to do if you think that the ventilator is not working right. 2. List what to do if the ventilator stops working. 3. List what to do if the ventilator begins alarming and you can't figure out why. 4. Explain what to do if power goes out during ventilator use. 5. Explain what to do if the low internal battery alarm begins sounding.		
e. Oxygen supply/ system problems	1. Explain what to do if the oxygen supply runs out. 2. Explain what to do if you think the oxygen flow is not right. 3. Explain what to do if you think the oxygen container may be damaged.		
f. Cardiopulmonary resuscitation	1. Explain why CPR is important. 2. Explain the purpose of CPR and how it works. 3. Demonstrate CPR.		

(continued)

Learning Objectives	**EMERGENCIES** *(continued)*		
Topic	**Objective**	**P**	**R/D**
g. Tracheostomy tube problems	1. Describe how to recognize and what to do for: • a tracheostomy cuff that has a leak • aspiration • bloody sputum • an air leak around the cuff • a leaky pilot balloon or valve • a blocked tracheostomy tube • a tracheostomy tube that slips out of the neck • bleeding from or around the tracheostomy tube • signs of infection around the tracheostomy tube 2. Explain what to do if different parts of the tracheostomy tube break or crack. 3. Explain what to do if the tracheostomy tube will not slip back into the neck. 4. Explain what to do if the tracheostomy tube will not slip out of the neck. 5. Explain what to do if food is suctioned from the tracheostomy tube.		
h. Vomiting and aspiration	1. Explain why vomiting adds special risks when a tracheostomy tube is present. 2. Demonstrate proper positioning if vomiting begins. 3. List what to do if aspiration may have happened: • with a tracheostomy tube in place • without a tracheostomy tube 4. Describe when to use the Heimlich maneuver. 5. Demonstrate the Heimlich maneuver.		
i. Use of deLee suction	1. Identify a deLee suction catheter. 2. Explain why a deLee suction catheter could be useful. 3. Demonstrate how to use a deLee catheter.		

Learning Objectives	**OTHER PATIENT AND CAREGIVER ISSUES**		
Topic	**Objective**	**P**	**R/D**
a. Coordination of care	1. Explain the importance of open communication between the ventilator-assisted individual and caregivers. 2. Identify community resources available for transportation, financial assistance, or additional care needs.		
b. Respite care	1. Identify signs of caregiver burnout. 2. Identify community or other resources available for respite care.		

(continued)

Learning Objectives	OTHER PATIENT AND CAREGIVER ISSUES *(continued)*		
Topic	**Objective**	**P**	**R/D**
c. Future care	1. Discuss convictions and choices about future medical care, including: • tracheostomy • CPR • feedings and fluids given by tube into a vein or the stomach		
d. Advanced directives	1. Explain an advanced directive. 2. Discuss any specific wishes with family members, caregivers, physicians, and medical personnel. 3. Prepare an advanced directive, if desired. Inform family, caregivers, and health providers of this directive, where it is kept, and its contents. Give copies to the physician and hospital.		

─────────────────── **SUMMARY** ───────────────────

Mechanical ventilation has been used effectively to support patients suffering from ventilatory or oxygenation failure. Many of these patients require continuing ventilatory support due to irreversible problems such as high cervical or head injuries. As a result, they are required to stay in an acute care setting longer than other patients. Since acute care settings are traditionally more costly, home mechanical ventilation has gained popularity in caring for patients requiring prolonged ventilatory assistance.

The successful management of a patient on a home mechanical ventilator demands proper patient selection, careful planning, detailed home instruction, and a programmatic follow up by the health care team. The team approach is probably the most critical element of successful ventilator care in the home. The health care professionals and especially the family members must be able and willing to make a long-term commitment in caring for the patient in the home.

A set of learning objectives provided by the National Center for Home Mechanical Ventilation and National Jewish Center for Immunology and Respiratory Medicine (Glenn et al., 1993) can be a very useful resource for all individuals who work closely with the patient and ventilator outside an acute care setting. These objectives may be modified to suit individual patient needs.

Self-Assessment Questions

1. Which of the following is *not* a goal of mechanical ventilation provided in the home?

   A. extension of the patient's life and quality of life

   B. development and improvement of the patient's body functions

   C. elimination of staff positions in an acute care setting

   D. reduction of the cost for acute ventilator care

2. Providing or receiving mechanical ventilation in the home:

   A. needs careful evaluation in selecting a suitable patient.

   B. gives the patient less time to interact with family members and friends.

   C. requires little or no commitment from family members.

   D. is more costly than one provided in an acute care setting.

3. Some essential team members for a successful home ventilator program should include all of the following *except*:

   A. physician.

   B. insurance clerk.

   C. respiratory therapist.

   D. nurse.

4. Dr. Kingston asks you to evaluate Mr. Lange, a patient who has been on the ventilator for three weeks, for continuation of ventilator care in the home. You would evaluate all of the following *except*:

A. age of patient.

B. clinical stability of the patient.

C. type of ventilator suitable for the patient.

D. laboratory and clinical assessment of the patient.

5 to 8. Match the type of pulmonary problem with the respective clinical characteristics. Use each answer once.

Pulmonary Problem	Characteristics
5. COPD	A. Apnea and chronic hypoventilation
6. Restrictive lung disease	B. Inefficient ventilation, atelectasis, and pneumonia
7. Ventilatory muscle dysfunction	C. Air flow obstruction and air trapping
8. Central hypoventilation syndrome	D. Reduction of lung volumes/capacities and deadspace ventilation

9. A COPD patient has an admitting diagnosis of lobar pneumonia affecting three of five lobes. When this pulmonary problem triggers a rapid deterioration of the patient's clinical status, it is called:

A. acute bronchitis and COPD.

B. acute exacerbation of COPD.

C. chronic ventilatory failure with metabolic acidosis.

D. respiratory failure of COPD.

10. Which of the following blood gas reports illustrates the condition in Question #9?

Blood Gas Report
A. pH = 7.26, $PaCO_2$ = 77 mm Hg, PaO_2 = 44 mm Hg, HCO_3^- = 35 mEq/L
B. pH = 7.40, $PaCO_2$ = 45 mm Hg, PaO_2 = 81 mm Hg, HCO_3^- = 27 mEq/L
C. pH = 7.39, $PaCO_2$ = 52 mm Hg, PaO_2 = 56 mm Hg, HCO_3^- = 31 mEq/L
D. pH = 7.49, $PaCO_2$ = 30 mm Hg, PaO_2 = 43 mm Hg, HCO_3^- = 22 mEq/L

11. In addition to V/Q mismatch and pulmonary hypertension, COPD patients usually have:

A. low lung compliance.
B. high elastic recoil of lung tissues.

C. air trapping.
D. reduced lung volumes and capacities.

12. Mechanical ventilation may be necessary for patients with restrictive lung disease because they have:

A. high lung compliance.

C. low lung inflating pressure requirement.

B. increased lung volumes and capacities.

D. increased work of breathing.

13. Apnea, hypoventilation, infection, and atelectasis are some signs of patients diagnosed with:

A. central hypoventilation syndrome.

C. restrictive lung disease.

B. COPD.

D. spinal cord injury at the C-5 level.

14. Selection of patient for a home mechanical ventilation program should be based on all of the following considerations *except* the:

A. desires of the patient.

C. available equipment and financial resources.

B. desires of the physician.

D. cost for the home care program.

15. Ms. Lange has been receiving around-the-clock mechanical ventilation for two months due to a head injury sustained in an automobile accident. Prior to transfer to her home for ventilator care, which of the following is the most essential safety feature based on her condition?

A. insurance coverage

C. live-in health care assistance

B. high and low pressure alarms

D. backup ventilator

References

Eigen, H. et al. (1990). Home mechanical ventilation of pediatric patients. *Am Rev Respir Dis, 141*(1), 258–259.

Ferns, T. (1994). Home mechanical ventilation in a changing health service. *Nurs Times, 90*(40), 43–45.

Glass, C. A. (1993). The impact of home based ventilator dependence on family life. *Paraplegia, 31*(2), 93–101.

Glenn, K. A. et al. (1993). Learning objectives for positive pressure ventilation in the home. National Center for Home Mechanical Ventilation, Denver, CO.

Goldstein, R. S. et al. (1995). Home mechanical ventilation: Demographics and user perspectives. *Chest, 108*(6), 1581–1586.

Gower, D. J. et al. (1985). Home ventilator dependence after high cervical cord injury. *South Med J, 78*(8), 1010–1011.

Hazlett, D. E. (1989). A study of pediatric home ventilator management: Medical, psychosocial, and financial aspects. *J Pediatr Nurs, 4*(4), 284–294.

Hill, N. S. (1994). Use of negative pressure ventilation, rocking beds, and pneumobelts. *Respir Care, 39,* 532–549.

Ilbawi, M. N. et al. (1985). Diaphragm pacing in infants: Techniques and results. *Ann Thorac Surg, 40,* 323–329.

Malley, W. J. (1990). *Clinical blood gases: Application and noninvasive alternatives.* Philadelphia: W.B. Saunders Co.

Murray, J. E. (1989, October). Payment mechanisms for pediatric home care. *Caring,* 33–35.

O'Donohue, W. J. et al. (1986). Long-term mechanical ventilation: Guidelines for management in the home and at alternate community sites (Report of the ad hoc committee, Respiratory Care Section, American College of Chest Physicians). *Chest,* (Suppl. 90, 1), 1S–37S.

Smith, C. E. (1994). Caregiver learning needs and reactions to managing home mechanical ventilation. *Heart Lung, 23*(2), 157–163.

Votroubek, W. L. (1995). Home mechanical ventilation: What are all the options? *J Home Health Care Prac, 7*(3), 21–26.

Suggested Reading

Banaszak, E. F. et al. (1981). Home ventilator care. *Respir Care, 26*(12), 1262–1268.

Carroll, P. F. (1987). Home care for the ventilator patient: A check list you can use. *Nursing, 17*(10), 82–83.

Feldman, J. et al. (1982, March/April). Mechanical ventilation: From hospital intensive care to home. *Heart Lung, 11,* 162.

Goldberg, A . I. (1989). Home care for life-supported persons: The French system of quality control, technology assessment, and cost containment. *Public Health Rep, 104*(4), 329–335.

Hughes, S. L. et al. (1987). Impact of long-term home care on hospital and nursing home use and cost. *Health Serv Res, 22*(1), 19–47.

Hughes, S. L. et al. (1992). A randomized trial of the cost effectiveness of VA hospital-based home care for the terminally ill. *Health Serv Res, 26*(6), 801–817.

Sivak, E. et al. (1983, August). Home care ventilation. *Chest, 84,* 239.

Smith, J. E., & Shneerson, J. M. (1996). A laboratory comparison of four positive pressure ventilators used in the home. *Eur Respir J, 9*(11): 2410–2415.

White, K. D. et al. (1986). Your ventilator patient can go home again. *Nursing, 16*(12), 54–56.

CHAPTER SEVENTEEN

CASE STUDIES

CASE 1: COPD

INTRODUCTION

A 74-year-old Caucasian male with a diagnosis of pulmonary emphysema, made six years prior, was seen in the emergency department with a complaint of shortness of breath. He has had respiratory problems on and off since diagnosis, including two hospital admissions, each of several days duration. He stated he caught a cold the previous week that moved down into his chest, and since that time breathing has become increasingly more difficult. He related that in his usual state of health, he was able to move freely about his home and yard and enjoyed his hobby of gardening, but now was unable to do either. Sleeping in bed had become such a problem that for the previous two nights he slept sitting back in his easy chair. His normal sputum production of about a tablespoon per day had increased to about 1/4 cup a day and had turned from white to yellow in color. He gained 6 pounds in the past four days and noticed that his ankles were swollen by the end of the day. When questioned about his smoking history, he stated that he had smoked two packs per day for 40 years, and had tried unsuccessfully to quit after his diagnosis of emphysema was made. He now smokes a half pack per day of a "lighter" brand. His home medications include an albuterol MDI, 1–2 puffs every 2–6 hours, as needed.

✓ The inability to breathe comfortably unless standing or sitting up is termed orthopnea and is a common clinical manifestation of pulmonary disease.

✓ Sudden weight gain with dependent edema in a COPD patient is a sign of cor pulmonale.

PHYSICAL EXAMINATION

General. The patient is a mildly obese male, weight 100 kg, height 72 inches, in moderately severe respiratory distress, sitting on the edge of the bed leaning forward supporting his weight with his palms and breathing through pursed lips.

Vital Signs.   Heart rate 124/minute, blood pressure 150/90 mm Hg, respiratory rate 28/minute, and temperature 100.5°F.

HEENT.   Some cyanosis of the lips, otherwise unremarkable.

Neck.   Trachea in the midline, no masses, stridor, lymphadenopathy, or thyromegaly. Carotid pulses ++ without bruit. There is marked use of accessory muscles of the neck with mild jugular venous distention.

☑ Paradoxical motion of the abdomen during ventilation is an indication diaphragmatic muscle fatigue.

Chest.   The anteroposterior diameter of the chest is increased with a deep suprasternal notch and some paradoxical motion of the abdomen. Decreased tactile fremitus and absent point of maximal impulse (PMI) are noted with hyperresonance to percussion bilaterally.

Heart.   Sounds are distant with no irregularity in rate or rhythm noted, no gallops or murmurs.

Lungs.   Bilaterally diminished with scattered expiratory wheezing, bibasilar rhonchi, and a prolonged expiratory phase.

Abdomen.   Mild hepatomegaly, paradoxical movement with breathing, otherwise unremarkable.

Extremities.   Slight digital cyanosis with +2 pitting edema in both ankles.

INITIAL ASSESSMENT AND TREATMENT

In the emergency room, a portable chest radiograph and arterial blood gas with co-oximetry were obtained, the patient was placed on a 2 lpm nasal cannula and given an aerosol treatment with 2.5 mg albuterol sulfate in NS. Room air blood gas results revealed:

pH	7.32
$PaCO_2$	70 mm Hg
PaO_2	44 mm Hg
HCO_3^-	35 mEq/L
BE	+6
SaO_2	85%
Hb	16 gm/dl
HBCO	3%

☑ Acute on chronic ventilatory failure in the COPD patient is an indication for admission to the ICU.

The chest radiograph revealed evidence of hyperinflation, an increase in vascular markings, and an infiltrate in the RLL. Because of the patient's clinical condition, chest radiograph findings, and the acute imposed-on chronic ventilatory failure indicated by the blood gas, the patient was transferred immediately to the medical intensive care unit for further evaluation and treatment. The patient was then

☑ Aminophylline (theophylline) improves diaphragmatic function in the COPD patient.

☑ Corticosteroids are only useful in the treatment of COPD if the patient has evidence of reversible airway disease.

started on the following regimen: supplemental oxygen at 2 lpm by nasal cannula, nebulized albuterol sulfate, 2.5 mg in NS Q2H, 2.5 mg/kg loading dose of aminophylline over 30 minutes, followed by a maintenance dose of 0.5 mg/kg per hour IV (titrated according to serum levels), furosemide, 40 mg, IV push, and methylprednisolone, 120 mg IV, Q6H. Sputum for Gram stain and culture was obtained and sent to the lab. The patient was also started on a prophylatic broad-spectrum antibiotic. The report on the Gram stain came back later and showed numerous Gram positive diplococci.

INDICATIONS

Over the next hour, the patient's respiratory status continued to deteriorate despite intervention. Respiratory rate rose to 36/minute and paradoxical abdominal motion became more pronounced. The rising respiratory rate in conjunction with the abdominal paradox and the increasing $PaCO_2$ from the first blood gas are indicative of increasing ventilatory fatigue. Impending acute ventilatory failure must be assumed.

INITIAL SETTINGS

☑ In the alert and cooperative patient with intact airway defenses, noninvasive ventilation can provide ventilatory support without the risks associated with intubation.

On the basis of clinical and laboratory data, a decision was made to assist the patient's ventilation. In lieu of endotracheal intubation, bilevel positive airway pressure (bilevel PAP) was initiated via nasal mask at the settings below. The IPAP and EPAP levels were titrated to 15/5 resulting in an SpO_2 endpoint of around 90%.

Mode	Spontaneous
IPAP	15 cm H_2O
EPAP	5 cm H_2O
Sup. O_2	2 lpm

The patient was poorly compliant with the therapy, removing the mask at regular intervals, complaining of not being able to get enough air. After one hour, an arterial blood gas was obtained and revealed the following:

pH	7.25
$PaCO_2$	80 mm Hg
PaO_2	56 mm Hg
HCO_3^-	34 mEq/L
BE	+3
SaO_2	89%
Hb	16 gm/dl
HBCO	2%

On the basis of the worsening ventilatory failure despite noninvasive ventilatory assistance, the patient was intubated with a size 8.5 endotracheal tube, and volume-targeted mechanical ventilation was initiated on the following settings:

Mode	CMV
V_T	750 ml
f	10/min
PIF	55 lpm, resulting in an I:E ratio = 1:4
F_IO_2	0.40
PEEP	5 cm H_2O
Flow Trigger	3 lpm

After thirty minutes, an arterial blood gas was obtained and revealed the following:

ph	7.35
$PaCO_2$	65 mm Hg
PaO_2	88 mm Hg
HCO_3^-	36 mEq/L
BE	+6
SaO_2	96%
Hb	16 gm/dl
HBCO	1%

On the basis of the blood gas, an order was written to titrate the patient's F_IO_2 to maintain the $SpO_2 \geq 92\%$. No other changes were made to the ventilatory parameters. Albuterol orders were changed to MDI, 8 puffs in-line Q4H. The patient was suctioned PRN for moderate amounts of thick pale yellow secretions.

PATIENT MONITORING

Over the course of the next 72 hours the patient was rested on the ventilator and treated appropriately for his pneumonia and right heart failure. The patient remained alert and cooperative with his care. A chest radiograph done on day three of ICU admission demonstrated clearing of the pneumonic process in the RLL. Findings characteristic of emphysema were also present including hyperlucent lung fields, flattened diaphragm, widely spaced ribs, and a narrow heart shadow. Serum theophylline levels were monitored daily, averaging 9 µg/ml.

The ventilator settings were adjusted appropriately and currently are:

Mode	SIMV
V_T	750 ml
f	6
PIF	55 lpm, resulting in an I:E ratio = 1:4
F_IO_2	0.35
PEEP	5 cm H_2O

☑ In order to minimize theophylline toxicity, the therapeutic range for serum theophylline level should be kept from 8 to 12 µg/ml.

PSV	7 cm H_2O
Flow Tr.	3 lpm

Spontaneous Parameters

Spont. f	12
Spont. V_T	550 ml
VC	2.21 L
MIP	−36 cm H_2O

The arterial blood gas drawn on the current ventilator settings shows:

pH	7.39
$PaCO_2$	56 mm Hg
PaO_2	74 mm HG
HCO_3^-	34 mEq/L
BE	+7
SaO_2	94%
Hb	15.5 gm/dl
HBCO	1%

PATIENT MANAGEMENT

The patient's vital signs have normalized and along with ventilator care, fluid status was normalized and bronchodilator therapy was continued to relieve bronchospasm and help promote mucociliary clearance. Antibiotic therapy was continued and adjusted on the basis of the culture and sensitivity report. Secretion volume and consistency have decreased and color has changed from yellow to white.

WEANING

As the patient's condition continued to improve, ventilatory support was gradually withdrawn over the next three days. He was placed on the spontaneous breathing mode (CPAP mode) at an F_IO_2 of 0.35 with a pressure support of 5 cm H_2O and CPAP of 5 cm H_2O. After four hours, spontaneous ventilatory parameters were measured and an arterial blood gas was obtained. The results are as follows:

✓ f/V_T ratio < 100/min/L is predicative of weaning success.

f	18
V_T	525 ml
VE	9.45 L
f/V_T	34/min/L
VC	2.85 L
MIP	−44 cm H_2O
pH	7.38
$PaCO_2$	58 mm Hg
PaO_2	68 mm Hg

HCO_3^-	34 mEq/L
BE	+7
SaO_2	92%
Hb	15.1 gm/dl
HBCO	1%

COMPLICATIONS

On the basis of the patient's clinical condition and diagnostic results, he was extubated and placed on 2 lpm O_2 via nasal cannula. He was moved to the medical floor later that day, and was subsequently discharged two days later after being enrolled in the hospital's comprehensive outpatient rehabilitation program. His home medications included albuterol viai MDI, ipratropium via MDI, and oral theophylline.

☑ A comprehensive rehabilitation program teaches the patient about his or her disease, self-care, maintenance of an active lifestyle, and smoking cessation.

CASE 2: STATUS ASTHMATICUS

INTRODUCTION

P.W., a 32-year-old, 48-kg female, was gravida 14, para 0-4-9-4, and about 21½ weeks pregnant at the time of her admission. She was evaluated for acute exacerbation of asthma with upper respiratory tract infection. The patient stated that she was "doing fine" until approximately midnight at which time she began having difficulty breathing. Her shortness of breath continued despite taking her bronchodilator inhalers.

In the emergency room, she was tachypneic with inspiratory and expiratory wheezes, rhonchi, and dry crackles throughout all lung fields. She was placed on oxygen with a nonrebreathing mask at 10 LPM and given one Proventil nebulizer treatment. A stat blood gas was done and she was started on IV aminophylline. Her respiratory rate at that time was 28/min., with the following blood gas results:

☑ Aminophylline is commonly used to reverse severe bronchospasm in acute asthma that has not responded to epinephrine.

☑ Hypoxemia is severe since the PaO_2 is only 59 mm Hg with a nonrebreathing mask.

pH	7.42
$PaCO_2$	34 mm Hg
PaO_2	59 mm Hg
HCO_3^-	24.2 mEq/L
Hb	12.8 gm%
SpO_2	91%
Mode	Nonrebreathing mask
Oxygen	10 LPM
RR	Spontaneous 28/min

☑ $PaCO_2$ of 34 mm Hg indicates the work of breathing is excessive in order to maintain borderline oxygenation.

Four hours later her respiratory rate had increased to 36/min. and she had received medication nebulizer treatments every hour with Proventil. However, inspiratory and expiratory wheezes persisted. A follow-up blood gas revealed:

☑ Increase in respiratory rate from 28 to 36/min. is an ominous sign in the progression of acute asthma.

☑ PaO$_2$ does not show much improvement in spite of increase in spontaneous respiratory rate.

pH	7.42
PaCO$_2$	36 mm Hg
PaO$_2$	58 mm Hg
HCO$_3^-$	23.2 mEq/L
Hb	12.8 gm%
SpO$_2$	91%
Mode	Nonrebreathing mask
Oxygen	10 LPM
RR	Spontaneous 36/min

INDICATIONS

Subsequent blood gases indicated that the patient's ventilatory status quickly deteriorated and she became unable to maintain hyperventilation. Her PaCO$_2$ began rising toward normal.

Rising PaCO$_2$ from a low level (hyperventilation) toward normal is indicative of muscle fatigue. Impending ventilatory failure is likely if not treated aggressively.

In asthma, the increased work of breathing is related to a combination of bronchospasm, airway inflammation, and mucus accumulation. This condition increases the airway resistance and work of breathing, which perpetuates the degranulation of mast cells. Asthmatic patients may not respond to bronchodilators and eventually may show signs of exhaustion and progressive somnolence with hypoxemia and hypercapnea. At that point, intubation and mechanical ventilation are indicated.

INITIAL SETTINGS

The patient was initially set on Assist/Control mode at rate of 10/min., V$_T$ of 600 ml, F$_I$O$_2$ of 90%, and PEEP of 5 cm H$_2$O. The peak flow was increased to match her inspiratory demand, approaching 110 LPM. Every effort was made to reduce the work of breathing and decrease her anxiety level from a ventilatory standpoint. Blood gases obtained revealed the following:

pH	7.42
PaCO$_2$	33 mm Hg
PaO$_2$	55 mm Hg
HCO$_3^-$	21.3 mEq/L
Hb	12.4 gm%
SpO$_2$	90%
Mode	A/C
RR	10/min
V$_T$	600 ml
F$_I$O$_2$	90%
PEEP	5 cm H$_2$O

☑ PC-IRV may improve oxygenation and minimize occurrence of barotrauma.

Although pharmacologic sedation is generally not recommended for asthmatic patients, she was medicated and changed to inverse I:E ratio ventilation on pressure control (PC-IRV) mode at a 2:1 ratio to improve oxygenation and prevent barotrauma related to positive pressure ventilation. She was started at a rate of 20/min., an inspiratory pressure of 40 cm H_2O, T_I of 0.5 seconds, F_IO_2 of 60%, and PEEP of 10 cm H_2O. Blood gases were as follows:

pH	7.36
$PaCO_2$	44 mm Hg
PaO_2	64 mm Hg
HCO_3^-	24 mEq/L
Hb	11.8 gm%
SpO_2	92%
Mode	PC-IRV
T_I	0.5 sec
I:E ratio	2:1
Rate	20/min
P_{INSP}	40 cm H_2O
F_IO_2	60%
PEEP	10 cm H_2O

No changes in her care or ventilator parameters were made at that time. Breath sounds revealed wheezes and coarse rhonchi throughout all lung fields. She continued with her bronchodilator therapy and was suctioned appropriately.

PATIENT MONITORING

The chest radiograph shows the characteristic hyperinflation of the lungs. The distance between the adjacent ribs is widened and the diaphragm is depressed. Infiltrates or areas of edema are also noted on the chest radiograph (Figure 17-1). Other than these signs, the chest radiograph is normal.

Over the next three days, the ventilator settings were changed accordingly and the latest settings were: pressure control at 30 cm H_2O, T_I of 0.7 seconds for a 2:1 ratio, F_IO_2 of 50%, and PEEP of 10 cm H_2O. She was beginning to show signs of reduced inflammation of her airway with only occasional inspiratory and expiratory wheezes. Small amounts of cloudy, clear secretions were suctioned from her endotracheal tube. Peak and trough levels of serum theophylline were drawn to monitor possible toxicity. Blood gas results were as follows:

☑ The therapeutic range of serum theophylline is between 5 to 20 µg/ml.

pH	7.43
$PaCO_2$	36 mm Hg
PaO_2	78 mm Hg
HCO_3^-	23 mEq/L
Hb	12 gm%
SpO_2	93%

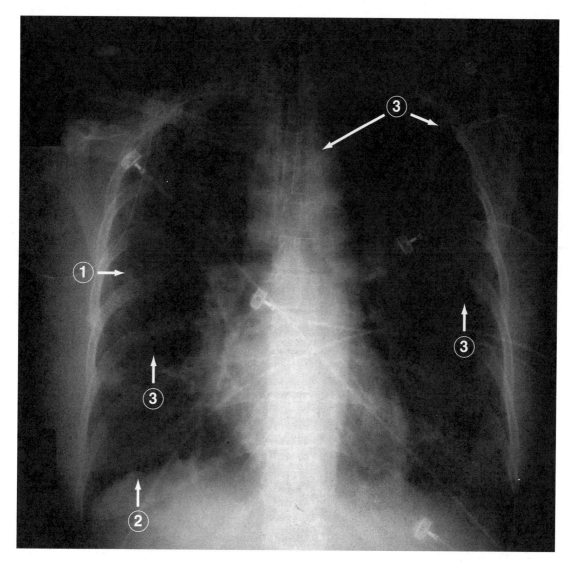

Figure 17-1 Status asthmaticus. Hyperinflation is evident on this chest radiograph since the distance between the adjacent ribs is widened (1) and the diaphragm is depressed (2). Infiltrates or areas of edema are noted (3). The central venous line (4) is also visible on this chest radiograph.

Mode	IR-PCV
T_I	0.7 sec
I:E ratio	2:1
Rate	20/min
P_{INSP}	30 cm H_2O
F_IO_2	50%
PEEP	10 cm H_2O

She was becoming more alert and subsequently changed to SIMV with pressure support to supplement her own efforts to breathe. She appeared calm at first but became increasingly restless and combative over the afternoon and evening. She frequently motioned for the endotracheal tube to be removed and was frustrated about her inability to talk.

PATIENT MANAGEMENT

☑ Intal is not given in acute asthma episodes but is used as a prophylactic measure to control airway hyperreactivity.

In addition to the ventilator management strategies, adequate hydration was provided to promote mucociliary clearance and bronchopulmonary hygiene. Bronchodilators, glucocorticosteroids, and mast cell stabilizers were used to bring the bronchospasm under control.

KEY MEDICATIONS

The patient was treated with aminophylline given intravenously, sympathomimetic beta adrenergics (Proventil and Serevent) via MDI and given in-line through the ventilator circuit every three to four hours. These served to control the symptoms associated with asthma while she was started on triacinolone acetonide (Azmacort), a corticosteroid inhaler to control the inflammation. She was also started on two puffs of cromolyn sodium (Intal) to help prevent the degranulation of mast cell mediators responsible for reactive airway disease.

WEANING

The weaning process was uneventful as the patient continued to improve. She was eventually placed on CPAP without pressure support or PEEP for assessment of possible extubation. Her spontaneous ventilatory parameters revealed the following results:

☑ An f/V_T ratio of less than 100/min/L is highly predictive of weaning success.

$f = 15 \quad V_E = 8.1$ L $\quad V_T = 0.54$ L $\quad$ VC $= 2.19$ L $\quad$ MIF $= -43$
$f/V_T = 28$/min/L

She eventually extubated herself, while restrained, and was placed on a nasal cannula at 6 LPM, which maintained saturations above 90%.

COMPLICATIONS

Her oxygen demands decreased over several days where she continued on her bronchodilators, weaned to room air, and was discharged after six days. There were no apparent complications throughout her hospital stay and she was advised to seek and follow medical care through her primary care provider. She remained on an oral steroid (Prednisone) and an antibiotic (Erythromycin) for an additional ten days after discharge from the hospital.

Note: This case study on status asthmaticus describes the evaluative, diagnostic, and ventilatory management techniques employed at the time it was first written. For additional information, please refer to the guidelines outlined by the National Institute of Health (1997, Oct). *Practical guide for the diagnosis and management of asthma. NIH Publication No. 97-4053.*

CASE 3: POSTABDOMINAL SURGERY

INTRODUCTION

C.T., a 78-year-old, 90-kg, 5'4" female, was admitted to the emergency room (ER) with complaints of the following ailments that had persisted for the past several days: abdominal pain, nausea, fatigue, weakness, shortness of breath, decreased exercise tolerance, vomiting, and black tarry stools.

She had a history of steroid-dependent asthma, COPD, coronary artery disease, diabetes, and arthritis. Her medications at home included Lasix, Diabeta, nitroglycerin, aspirin, Prozac, potassium, Proventil, Intal, Azmacort, and oxygen at 2 to 3 LPM.

In the ER her abdominal exam revealed severe pain in all quadrants and her abdominal radiograph showed free air in all areas. Respiratory assessments showed severe peripheral cyanosis, respiratory rate 32/min., heart rate 120/min., decreased breath sounds in all lobes with fine inspiratory crackles in the lower lobes, and accessory muscle use during inspiration.

Laboratory studies were done upon admission with the following results: WBC 22.2×10^3 (*normal 3.2 to 9.8 $\times 10^3$*), hematocrit (Hct) 25% (*female average 42%*), platelets 34.2×10^3 (*normal 130 to 400 $\times 10^3$*). The electrocardiograph (ECG) showed sinus tachycardia with nonspecific ST and T wave changes.

Other medical history was not significant. The patient's last hospitalization was three years ago for asthma. Upon discharge from the hospital, her room air blood gases were: pH 7.43, $PaCO_2$ 50 mm Hg, PaO_2 42 mm Hg, HCO_3^- 32 mEq/L, and SaO_2 77%. She was placed on supplemental O_2 at home at that time.

After her exam the patient received two units of packed red blood cells (RBC) and one unit of plasma to treat her low hematocrit. Due to her acute and severe condition, she was taken to the operating room for abdominal exploratory surgery.

Sidebar:

☑ Leukocytosis (↑WBC) is generally caused by infection and is usually transient. It may also occur after hemorrhage.

☑ Low hematocrit leads to tissue hypoxia and it may account for her symptoms of shortness of breath, fatigability, weakness, and decreased exercise tolerance.

☑ Thrombocytopenia (↓platelets) occurs in acute infections, anaphylactic shock, and some hemorrhagic diseases and anemias.

☑ Discharge $PaCO_2$ (50 mm Hg) will serve as the target value in subsequent weaning attempts.

☑ Blood transfusion is indicated because of ↓ hematocrit and ↓ platelets.

INDICATIONS

The patient was heavily sedated during her abdominal exploratory surgery and required large amounts of IV fluids, including blood products to maintain her blood pressure during surgery and to increase her low hematocrit level. A bleeding gastric ulcer and a perforated duodenal ulcer were found and repaired without complications. The patient was returned to the ICU, intubated, and placed on mechanical ventilation for postanesthesia recovery.

INITIAL SETTINGS

The patient was intubated with a size 8.0 cuffed endotracheal tube secured at the 23 cm mark at the lips. The cuff pressure was maintained at 35 cm H_2O to prevent air leak around the cuff. The settings on the Puritan-Bennett 7200 ventilator were: SIMV mode, rate 10/min., V_T 800 ml, F_IO_2 100%, no PEEP, peak flow 45 LPM, sensitivity –2 cm H_2O. Her initial static compliance was 74 ml/cm H_2O. Breath sounds were equal bilaterally with fine inspiratory crackles in both lower lobes. Blood gases showed:

pH	7.44
$PaCO_2$	36 mm Hg
PaO_2	102 mm Hg
SaO_2	97%
HCO_3^-	24 mEq/L
Mode	SIMV
Rate	10/min
V_T	800 ml
F_IO_2	100%
PEEP	0 cm H_2O
Peak Flow	45 LPM
Sensitivity	–2 cm H_2O
C_{ST}	74 ml/cm H_2O

PATIENT MONITORING

The major monitoring tools used during her recovery were pulse oximetry, end-tidal CO_2 monitor, and central venous pressure (CVP). Her SpO_2 was 96%. The $P_{ET}CO_2$ was about 33 to 35 mm Hg (*normal 2 mm Hg below PaCO_2*), and her CVP was consistently between 10 and 12 mm Hg (*normal 1 to 7 mm Hg*).

PATIENT MANAGEMENT

The patient was maintained for several hours on SIMV, rate 10, V_T 800 ml, F_IO_2 40%, peak flow 45 LPM. The patient had no spontaneous ventilation after six hours despite being fully alert and oriented. After the F_IO_2 was decreased to 40%, the blood gas results were:

☑ Normal cuff pressure is between 27 to 40 cm H_2O, lower for patients with hypotension.

☑ The PaO_2 is too high and the F_IO_2 should be reduced.

☑ SpO_2 (96%) correlates well with the SaO_2 (97%).

☑ CVP is higher than normal. The systemic venous volume status should be monitored closely.

☑ Since the patient was a chronic CO_2 retainer, the target $PaCO_2$ (50 mm Hg) should be used to manage this patient.

☑ The $PaCO_2$ can be increased (from the current 38 mm Hg to patient's target 50 mm Hg) by decreasing the SIMV rate or changing to CPAP mode.

☑ Preexisting asthma, postanesthesia, and tissue hypoxia are three major factors that lead to failure of CPAP trial.

☑ Since the rate (f) and V_T are 16/min and 0.476 L (476 ml), respectively, the f/V_T ratio is 34/min/L (16/0.476).

☑ An f/V_T ratio of less than 100/min/L is highly predictive of weaning success.

pH	7.40
$PaCO_2$	38 mm Hg
PaO_2	65 mm Hg
SaO_2	92%
HCO_3^-	23 mEq/L
Mode	SIMV
Rate	10/min
V_T	800 ml
F_IO_2	40%
PEEP	0 cm H_2O
Peak Flow	45 LPM

Fluid intake was adjusted to maintain a CVP reading between 10 and 12 mm Hg. Other vital signs were within normal limits for her age. Proventil and Intal treatments were started for her asthma and her static compliance remained in the 70s.

The spontaneous respiratory parameters measured eight hours post-surgery showed: MIP –22 cm H_2O, vital capacity 700 ml. A trial of CPAP of 5 cmH_2O at an F_IO_2 of 40% was unsuccessful as she developed periods of apnea with intermittent tidal volumes of between 300 and 350 ml.

Over the next several hours, her cardiopulmonary status showed steady improvement from the anesthesia effects and the patient was again tried on CPAP. She tolerated the procedure very well this time, and her spontaneous respiratory parameters at the end of the CPAP trial were: MIP –40 cm H_2O, vital capacity 1,500 ml, spontaneous rate 16 and average V_T of 476 ml. She was successfully extubated and placed on a 50% venturi mask and eventually weaned to nasal cannula at 3 LPM later that evening.

Some minor complications with the patient's oxygenation and perfusion status were adequately managed using oxygen, blood, and fluids. Her recovery from the abdominal exploratory surgery was gradual but uneventful, and she was discharged from the hospital a few days later.

COMPLICATIONS

The chest radiograph done 16 hours postextubation revealed increasing atelectasis and pneumonia in both bases with bilateral pleural effusions. Breath sounds showed increasing crackles with occasional rhonchi and wheezing. Aerosol treatments were started with Proventil TID and Intal BID. Her SpO_2 on 3 LPM of oxygen was consistently in the mid- to low-80s and she was placed back on a Venturi mask at 40% during the night. The F_IO_2 was increased to 50% at times during periods of desaturation on 40% oxygen.

Her hematocrit increased from 25% to 30% (*female average 42%*) after several transfusions of Hespan, plasma, and packed red blood cells. Her most recent vital signs before discharge were: SpO_2 90%, heart rate 95/min., blood pressure 140/90 mm Hg, and CVP 20 mm Hg (*normal 1 to 7 mm Hg*).

CASE 4: HEAD INJURY

INTRODUCTION

T.A., a 16-year-old, 52-kg female, was brought to the emergency department after sustaining multiple trauma from a moving vehicle accident. She was a passenger in a small car involved in a high-speed collision with a truck. It was unknown if she was restrained prior to the accident but paramedics required approximately 30 to 45 minutes to extract her from the vehicle. She was reportedly conscious at the scene but became combative and hysterical when she arrived at the hospital. Her blood pressure (BP) was 149/87 mm Hg, pulse 104/min., temperature 34.8°C, and she was able to move all of her extremities.

Due to the extent of her injuries, she was orally intubated and maintained by sedation. The routine trauma laboratory studies revealed the following results: WBC count of 2.3×10^3 (*normal 3.2 to 9.8 $\times$ 10^3*), hematocrit (Hct) 37% (*female average 42%*), platelets of 269×10^3 (*normal 130 to 400 $\times$ 10^3*), prothrombin time (PT) of 13 seconds (*normal 9 to 12 sec.*), and partial thromboplastin time (PTT) of 27 seconds (*normal 22 to 37 sec.*). Radiographs of the abdomen and chest were unremarkable. However, due to the extent of her head injuries, she was flown by Lifeflight and transferred to a nearby trauma center.

Throughout transport, she was reportedly in and out of consciousness, and upon her arrival to the trauma center her BP was 119/70 mm Hg, pulse 92/min., Glasgow coma score of 3 with no spontaneous eye opening, no movement of her arms or legs. During assessment, she was nonverbal and noted to have a cephalhematoma in the right frontal region with a large laceration in the occipital area. Pupils were equal, round, and reactive to light. She was in a normal sinus rhythm, had equal breath sounds, and her SpO$_2$ was 100% while being manually ventilated.

INDICATIONS

A computerized tomography (CT) scan of her head revealed an occipital condylar fracture on the right with a small intrahemispheric subdural hematoma that did not require surgical intervention. Radiographs of her spine were unremarkable and there was no evidence of spleen or liver injury. The chest radiograph was also normal (Figure 17-2). She was transported to the ICU in critical condition and placed on a mechanical ventilator due to her extensive head injuries and therapeutic drug-induced coma.

INITIAL SETTINGS

Since heavy sedation and sustained hyperventilation were desired, the initial ventilator settings on the Puritan-Bennett 7200 consisted of

☑ Leukopenia (decrease in WBC) may be due to the trauma or adverse effects of drugs.

☑ Glasgow coma score of ≤7 indicates coma. A score of 3 reflects a severe coma state.

☑ Pupils that are reactive to light mean that cerebral circulation and oxygenation are adequate.

☑ CT scan of the head and radiographs of the spine and major organs are indicated for head trauma patients.

☑ In head injury, the lungs are not affected unless there are coexisting complications (e.g., aspiration).

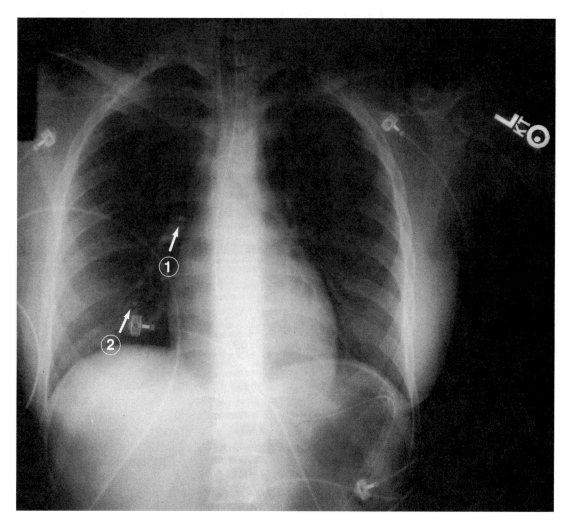

Figure 17-2   Head injury. The chest radiograph is normal. The small round markings (1 and 2) are the pulmonary blood vessels running parallel to the roentgen ray (X ray).

☑ Drug-induced coma is done to reduce metabolic rate and minimize intracranial pressure (ICP).

☑ Hyperventilation (e.g., $PaCO_2$ 29 mm Hg) should be done to reduce intracranial pressure in the initial stage of management.

☑ An ICP of less than 10 mmHg is the desirable target for patients with head injury.

☑ Hyperventilation is used to maintain a $PaCO_2$ between 25 and 35 mm Hg.

☑ Cerebrospinal fluid may also be drained to minimize the rise of intracranial pressure from subsequent swelling of the brain.

☑ PEEP is contraindicated in head injuries unless severe hypoxemia is present.

assist/control (A/C) mode at a rate of 14/min., V_T of 600 ml, F_IO_2 of 60%, and no PEEP.

PATIENT MONITORING

The initial blood gas analysis after twenty minutes of mechanical ventilation showed:

pH	7.30
$PaCO_2$	29 mm Hg
PaO_2	256 mm Hg
HCO_3^-	13.9 mEq/L
Hb	11 gm%
Mode	A/C
Rate	14
V_T	600 mL
F_IO_2	60%
PEEP	0 cm H_2O

The patient was closely monitored using continuous intracranial pressure (ICP) measurements between 6 to 8 mm Hg, hemodynamics with indwelling pulmonary artery and arterial catheters revealed a heart rate of 118/min, BP of 116/84 mm Hg, and a pulmonary capillary wedge pressure (PCWP) of 11 mm Hg.

PATIENT MANAGEMENT

Carbon dioxide in the blood is a very potent vasodilator. This serves to promote swelling and edema following an acute injury to the brain. Blood flow to the area, and the subsequent swelling, may be reduced during the first 24 hours by maintaining the $PaCO_2$ between 25 and 35 mm Hg while monitoring the ensuing edema with an ICP monitor.

Consequently, hyperventilation is used as a means to reduce the $PaCO_2$ level in the blood as well as to regulate the pressure resulting from swelling of the brain after the injury. Following the insertion of the ICP monitor, the level of hyperventilation can be assessed and titrated to maintain that pressure preferentially below 10 mm Hg to minimize further injury.

The PEEP level is usually maintained at or below 5 cm H_2O because the lungs are generally not affected by head injury, and that additional pressure is transmitted to the head by the use of positive pressure to ventilate the patient. This level is desirable unless the patient's oxygen requirements exceed 60% F_IO_2 when higher levels of PEEP may be indicated.

The ventilator settings were adjusted during the next several hours and the patient was weaned to a rate of 12/min. resulting in a pH of 7.46 and $PaCO_2$ of 28 mm Hg.

KEY MEDICATIONS

☑ Neurological assessment should be done after recovery from drug-induced sedation.

The patient remained sedated with Phenytoin, Phenobarbital, Diazepam, and Midazolam during the acute phase (i.e., 24 to 48 hours following the accident) of her hospitalization to minimize the risk of further injury. She was then allowed to awaken for neurological assessment.

Since the lungs were relatively unaffected, she was not given bronchodilator therapy, but was monitored for complications including atelectasis and consolidation resulting from inactivity, oral intubation, and subsequent ventilation. She was suctioned appropriately as necessary and was given periodic oral care to minimize the occurrence of infection.

WEANING

The patient was allowed to awaken fully and was changed to SIMV mode at 10/min. with a pressure support level at 15 cm H_2O in an attempt to begin the weaning process. Blood gas analysis revealed the following:

pH	7.39
$PaCO_2$	40 mm Hg
PaO_2	83 mm Hg
HCO_3^-	23.3 mEq/L
Hb	13.8 gm%
Mode	SIMV
Rate	10
V_T	600 mL
F_IO_2	60%
Pressure Support	15 cm H_2O

Weaning parameters done each morning included respiratory rate, minute volume, tidal volume, vital capacity, maximum inspiratory pressure, and frequency to tidal volume ratio. The weaning criteria done on the second day after admission showed that her ventilatory effort was adequate and she was weaned off the ventilator only with minor neurological deficit.

She was alert and oriented to time and place but without memory of the accident. She appeared comfortable, cooperative, able to follow commands, and was not diaphoretic or febrile. She was not anxious and was spontaneously breathing on CPAP with 10 cm H_2O of pressure support at a RR of 14/min., HR of 88/min., BP of 112/78 mm Hg, SpO_2 of 96% on 35% F_IO_2 with satisfactory blood gases.

She was extubated and placed on a nasal cannula at 3 LPM of O_2. She was weaned off oxygen and discharged from the hospital six days after admission.

COMPLICATIONS

The patient had no apparent pulmonary complications, however, there were minor neuromotor obstacles to overcome including the loss of short-term memory and minimal motor sensory perception to the left. She will undergo physical and occupational therapy regimens after her release from the hospital to rehabilitate her injuries.

CASE 5: SMOKE INHALATION

INTRODUCTION

F.H. was a 64-year-old, 76-kg male admitted to the emergency department from his home where he was found in a smoke-filled room. He was unable to communicate with rescuers, appeared confused, and presented with first- and second-degree burns over 50% of his upper torso. His facial features contained dark smoke and soot about his nose and mouth, a singed mustache, and he had a strong odor of alcohol on his breath.

The initial blood pressure was 139/100 mm Hg, temperature was 35.8°C with a pulse of 102/min., and respirations of 24/min. while breathing on a nonrebreathing mask at 15 LPM. He was immediately fluid resuscitated with 1,000 ml of D_5W, and treated empirically for cyanide toxicity, which interferes with oxidative metabolism at the cellular level by impairing the utilization of oxygen.

The clinical signs of cyanide poisoning may include the following:

Blood cyanide concentration 0.2 to 0.3 mg/L	↑ HR, ↑ RR, dizziness
Blood cyanide concentration 0.3 to 1 mg/L	↑ lethargy, arrhythmias, apnea
Blood cyanide concentration >1 mg/L	Death

Upon admission into the hospital, the chest radiograph was normal (Figure 17-3). His breath sounds were mostly clear but dramatically changed following IV fluids to basilar crackles with expiratory wheezes throughout, and a prolonged expiratory phase. Although the patient maintained an SpO_2 of 99% per pulse oximetry, he did not appear short of breath. A stat blood gas was ordered in the emergency room followed immediately by a nebulizer treatment with 0.5 ml of 0.5% Proventil in 2.5 ml of normal saline. The results of the blood gases were as follows:

pH	7.29
$PaCO_2$	41 mm Hg
PaO_2	155 mm Hg
HCO_3^-	19.4 mEq/L

☑ Patient history suggests potential complications of burn and smoke inhalation: infection, bronchospasm, carbon monoxide (CO), and cyanide poisoning.

☑ Cyanide is one of the by-products of combustion.

☑ With adequate spontaneous ventilation, the initial supportive measure for smoke inhalation is 100% O_2.

☑ Pulse oximetry should not be used in smoke inhalation because it cannot distinguish carboxyhemoglobin and provides false high SpO_2 readings.

☑ Blood gases with carboxyhemoglobin (HbCO) capability must be done in managing patients with smoke inhalation.

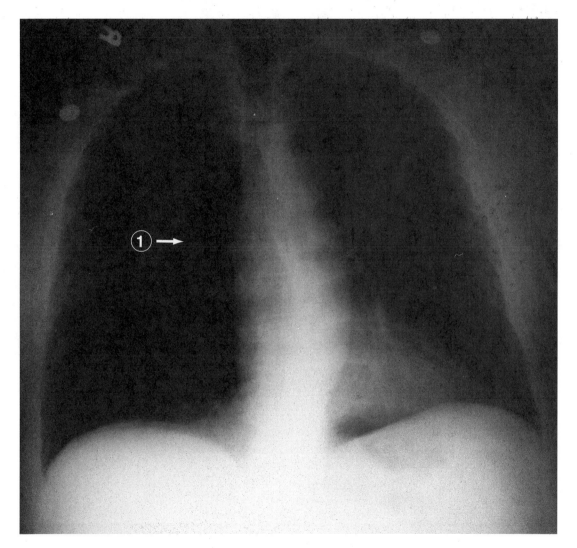

Figure 17-3   Smoke inhalation. The chest radiograph is normal. The lungs typically are not affected unless there is edema formation secondary to smoke inhalation. The small round marking (1) represents a pulmonary blood vessel running parallel to the roentgen ray (X ray).

HbCO	21.2 gm %
Hb	14.4 gm %
CaO_2	12.7 vol %
SaO_2	92%
Mode	Nonrebreathing mask
Flow	15 LPM

The patient was then transported to the intensive care unit for further evaluation and treatment.

INDICATIONS

Physical examination revealed that the patient had received a moderate thermal burn to the airway as well as to his torso and extremities. He was electively intubated to maintain an adequate airway and as expected, he became edematous to the point that his facial features were no longer recognizable.

INITIAL SETTINGS

He was lightly sedated and placed on CPAP with pressure support of 15 cm H_2O and the spontaneous rate was 16/min. He maintained a spontaneous V_T of 550 ml at an F_IO_2 of 100% and PEEP of 6 cm H_2O. After thirty minutes, blood gases revealed:

pH	7.42
$PaCO_2$	36 mm Hg
PaO_2	255 mm Hg
HCO_3^-	22.8 mEq/L
HbCO	19.2 gm %
Hb	14.4 gm %
CaO_2	14.7 vol %
SaO_2	94%
Mode	CPAP
PEEP	6 cm H_2O
Pressure Support	15 cm H_2O
RR (spontaneous)	16/min
V_T (spontaneous)	550 ml
F_IO_2	100%

The patient was maintained on the same ventilator settings as he had normal acid-base balance and was breathing spontaneously. A high F_IO_2 was maintained to reduce the half-life of HbCO.

The half-life of HbCO is as follows:

F_IO_2 of 100% and one atmospheric pressure	80 to 90 min
F_IO_2 of 21% (air) and one atmospheric pressure	280 to 320 min

---

☑ In CO poisoning, the CaO_2 should be used to evaluate the patient's oxygenation status.

☑ In spite of normal Hb and satisfactory SaO_2, the measured CaO_2 is low (12.7 vol%) because of the high HbCO level (21.2 gm %).

☑ Elective intubation is done to maintain a patent airway in anticipation of airway edema and obstruction.

☑ The measured CaO_2 showed improvement (from 12.7 to 14.7 vol %) after initiation of CPAP, PS and 100% O_2.

PATIENT MONITORING

Careful observation should be carried out to assess any evidence of pulmonary complications such as thermal injuries to the airway or pulmonary edema. These injuries also increase the incidence and severity of ARDS. Impaired gas exchange or hypoxia caused by increased levels of CO may be treated by the use of PEEP. The patient's mental functions should be monitored to prevent CO-induced anoxic brain syndrome.

PATIENT MANAGEMENT

The patient was closely monitored for two days while on mechanical ventilation for evidence of further injuries (i.e., decreasing lung compliance, thermal airway injuries, and hypoxia).

KEY MEDICATIONS

The patient was given MDI treatments with 10 puffs of Proventil given in-line through the ventilator circuit and continued with medication nebulizer treatments with Proventil after extubation.

WEANING

The swelling to the airway was significantly reduced and the patient was extubated after the return of adequate ventilation. He was immediately given an aerosol treatment of 0.5 ml racemic epinephrine (Micronephrine) in distilled water to minimize stridor and edema to the upper airway. Blood gases after extubation revealed:

☑ Reduction of peak airway pressure, improvement of breath sounds, and dynamic compliance are signs that the swelling to the airway has improved.

pH	7.43
$PaCO_2$	38 mm Hg
PaO_2	104 mm Hg
HCO_3^-	23.6 mEq/L
HbCO	2.8 gm %
Hb	14.1 gm %
CaO_2	18.8 vol %
SaO_2	96%
Mode	Cool aerosol mask
RR (spontaneous)	16/min
F_IO_2	28%

The patient remained in the hospital for three more days where he was weaned from the oxygen and required fewer medication nebulizer treatments to control intermittent wheezing.

COMPLICATIONS

The patient experienced no lasting complications from his injuries. He was weaned to room air and discharged from the hospital after a six-day convalescence period.

CASE 6: DRUG OVERDOSE

INTRODUCTION

K.L. was a 78-year-old white male, 5' 8", medium build who weighed about 73 kg (160 lb). Upon admission to the 200-bed community hospital, his respiratory rate was 6/min. and shallow. His skin color was pale but showed no cyanosis.

The paramedics stated that the patient was found by his neighbors in the bathroom on his back next to a pool of vomitus. The neighbors told the paramedics that the patient had a history of asthma and that he had been depressed since his girlfriend left him two weeks ago. An albuterol inhaler was found next to the patient and two empty bottles of tricyclic antidepressants were found on the kitchen table. Additional medical history revealed that the patient smoked about one pack of cigarettes each day.

The paramedics used a bag/mask resuscitator to ventilate the patient with O_2 at a rate of about 20/min. They suctioned and removed large amounts of vomitus from his airway en route to the hospital.

Upon arrival at the emergency room, the respiratory therapist provided bag/mask ventilation. A nasogastric tube was inserted to prevent gastric distention and aspiration.

Cardiopulmonary assessments provided the following information: heart rate 45/min., weak pulses, systolic blood pressure 90 mm Hg, SpO_2 90%, spontaneous respiratory rate 8/min. and shallow breath sounds with crackles and wheezes bilaterally.

Arterial blood gases on 100% O_2 revealed: pH 7.08, $PaCO_2$ 70 mm Hg, PaO_2 54 mm Hg, SaO_2 85%, and HCO_3^- 20 mEq/L.

☑ Blood gases show acute ventilatory failure with moderate hypoxemia.

INDICATIONS

The patient was intubated with a size 8.0 endotracheal (ET) tube. After checking for bilateral breath sounds, the ET tube was secured at the 24 cm mark at the lips. The end-tidal CO_2 reading was 20 mm Hg. During intubation, large amounts of watery brown secretions were suctioned from the airway and a sample was collected and sent to the laboratory for analysis.

☑ An end-tidal CO_2 reading of 20 mm Hg confirms placement of an ET tube in the airway.

After the ET tube cuff was properly inflated, activated charcoal was put into the stomach via the nasogastric tube in order to absorb the remaining tricycles.

While the activated charcoal was being administered, the airways and lungs were lavaged with normal saline and suctioned. This procedure was repeated until the return solution became clear.

Chest radiograph done later showed that the ET tube was 4 cm above the carina. Hazy infiltrates were noted in both lungs indicating that the patient had aspirated.

☑ Repeat suctioning is indicated because watery brown secretions (stomach content) have been suctioned from the ET tube.

Another blood gas was drawn with the patient intubated and being bagged at a rate of 20/min. The results were: pH 7.34, PCO_2 35 mm Hg, PO_2 350 mm Hg.

INITIAL SETTINGS

The patient was transferred to the adult ICU and placed on a Puritan-Bennett 7200 ventilator. The initial settings were CMV, RR 20/min., V_T 720 ml, F_IO_2 100%, PEEP 5 cm H_2O, peak flow 60 LPM, and square flow pattern. With these settings, the peak airway pressure was 25 cm H_2O, plateau pressure was 20 cm H_2O, and corrected V_T was 710 ml. All alarms were set appropriately.

pH	7.42
$PaCO_2$	32 mm Hg
PaO_2	264 mm Hg
HCO_3^-	16 mEq/L
SpO_2	98%
Mode	CMV
Rate	20/min
V_T	720 ml
F_IO_2	100%
PEEP	5 cm H_2O
P_{PEAK}	25 cm H_2O
$P_{PLATEAU}$	20 cm H_2O

> ✓ Since aspiration is likely to have occurred, PEEP of 5 cm H_2O is used to prevent atelectasis.

> ✓ Alarms should include low minute volume, low tidal volume, PEEP, high pressure, low pressure, high respiratory rate and apnea alarms.

PATIENT MONITORING

A continuous SpO_2 monitor was placed on the patient with the low alarm set at 90%. A good waveform was noted, and the heart rate matched that on the cardiac monitor.

Respiratory monitoring of the patient consisted of Q 2° ventilator checks to include the peak and plateau pressures, returned volumes, minute volumes, F_IO_2 and compliance. Other clinical information and procedures included RR, breath sounds, suctioning, and ET tube cuff pressure.

Due to the potential complications of aspiration, of particular importance was the monitoring of high peak and plateau pressure, F_IO_2, and PaO_2. A Swan-Ganz catheter and an arterial line were used to monitor the patient's hemodynamic status (i.e., arterial blood pressure, central venous pressure, pulmonary artery pressure, pulmonary capillary wedge pressure, cardiac output, and mixed venous saturation). Laboratory studies included serum electrolytes.

> ✓ Potential complications of aspiration may include aspirations pneumonia and ARDS.

> ✓ ARDS is usually preceded by increasing peak and plateau pressures (due to decreasing lung compliance), and increasing F_IO_2 requirement (due to intrapulmonary shunting).

PATIENT MANAGEMENT

Initially, the patient's respiratory status was stable but it began to deteriorate on the second day. The ventilator settings were changed to accommodate the patient's needs. The ventilator settings were: CMV mode, RR 35/min., V_T 720 ml, F_IO_2 100%, 20 cm H_2O PEEP. The peak airway pressure was 80 cm H_2O and plateau pressure was 70 cm H_2O. The blood gas results were:

pH	7.33
$PaCO_2$	43 mm Hg
PaO_2	72 mm Hg
HCO_3^-	19 mEq/L
SpO_2	92%
Mode	CMV
Rate	35/min
V_T	720 ml
F_IO_2	100%
PEEP	20 cm H_2O
P_{PEAK}	80 cm H_2O
$P_{PLATEAU}$	70 cm H_2O

☑ In PCV, the initial pressure may be set at 10 cm H_2O below the peak airway pressure on CMV.

Because of the increasing pressure requirement, pressure control ventilation (PCV) was started so as to minimize the occurrence of volume- or pressure-induced lung injuries. The pressure on PCV was initially set at 70 cm H_2O (10 cm H_2O below the peak airway pressure on CMV). Other ventilator parameters for PCV were: inspiratory time 1 sec, RR 35/min., F_IO_2 100%, 20 cm H_2O PEEP. The blood gases were as follows:

pH	7.32
$PaCO_2$	41 mm Hg
PaO_2	56 mm Hg
HCO_3^-	20 mEq/L
SpO_2	88%
Mode	PCV
Pressure	70 cm H_2O
Rate	35/min
F_IO_2	100%
PEEP	20 cm H_2O

☑ In PCV, the minute volume is primarily determined by the pressure, inspiratory time, and lung compliance.

☑ In ARDS, the lungs will heal faster with lower airway pressures.

The inspiratory time was then increased to 2 sec. to keep the PaO_2 in the 70s. The I:E ratio was changed to 4:1 to provide longer inspiratory time. Subsequently the minute volume was increased with these settings and the pressure was lowered to 50 cm H_2O. Blood gases on these settings were satisfactory. The minute volume of the patient was trended carefully during the use of PCV.

The patient was placed on a Roto-bed and was administered neuromuscular and sedative agents to minimize agitation and oxygen consumption. For proper airway management, a tracheostomy was performed because extended mechanical ventilation was anticipated.

To further minimize pressure-induced lung injuries, the pressure on PCV was further decreased until the tidal volume was about 450 ml. The $PaCO_2$ was allowed to reach 80 mm Hg (permissive hypercapnia) while the pH was maintained near 7.35 by bicarbonate infusion and kidney compensation.

✓ Permissive hypercapnia is used to reduce the pressure and volume requirement for ventilation.

KEY MEDICATIONS

No medication was needed for intubation because the patient was unconscious at the time of intubation. Additional medications were withheld because of the uncertain drug interaction with other unknown drugs that the patient might have taken.

The patient was given neuromuscular blocking agents and sedatives while on mechanical ventilation. As the respiratory status improved, the patient was weaned from these drugs. Albuterol was given PRN for wheezing.

WEANING

Over the next two weeks, the patient continued to improve. Weaning was done by alternating CPAP with pressure support (during day) and SIMV (during night). Both modes of ventilation were supported with flow triggering. The SIMV mode allowed the patient to rest. He was also ambulated daily to strengthen his respiratory muscles and exercise endurance.

✓ An f/V_T ratio of less than 100/min/L is highly predictive of weaning success.

As he regained strength, the following spontaneous respiratory parameters were obtained: RR < 35/min., minute volume around 9 liters, vital capacity > 1 liter, MIF > –30 cm H_2O and f/V_T < 100/min./L.

Eventually, the patient was weaned to CPAP of 5 cm H_2O, F_IO_2 35%, and pressure support of 5 cm H_2O. A spontaneous rate of 16–20/min yielded these ABG results:

pH	7.37
$PaCO_2$	43 mm Hg
PaO_2	80 mm Hg
HCO_3^-	24 mEq/L
SpO_2	95%
Mode	CPAP
PEEP	5 cm H_2O
F_IO_2	35%
Pressure support	5 cm H_2O
Spontaneous rate	16 to 20/min

After two days of CPAP, the patient continued to improve and he was placed on a nasal cannula at 4 LPM and his fenestrated tracheostomy tube was buttoned allowing the patient to breathe through his upper airway. He tolerated the closure of his tracheostomy very well, and it was left this way for two days. Two more days later, he was transferred to the rehabilitation floor.

✓ Tension pneumothorax was probably caused by excessive airway and pulmonary pressures.

COMPLICATIONS

During the course of mechanical ventilation, a left-sided tension pneumothorax occurred and this led to: decreased lung compliance, decreased O_2 saturation, and decreased breath sounds on the left side. Chest radiograph showed shift of the mediatinum to the right side.

☑️ To prevent self-extubation, neuromuscular blocking agents and sedatives may be used to provide comfort. An alternative is to use active restraints.

☑️ Chest tube is used to remove air, blood, or fluid accumulated in the pleural space.

☑️ Hypotension and tachycardia are two common signs of inadequate blood volume.

☑️ Tension pneumothorax or hemopneumothorax shifts the mediastinum to the unaffected (opposite) side.

☑️ Colloids are used to enhance fluid balance in the early phase of volume replacement.

☑️ Hemodynamic instability is mainly due to blood loss.

☑️ Reduction of lung volumes is caused by compression of the lungs by blood and air in the pleural space.

The tension pneumothorax gradually resolved with the placement of a chest tube.

At one point during weaning the patient became very combative and he self extubated. He was reintubated without delay. Cloth restraints were then used to secure his extremities.

CASE 7: TENSION HEMOPNEUMOTHORAX

INTRODUCTION

P.S. was a 50-year-old, 96-kg male transferred from another hospital with a complicating right-sided pneumonia and hemothorax. At the onset, a small right pleural effusion was found that required drainage via a needle thoracentesis. This effusion again reaccumulated and a second thoracentesis was performed that was productive of over 400 ml of thin, cloudy fluid. A chest tube was placed following the procedure, which continued to drain thin, cloudy fluid followed by frank blood. This output continued throughout the day requiring massive transfusions to maintain his blood pressure, thus, he was transferred to a tertiary care facility for definitive therapy. Prior to Lifeflight, the patient was volume resuscitated with both blood and fluid, nasally intubated, and noted to have inadequate drainage of the right hemothorax.

Upon arrival to the ICU, the patient developed further hemodynamic instability with a systolic pressure of 70 mm Hg (*normal 120 mm Hg*) and a heart rate of 120/min. (*normal 60 to 100/min.*). He had weak pulses bilaterally, dullness to percussion of the right hemithorax, expiratory wheezes, and coarse rhonchi with the left being greater than the right. The chest tube drained about 950 ml of bloody fluid. The patient was resuscitated with colloids followed by blood transfusions. A chest radiograph revealed a complete opacification on the right with concurrent mediastinal shift to the left side (Figure 17-4).

INDICATIONS

The patient was electively intubated prior to transport to establish and maintain an adequate airway. Mechanical ventilation was established because of hemodynamic instability, reduction of lung volumes, and increased work of breathing.

INITIAL SETTINGS

The patient was lightly sedated and placed on a Puritan-Bennett 7200 ventilator in the assist/control mode at 16/min. with V_T of 800 ml, F_IO_2

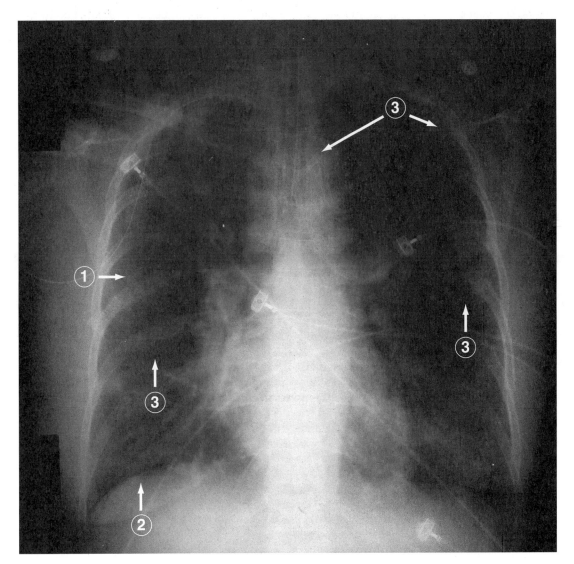

Figure 17-4 Tension hemopneumothorax. Right-sided hemopneumothorax shifts the mediastinum and trachea (1) to the left. The shift is not significant, possibly due to patient rotation when the radiograph was taken. The white area (2) on the radiograph is caused by the blood in the pleural space (Note: air in pleural space would appear dark). Compression of the left lung is noted (3). Chest tube (4) can be seen on the right side.

☑ Increase in work of breathing is caused by reduction of lung compliance and/or increase of airway resistance.

☑ The peak inspiratory pressure was high (> 70 cm H_2O) because of low lung compliance (due to compression of lung parenchyma by blood and air in the pleural space).

of 100%, and PEEP of 5 cm H_2O. There was no spontaneous respiratory effort.

The peak inspiratory pressures exceeded 70 cm H_2O with each breath and the tidal volume delivered was about 8 ml/kg of body weight. This low volume maintained adequate ventilation without excessive cardiovascular compromise induced by positive pressure ventilation.

The patient was hemodynamically stabilized using stored blood and clinically evaluated with a chest radiograph and arterial blood gas analysis. The initial blood gas results were as follows:

pH	7.30
$PaCO_2$	40 mm Hg
PaO_2	83 mm Hg
HCO_3^-	18.9 mEq/L
B.E.	−6.8 mEq/L
Hb	15.8 gm %
CaO_2	20.9 vol %
SaO_2	94%
SpO_2	89%
Mode	A/C
RR	16/min
V_T	800 ml
F_IO_2	100%
PEEP	5 cm H_2O

Twenty-five minutes later, the patient remained in critical but stable condition while continuing to bleed into the chest tube. The endotracheal tube position was noted and secured in the airway awaiting visualization on the chest radiograph. Blood gases were drawn to evaluate his acidosis and quantify the degree of blood loss from the tension hemothorax. These were outlined as follows:

☑ Change in the hemoglobin level (from 15.8 to 10.7 gm %) greatly diminishes the patient's arterial oxygen content (from 20.9 to 15 vol %).

pH	7.40
$PaCO_2$	33 mm Hg
PaO_2	196 mm Hg
HCO_3^-	19.6 mEq/L
B.E.	−4.2 mEq/L
Hb	10.7 gm %
CaO_2	15 vol %
SaO_2	96%
SpO_2	95%
Mode	A/C
RR	16/min
V_T	800 ml
F_IO_2	100%
PEEP	5 cm H_2O

☑ The F_1O_2 was reduced to 60% because the PaO_2 (196 mm Hg) was excessive.

The F_1O_2 was reduced to 60%. Chest radiograph confirmed proper placement of the endotracheal tube and noted a tension hemothorax on the right side. He was taken to the operating room for an emergency thoracotomy and relief of the tension hemothorax resulting from a spontaneous intercostal bleed.

By the end of thoracotomy and repair of the bleed, he received eleven units of blood prior to returning to the ICU. Later, he received nine more units of blood in the ICU.

PATIENT MONITORING

Upon return from the OR, the patient was placed back on mechanical ventilation at 1,000 ml tidal volume on assist/control with a rate of 12/min., F_1O_2 of 60%, and 5 cm H_2O of PEEP. Peak inspiratory pressures returned to 36 cm H_2O, he was hemodynamically stable, and allowed to awaken from the anesthesia. Blood gases ten minutes after returning from surgery revealed the following:

pH	7.41
$PaCO_2$	39 mm Hg
PaO_2	55 mm Hg
HCO_3^-	24.1 mEq/L
B.E.	–2.7 mEq/L
Hb	11.4 gm %
CaO_2	17.7 vol %
SaO_2	90.5%
SpO_2	87%
Mode	A/C
RR	12/min
V_T	1,000 ml
F_1O_2	60%
PEEP	5 cm H_2O

In an effort to minimize the effects of oxygen toxicity, the ventilator was adjusted by increasing the PEEP to 8 cm H_2O to increase the PaO_2 without raising the F_1O_2 past 60%.

PATIENT MANAGEMENT

☑ Cardiac output and pulmonary wedge pressures are used to monitor the adequacy of circulating blood volume.

This patient was recovered from surgery in the ICU on mechanical ventilation in an effort to minimize any postsurgical complications associated with continued blood loss and to guard against the development of respiratory distress.

Following rapid infusion of twenty units of blood to cover his losses, hemodynamic measurements including cardiac output and pulmonary wedge pressures help to assure adequate perfusion to the tissues. Oxygenation, under the conditions presented, may be complicated by the use of stored blood used for volume replacement.

Of particular importance is the fact that stored blood contains limited amounts of 2,3 diphosphoglycerate (DPG), which effectively shifts the oxyhemoglobin dissociation curve to the left. Thus, stored blood reduces the unloading of oxygen at the tissues causing hypoxia, necrosis, and possibly sepsis if not managed properly. As a result, the patient's PaO_2 was closely monitored to maintain adequate oxygenation and saturation. He was also monitored for clinical signs of tissue hypoxia. At that time, follow-up blood gases revealed these results:

pH	7.46
$PaCO_2$	34 mm Hg
PaO_2	124 mm Hg
HCO_3^-	24.1 mEq/L
B.E.	−1.7 mEq/L
Hb	11.4 gm %
CaO_2	15.5 vol %
SaO_2	95.7%
SpO_2	94%
Mode	A/C
RR	12/min
V_T	1,000 ml
F_IO_2	60%
PEEP	8 cm H_2O

☑ Reduce F_IO_2 when PaO_2 is too high.

The F_IO_2 was reduced to 50% and the patient was continuously monitored by the SpO_2 and SvO_2 measurements.

RESPIRATORY CARE PROCEDURES

Based on the preadmission diagnosis of complicating pneumonia, the patient was aggressively treated with frequent suctioning and a moderate amount of cloudy secretions was removed. Bronchopulmonary toilet was initiated and he was immediately started on bronchodilator therapy with 20 puffs of Proventil via a metered dose inhaler (MDI) given in-line through the ventilator circuit via Aerochamber®, and he was frequently turned from side-to-side to help prevent atelectasis.

WEANING

Two days following surgery, the patient began to breathe spontaneously and he was changed to SIMV in an attempt to wean him from the ventilator. Initially, his rate was decreased to 8/min., and all spontaneous breaths were supported by 10 cm H_2O of pressure support. He was able to initiate twenty breaths above the set rate and maintained a tidal volume of 400 to 600 ml at this level of support. His machine breaths were set at 1,000 ml tidal volume and over that time, his PEEP was reduced to 5 cm H_2O and his F_IO_2 was reduced to 40%. As his muscular effort improved, the tidal volume increased and his pressure support was quickly weaned to 6 cm H_2O while maintaining the same tidal volume. He remained at that level throughout the day without signs of fatigue, hypoxemia, tachypnea, hypertension, evidence of desaturation, or excessive tachycardia.

That night he was placed on assist/control in an effort to rest the muscles of inspiration. Weaning began at six o'clock the next morning on CPAP with pressure support of 12 cm H_2O, PEEP of 5 cm H_2O, and F_IO_2 of 40%. Spontaneous parameters obtained two hours later revealed:

> ✔ An f/V_T ratio of less than 100/min/L is highly predictive of weaning success.

$$f = 26 \quad V_E = 12.4\ L \quad V_T = 0.47\ L \quad VC = 1.09\ L \quad MIP = -52\ cm\ H_2O$$
$$f/V_T = 55/min/L$$

Based on stable spontaneous parameters and clinical condition, he was removed from the ventilator and allowed to breathe on a "T-piece" at 40% F_IO_2 for four hours. Subsequent evaluations led to successful weaning and extubation. He was placed on a nasal cannula at 6 LPM and continued to improve.

COMPLICATIONS

Besides the tension hemopneumothorax, there were no apparent complications from either the right-sided pneumonia or throughout the postoperative period resulting from the mechanical ventilation. He was followed throughout his hospital stay with respiratory therapy and continued treatments with deep breathing regimens and with bronchodilator therapy for wheezing. His oxygen demands were monitored with daily pulse oximetry and the oxygen cannula was titrated to maintain the SpO_2's above 90%. He was discharged on the eighth postsurgical day from the tertiary care facility on room air and without further complications.

CASE 8: CHEST TRAUMA

INTRODUCTION

A.P. was a 24-year-old, 56-kg female involved in a moving vehicle accident. The patient was unrestrained and was struck on her side of the vehicle. She was thrown from the vehicle but her car was found to contain multiple prescription pain medication bottles. She was apparently comatose at the scene with no spontaneous breathing or pulse. However, her vital signs returned to normal en route to the hospital.

Upon arrival to the emergency department, her vital signs revealed a blood pressure (BP) of 122/80 mm Hg, pulse of 80/min., normal sinus rhythm, and temperature of 35.8°C. Her breathing was assisted by the respiratory care practitioner (RCP) with a manual resuscitator

☑ The white blood count is significantly elevated.

☑ Pulmonary contusion is an internal injury of the lung parenchyma in which the skin is not broken.

☑ Bilateral rib fractures and pneumothoraces with blood accumulation limit chest expansion and hinder ventilation and oxygenation.

☑ History of smoking and chronic bronchitis limit the patient's lung functions.

☑ Chest trauma, unstable and worsening cardiopulmonary and hemodynamic status are the primary indications for mechanical ventilation.

☑ $PaCO_2$ of 25 mm Hg shows alveolar hyperventilation and it indicates ventilatory insufficiency (i.e., hyperventilation to maintain a PaO_2 of 83 mm Hg).

bag. Breath sounds revealed diffuse coarse rhonchi bilaterally without wheezing.

Laboratory and radiology results revealed a white blood cell count (WBC) of 17.5×10^3 (*normal 3.2 to 9.8 $\times 10^3$*), hemoglobin (Hb) of 12.7 gm% (*normal 12 to 15 gm%*), platelets of 195×10^3 (*normal 130 to 400 $\times 10^3$*), prothrombin time (PT) of 13 seconds (*normal 9 to 12 sec.*), and a partial thromboplastin time (PTT) of 30 seconds (*normal 22 to 37 sec.*). A portable chest radiograph (Figure 17-5) revealed rib fracture on the right and bilateral infiltrates in which the left were greater than the right. The left hemidiaphragm, heart border, and parenchymal changes were consistent with pulmonary contusion or possible aspiration pneumonitis.

The patient underwent an extensive evaluation of her injuries including a computerized tomography (CT) of her head that was essentially normal. Scans of her chest and abdomen revealed bilateral rib fractures, pneumothoraces with blood accumulation, and rupture of her spleen with evidence of free peritoneal fluid. Also noted was an apparent transverse process fracture of the lumbar spine as well as possible posterior element fractures of the T1 vertebrae. She also had multiple contusions and lacerations including a large laceration to the right axilla and in the right wrist region.

Her previous history included smoking one pack of cigarettes per day and chronic bronchitis.

INDICATIONS

Due to the extent of her injuries, she was hemodynamically stabilized with a transfusion of four units of blood, paralyzed with a short-acting paralytic (Succinylcholine), and intubated with a 8.0 mm endotracheal tube. She was subsequently transferred to the intensive care unit (ICU) in critical but stable condition requiring mechanical ventilation.

INITIAL SETTINGS

She was immediately placed on a Puritan-Bennett 7200 ventilator on assist/control at 15/min control rate, V_T 600 ml, F_IO_2 60%, and PEEP 5 cm H_2O. Chest tubes were placed to evacuate the pleural space of blood and air. Her initial blood gases after ten minutes on the ventilator were:

pH	7.45
$PaCO_2$	25 mm Hg
PaO_2	83 mm Hg
HCO_3^-	17.3 mEq/L
Hb	13.7 gm %
Mode	A/C
Rate	15
V_T	600 mL
F_IO_2	60%
PEEP	5 cm H_2O

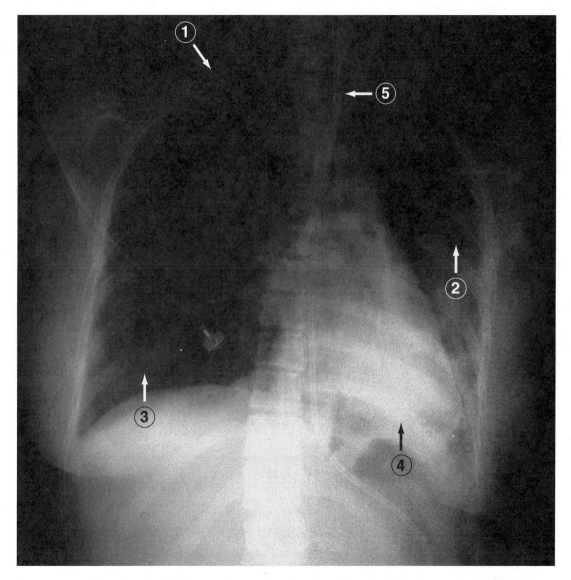

Figure 17-5   Chest Trauma. Rib fracture is noted on the right side (1) of this chest radiograph. Infiltrates on the left side (2) cause a greater density than the right side (3). The diaphragm shadow on the left is lost (4) likely due to pulmonary contusion or possible aspiration pneumonitis. Left-sided atelectasis pulls the mediastinum and trachea (5) to the left. The shift does not appear to be significant, possibly due to patient rotation when the radiograph was taken.

✓ When the patient fatigues, it leads to deteriorating ventilation and oxygenation status.

✓ Pressure Control-Inverse Ratio Ventilation (PC-IRV) uses a predetermined inspiratory pressure to minimize the occurrence of pressure-induced barotrauma.

✓ PC-IRV increases the mean airway pressure, central venous pressure, and pulmonary artery pressure.

Over the next 24 hours, her condition quickly deteriorated requiring 100% F_IO_2 and increasing levels of PEEP to maintain adequate oxygenation.

PATIENT MONITORING

The increasing pressure required to ventilate her lungs began to compromise her cardiac output and, as such, limit perfusion to her tissues. As a result, she was heavily sedated and changed to Pressure Control-Inversed Ratio Ventilation (PC-IRV) mode at a rate of 12/min. and an inspiratory pressure of 30 cm H_2O. Her inspiratory time (T_I) was set at 1.0 sec. resulting in a 3:1 I:E ratio. Her PEEP and F_IO_2 requirements were 8 cm H_2O and 100%, respectively. These settings provided hyperexpansion of the chest in order to stabilize the thorax and limit movement of the rib fractures. She was monitored by an end-tidal CO_2 monitor. Frequent blood gases were ordered to evaluate her ventilatory and oxygenation status. Blood gases drawn at this time revealed the following:

pH	7.36
$PaCO_2$	42 mm Hg
PaO_2	62 mm Hg
SaO_2	90%
HCO_3^-	22.9 mEq/L
Hb	11.2 gm %
Mode	PC-IRV
T_I	1.0 sec
I:E ratio	3:1
Rate	12
P_{INSP}	30 cm H_2O
F_IO_2	100%
PEEP	8 cm H_2O

✓ Increase in central venous pressure lowers the systemic arterial and venous pressure gradient. Decreased venous return to the heart causes a lower cardiac output.

The patient appeared to tolerate these changes well. However, within one hour her hemodynamic values (including cardiac output) were reduced as a result of pressure ventilation. The T_I was decreased to 0.82 seconds (2:1 ratio) and respiratory rate was increased to 24/minute. The PEEP was increased to 15 cm H_2O. Arterial and mixed venous blood gases revealed the following:

Arterial	
pH	7.38
$PaCO_2$	38 mm Hg
PaO_2	90 mm Hg
SaO_2	95%
HCO_3^-	21.8 mEq/L
B.E.	−2.4 mEq/L
Hb	11.1 gm %
CaO_2	14.9 vol %

Mixed Venous
pH	7.36
PvO_2	47 mm Hg
SvO_2	78%
$A\text{-}aDO_2$	462 mm Hg
Qs/QT	42%

Ventilator Settings
Mode	PC-IRV
T_I	0.82 sec
I:E ratio	2:1
Rate	24
P_{INSP}	30 cm H_2O
F_IO_2	100%
PEEP	15 cm H_2O

✓ Ventilator settings should be adjusted based on the patient's ventilation and oxygenation requirement, as well as the patient's hemodynamic status.

The patient remained on a 2:1 I:E ratio and other ventilator settings were manipulated to normalize ventilation and oxygenation. To maintain a PaO_2 greater than 65 mm Hg, the required settings were: inspiratory pressure 30 cm H_2O, PEEP 18 cm H_2O, and F_IO_2 70%.

PATIENT MANAGEMENT

For the next 14 days, the patient was monitored closely for adverse signs while in a drug-induced coma. She was placed on a fentanyl citrate drip to manage her pain and was given narcotic medications to limit her movements while on pressure control ventilation. Vigorous pulmonary toilet was begun and she was suctioned with a closed directional tip catheter to the main-stem bronchi. This produced a large amount of thick, yellow secretions. She also received frequent acetylcystine (Mucomyst) lavage every four hours and was confined to a Rotorest® bed to help prevent pulmonary complications associated with atelectasis.

✓ Aggressive pulmonary hygiene is important in managing patients who are intubated and receiving prolonged mechanical ventilation.

KEY MEDICATIONS

She was given nebulizer treatments with 0.5 ml of 0.5% albuterol sulfate (Proventil) and 0.5 mg ipratropium bromide (Atrovent) every four hours for wheezing. Broad spectrum antibiotics including a fourth generation cephalosporin were used to treat pneumonia from long-term ventilation.

WEANING

Several days later, the patient's oxygen was weaned to 45% and respiratory rate of 22/min. Her condition continued to improve over time and the RCPs were also able to wean the PEEP to 15 cm H_2O. Blood gases on these settings revealed:

✓ For ventilator patients requiring high F_IO_2 and PEEP, wean F_IO_2 first to about 40% before weaning PEEP.

pH	7.58
$PaCO_2$	26 mm Hg
PaO_2	87 mm Hg
SaO_2	96%
HCO_3^-	23.5 mEq/L
B.E.	3.3 mEq/L
Hb	11.7 gm %
CaO_2	15.8 vol %
Mode	IR-PCV
Rate	22
P_{INSP}	30 cm H_2O
F_IO_2	45%
PEEP	15 cm H_2O

At this point, she was removed from pressure control ventilation and allowed to awaken. As her spontaneous breathing resumed, she was quickly weaned to continuous positive airway pressure (CPAP) with 5 cm H_2O of PEEP and pressure support of 20 cm H_2O without difficulty. She maintained a respiratory rate of less than 24/min. with tidal volumes of about 300 ml. As her muscular effort improved, tidal volume increased and her pressure support was titrated to maintain the same tidal volume and assure adequate alveolar ventilation and lung expansion.

> ☑ During weaning attempt, the pressure support level should be titrated based on the appropriate tidal volume and respiratory rate.

At night, she was rested on assist/control at a V_T of 600 ml, backup rate of 12/min. She maintained a spontaneous rate of 14/min. This regimen continued for the next three days where she was placed on CPAP with pressure support titrated to assist her spontaneous tidal volumes during the day, and rested during the night. Spontaneous parameters were obtained each morning to determine suitability to wean and monitor her effort to breathe on her own. Eventually, rather that returning to assist/control, she was able to tolerate synchronized intermittent mandatory ventilation (SIMV) mode with pressure support of 15 cm H_2O during the night. The following day, she remained on CPAP with 20 cm H_2O of pressure support throughout the next 36 hours without signs of respiratory insufficiency or distress.

She was evaluated for extubation, and her spontaneous respiratory parameters over the last five days were:

Day 1: f = 50 V_E = 14.8 L V_T = 0.3 L   VC = 0.80 L   MIP = −46
f/V_T = 167

Day 2: f = 40 V_E = 10.6 L V_T = 0.27 L   VC = 0.85 L   MIP = −48
f/V_T = 148

Day 3: f = 37 V_E = 9.5 L V_T = 0.26 L   VC = 0.87 L   MIP = −56
f/V_T = 142

Day 4: $f = 33$ $V_E = 8.2$ L $V_T = 0.3$ L VC = 1.02 L MIP = –57
$f/V_T = 110$

Day 5: $f = 32$ $V_E = 10.3$ L $V_T = 0.32$ L VC = 1.14 L MIP = –42
$f/V_T = 100$

✓ The weaning criteria on day 5 are satisfactory. See other weaning criteria in Chapter 14.

✓ An f/V_T ratio of less than 100 is highly predictive of weaning success.

Extubation decisions are frequently made in conjunction with spontaneous breathing parameters as well as other clinical indicators that may predict success. Ideally, every member of the patient care team may give input concerning this important decision. The frequency (f) should be below 30/min. The minute volume (V_E) should be around 10 liters with a tidal volume of > 5 to 8 ml/kg and a vital capacity > 10 to 15 ml/kg. The maximum inspiratory pressure (MIP) should be greater than –20 to –30 cm H_2O where muscle strength is directly proportional to the volume generated for inspiration. The frequency to tidal volume ratio (f/V_T), sometimes called the rapid, shallow breathing test, measures the patient's volume as compared to the respiratory rate. Patients breathing rapidly with shallow volumes may only ventilate the anatomic deadspace (i.e., conducting zones within the lungs without effective alveolar ventilation). This ratio, then, should be below 100/min/L before effective weaning may take place.

Realize, however, that these indicators are only idealistic values and should not be taken individually as predictors of success. Other clinical signs such as level of consciousness, sensorium, ability to follow commands, character and volume of secretions, and hemodynamics may also help in predicting a successful postextubation course.

COMPLICATIONS

The patient followed a gradual resolution of her multiorgan dysfunction and severe refractory pulmonary difficulties after an eighteen-day ventilator course. She was recovered and discharged to a home health agency where she was advised to abstain from prescription narcotics, continued on Gentamicin 360 mg IV once per day, and Ciprofloxacin 750 mg twice daily for ten days. Her SpO_2 at discharge was 90% on room air while walking.

CASE 9: ADULT RESPIRATORY DISTRESS SYNDROME

INTRODUCTION

M.I. was a 22-year-old, 54-kg female with a history of systemic lupus erythematosus, congenital mitral regurgitation, and syncopes. For the past several months, she complained of mild productive cough while lying down. One week prior to her admission she developed severe cough, progressive dyspnea without the use of accessory muscles, and associated pain throughout her chest wall and into her upper abdomen.

Her medical history also included chronic anemia (hemoglobin 8.7 gm %, *normal 12 to 15 gm %*) and was on iron supplement at the time. Her white blood cell count (WBC) was 21×10^3 (*normal 3.2 to 9.8 $\times 10^3$*), hematocrit (Hct) 27% (*female average 42%*) without evidence of blood loss. Blood pressure was 93/59 mm Hg (*normal 120/80 mm Hg*), pulse 114, respirations were shallow and guarded at 20 breaths per minute. Tenderness was noted across the upper abdomen and the lower ribs without organomegally or other masses present.

She was four months postpartum with gradual onset abdominal pain, progressive dyspnea with nonproductive coughs, and was admitted to the hospital for further evaluations.

The patient's nonspecific symptoms led to a wide range of diagnostic tests for her condition which included lupus, mitral regurgitation, and pulmonary insufficiency. Initial blood gases on room air were obtained in the emergency room, the patient was admitted to the medical floor, and a sputum culture was ordered to evaluate pathology concerning the respiratory tract.

The initial blood gases were as follows:

pH	7.49
$PaCO_2$	31 mm Hg
PaO_2	67 mm Hg
HCO_3^-	22.7 mEq/L
Hb	8.4 gm %
Mode	Spontaneous
F_IO_2	21%

Her breath sounds were unremarkable but she was moderately fatigued and continued to be short of breath. She was started on a nasal cannula at 2 LPM and was encouraged to deep breathe and cough. At this point, the patient was still able to adequately ventilate as evidenced by the $PaCO_2$. However, her condition deteriorated during the course of her evaluation and workup. Shortly thereafter, she developed intermittent wheezing for which albuterol nebulizer treatments were ordered.

INDICATIONS

Her blood gases continued to deteriorate, and six days later she required a nonrebreathing mask to maintain her SpO_2 above 90%. She showed signs of impending ventilatory failure evidenced by the rising $PaCO_2$s and acidotic pH on blood gases. A chest radiograph showed areas of bibasilar atelectasis and haziness with bilateral infiltrates. No pulmonary consolidation was noted. Postural drainage and chest

---

Margin notes:

✓ Iron supplement is used to increase the O_2-carrying capacity of hemoglobin.

✓ Hemoglobin, WBC, Hct, and blood pressure are all outside normal limits.

✓ Alveolar hyperventilation ($PaCO_2$ 31 mm Hg) with moderate hypoxemia (PaO_2 67 mm Hg) could lead to fatigue of respiratory muscles if causes of hypoxemia are not identified and treated promptly.

✓ Impending ventilatory failure typically shows increasing $PaCO_2$ and decreasing PaO_2.

✓ Postural drain-
age and chest
physiotherapy were
done to facilitate
loosening and re-
moval of secretions.

✓ CPAP requires
adequate spon-
taneous breathing.
Development of
respiratory muscle
fatigue is the pri-
mary concern for
prolonged CPAP
usage in critically ill
patients.

physiotherapy were started but she was too weak to generate a productive cough.

Family members refused permission to obtain a diagnostic bronchoscopy or any attempts at percutaneous biopsies. Three days later,
her oxygen requirements had increased to the point where she required
a heated nebulizer analyzed at an F_IO_2 of 95% bled into her nonrebreathing mask at 15 LPM, and a nasal cannula at 6 LPM simply to maintain
oxygen saturation of 86 to 92%. Practitioners were able to convince the
family to utilize free standing CPAP at 12 cm H_2O and F_IO_2 of 50% to
improve oxygenation, but the patient became fatigued to the extent that
she was only able to tolerate the procedure 20 minutes every two hours.
At that time she had a vital capacity of 0.9 L and MIP of −75 cm H_2O.
This continued for two days as she became refractory to oxygen therapy
and was unable to maintain adequate oxygen saturation.

INITIAL SETTINGS

Every attempt was made to forestall ventilatory failure and prevent
intubation but the patient's condition continued to deteriorate, and
she became progressively fatigued. Her age and previous health were
positive factors in postponing ventilatory failure, but she eventually
became overwhelmed by fatigue. She was moderately sedated,
intubated with a 7.5 mm endotracheal tube, and placed on a Puritan-
Bennett 7200 for mechanical ventilation. Initially, she was set on
assist/control at 25/min., V_T of 800 ml, F_IO_2 of 100%, and PEEP of
8 cm H_2O. Arterial and mixed venous blood gases on these settings
revealed the following:

Arterial
pH	7.40
$PaCO_2$	33 mm Hg
PaO_2	58 mm Hg
SaO_2	88%
HCO_3^-	29.5 mEq/L
Hb	10.1 gm %

Mixed Venous
pH	7.38
PvO_2	33 mm Hg
SvO_2	58%
$C(a-v)O_2$	4.6 vol %
Qs/QT	37%

Ventilator Settings
Mode	AC
Rate	25/min
V_T	800 ml
F_IO_2	100%
PEEP	8 cm H_2O

✓ The ventilator
rate was de-
creased because
of the low $PaCO_2$
(33 mm Hg).

✓ The PEEP was
increased be-
cause of the low
PaO_2 (58 mm Hg).

Her ventilator rate was reduced to 14/min., and her PEEP was increased to 10 cm H_2O.

PATIENT MONITORING

☑ With cardiogenic pulmonary edema, the PCWP is usually elevated (> 18 mm Hg).

In addition to blood gases and vital signs, other cardiopulmonary monitoring included chest radiograph and hemodynamic measurements. Her chest radiograph at that time revealed initial findings consistent with adult respiratory distress syndrome (ARDS), including a uniform reticulogranular pattern or ground glass appearance throughout both lung fields. Arterial and pulmonary artery catheters were used to monitor the cardiac output and hemodynamic status. Cardiac output was stable at 4.2 liters. The pulmonary capillary wedge pressure (PCWP) was around 11 mm Hg and thus ruled out cardiogenic edema.

☑ Pulmonary edema with normal PCWP is likely caused by lung parenchymal changes (e.g., ARDS).

For unknown reasons, the patient developed a parenchymal injury causing progressive inflammation, alveolar collapse, and hypoxemia.

Hypoxemia in ARDS may be summarized as follows:
Hypoxic vasoconstriction in ARDS increases the vascular resistance and diminishes the cardiac output. The lack of oxygen in the pulmonary circulation also causes necrosis of the tissue lining of the alveolar-capillary membrane that, in turn, induces capillary leak into the interstitium (third spacing) and hence, impairs gas exchange. This eventually causes a severe V/Q mismatch and further hypoxemia. As a result of these factors, perfusion must be maintained and oxygenation restored for effective management of ARDS.

PATIENT MANAGEMENT

☑ Hypoxemia caused by intrapulmonary shunting may be supported by PEEP (with mechanical ventilation) or CPAP (with spontaneous breathing).

Management strategies for ARDS include correcting hypoxemia and acid-base disturbance, restoring cardiac function, and treating the underlying disease or other precipitating factors. This is generally accomplished with mechanical ventilation at 10 to 15 ml/kg of body weight and the application of PEEP or CPAP to correct refractory hypoxemia.

☑ Pressure control ventilation limits the inspiratory pressure during mechanical ventilation.

High level of positive pressure may be required to produce adequate ventilation and oxygenation, but its adverse effect on cardiac function must be monitored carefully. Some patients may benefit from pressure control (PC) ventilation to minimize the mean airway and parenchymal pressures. In PC mode the inspiratory time is increased and pressures are generally reduced, but the mean airway pressure may remain nearly the same or slightly increased. This ultimately shortens the expiratory time, inverts the I:E ratio, and potentially increases alveolar ventilation. As inspiratory time increases, and the elastic limit of the lung is reached, intrinsic PEEP increases air trapping and thus, may increase the $PaCO_2$ while also increasing the occurrence of pneumothorax in an already stiff lung. These important considerations must be kept in fine balance with each factor receiving equal attention.

In an attempt to decrease the pressures exerted within the thorax, the patient was placed on pressure control ventilation with an inverse ratio of 2:1 at pressure of 30 cm H_2O, T_I of 0.84 sec., F_IO_2 of 60%, and PEEP of 10 cm H_2O. Blood gases taken at the time revealed:

pH	7.42
$PaCO_2$	47 mm Hg
PaO_2	60 mm Hg
HCO_3^-	30 mEq/L
Hb	11.1 gm %
SpO_2	90%
Mode	PC-IRV
T_I	0.84 sec
I:E ratio	2:1
Rate	14
P_{INSP}	30 cm H_2O
F_IO_2	60%
PEEP	10 cm H_2O

The pressures were then titrated in an effort to improve oxygenation and normalize her condition, but without success.

KEY MEDICATIONS

☑ As in IPPB, the tidal volume delivered by pressure control ventilation is directly related to the inspiratory pressure.

☑ Mucomyst and Pulmozyme are used to mobilize thick, retained secretions.

The patient was placed in a Rotorest® bed to prevent development of atelectasis. She was also heavily sedated and maintained in a medicated coma for over thirty days but without significant improvement. She was given medication nebulizers with Proventil every four hours, lavaged with a combination of 2.0 ml normal saline (NS), 0.5 ml of 0.5% Proventil, and 4.0 ml of 10% Mucomyst solution, and suctioned every four hours with her treatment to improve bronchopulmonary hygiene. By this time she had a large amount of thick, yellow secretions and 0.5 ml of Dornase Alpha (Pulmozyme) in NS was used to loosen and remove her retained secretions.

WEANING

☑ Low V_T is used to minimize the airway pressures.

The deteriorating hemodynamic status prevented continuing use of inverse I:E ratio ventilation. She was returned to conventional methods throughout the remainder of her hospitalization. This included ventilation in the assist/control mode at a rate of 24/min. The patient initiated inspiratory effort to 28/min. She was set to a V_T of 500 ml, F_IO_2 of 80%, and PEEP of 8 cm H_2O. Arterial blood gases on these settings produced these results:

pH	7.43
$PaCO_2$	48 mm Hg
PaO_2	64 mm Hg
HCO_3^-	31 mEq/L
Hb	11.1 gm %
CaO_2	13.9 vol %
SpO_2	91%
Mode	A/C
RR	24/min
V_T	500 ml
F_IO_2	80%
PEEP	8 cm H_2O

The respiratory rate was increased to 30 breaths per minute to override her excessive and demanding respiratory efforts. PEEP was increased to 10 cm H_2O, and F_IO_2 was reduced to 70%.

Blood gases were drawn thirty minutes later with the following results:

pH	7.50
$PaCO_2$	47 mm Hg
PaO_2	59 mm Hg
HCO_3^-	36.4 mEq/L
B.E.	12.4 mEq/L
Hb	9.6 gm %
CaO_2	12.4 vol %
SpO_2	91%
Mode	A/C
RR	30/min
V_T	500 ml
F_IO_2	70%
PEEP	10 cm H_2O

Several unsuccessful weaning attempts were made. Over several days she was weaned to a rate of 24/min. on assist/control with a V_T of 380 ml, F_IO_2 of 50%, and PEEP of 8 cm H_2O and remained on those settings for nearly one week. Due to her deteriorating condition and persistent complications, it was decided to remove her from ventilatory support, and she died a short time later.

COMPLICATIONS

Through the course of her hospitalization the patient experienced many complicating injuries which contributed to her failure to recover. These included barotrauma to the lung parenchyma (pneumothorax was corrected with a chest tube), pneumomediastinum, and interstitial emphysema verified through serial chest radiographs,

✓ Complicating
ARDS carries a
50% mortality rate.

subcutaneous emphysema, and ultimately death. Many of these complications could have been expected as a result of her hospital course because ARDS, even without her related complicating factors, carries a 50% mortality rate.

Note: This case study on ARDS describes the evaluative, diagnostic, and ventilatory management techniques employed at the time it was first written. Recently, however, the National Heart, Lung, and Blood Institute of the National Institute of Health has released a statement concerning the ARDS Network Clinical Trial. This included research at a consortium of 10 clinical centers conducted at 24 hospitals across the United States. For further information, please refer to this statement outlined by the NIH (1999, Mar). *NHLBI Clinical Trial Stopped Early: Successful Ventilator Strategy Found for Intensive Care Patients on Life Support.* NIH Press Release @ http://www.nih.gov/news/pr/mar99/nhlbi-15.htm

Data from this clinical trial on the first 800 patients showed approximately 25 percent fewer deaths among patients receiving small, rather than large, tidal volumes from a mechanical ventilator. Patient tidal volume is based on an ideal body weight calculation. This is calculated from the following equation:

Male: $50 + 2.3$ (height in inches $- 60) \times 6cc's$

Female: $45.5 + 2.3$ (height in inches $- 60) \times 6$ cc's

Although the patient in this case study was not on this protocol, it seems worth mentioning that these new guidelines have proved to be useful in clinical practice. This is especially true with the ARDS protocol.

CASE 10: MYASTHENIA GRAVIS

INTRODUCTION

G.L. was a 72-year-old Caucasian male (6'1", 74 kg) with a history of myasthenia gravis for 25 years, but it had been in remission until about 6 months ago. His last hospitalization was 2 months ago because of ongoing shortness of breath, easy fatigability, inability to complete a sentence without taking a breath, chronic cough, malaise, yellow sputum production and difficulty in swallowing. The diagnosis was pneumonia and he required mechanical ventilation for 17 days. He was eventually weaned off mechanical ventilation and discharged. During that hospitalization, he had repeated guaiac positive stool samples indicative of the presence of occult blood in the feces.

✓ Barium study is done to evaluate the cause of guaiac positive stools.

✓ Chest radiograph is done to evaluate the residual effects of pneumonia.

✓ Blood gas report indicates that the primary problem is acute ventilatory failure imposed on chronic ventilatory failure.

✓ $PaCO_2$ indicates that the bag/mask system in the ambulance was not ventilating the patient.

✓ HCO_3^- is elevated as a compensatory mechanism of the patient's pre-existing ventilatory failure.

✓ Glasgow coma score of ≤7 indicates coma. A score of 15 rules out coma.

✓ Chest radiograph shows aspiration of barium in the left lower lobe.

✓ PaO_2 168 mm Hg is too high and the F_IO_2 should be decreased.

He had been home for four weeks and continued to have shortness of breath, fatigability, muscle weakness, orthopnea, and had to sleep sitting up in his recliner. He came to the outpatient radiology clinic for barium and chest radiograph studies. Upon arrival to the radiology department he was extremely short of breath and after his exams were completed he was referred to the emergency room. The patient declined to be seen and went home with his wife.

Within five minutes of arrival home the patient suffered a respiratory arrest. His wife reported that he just stopped breathing and turned blue. The paramedics arrived and attempted to intubate but were unsuccessful after three attempts. While being transported to the ER, the patient had some spontaneous respirations but poor diaphragmatic movement.

The initial blood gas analysis done upon arrival to the ER revealed the following results:

pH	6.95
$PaCO_2$	143 mm Hg
PaO_2	115 mm Hg
SaO_2	96%
HCO_3^-	30 mEq/L
Mode	Ambu bag and mask
F_IO_2	About 100%
Notes	Poor ventilation

INDICATIONS

The patient was intubated in the ER and bagged at a rate of 20/min. and F_IO_2 of 100%. Vital signs included: blood pressure 138/40 mm Hg, heart rate 60/min., temperature 95.2°F, SpO_2 97%, and Glasgow coma score 15. Bilateral breath sounds were present. Chest radiograph (Figure 17-6) showed proper ET tube position, good thoracic expansion, but barium in the left lower lobe.

INITIAL SETTINGS

The patient was initially placed on a Puritan-Bennett 7200ae ventilator with the following settings: CMV 16/min., V_T 750 ml, F_IO_2 80%, PEEP 0 cmH₂O. The patient had the following ABG results:

pH	7.47
$PaCO_2$	43 mm Hg
PaO_2	168 mm Hg
SaO_2	97%
HCO_3^-	30.5 mEq/L
Mode	CMV
Rate	16
V_T	750 mL
F_IO_2	80%
PEEP	0 cm H₂O

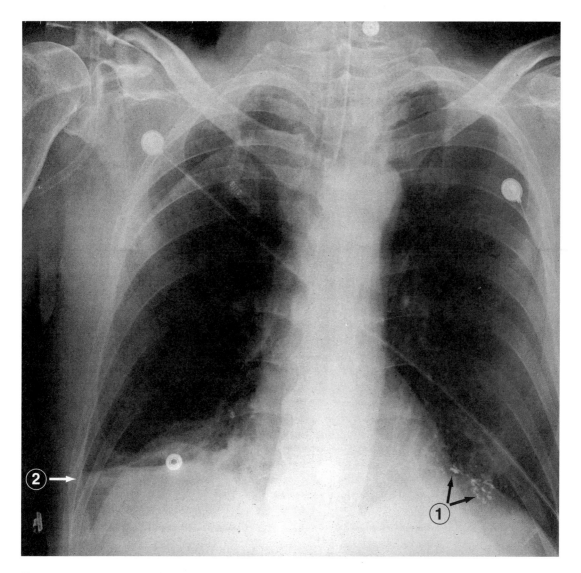

Figure 17-6 Myasthenia Gravis. Aspiration of barium on the left side (1) is seen. The right hemidiaphragm shadow is flat with a poorly defined costophrenic angle (2). This condition may be caused by pleural effusion.

PATIENT MANAGEMENT

(Day 1) The patient was continued on mechanical ventilation and the F_IO_2 was weaned to 40% with the following results:

☑ **PaCO₂ 21 mm Hg is too low and the rate should be decreased.**

pH	7.58
PaCO₂	21 mm Hg
PaO₂	122 mm Hg
SaO₂	96%
HCO₃⁻	19.1 mEq/L
Mode	CMV
Rate	16
V_T	750 mL
F_IO₂	40%
PEEP	0 cm H₂O

The patient's set respiratory rate was decreased to 12 and the blood gas results were:

☑ **PaCO₂ 25 mm Hg is still too low and the rate should be decreased again.**

pH	7.52
PaCO₂	25 mm Hg
PaO₂	128 mm Hg
SaO₂	97%
HCO₃⁻	20 mEq/L
Mode	CMV
Rate	12
V_T	750 mL
F_IO₂	40%
PEEP	0 cm H₂O

The CMV rate was further decreased to 8/min. for the rest of Day 1.

(Day 2) The next morning the patient was on CMV of 8/min., V_T 750 ml, F_IO_2 40%, and no PEEP. He had the following spontaneous parameters: V_E 9.7 L, V_T 660 ml, rate 15/min., MIP -24 cm H₂O, and a vital capacity of 2,080 ml. The patient was alert and responsive. A CPAP/pressure support (CPAP/PS) trial was done with PS of 5 cm H₂O, base flow of 2 LPM, PEEP of 5 cm H₂O, and an F_IO_2 of 40%. The patient tolerated this for four hours with spontaneous tidal volumes of 600 to 700 ml and a spontaneous rate of 16 to 21/min. Breath sounds showed fine inspiratory crackles throughout the anterior bases. All vital signs were within normal limits.

☑ **The increased WBC may be due to aspiration of barium and subsequent aspiration pneumonitis.**

(Day 3) The patient was rested on CMV overnight. Spontaneous parameters were: V_E 7.8 L, V_T 720 ml, rate 12/min., MIP –12 cm H₂O, and a vital capacity of 4,020 ml. Heart rate, blood pressure, and temperature were all within normal limits. The patient's WBC spiked at a high of 16.2×10^3 (*normal 3.2 to 9.8 × 10³*), chest radiograph showed the endotracheal tube was in proper position, and the bilateral opacities were consistent with barium aspiration.

He tolerated the previous CPAP/PS settings for four hours and was taken off CPAP/PS when he began to show extreme accessory muscle use. Blood gases during spontaneous breathing revealed:

pH	7.38
PaCO$_2$	34 mm Hg
PaO$_2$	87 mm Hg
SaO$_2$	97%
Mode	Spontaneous breathing
F$_I$O$_2$	40%

☑ PaCO$_2$ 34 mm Hg indicates hyperventilation. It may lead to fatigue of respiratory muscles.

(Day 4) The patient was rested overnight on CMV, spontaneous parameters were: V$_E$ 9.9 L, V$_T$ 550 ml, rate 18, MIP –26 cm H$_2$O and a vital capacity of 3 L. Vital signs revealed: heart rate 76/min., temperature 38°C, blood pressure 120/74 mm Hg. The patient tolerated two trials of CPAP/PS at previous settings for two hours each time. Breath sounds were markedly decreased in both lower lobes. Patient was very anxious, restless, and had difficulty sleeping at night. He was started on Ativan for his anxiety. The patient had a feeding tube placed today for total nutrition.

(Day 5) He was rested overnight on CMV. Spontaneous parameters were: V$_E$ 12.9 L, V$_T$ 720 ml, rate 18/min., MIP –29 cm H$_2$O, and a vital capacity of 3.4 L. Patient had a repeat endoscopy and was heavily sedated. One CPAP/PS trial was done before the patient was sedated. The spontaneous respiratory rate was between 15 to 17/min. and the spontaneous tidal volume was in the low 400 ml range. Patient's vital signs were: heart rate 73/min., temperature 36.8°C, and blood pressure 120/59 mm Hg. The patient's endoscopy biopsy was positive for Cytomegalovirus and he was started on Ganciclovir and Prilosec.

(Day 6) The patient was again rested on CMV overnight. He was only able to tolerate partial spontaneous parameters and the results were: MIP –28 cm H$_2$O and a vital capacity of 1.1 L. The patient tolerated 90 minutes on CPAP/PS before he was extremely short of breath and exhibited an increased work of breathing with marked accessory muscle use. The patient's daily chest radiograph showed increasing bilateral infiltrates consistent with pneumonia/aspiration and the presence of barium in the left lower lobe. The patient had bilateral lower lobe rhonchi and was being suctioned for copious amounts of light yellow secretions. The patient also spiked a temperature to 39°C. Pulmonary consultation was obtained at this time.

PATIENT MONITORING

The patient's spontaneous breathing parameters from Day 2 through Day 6 are summarized as follows. On Day 6, the patient could perform only part of the breathing parameters.

☑ The overall breathing parameters are not satisfactory for a weaning attempt.

Day	V_E (L)	V_T (ml)	Rate (min)	MIP (cm H_2O)	VC (L)
2	9.7	660	15	−24	2.08
3	7.8	720	12	−12	4.02
4	9.9	550	18	−26	3.0
5	12.9	720	18	29	3.4
6	N/A	N/A	N/A	−28	1.1

WEANING

This patient was eventually weaned from mechanical ventilation after 25 days. He was weaned by using SIMV ventilation to build up his respiratory muscle strength before weaning to CPAP/PS again. The PS level was much higher than with previous attempts. The PS level was gradually weaned down each day as the patient's own spontaneous tidal volumes increased. He was then weaned to CPAP only and eventually extubated from CPAP to a face mask at 30%.

A vigorous program of physical therapy was started to assist the patient with overall strengthening of his weakened muscle. A dietary consult was obtained and a metabolic study performed in order to adjust his feedings to appropriate nutritional levels needed for successful weaning.

Notes: Adequate nutrition prior to and during weaning is necessary for a successful outcome. Appropriate nutrition helps to maintain and build respiratory muscle mass and strength, which enhances the likelihood of weaning.

☑ Neostigmine (Prostigmin) is a cholinergic drug used to treat myasthenia gravis.

The patient was also started on albuterol Q 4° with postural drainage and percussion. Antibiotics were used to treat the pneumonia. The patient was given Neostigmine for his myasthenia gravis crisis.

COMPLICATIONS

Weaning attempts on this patient were complicated by three major factors:

(1) myasthenia gravis, (2) aspiration pneumonia, (3) premature weaning attempts.

The history of myasthenia gravis (a neuromuscular disease) inhibits the transmission of nerve impulses at the myoneural junction. These patients typically have chronic fatigability and weak muscles in the face and throat. They can also suffer what is known as a myasthenia gravis crisis—an acute exacerbation of muscle weakness that leads to respiratory distress and periods of apnea.

☑ Myasthenia gravis, aspiration pneumonia, and poor nutritional intake all contributed to the failure of earlier weaning attempts.

Aspiration pneumonia from the barium study increased the work of breathing and made it difficult for him to tolerate weaning procedures.

Premature and inconsistent weaning attempts during the first three days of his hospitalization made subsequent weaning attempts more diffcult.

CASE 11: GUILLAIN-BARRE

INTRODUCTION

K.D. was a 14-year-old, 49-kg, right-handed male who sustained two minor head injuries at school over a period of one week. One injury occurred while playing basketball when a heavier student fell on him and the other occurred in an altercation during a break. Neither injury resulted in the loss of consciousness. He presented to the clinic complaining of headache and back pain but did not complain of slurred speech until being started on pain medication (Dolobid®) one day prior to admission. His medical history is noncontributory and consists of one hospitalization for a hernia repair in the distant past. He denied blurred vision but admitted to having transient nausea and had recently refused food. Since his slurred speech had become more pronounced he was admitted for further evaluation.

On examination, the patient was afibrile and had these vital signs: BP 110/70 mm Hg, pulse 78/min, respirations 14/min (up to 40/min on occasion). His facial muscles showed symmetry. He had trouble sitting up due to excessive pain in his lower extremities, especially on the left. Lung sounds revealed basilar crackles on the right with decreased aeration on the left. A chest radiograph showed left lower lobe atelectasis. The cranial nerves 2–12 appeared intact and motor strength showed marked weakness. The patient was able to lift his right heel 2 to 3 inches with great difficulty but was unable to lift his left heel at all. His deep tendon reflexes were completely absent.

Laboratory results revealed WBCs of 14,000 with 84 segs. The electrolytes and urinalysis were normal. His FEV_1 and FVC were 1.4 liters and 1.7 liters, respectively. The FEV_1/FVC ratio was 82%. CT scan of the brain revealed a normal study. Chest radiograph at the time showed bilateral consolidation secondary to muscle weakness and left lower lobe atelectasis.

INDICATIONS

☑ Restrictive lung disease typically shows reduction in FEV_1 and FVC, resulting in a normal FEV_1/FVC%.

The patient had a five-day history of progressive muscular weakness. For this reason, simple spirometry studies were done Q4 hours through the night. His predicted forced vital capacity (FVC) was 3.38 liters and his initial vital capacity was 1.7 liters (50% of the predicted value), which he maintained through the early evening. His predicted FEV_1 was 3.12 liters and his initial measurement revealed 1.4 liters

☑ Mechanical ventilation is indicated when the vital capacity falls below 1 L or twice the patient's predicted tidal volume.

☑ Bilateral breath sounds suggests proper endotracheal intubation. This sign should coincide with absence of respiratory distress, presence of adequate SpO_2, and stable vital signs.

☑ Chest radiograph is done to confirm proper placement of endotracheal tube and to rule out inadvertent mainstem intubation.

(48% of predicted) for an 82% FEV_1/FVC ratio. By 03:30am, the patient's vital capacity had dropped to 1.2 liters (35% of predicted) and an arterial blood gas (ABG) at that time, on room air, revealed the following:

pH	7.42
$PaCO_2$	45 mm Hg
PaO_2	46 mm Hg
SaO_2	76%
HCO_3^-	24.9 mEq/L
RR	24/min
F_IO_2	21%

Oxygen therapy was initiated at 2 lpm per nasal cannula. He rested well until 08:22 the next morning. The vital capacity at that time was slightly over one liter (30% of predicted) and the ABG's revealed:

pH	7.44
$PaCO_2$	43 mm Hg
PaO_2	52 mm Hg
SaO_2	86%
HCO_3^-	25.2 mEq/L
RR	22/min

Every attempt was made to forestall clinical deterioration. Trends of spirometry and blood gases showed that the patient was going into ventilatory failure. By 10:30, the patient's vital capacity had dropped to 0.7 liter (20% of predicted) and maintaining adequate oxygenation was becoming more difficult. Consequently, a decision was made to perform elective intubation. Preparation was made to notify family members of the impending ventilatory compromise, and the respiratory therapist gathered the necessary equipment for a controlled intubation. The patient was mildly sedated and intubated with a 7.5mm endotracheal tube without difficulty. Bilateral breath sounds were heard and a portable chest radiograph was ordered.

INITIAL SETTINGS

Following intubation and confirmation of proper tube placement, the patient was placed on a Puritan-Bennett 7200a ventilator in A/C mode, backup rate of 12, tidal volume of 600 ml, and F_IO_2 of 40%. PEEP was not initiated at that time. ABGs revealed the following:

pH	7.43
$PaCO_2$	43 mm Hg
PaO_2	53 mm Hg
SaO_2	86%
HCO_3^-	23.7 mEq/L
Mode	A/C

Rate	12/min
Spont. Rate	17 min
V_T	600 ml
F_IO_2	40%

The ventilator settings were changed accordingly to a backup rate of 14/min, F_IO_2 of 50%, and PEEP of 5 cm H_2O. Follow-up ABGs showed:

pH	7.45
$PaCO_2$	42 mm Hg
PaO_2	73 mm Hg
SaO_2	94%
HCO_3^-	28 mEq/L
Mode	A/C
Rate	14/min
V_T	600 ml
F_IO_2	50%
PEEP	5 cm H_2O

The patient remained relatively stable and was monitored closely for signs of respiratory distress. The ventilator peak flow was adjusted to meet the patient's inspiratory demand without compromise to alveolar ventilation. By the third ventilator day, the F_IO_2 was increased to 60% and the PEEP was increased to 8 cm H_2O. These changes were made to prevent atelectasis and improve alveolar ventilation as evidenced by a declining PaO_2 on his morning blood gas. These revealed the following:

pH	7.48
$PaCO_2$	35 mm Hg
PaO_2	57 mm Hg
SaO_2	87%
HCO_3^-	22.5 mEq/L
Mode	A/C
Rate	14/min
V_T	600 ml
F_IO_2	60%
PEEP	8 cm H_2O

The patient's PEEP was subsequently increased to 10 cm H_2O without cardiac or hemodynamic compromise. F_IO_2 was decreased to 50% because of improving SpO_2 values. Follow-up ABGs revealed:

pH	7.48
$PaCO_2$	35 mm Hg
PaO_2	132 mm Hg

SaO_2	97%
HCO_3^-	23.5 mEq/L
Mode	A/C
Rate	14/min
V_T	600 ml
F_IO_2	50%
PEEP	10 cm H_2O

The F_IO_2 was again lowered to 40% and he remained stable for the next two days.

KEY MEDICATIONS

On day four of mechanical ventilation, a persistent low-grade fever and thick tenacious secretions necessitated initiation of vigorous pulmonary toilet. Albuterol with Mucomyst via small volume nebulizer was started Q4 hours in-line with the ventilator circuit as well as postural drainage and percussion to the bilateral lower lobes. Broncho-alveolar lavage with 4 ml of 10% Mucomyst, 0.5 ml of 0.5% albuterol and 5 ml of normal saline facilitated suction of moderate to large amounts of thick secretions. Gradual clearing of retained secretions aand atelectasis became evident by follow-up chest radiographs. These management strategies in pulmonary toilet were continued for the remainder of the ventilatory period.

Immobility was a major factor in the patient's clinical deterioration. Extensive physical therapy was begun with range of motion and activity as tolerated. However, extreme pain made these sessions almost unbearable to the patient.

☑ Each week of muscle immobility requires four weeks of rehabilitation of his diminished muscle mass.

PATIENT MONITORING

Respiratory parameters were obtained every morning in an effort to trend his ventilatory mechanics. The parameters listed in Table 17-1 were obtained on representative days and are not necessarily concurrent (please note on ventilator day 6 through 26 the patient was mainly unable to breathe on his own):

PATIENT MANAGEMENT

Management strategy for Guillain-Barre was mainly supportive as the ascending paralysis typically runs its course. Being predominantly idiopathic in nature, treatment included plasma phoresis in an attempt to reverse the pathology. However, by the sixth ventilator day it was apparent that long-term management strategies would be necessary. As such, a pediatric feeding tube was inserted and tracheostomy was performed in an effort to facilitate removal of secretions and to make oral care more accessible. A metabolic study was performed to ascertain the patient's nutritional status and feedings were adjusted in terms of optimizing the resulting V/Q ratio and total caloric intake.

TABLE 17-1   Respiratory Parameters

VENT DAY	RR (f)	V_T (ml)	FVC (L)	V_E (L)	f/VT	MIP (cm H_2O)	COMPLIANCE (ml/cm H_2O)
2	37	140	0.67	5.30	264	−20	28
3	50	60	0.32	5.30	833	−15	32
4	25	80	0.69	2.60	312	−13	38
5	23	80	0.10	5.40	287	−2	62
26	6	410	0.41	4.90	15	−15	45
28	10	440	0.45	5.00	23	−15	52
32	23	70	0.65	1.03	328	−10	34
36	30	135	0.55	4.00	222	−26	48
42	29	110	0.54	3.10	263	−11	41
46	32	85	0.25	2.73	376	−10	44
52	27	200	0.36	4.20	135	−14	51
54	23	210	0.57	4.83	1.09	−17	53
56	32	115	0.52	3.70	278	−17	55
58	21	240	0.68	4.60	88	−15	64
60	25	250	0.96	6.22	100	−23	70
62	29	175	1.02	5.09	165	−24	58
64	25	240	0.68	5.89	104	−26	55
66	19	210	1.15	4.91	90	−30	54
68	18	200	1.07	6.11	90	−37	54

He was placed in a Rotorest bed and continuously turned from side to side and kept comfortable with antianxiolytics. The patient was closely monitored for signs of hypercapnea, hypoxia, and respiratory distress. It is important to note that the patient was not able to initiate any significant spontaneous tidal volume. The ventilator was thus completely responsible for his total alveolar ventilation. Blood gas analysis after tracheostomy by general anesthesia revealed the following:

pH	7.40
$PaCO_2$	52 mm Hg
PaO_2	122 mm Hg
SaO_2	96%
HCO_3^-	31 mEq/L
Mode	A/C
Rate	14/min
V_T	600 ml
F_IO_2	40%
PEEP	10 cm H_2O

In order to improve alveolar ventilation, the rate was increased to 16/min and the tidal volume was increased to 670 ml as he was still unable to initiate spontaneous ventilation. Due to his unstable ventilatory status, blood gas results from the following morning revealed:

pH	7.39
$PaCO_2$	48 mm Hg
PaO_2	90 mm Hg
SaO_2	94%
HCO_3^-	28 mEq/L
Mode	A/C
Rate	16/min
V_T	670 ml
F_IO_2	40%
PEEP	10 cm H_2O

In order to minimize airway pressures and risk of barotrauma, the $PaCO_2$ was allowed to stay in the mid to upper 40s. The patient appeared to rest comfortably. Blood gases obtained on the eighteenth ventilator day revealed:

pH	7.48
$PaCO_2$	47 mm Hg
PaO_2	114 mm Hg
SaO_2	97%
HCO_3^-	34 mEq/L
Mode	A/C
Rate	18/min
V_T	670 ml
F_IO_2	40%
PEEP	10 cm H_2O

These parameters were maintained until the 24 ventilator day when the patient appeared to improve clinically and began to breathe significantly on his own. Although he became increasingly uneasy about his breathlessness and, as a result, was changed to SIMV mode, rate of 18 breaths per minute, tidal volume of 750 ml, and F_IO_2 of 40%. PEEP was reduced to 5 cm H_2O and pressure support was initiated to augment his spontaneous volume. Blood gases taken after these changes indicated marked improvement in oxygenation and acid-base balance:

pH	7.47
$PaCO_2$	38 mm Hg
PaO_2	117 mm Hg
SaO_2	94%
HCO_3^-	27 mEq/L
Mode	SIMV
Rate	18/min
V_T	750 ml

F$_I$O$_2$ 40%
PEEP   5 cm H$_2$O
Press. Support   15 cm H$_2$O

At this point, the F$_I$O$_2$ was reduced to 35% and remained relatively stable for the next nineteen days. A bronchoscopy was performed on ventilator day 32 to clear an obstructed left lower lobe bronchus. This was achieved without difficulty and by ventilator day 39, the rate was decreased from 18 to 12/min. The following day, the rate was decreased to 10/min. His spontaneous rate ranged between 29 and 32/min.

WEANING

On ventilator day 40, the patient continued to show evidence of improved alveolar ventilation. Brief trials of ventilator discontinuance, as little as 10 to 15 minutes every 2 to 4 hours were initiated to encourage the use of respiratory muscles. Gradually, by the 54th ventilator day, he was able to tolerate short periods of ventilator discontinuance of 30 minutes to an hour twice a day on CPAP with minimal pressure support (10 to 15 cm H$_2$O). At this pressure support range, the patient was able to achieve an alveolar tidal volume of 300 to 400 ml. As muscle strength returned and gradually improved, less pressure support was necessary to maintain an adequate volume. The patient was allowed to rest completly at night on A/C mode and weaning was resumed each morning to CPAP with low level of pressure support.

By day 59, the patient progressed to 40 minutes to an hour of ventilator discontinuance every 2 hours during the day while resting at night. Each day brought the same monotonous routine but he continued to improve. On ventilator day 68 he was able to remain off the ventilator 24 hours per day. Real rehabilitation had just begun!

☑ The pressure support level is titrated and subsequently adjusted until spontaneous tidal volume = 10 to 15 ml/kg or spontaneous respiratory rate <25/min.

COMPLICATIONS

This patient encountered almost complete paralysis in the acute pathologic phase of his disease as he was only able to blink his eyes. He was under severe emotional and psychological stress throughout his hospitalization. He developed GI bleeding from a duodenal ulcer for which he was treated with Zantac via his feeding tube. Otitis media developed and was treated with broad spectrum antibiotics, and a persistent left lower lobe pneumonitis requiring bronchoscopy. Rehabilitation was begun and he was transferred out of the intensive care unit with humidified O$_2$ at an F$_I$O$_2$ of 30%. The tracheostomy was gradually buttoned. He required only 2 lpm of oxygen via nasal cannula while recovering in rehab. The patient was discharged after 154 days of hospital stay (last 94 days in extensive rehabilitation) on room air requiring only 25 mg of prednisone and follow-up physical therapy. He continued to progress and, eventually, demonstrated no residual effects from this debilitating illness.

CASE 12: BOTULISM

INTRODUCTION

J.D. was a 66-year-old, 50-kg female in her usual state of health until she consumed a partial jar of home-canned salsa. The following day she developed abdominal cramping thought to be the flu. Her intermittent cramping continued for 48 hours postingestion, then she deloped slurred speech and blurred vision. In addition to these symptoms, the patient experienced vertigo and diplopia at times and sought medical attention when diffuse upper motor weakness appeared. Her bulbar weakness and generalized fatigue necessitated admission for close observation in the ICU. *Clostridium botulism* was cultured from the salsa and also found to be present in the patient's stool. Community and state health officials were contacted for an antitoxin and subsequently this case was reported to the Centers for Disease Control and Prevention (CDCP) in Atlanta. Within 24 hours of admission the patient received trivalent botulism antitoxin but she encountered progressive deterioration with concomitant respiratory compromise.

INDICATIONS

On examination, the patient exhibited no evidence of distress. She did, however, manifest bilateral ptosis (drooping of eyelids) with decreased facial expression. Neck was supple, lungs were clear, and her mental status appeared normal. Pupillary light reflexes revealed sluggish reactions bilaterally. The tongue was midline with evidence of slurred speech. Motor examination revealed diffuse weakness of the upper extremities. Symmetrical fatigability of the biceps, deltoids, and grips were also noted. Gait revealed mild weakness, and electromyogram (EMG) studies showed decreased amplitude of repetitive nerve action potentials.

The patient was admitted for close observation. Vital capacities and maximum inspiratory pressure (MIP) were done Q2 hours. Her white blood cell count was 6,900 on admission and 12,500 (*normal 3.2 to 9.8 ×* 10^3) 48 hours later. Vital signs revealed blood pressure of 168/56 mm Hg, heart rate of 88/min, temperature of 36.4°C, and respirations of 24/min. Her initial arterial blood gases on room air revealed:

pH	7.43
$PaCO_2$	36 mm Hg
PaO_2	72 mm Hg
SaO_2	95%
HCO_3^-	24.5 mEq/L
RR	24/min
F_1O_2	21%

Her vital capacity at 03:30 was 1.6 liters (62% of predicted) with a MIP of –18 cm H_2O. By 08:00, the condition of the patient remained relatively unchanged except that her MIP had decreased to –12 cm H_2O. Due to progressive fatigue of respiratory muscles, she was nasally intubated at 10:00 with a 7.5 mm nasotracheal tube for mechanical ventilation.

In spite of normal $PaCO_2$, mechanical ventilation is indicated because of progressive muscle weakness (decreasing MIP) and anticipated outcome of botulism.

INITIAL SETTINGS

She was started on a Puritan-Bennett 7200a ventilator in assist/control (A/C) mode, backup rate of 12/min, tidal volume of 400 ml/PEEP of 5 cm H_2O, and F_IO_2 of 35%. ABGs drawn 30 minutes later revealed the following:

pH	7.54
$PaCO_2$	25 mm Hg
PaO_2	120 mm Hg
SaO_2	96%
HCO_3^-	21.1 mEq/L
Mode	A/C
Rate	12/min
Spont. Rate	22/min
V_T	400 ml
F_IO_2	35%
PEEP	5 cm H_2O

Based on these results, the rate was decreased to 8/min and the F_IO_2 was reduced to 30%. ABGs were ordered for the following morning. The results showed:

pH	7.42
$PaCO_2$	37 mm Hg
PaO_2	110 mm Hg
SaO_2	97%
HCO_3^-	23.6 mEq/L
Mode	A/C
Rate	8/min
Spont. Rate	12/min
V_T	400 ml
F_IO_2	30%
PEEP	5 cm H_2O

The patient remained febrile and weak as manifested by serial MIPs performed on the ventilator and on the fifth ventilator day, the patient underwent an elective tracheostomy for comfort and to prevent development of septic sinusitis from prolonged nasal intubation. She tolerated the procedure well.

PATIENT MONITORING

Her respiratory mechanics showed no signs of improvement initially but gradually improved over time. She was monitored for progressive muscle strength. Serial vital capacities and maximum inspiratory pressure (MIP) measurements while on CPAP every morning indicated gradual improvement. The serial measurements are are listed in Table 17-2. The patient continued to improve over the latter half of her hospitalization and after 14 days of mechanical ventilation, she exhibited evidence that she could support her own respiratory status without assistance.

PATIENT MANAGEMENT

☑ Management strategy for botulism consists mainly of supportive measures.

Management strategy for botulism consists mainly of supportive measures as she was mechanically ventilated for 14 days. Patient supportive measures included turning the patient from side to side, assisting the patient to an Ortho chair at the bedside, and using medications for comfort. Her nutritional status was maintained through I.V. fluids alone. The patient continued to improve and on the seventh ventilator day she was transferred to a subacute unit for further recovery and monitoring.

TABLE 17-2 Serial Vital Capacities and Maximum Inspiratory Pressure

VENT DAY	RESPIRATORY RATE (f)	FORCED VITAL CAPACITY (VC) L	MAXIMUM INSPIRATORY FORCE (MIP) cm H_2O
1	18	1.03	−30
2	22	1.30	−30
3	28	1.11	−33
4	32	1.13	−36
5	34	1.06	−35
6	30	1.45	−39
7	28	1.42	−36
8	28	1.21	−50
9	24	1.40	−38
10	20	1.80	−34
11	24	1.70	−38
12	24	1.60	−40
13	18	1.65	−43
14	18	2.10	−46

KEY MEDICATIONS

The patient's lungs remained diminished but clear throughout. There were no abnormal secretions when she was suctioned. However, vigorous pulmonary toilet was done to prevent lung pathology while in the step-down ICU. She was treated, prophylactically, on small volume nebulizer therapy with 0.5 ml of 0.5% albuterol in 2.0 ml of saline Q4 hours in-line with the ventilator circuit. These were discontinued after her removal from the ventilator.

WEANING

Beginning on the tenth day of mechanical ventilation, the patient began CPAP trials. She tolerated this procedure well for up to eight to ten hours at a time. She was then returned to SIMV mode with a backup rate of 6/min, tidal volume of 400ml, PEEP of 5 cm H_2O, F_IO_2 of 30%, and pressure support of 10 cm H_2O to rest for the night. Her respiratory rate remained in the mid to high 20s and her return volume was consistently between 350 ml to 450 ml. She did not complain of shortness of breath, difficulty breathing, or discomfort, and appeared to rest comfortably. By the twelfth day of continuous mechanical ventilation, the patient was able to tolerate CPAP of 5 cm H_2O and F_IO_2 of 30% 24hours/day. Her ABGs revealed the following:

pH	7.42
$PaCO_2$	46 mm Hg
PaO_2	91 mm Hg
SaO_2	96%
HCO_3^-	29.9 mEq/L
Mode	CPAP
Spont. Rate	28/min
F_IO_2	30%
PEEP	5 cm H_2O

At that point, she was removed from the ventilator and placed on a humidified T-piece (Briggs "T" adapter) at an F_IO_2 of 30%. She was monitored via a continuous pulse oximeter that revealed SpO_2 between 92% and 94%. Her respiratory rate remained in the low 20s. She was closely observed for signs of respiratory distress or tachypnea (>30/min). Three days later, ABGs again were obtained while on the T-piece at an F_IO_2 of 30%. These revealed:

pH	7.44
$PaCO_2$	45 mm Hg
PaO_2	87 mm Hg
SaO_2	96%
HCO_3^-	30.9 mEq/L
RR	24/min

On the fourteenth day, her tracheostomy was buttoned and she was placed on a nasal cannula at 2 lpm without complications.

COMPLICATIONS

The patient showed no serious and lasting complications from this episode of botulism and was discharged from the hospital on room air 21 days following her admission. She did exhibit some generalized weakness and mild ptosis that continued to improve after discharge.

CASE 13: MECONIUM ASPIRATION/ PATENT DUCTUS ARTERIOSUS

INTRODUCTION

L.F. was a 42-week (normal 40-week) gestation female Caucasian baby born to a 24-year-old gravida III mother. The birthweight was 3,054-gm (6.7 lb). All previous births were normal. The mother experienced spotting and early labor at four months, but the labor was halted at that time with terbutaline.

Shortly before delivery, the amniotic membrane ruptured and thick meconium was noted in the amniotic fluid. Upon delivery, the infant initiated her first breath and cried before visualization of the cords and suctioning could be performed. Immediately thereafter, the respiratory therapist visualized the cords and found meconium staining present at and below the vocal cords. Suctioning was performed immediately to remove as much meconium as possible.

The Apgar scores were 7 and 8 at one and five minutes, respectively. They were scored as shown below.

☑ Long gestational age has a higher incidence of meconium aspiration syndrome.

☑ Visualization of the vocal cords helps to determine if meconium is present in the upper airway. If the vocal cords are stained green, suction should be done prior to the first breath so as to prevent or minimize meconium aspiration.

	0	1	2	1 min	5 min
Heart rate	None	Slow Irregular	Over 100	2	2
Respiratory effort	Apnea	Irregular shallow Gasping	Yelling, crying	1	1
Muscle tone	Flaccid	Some flexion of extremities	Well flexed	2	2
Reflex	No response to stimulus	Grimace	Crying	2	2
Color	Pale blue	Blue extremities Body pink	Pink all over	0	1
Total				7	8

INDICATIONS

After stabilization at the delivery room, the infant female was admitted to the regular nursery with blow-by oxygen. Within a few hours of arrival, she became dusky and presented with moderate to severe intercostal and substernal retractions. As her condition continued to deteriorate, she was transferred to the NICU for further evaluation and treatment. Umbilical artery catheter (UAC) and orogastric (OG) tube were placed and mask CPAP on an F_IO_2 of 100% was initiated. Phenobarbital was begun to improve oxygenation. UAC blood gas results were:

☑ **Phenobarbital is used to reduce seizure activity and facilitate ventilation and oxygenation.**

pH	7.32
PaCO$_2$	40 mm Hg
PaO$_2$	43 mm Hg
HCO$_3^-$	20 mEq/L
B.E.	–6 mEq/L
Hct	41%
Mode	Mask CPAP
F$_I$O$_2$	100%

☑ **Increased capillary refill indicates shunting of blood flow from the extremities or increased peripheral vascular resistance.**

In spite of CPAP and 100% oxygen, the infant's oxygenation status continued to deteriorate. Her respiratory rate increased as she tried to compensate for the hypoxia. Capillary refill time was increased from 4 to 5 seconds. Her extremities were cold and the mean arterial pressure was 35 mm Hg.

Based on the condition and prognosis of this infant, she was electively intubated with a 3.5 mm endotracheal (ET) tube and placed on a pressure-limited ventilator. During the initial hours of mechanical ventilation, large amounts of bright red secretions were suctioned from the ET tube.

INITIAL SETTINGS

The initial settings of the pressure-limited ventilator were: A/C, rate 60/min., PIP/PEEP 28/5 cm H$_2$O, T$_{INSP}$ 0.5 sec, F$_I$O$_2$ 100%. At these settings, the mean airway pressure was 14.5 cm H$_2$O and blood gases from a UAC sample showed:

☑ **PIP of 28 cmH$_2$O should be increased to enhance alveolar recruitment and oxygenation.**

pH	7.30
PaCO$_2$	44 mm Hg
PaO$_2$	39 mm Hg
HCO$_3^-$	21.2 mEq/L
B.E.	–5.9 mEq/L
Mode	A/C
PIP/PEEP	28/5 cm H$_2$O
Rate	60/min
T$_{INSP}$	0.5 sec
F$_I$O$_2$	100%
Mean Airway Pressure	14.5 cm H$_2$O

☑ Since the initial rate is 60/min (or 1/sec), the T_{EXP} is $1 - T_{INSP} = 1 - 0.5$ sec = 0.5 sec. The I:E ratio is 1:1.

☑ The rate should be reduced to allow more time for expiration.

☑ The increase in PIP and PEEP causes a higher mean airway pressure (from 14.5 to 16.5 cm H_2O). This may (1) lower the production of natural surfactant, (2) cause patent ductus arteriosus, and (3) increase the risk of barotrauma.

The PIP/PEEP were changed to 32/6 cm H_2O and the rate was changed to 50/min. At these settings, blood gases and transcutaneous gas tension showed:

pH	7.43
$PaCO_2$	32 mm Hg
PaO_2	43 mm Hg
HCO_3^-	21.1 mEq/L
B.E.	–2.7 mEq/L
SpO_2	86%
$P_{tc}O_2$	28 mm Hg
$P_{tc}CO_2$	30 mm Hg
Mode	A/C
PIP/PEEP	32/6 cm H_2O
Rate	50/min
T_{INSP}	0.5 sec
F_IO_2	100%
Mean Airway Pressure	16.5 cm H_2O

An echocardiogram was performed at this time that showed a patent ductus arteriosus (PDA) with a right-to-left shunt and evidence of persistent pulmonary hypertension of the newborn. The patient was started on dopamine and dobutamine.

Ninety minutes after dopamine and dobutamine administration, the blood gases showed:

pH	7.58
$PaCO_2$	27 mm Hg
PaO_2	66 mm Hg
HCO_3^-	24.9 mEq/L
B.E.	3.1 mEq/L
SpO_2	96%
$P_{tc}O_2$	53 mm Hg
$P_{tc}CO_2$	28 mm Hg
Mode	A/C
PIP/PEEP	38/6 cm H_2O
Rate	60/min
T_{INSP}	0.3 sec
F_IO_2	100%
Mean Airway Pressure	16.5 cm H_2O

Over the course of the next 12 hours, three doses of artificial surfactant were needed. The following results were obtained after the third dose:

pH	7.37
$PaCO_2$	42 mm Hg

✓ The PDA has partially closed allowing a decrease of the right to left shunt. This lowers the peak inspiratory pressure and improves gas exchange. The risk of barotrauma is therefore lowered.

✓ The administration of surfactant helps to increase the pulmonary compliance and to lower the peak inspiratory pressure, F_IO_2, and mean airway pressure requirements.

✓ An important aspect of weaning in this case is to maintain the PaO_2 at a safe level (50s mm Hg) so as to prevent increase of PVR and reopening of PDA.

PaO_2	56 mm Hg
HCO_3^-	24.2 mEq/L
B.E.	–0.9 mEq/L
SpO_2	90%
$P_{tc}O_2$	47 mm Hg
$P_{tc}CO_2$	66 mm Hg
Mode	A/C
PIP/PEEP	25/6 cm H_2O
Rate	36/min
T_{INSP}	0.4 sec
F_IO_2	51%
Mean Airway Pressure	12 cm H_2O

Over the next two days the ventilator was weaned by gradually decreasing the PIP, PEEP, rate, and F_IO_2. The patient continued to improve and was finally extubated to an oxyhood at 36% F_IO_2.

KEY MEDICATIONS

Medication	Main Purpose
Decadron	Improves lung function in infants requiring prolonged ventilation. It also decreases tracheal edema to facilitate extubation.
Dopamine	Improves cardiac output and blood pressure.
Dobutamine	Decreases pulmonary vascular resistance.
Phenobarbital	May have some value in preventing intraventricular hemorrhage (IVH). Aids in sedation to improve mechanical ventilation. Limits seizure activity.
Albumin	Used for volume expansion when treating RDS. Shock may be seen after correction of acidosis or hypoxia (due to ↓ systemic vascular resistance and ↓ blood pressure).
Ampicillin	Broad spectrum antibiotic.
Surfactant	Prevention and treatment of RDS by increasing the lung compliance and decreasing the alveolar surface tension.

SPECIAL CONSIDERATIONS

Meconium aspiration is most likely to occur in term or postterm infants who have intrauterine distress or hypoxia. When meconium is seen in the amniotic fluid, vigorous suctioning of the oral cavity and upper airway should be done, preferably before the first breath. This is done to prevent aspiration of meconium and airway obstruction by these particles.

An infant diagnosed with meconium aspiration runs a high risk of barotrauma when mechanical ventilation is instituted. Ongoing assessment of the chest is of vital importance. Monitoring the MAWP is the best indicator of impending barotraumatic events. It is important to keep the MAWP as low as possible.

With the presence of PDA revealed by the echocardiogram, an adequate PaO_2 should be provided and maintained in an attempt to minimize an increase of the pulmonary vascular resistance (PVR). Surely we will try to reduce the F_IO_2 requirement, but this must be done slowly to prevent the PVR from increasing.

☑ Excessive PaO_2 may cause oxygen toxicity and related problems.

☑ Insufficient PaO_2 may cause hypoxemia and an increase of the PVR.

CASE 14: PERSISTENT PULMONARY HYPERTENSION OF THE NEWBORN

INTRODUCTION

B.G. was a 30-week gestation, 1,398-gm male infant born without prenatal care. The one- and three-minute Apgar scores were 5 and 6, respectively.

Inspite of an Apgar score of 6 at three minutes, the cardiopulmonary status of the infant continued to deteriorate and cardiopulmonary resuscitation (CPR) became necessary. CPR was started using 100% oxygen via a resuscitation bag with pressure manometer attached. The infant was subsequently intubated with a 3.0 mm endotracheal tube and placed on a pressure-limited ventilator without complications.

An umbilical artery catheter (UAC) was inserted and secured. After a period of stabilization on the ventilator, the infant still appeared dusky. His capillary refill was slow indicating poor peripheral perfusion but the extremities were warm. The anterior fontanel was soft with slightly overlapping sutures. Breath sounds were diminished bilaterally.

Arterial blood was drawn from the UAC while using a resuscitation bag and 100% oxygen with pressures of 28/4 mm Hg at a rate of 40/min. The results were:

☑ The three-minute Apgar score should show significant improvement over the one-minute score.

☑ Peripheral perfusion status is a gross indicator of cardiac output or tissue perfusion.

☑ The blood gases show oxygenation failure because the PaO_2 is much lower than one that can be caused by a $PaCO_2$ of 48 mm Hg.

UAC Sample
pH   7.26
$PaCO_2$ 48 mm Hg

PaO$_2$ 22 mm Hg
HCO$_3^-$ 21.6 mEq/L
B.E.   −7.2 mEq/L
Mode   Bag/mask ventilation
F$_I$O$_2$ 100%
P$_{INSP}$ 28 mm Hg
PEEP   4 mm Hg
Rate   40/min

✓ If hyperventilation (to pH 7.5 and PaCO$_2$ between 20 and 25 mm Hg) provides significant improvement to the PaO$_2$, PPHN is likely the cause of hypoxemia.

✓ PaO$_2$ shows significant improvement (from 22 to 95 mm Hg) after 3 minutes of hyperventilation.

✓ Hyperventilation reduces the PaCO$_2$. In turn, it lowers the pulmonary vascular resistance and improves the pulmonary circulation and V/Q matching.

✓ Since the patient's condition is responsive to hyperventilation, pulmonary hypertension is likely the cause of hypoxemia. He is a candidate for trial of NO therapy.

While using the resuscitation bag/mask system, it was decided to hyperventilate the infant at a rate of 100/min. with pressures of 28/4 mm Hg on 100% oxygen. This was done to rule out the presence of persistent pulmonary hypertension of the newborn (PPHN). The blood gases after three minutes of hyperventilation showed:

UAC Sample
pH   7.48
PaCO$_2$ 23 mm Hg
PaO$_2$ 95 mm Hg
Mode   Bag/mask ventilation
F$_I$O$_2$ 100%
P$_{INSP}$ 28 mm Hg
PEEP   4 mm Hg
Rate   100/min

Based on the information obtained from the last blood gases, it was decided to continue hyperventilation using conventional ventilation. After 24 hours, the following results were obtained.

UAC Sample
pH   7.46
PaCO$_2$ 26 mm Hg
PaO$_2$ 89 mm Hg
Mode   A/C
PIP/PEEP   32/6 cm H$_2$O
Rate   100/min
T$_{INSP}$ 0.24 sec
F$_I$O$_2$ 98%

During this 24-hour period, unsuccessful attempts were made to decrease the oxygen requirement. Very little progress was seen in the patient as the pulmonary hypertension was not resolved using the hyperventilation strategy. Nitric oxide (NO) therapy was started in hope of reversing the pulmonary hypertension.

The patient received 55 ppm (parts per million) of NO, and the blood gases after one hour of NO therapy showed:

☑ The PaO_2 improved from 89 to 105 mm Hg at a lower F_IO_2 (from 98 to 85%).

UAC Sample
pH	7.50
$PaCO_2$	21 mm Hg
PaO_2	105 mm Hg
Mode	A/C
PIP/PEEP	32/6 cm H_2O
Rate	100/min
T_{INSP}	0.24 sec
F_IO_2	85%

The infant's F_IO_2 requirement continued to decrease over the next 48 hours. NO therapy was discontinued and the F_IO_2 was weaned to 45%. Conventional ventilation continued at a rate of 55/min.

PATIENT MANAGEMENT

The pulmonary vascular resistance of the infant was increased due to severe hypoxemia and hypoxic vasoconstriction. Since hypoxemia could not be reversed with oxygen and ventilation, long-standing hypoxemia caused a persistent increase in PVR, thus the name persistent pulmonary hypertension of the newborn (PPHN).

Test to Rule Out PPHN. Persistent pulmonary hypertension of the newborn can be tested by hyperventilating the patient to an arterial pH of 7.5 and a $PaCO_2$ of between 20 and 25 mm Hg. The alkalotic condition reduces the pulmonary vascular resistance, thereby enhancing pulmonary perfusion and oxygen content. If PPHN is the cause of hypoxemia, the patient's oxygenation should show drastic improvement following hyperventilation.

Nitric Oxide to Treat PPHN. Nitric oxide therapy is done to lower pulmonary vascular resistance. The walls of the pulmonary arteries are lined with endothelial cells that release a substance known as endothelium-derived relaxing factor (EDRF, which has been identified as nitric oxide). This substance is responsible for vasodilation in vascular smooth muscle. EDRF has been found to be an essential link in the transition from fetal to neonatal circulation. Because NO dilates the pulmonary arteries, it decreases the pulmonary vascular resistance and its associated hypertension. Once the pulmonary vessels are dilated, this change should improve the patient's pulmonary circulation, V/Q ratio, and oxygenation status.

CASE 15: HOME CARE AND DISEASE MANAGEMENT

INTRODUCTION

F.W. was a 66-year-old moderately obese (weight 240 lbs.) white female. She was brought to the emergency department by her husband and their 17-year-old daughter on a Saturday morning because they "couldn't keep her awake and her breathing sounded funny." Upon further questioning, the doctor was told by the patient's husband that she had no fever, but did have a productive cough with thick greenish sputum for the past five days. The patient had a history of COPD/asthma, cor pulmonale, hypoatremia, and hyperkalemia. She had no chest pain, except when coughing, but did have difficulty breathing when lying down (orthopnea). F.W.'s husband reported that she had no nausea and vomiting, and had not complained of pain other than when coughing.

Social history revealed that F.W. smoked one pack of cigarettes per day for 25 years, but quit 10 years ago. She did not drink alcohol. She lived with her spouse of 25 years and a 17-year-old daughter. Two other grown children from a previous marriage no longer lived at home.

> ☑ At the onset or worsening of dyspnea due to congestive heart failure or pulmonary congestion, breathing in an upright position reduces pulmonary congestion and work of breathing.

INDICATION

Physical assessment revealed an obese white female, lethargic, with central cyanosis and in respiratory distress. From the information provided by her husband, the physician determined that the patient had experienced paroxysmal nocturnal dyspnea in addition to orthopnea. She was placed on a monitor that revealed these vital signs: blood pressure of 160/80 mm Hg, heart rate of 128/min, respiratory rate of 28/min and labored, and SpO₂ of 85% on room air.

Further assessment showed 1 to 2+ pedal edema, jugular vein distension, bibasilar crackles and wheezes throughout.

Arterial blood gases on rom air revealed:

> ☑ Paroxysmal nocturnal dyspnea and orthopnea are signs of congestive heart failure.

pH	7.26
$PaCO_2$	88 mm Hg
PaO_2	38 mm Hg
HCO_3^-	38 mEq/L
SaO_2	80%

Pertinent lab work results were as follows:

WBC: 7400 (*normal 3.2 to 9.8 × 10³*)
H&H: 16/49.3 (*normal for women: hemoglobin 12 to 16 g/100ml hematocrit 37 to 47%*)
Na+: 119 (*normal 140 mEq/L*)

> ☑ Blood gases show acute ventilatory failure superimposed on chronic ventilatory failure. Noninvasive positive pressure ventilation is indicated for this patient.

✓ IPAP provides mechanical ventilation and reduces the patient's work of breathing.

INITIAL SETTINGS

The patient was stabilized in the emergency department prior to transfer to the telemetry unit. For her severe hypercapnia and hypoxemia, she was placed on nasal bilevel PAP at 12/6 cm H_2O with 5 LPM of oxygen. IPAP of 12 cm H_2O was used to augment the patient's ventilatory effort. EPAP of 6 cm H_2O and 5 lpm of oxygen were used to maintain oxygenation and minimize auto-PEEP due to air trapping.

PATIENT MANAGEMENT

For ther excessive fluid buildup due to cor pulmonale, 60 mg of Lasix were given via an intravenous line. Blood was drawn for lab workup. Chest radiograph and repeat ABG on bilevel PAP were done. Lab reports showed normal WBC, hemoglobin, and hematocrit, and low sodium, which could explain some of her confusion. Chest radiograph showed enlarged heart (cardiomegaly) with pulmonary vascular congestion and bilateral infiltrates especially on the left side. (See Figure 17-7.)

✓ IPAP of 12 cm H_2O is primarily responsible for the improvement of ventilation ($PaCO_2$ from 88 mmHg to 68 mmHg).

Repeat ABG two hours after initiation of bilevel PAP showed:

pH	7.34
$PaCO_2$	68 mm Hg
PaO_2	82 mm Hg
HCO_3^-	36 mEq/L
SaO_2	96%
Bilevel PAP	12/6 cm H_2O
F_IO_2	5 lpm

✓ EPAP of 6 cm H_2O and 5 LPM of oxygen is primarily responsible for the improvement of oxygenation (PaO_2 from 38 mmHg to 82 mmHg).

HOSPITAL COURSE

During the first two days of her hospital stay, F.W. was maintained on continuous nasal bilevel PAP at 12/6 cm H_2O with 2 lpm of oxygen. For the CHF and related conditions, she was treated with Lasix, Digoxin, and Cardizem. The pulmonologist ordered nebulizer treatments Q 4 hours with 2.5 mg albuterol and 0.5 mg ipratropium bromide in 3 cc of normal saline to relieve bronchospasm and promote secretion clearance. Prednisone (steroid) was ordered to decrease airway inflammation secondary to her asthma. Prophylactic antibiotics (Biaxin) were administered, used to address her probable pneumonia since sputum induction was unsuccessful.

Note: F.W.'s medical record retrieved shortly after admission indicated that PFTs had been done one year before and at that time her FEV_1 was 14% of predicted and her DLCO was 21%. Baseline room air blood gases were:

pH	7.37
$PaCO_2$	67 mm Hg

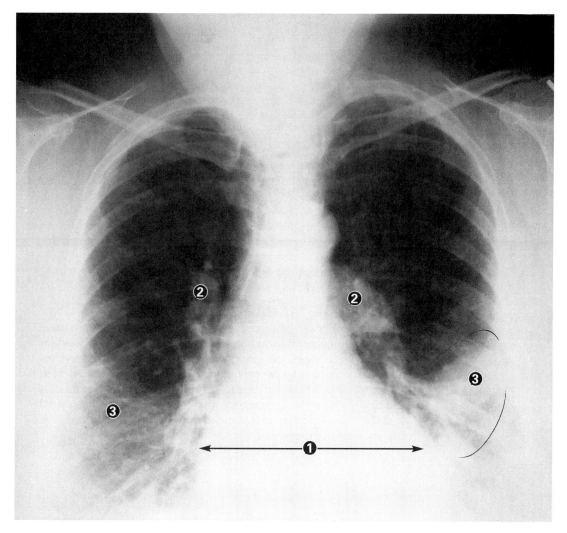

Figure 17-7 Chest radiograph shows cardiomegaly (1), pulmonary vascular congestion (2), and bilateral infiltrates (3).

PaO$_2$ 45 mm Hg
HCO$_3^-$ 38 mEq/L

✓ CPAP alone increases the work of breathing. Patient requires some mechanical assistance via bilevel PAP (i.e., IPAP)

On the third day following admission, the pulmonologist attempted to wean F.W. from bilevel PAP. She was placed on CPAP at 7.5 cm H$_2$O and ABGs were drawn an hour later; the results were as follows:

pH	7.16
PaCO$_2$	91 mm Hg
PaO$_2$	66 mm Hg
HCO$_3^-$	31 mEq/L
SaO$_2$	90%

As a result of her deteriorating blood gas results and clinical condition, F.W. was placed back on bilevel PAP at 12/6 cm H$_2$O for 24 hours. Over the next several days, she was gradually weaned to 1 lpm nasal cannula during the day and bilevel PAP at night. The physician discussed several options with F.W. and her family, and it was decided that upon discharge from the hospital she would use nocturnal ventilation at home. Her total hospital stay was 11 days.

HOME CARE MANAGEMENT

Twenty-four hours prior to discharge from the hospital, the case manager contacted a local home medical equipment provided for respiratory services and a home care agency for nursing services. Among other health care professionals, this case was reviewed with the respiratory therapist. Due to the complexity of her pulmonary condition and special management requirements, the physician decided to directly communicate with the respiratory therapist from the medical equipment company.

Arterial blood gases on day of discharge were as follows:

pH	7.32
PaCO$_2$	60 mm Hg
PaO$_2$	62 mm Hg
HCO$_3^-$	30 mEq/L
SaO$_2$	93%
Bilevel PAP	12/6 cm H$_2$O
Oxygen	1 lpm via nasal cannula during the day and bilevel PAP therapy at 12/6 cm

H$_2$O, F$_I$O$_2$ of 24% at night

ORDERS FOR HOME	EQUIPMENT
1. 1 lpm via nasal cannula continuously.	Oxygen concentrator
2. Portable oxygen	Conserving device with M-6 cylinders
3. Nebulizer treatments QID	Small air compressor
4. Nocturnal bilevel PAP 10/5 cm H_2O, 24%	NPPV with back-up rate of 6/min
5. Keep head of bed elevated 30 degrees	Hospital bed
6. 1200 calorie diet	
7. Ambulate as tolerated	
8. Incentive spirometry TID	Incentive spirometer (from hospital)

KEY MEDICATIONS

1. 2.5 mg albuterol and 0.5 mg atrovent in 3.0 ml of 0.9% NaCl QID and PRN for wheezing.
2. Lasix 20mg po BID
3. Prednisone po tapering dose
4. Cardizem po

HOME CARE PLAN

The plan was devised by the physician and respiratory therapist. The patient was informed of the home care plan, as follows:

1. Maintain SpO2 of 90% to 96%
2. Maintain tidal volume of 650 ml to 900 ml while on NPPV.
3. Use back-up rate of 6/min to ensure adequate ventilation if patient were to become apneic.
4. Closely monitor patient for signs of CHF, hypercapnia, and exacerbation of asthma/COPD.
5. Notify physician of complications secondary to withdrawal or tapering of medications; specifically Prednisone and Lasix.
6. Increase exercise level as tolerated.
7. Improve diet and continue to lose weight. (F. W.'s height and weight: 5 feet 2 inches and 235 lbs.)
8. Educate patient on disease and promote a healthier lifestyle (F.W. had already quit smoking 10 years ago).
9. Observe patient's attitude and family support and report to physician.

PATIENT MONITORING

F.W. required close monitoring for the first month. The same respiratory therapist visited her twice a week for the first four weeks and then once a week for the next four weeks. Routine monthly visits started in the third month. *NOTE:* Nursing services were present in the home once a day for two weeks, and communication was established between the nurse (from a home care agency) and the respiratory therapist (from a DME company). During each visit, patient assessment was done and respiratory equipment was checked by the therapist.

Parameters monitored were as follows:

1. Tidal volume delivered via NPPV.
2. Vital signs (BP, HR, RR, SpO_2, weight & breath sounds)
3. Bedside spirometry (PEFR, FVC, FEV_1) on initial visit, then every 6 months and prn.
4. Pedal edema (present or not)
5. Exercise tolerance—using vital signs and subjective response as indicators.
6. Saturation on room air—at rest and with exertion (walking with distance recorded)
7. Saturation on oxygen—at rest and with exertion (walking with distance recorded)
8. Sputum production—amount, color, and consistency.
9. Subjective response from patient and family members.
10. Patient compliance

NOTE: In order to have a successful outcome with home care, solid family support and proper emotional well-being of the patient are crucial. Motivation and positive attitude on the part of the patient are essential in order to achieve a positive outcome. Any signs of patient noncompliance, lack of family support, depression, lack of necessary resources, or other emotional problems should be promptly reported to the physician so that these issues may be addressed. If a home care nurse is also seeing the patient, then all information should be shared so that the patient may receive the best quality care.

PATIENT WEEKLY PROGRESS

Week 1. F.W. stayed in bed most of the time and got up only to go to the bathroom. Nocturnal bi-level ventilation was done at 10/5 cm H_2O with 1 lpm titrated through the nasal mask. Other parameters on the ventilator were: back-up rate 6/min, expired tidal volume between 535 ml and 700 ml. Nebulizer treatments were done QID and incentive spirometry was done TID. Patient was able to achieve 800 to 1000 ml on the incentive spirometry. Patient appeared to be compliant with her medications. Her weight was 235 lbs with no signs of pedal edema. Vital signs were BP 150/84 mmHg, RR 24/min, HR 82/min, resting SpO_2 91% on 1 lpm and 88% on room air.

Patient had a positive attitude and excellent family support. She was excited about getting better and used the nocturnal ventilator 6 to 8 hours every night. She claimed that she was still very tired and sore from her hospital stay.

Week 2. F.W. had improved a great deal. She was walking to the kitchen and watching television in the living room. She remained on 10/5 cm H_2O with 1 lpm O_2 at night and 1 lpm per nasal cannula continuously during the day. Vital signs were: BP 130/68 mmHg, RR 16/min, HR 84/min, SpO_2 94% on 1 lpm resting and 89% to 90% on room air. Her weight was 218 lb. No pedal edema noted.

F.W. was in good spirits and compliant with regime.

Week 3. The expired tidal volume was 800 ml to 1000 ml on 10/5 cm H_2O. This indicated an improvement of pulmonary mechanics. She also was able to reach 1600 ml on her incentive spirometer TID. Her weight was down to 208 lb and she was ambulating more every week. No pedal edema noted.

Vital signs were BP 128/68 mmHg, RR 18/min, HR 70/min, SpO_2 97% on 1 lpm and 93% resting on room air. Ambulating SpO_2 was 88% on room air after walking just 25 feet, indicating that she continued to desaturate upon mild exertion.

Auscultation revealed bilateral expiratory wheezes. Small amounts of brownish sputum was noted. Bedside spirometry showed: PEFR 88 lpm, VC 1.69L, FEV_1 0.709L. F.W. continued to improve and remained positive about improving the quality of her life.

Week 4. One month out of the hospital and F.W. remained stable. At this time she was able to go grocery shopping and have her hair done. She used her portable M-6 cylinders with a conserving device while she was out. According to both the patient and her spouse, her sleep had increased to 8 to 10 hours per night and she no longer took naps during the day. A decision was made to decrease her nocturnal ventilator pressures to 8/5 due to the increasing expired volumes (1,100 ml). On bilevel PAP 8/5 cm H_2O, F.W. was more comfortable and had volumes of 650 to 850 ml.

NOTE: Tidal volumes were obtained with patient in supine position and were monitored for 20 minutes. This allowed the patient to relax in order to obtain more accurate readings).

Vitals and physical signs: BP 100/50 mmHg, RR 20/min, HR 78/min, weight 211 lb, SpO_2 94% on 1 lpm. No pedal edema was noted. After ambulating 60 steps: HR 100, RR28, SpO_2 86%. SpO_2 recovering within 3 minutes upon administration of 1 lpm O_2.

COMPLICATIONS

F.W. remained stable with no significant complications other than sinusitis for 6 months. During a routine visit almost 7 months after discharge, the therapist notified the physician with this assessment:

Vitals: BP 165/85 mmHg, RR 22/min, HR 80/min, weight 224 lb., SpO_2 91% on 1 lpm, 1 to 2+ pedal edema.

Auscultation: inspiratory and expiratory wheezes bilaterally (audible); diminished in bases bilaterally.
Tidal volume on bilevel PAP of 8/5 cm H_2O = 500 to 600 ml.

Patient's husband reported that she was not sleeping well at night and with her legs "jittering" during the night. He also stated that F.W. was falling asleep during her meals and she frequently complained of headaches.

The respiratory therapist increased the nocturnal ventilator pressures to 10/5 cm H_2O (expired volume of 800 to 1000 ml) and notified the physician promptly. An appointment was made to see the physician on the following day. As a result of the office visit, the Lasix dosage was increased. She no longer experienced the signs and symptoms that were present prior to the visit, thus avoiding a possible hospital admission.

DISCUSSION

This case demonstrates one of the clinical indications for the use of nocturnal ventilation. F.W. was a COPD patient with hypercapnia and cor pulmonale. Is it also possible that F.W. suffered from a sleep disorder? Maybe; however, no sleep studies were ever done. F.W. qualified for nocturnal ventilation based on her $PaCO_2$ levels at the time of discharge from the hospital. Her pulmonary function studies indicated severe obstructive disease and poor diffusion capacity. Because of her obesity, F.W. also dealt with hypoventilation. The nocturnal ventilator assisted to overcome pressure placed on the diaphragm by her large abdomen, thereby increasing volumes when F.W. was in supine position.

Without nocturnal ventilation, home oxygen, bronchodilator therapies via nebulizer, and oral medications, F.W. would probably have had numerous physician visits and even hospital stays. In fact, she has avoided E.R. visits and hospital admissions for over one year. The home therapy allowed her greater independence and helped her "feel better;" therefore improving her quality of life. It is the responsibility of every home care provider to adequately assess patients, make sound clinical decisions, and report findings to the physician in a timely manner.

In this case the RCP quickly responded to signs and symptoms of hypercapnia and impending cardiac insufficiency. The pressure on the nocturnal ventilator was increased to improve minute ventilation and oxygenation and the physician was consulted to increase Lasix to eliminate pulmonary vascular congestion due to heart failure.

APPENDICES

APPENDIX 1: RESPIRATORY CARE CALCULATIONS

A AIRWAY RESISTANCE: ESTIMATED (R_{aw})

EQUATION

$$R_{aw} = \frac{(P_{max} - P_{st})}{Flow}$$

R_{aw} : Airway resistance in cm H_2O/L/sec.
P_{max} : Maximum airway pressure in cm H_2O (peak airway pressure).
P_{st} : Static airway pressure in cm H_2O (plateau airway pressure).
Flow : Flow rate in L/sec.

NORMAL VALUE

0.6 to 2.4 cm H_2O/L/sec at flow rate of 0.5 L/sec (30 L/min).
If the patient is intubated, use serial measurements to establish trend.

EXAMPLE

Calculate the estimated airway resistance of a patient whose peak airway pressure is 25 cm H_2O and whose plateau pressure is 10 cm H_2O. The ventilator flow rate is set at 60 L/min (1 L/sec).

$$R_{aw} = \frac{(P_{max} - P_{st})}{Flow}$$

$$= \frac{(25 - 10)}{1}$$

$$= \frac{15}{1}$$

$$= 15 \text{ cm } H_2O/L/sec$$

B ALVEOLAR–ARTERIAL OXYGEN TENSION GRADIENT: $P(A - a)O_2$

EQUATION

$$P(A - a)O_2 = P_AO_2 - P_aO_2$$

$P(A - a)O_2$: Alveolar–arterial oxygen tension gradient in mm Hg.
P_AO_2 : Alveolar oxygen tension in mm Hg.
P_aO_2 : Arterial oxygen tension in mm Hg.

NORMAL VALUE

(1) On *room air*, the $P(A - a)O_2$ should be less than 4 mm Hg for every 10 years in age. For example, the $P(A - a)O_2$ should be less than 24 mm Hg for a 60-year-old patient.
(2) On *100% oxygen*, every 50 mm Hg difference in $P(A - a)O_2$ approximates 2% shunt.

EXAMPLE 1

Given: $P_AO_2 = 100$ mm Hg
$\qquad P_aO_2 = 85$ mm Hg
$\qquad F_IO_2 = 21\%$
Patient age = 40 years
Calculate $P(A - a)O_2$. Is it normal or abnormal for this patient?
$$P(A - a)O_2 = P_AO_2 - P_aO_2$$
$$= (100 - 85) \text{ mm Hg}$$
$$= 15 \text{ mm Hg}$$
$P(A - a)O_2$ of 15 mm Hg is normal for a 40-year-old patient.

P_AO_2 AT SELECTED F_IO_2

F_IO_2*	CALCULATED PAO$_2$**
21%	100
25%	128
30%	164
35%	200
40%	235
45%	271
50%	307
55%	342
60%	388
65%	423
70%	459
75%	495
80%	530
85%	566
90%	602
95%	637
100%	673

*At F_IO_2 of 60% or higher, the factor 1.25 in the equation below is omitted.
**The calculated PAO_2 is based on a PCO_2 of 40 mm Hg, saturated at 37°C, P_B of 760 mm Hg. $PAO_2 = (P_B - 47) \times F_IO_2 - (PCO_2 \times 1.25)$.

C   ANION GAP

EQUATION

Anion gap = Na+ − (Cl⁻ + HCO₃⁻)

Na+ : Serum sodium concentration in mEq/L.
Cl⁻ : Serum chloride concentration in mEq/L.
HCO₃⁻ : Serum bicarbonate concentration in mEq/L.

NORMAL VALUE

10 to 14 mEq/L
15 to 20 mEq/L if potassium (K+) is included in the equation

EXAMPLE

Given: Na+ = 140 mEq/L
       Cl⁻ = 105 mEq/L
   HCO₃⁻ = 22 mEq/L
Calculate the anion gap.
Anion gap = Na+ − (Cl⁻ + HCO₃⁻)
           = 140 − (105 + 22)
           = 140 − 127
           = 13 mEq/L

D   COMPLIANCE: DYNAMIC (C_{dyn})

EQUATION

$$C_{dyn} = \frac{\Delta V}{\Delta P}$$

C_{dyn} : Dynamic compliance in mL/cm H_2O
ΔV : Corrected tidal volume in mL
ΔP : Pressure change (Peak airway pressure − PEEP) in cm H_2O

NORMAL VALUE

30 to 40 mL/cm H_2O
If the patient is intubated, use serial measurements to establish trend.

EXAMPLE

Given: ΔV = 500 mL
Peak airway pressure = 30 cm H_2O
PEEP = 10 cm H_2O
Calculate the dynamic compliance.

$$C_{dyn} = \frac{\Delta V}{\Delta P}$$

$$= \frac{500}{30 - 10}$$

$$= \frac{500}{20}$$

$$= 25 \text{ mL/cm H}_2\text{O}$$

E   COMPLIANCE: STATIC (C_{st})

EQUATION

$$C_{st} = \frac{\Delta V}{\Delta P}$$

C_{st} : Static compliance in mL/cm H_2O
ΔV : Corrected tidal volume in mL
ΔP : Pressure change (Plateau pressure − PEEP) in cm H_2O

NORMAL VALUE

40 to 60 mL/cm H_2O
If the patient is intubated, use serial measurements to establish trend.

EXAMPLE

Given: ΔV = 500 mL
Plateau pressure = 20 cm H_2O
PEEP = 5 cm H_2O
Calculate the static compliance.

$$C_{st} = \frac{\Delta V}{\Delta P}$$

$$= \frac{500}{20 - 5}$$

$$= \frac{500}{15}$$

$$= 33.3 \text{ or } 33 \text{ mL/cm H}_2\text{O}$$

F   CORRECTED TIDAL VOLUME (V_T)

EQUATION

Corrected V_T = Expired V_T − Tubing Volume

Expired V_T : Expired tidal volume in mL
Tubing volume : Volume "lost" in tubing during inspiratory phase
(Pressure change × 3 mL/cm H_2O)

EXAMPLE

$$\text{Expired } V_T = 650 \text{ mL}$$
$$\text{Peak airway pressure} = 25 \text{ cm H}_2\text{O}$$
$$\text{Positive end-expiratory pressure (PEEP)} = 5 \text{ cm H}_2\text{O}$$
$$\text{Tubing compression factor} = 3 \text{ mL/cm H}_2\text{O}$$

Calculate the corrected tidal volume.

Because

$$
\begin{aligned}
\text{Tubing volume} &= \text{Pressure change} \times 3 \text{ mL/cm H}_2\text{O} \\
&= (25 - 5) \text{ cm H}_2\text{O} \times 3 \text{ mL/cm H}_2\text{O} \\
&= 20 \times 3 \text{ mL} \\
&= 60 \text{ mL}
\end{aligned}
$$

then

$$
\begin{aligned}
\text{Corrected } V_T &= \text{Expired } V_T - \text{Tubing volume} \\
&= 650 - 60 \\
&= 590 \text{ mL}
\end{aligned}
$$

G DEADSPACE TO TIDAL VOLUME RATIO (V_D/V_T)

EQUATION

$$\frac{V_D}{V_T} = \frac{(P_a CO_2 - P_{\bar{E}} CO_2)}{P_a CO_2}$$

$\dfrac{V_D}{V_T}$: Deadspace to tidal volume ratio in %

$P_a CO_2$: Arterial carbon dioxide tension in mm Hg

$P_{\bar{E}} CO_2$: Mixed expired carbon dioxide tension in mm Hg

NORMAL VALUE

20 to 40% in patients breathing spontaneously
40 to 60% in patients receiving mechanical ventilation

EXAMPLE

Given: $P_a CO_2 = 40 \text{ mm Hg}$
$P_{\bar{E}} CO_2 = 30 \text{ mm Hg}$

Calculate the $\dfrac{V_D}{V_T}$ ratio.

$$
\begin{aligned}
\frac{V_D}{V_T} &= \frac{(P_a CO_2 - P_{\bar{E}} CO_2)}{P_a CO_2} \\[2mm]
&= \frac{40 - 30}{40} \\[2mm]
&= \frac{10}{40} \\[2mm]
&= 0.25 \text{ or } 25\%
\end{aligned}
$$

H   MEAN AIRWAY PRESSURE *(MAWP)*

EQUATION

$$MAWP = \left[\frac{RR \times I\,\text{time}}{60}\right] \times (PIP - PEEP) + PEEP$$

$MAWP$: Mean airway pressure in cm H_2O

RR : Respiratory rate/min

$I\,\text{time}$: Inspiratory time in sec

PIP : Peak inspiratory pressure in cm H_2O

PEEP : Positive end-expiratory pressure in cm H_2O

NORMAL VALUE

Below 30 cm H_2O (adults).

EXAMPLE 1

When PEEP is used.

Given: RR = 45/min

$\quad\quad I\,\text{time}$ = 0.5 sec

$\quad\quad\quad PIP$ = 35 cm H_2O

$\quad\quad$ PEEP = 5 cm H_2O

Calculate the mean airway pressure.

$$MAWP = \left[\frac{RR \times I\,\text{time}}{60}\right] \times (PIP - PEEP) + PEEP$$

$$= \left[\frac{45 \times 0.5}{60}\right] \times (35 - 5) + 5$$

$$= \left[\frac{22.5}{60}\right] \times 30 + 5$$

$$= \{0.375\} \times 30 + 5$$

$$= 11.25 + 5$$

$$= 16.25 \text{ or } 16 \text{ cm } H_2O$$

I   MINUTE VENTILATION: EXPIRED AND ALVEOLAR

EQUATION 1

$$\dot{V}_E = V_T \times RR$$

EQUATION 2

$$\dot{V}_A = (V_T - V_D) \times RR$$

$\dot{V}_E$: Expired minute ventilation in L/min

$\dot{V}_A$: Alveolar minute ventilation in L/min

V_T : Tidal volume in mL
V_D : Deadspace volume in mL
RR : Respiratory rate/min

EXAMPLE

Given: $V_T = 600$ mL
$\qquad V_D = 150$ mL
$\qquad RR = 12$/min

Calculate the expired minute ventilation ($\dot{V}_E$) and the alveolar minute ventilation ($\dot{V}_A$).

$\dot{V}_E = V_T \times RR$
$\quad = 600 \times 12$
$\quad = 7200$ mL/min or 7.2 L/min
$\dot{V}_A = (V_T - V_D) \times RR$
$\quad = (600 - 150) \times 12$
$\quad = 450 \times 12$
$\quad = 5400$ mL/min or 5.4 L/min

J   SHUNT EQUATION ($Q_{sp}/\dot{Q}_T$): CLASSIC PHYSIOLOGIC

EQUATION

$$\frac{Q_{sp}}{\dot{Q}_T} = \frac{C_cO_2 - C_aO_2}{C_cO_2 - C_{\bar{v}}O_2}$$

$Q_{sp}/\dot{Q}_T$: Physiologic shunt to total perfusion ratio in %
$\quad C_cO_2$: End-capillary oxygen content in vol%
$\quad C_aO_2$: Arterial oxygen content in vol%
$\quad C_{\bar{v}}O_2$: Mixed venous oxygen content in vol%

NORMAL VALUE

Less than 10%

EXAMPLE

Given: $C_cO_2 = 20.4$ vol%
$\qquad C_aO_2 = 19.8$ vol%
$\qquad C_{\bar{v}}O_2 = 13.4$ vol%

$$Q_{sp}/\dot{Q}_T = \frac{C_cO_2 - C_aO_2}{C_cO_2 - C_{\bar{v}}O_2}$$

$$= \frac{20.4 - 19.8}{20.4 - 13.4}$$

$$= \frac{0.6}{7}$$

$$= 0.086 \text{ or } 8.6\%$$

K SHUNT EQUATION ($Q_{sp}/\dot{Q}_T$): ESTIMATED

EQUATION 1

For normal individuals:

$$\frac{Q_{sp}}{\dot{Q}_T} = \frac{C_cO_2 - C_aO_2}{5 + (C_cO_2 - C_aO_2)}$$

EQUATION 2

For critically ill patients:

$$\frac{Q_{sp}}{\dot{Q}_T} = \frac{C_cO_2 - C_aO_2}{3.5 + (C_cO_2 - C_aO_2)}$$

$Q_{sp}/\dot{Q}_T$: Physiologic shunt to total perfusion ratio in %
  C_cO_2 : End-capillary oxygen content in vol%
  C_aO_2 : Arterial oxygen content in vol%

NORMAL VALUE

less than 10%

EXAMPLE 1

Given: Normal patient
$C_cO_2 = 20.4$ vol%
$C_aO_2 = 19.8$ vol%
Use 5 vol% as the estimated $C(a - \bar{v})O_2$ and calculate $Q_{sp}/\dot{Q}_T$.

$$\frac{Q_{sp}}{\dot{Q}_T} = \frac{C_cO_2 - C_aO_2}{5 + (C_cO_2 - C_aO_2)}$$

$$= \frac{20.4 - 19.8}{5 + (20.4 - 19.8)}$$

$$= \frac{0.6}{5 + 0.6}$$

$$= \frac{0.6}{5.6}$$

$$= 0.107 \text{ or } 10.7\%$$

L VENTILATOR RATE NEEDED FOR A DESIRED P_aCO_2

EQUATION 1

$$\text{New rate} = \frac{\text{Rate} \times P_aCO_2}{\text{Desired } P_aCO_2}$$

EQUATION 2

$$\text{New rate} = \frac{(\text{Rate} \times P_a CO_2) \times (V_T - V_D)}{\text{Desired } P_a CO_2 \times (\text{New } V_T - \text{New } V_D)}$$

New rate : Ventilator rate needed for a desired $P_a CO_2$
Rate : Original ventilator rate/min
$P_a CO_2$: Original arterial carbon dioxide tension in mm Hg
Desired $P_a CO_2$: Desired arterial carbon dioxide tension in mm Hg
V_T : Original tidal volume
V_D : Original deadspace volume
New V_T : New tidal volume
New V_D : New deadspace volume

NORMAL VALUE

Set rate to provide eucapnic (patient's normal) ventilation.

EXAMPLE 1

When tidal volume and deadspace volume remain unchanged. The $P_a CO_2$ of a patient is 55 mm Hg at a ventilator rate of 10/min. What should be the ventilator rate if a $P_a CO_2$ of 40 mm Hg is desired assuming the ventilator tidal volume and spontaneous ventilation are stable?

$$\text{New rate} = \frac{(\text{Rate} \times P_a CO_2)}{\text{Desired } P_a CO_2}$$

$$= \frac{(10 \times 55)}{40}$$

$$= \frac{550}{40}$$

$$= 13.75 \text{ or } 14/\text{min}$$

M WEANING INDEX: RAPID SHALLOW BREATHING

EQUATION

$$\text{Rapid Shallow Breathing Index} = \frac{f}{V_T}$$

f : Spontaneous respiratory rate/min
V_T : Spontaneous tidal volume (in liter)

NORMAL VALUE

< 100 breaths/min/L is predictive of weaning success

EXAMPLE

Calculate the rapid shallow breathing index given the spontaneous respiratory rate and tidal volume are 14 breaths/min and 0.5 L (500 mL), respectively. Does this index indicate successful weaning outcome?

$$\text{Rapid Shallow Breathing Index} = \frac{f}{V_T}$$

$$= 14/0.5$$
$$= 28 \text{ breaths/min/L}$$

Since the rapid breathing index is less than 100, it indicates a successful weaning outcome.

N   WEANING INDEX: SIMPLIFIED

EQUATION

$$\text{Simplified Weaning Index (SWI)} = \frac{f_{mv}\,(\text{PIP} - \text{PEEP})}{\text{MIP}} \times \frac{\text{PaCO}_{2\,mv}}{40}$$

SWI : Simplified Weaning Index/min
f_{mv} : Ventilator frequency
PIP : Peak inspiratory pressure
PEEP : Positive end-expiratory pressure
MIP : Maximal inspiratory pressure
$\text{PaCO}_{2\,mv}$: Arterial CO_2 tension while on ventilator

NORMAL VALUE

< 9/min. is predictive of weaning success
> 11/min. is predictive of weaning failure

EXAMPLE

Calculate the simplified weaning index given the following parameters and measurements. Does this index indicate a successful weaning outcome?

f_{mv} = 6/min, PIP = 40 cm H_2O, PEEP = 5 cm H_2O, MIP = 20 cm H_2O, $\text{PaCO}_{2\,mv}$ = 50 mm Hg.

$$\text{SWI} = \frac{f_{mv}\,(\text{PIP} - \text{PEEP})}{\text{MIP}} \times \frac{\text{PaCO}_{2\,mv}}{40}$$

$$= \frac{6\,(40 - 5)}{20} \times \frac{50}{40}$$

$$= \frac{6\,(35)}{20} \times 1.25$$

$$= \frac{210}{20} \times 1.25$$

$$= 10.5 \times 1.25$$

$$= 13.1/\text{min}$$

Since the SWI is greater than 11/min., it is predictive of weaning failure.

APPENDIX 2:
DUBOIS BODY SURFACE CHART

DIRECTIONS

To find the body surface of a patient, locate the height in inches (or centimeters) on Scale I and the weight in pounds (or kilograms) on Scale II and place a straight edge (ruler) between these two points which will intersect Scale III at the patient's surface area.

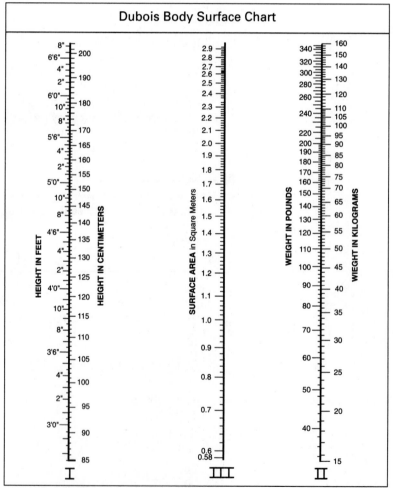

[From E. F. DuBois (1924). Basal metabolism in health and disease. Philadelphia: Lea & Febiger. Used with permission.]

APPENDIX 3:
PRESSURE CONVERSIONS

Pressure Conversions

cm H$_2$O	mm Hg	psig	kPa
1	0.735	0.0142	0.09806
1.36	1	0.0193	0.1333
70.31	51.7	1	6.895
10.197	7.501	0.145	1

EXAMPLES

To convert cm H$_2$O to mm Hg, multiply cm H$_2$O by 0.735. For example, a central venous pressure reading of 9 cm H$_2$O is about 6.6 mm Hg ($9 \times 0.735 = 6.615$).

To convert mm Hg to cm H$_2$O, multiply mm Hg by 1.36. For example, sea-level barometric pressure of 760 mm Hg is about 1034 cm H$_2$O ($760 \times 1.36 = 1033.6$).

To convert psig to mm Hg, multiply psig by 51.7. For example, a piped-in oxygen gas source of 50 psig equals 2585 mm Hg ($50 \times 51.7 = 2585$).

APPENDIX 4:
FRENCH (FR) AND MILLIMETER
(MM) CONVERSIONS

French (Fr) and Millimeter (mm) Conversions

French (Fr)	Millimeter (mm)
(4) mm + 2	1
1	$\dfrac{Fr - 2}{4}$

EXAMPLES

To convert mm to Fr, multiply mm by 4, then add 2. For example, an endotracheal tube with an internal diameter (*ID*) of 2.5 mm equals 12 Fr {(4) 2.5 + 2 = 10 + 2 = 12}.

To convert Fr to mm, subtract 2 from Fr, then divide by 4. For example, an 8-Fr suction catheter equals 1.5 mm $\left(\dfrac{8 - 2}{4} = \dfrac{6}{4} = 1.5 \right)$.

APPENDIX 5:
NORMAL ELECTROLYTE
CONCENTRATIONS IN PLASMA

Normal Electrolyte Concentrations in Plasma

Cations	Concentration (Range) mEq/L	Anions	Concentration (Range) mEq/L
Na^+	140 (138 to 142)	Cl^-	103 (101 to 105)
K^+	4 (3 to 5)	HCO_3^-	25 (23 to 27)
Ca^{++}	5 (4.5 to 5.5)	Protein	16 (14 to 18)
Mg^{++}	2 (1.5 to 2.5)	HPO_4^{2-}, $H_2PO_4^-$	2 (1.5 to 2.5)
		SO_4^{2-}	1 (0.8 to 1.2)
		Organic acids	4 (3.5 to 4.5)
Total	151	Total	151

APPENDIX 6:
OXYGEN TRANSPORT NORMAL RANGES

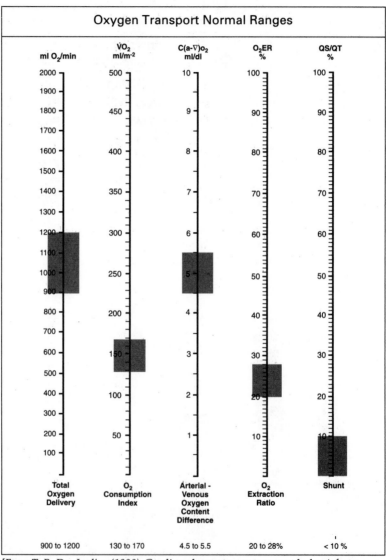

[From T. R. Des Jardins (1998). Cardiopulmonary anatomy and physiology—
Essentials for respiratory care (3rd ed.). Albany, NY: Delmar Publishers, Inc.
Used with permission.]

APPENDIX 7:
HEMODYNAMIC NORMAL RANGES

Hemodynamic Values Directly Obtained by Means of the Pulmonary Artery Catheter

Hemodynamic Value	Abbreviation	Normal Range
Central venous pressure	CVP	1 to 7 mm Hg
Right atrial pressure	RAP	1 to 7 mm Hg
Mean pulmonary artery pressure	PA	15 mm Hg
Pulmonary capillary wedge pressure (also called pulmonary artery wedge; pulmonary artery occlusion)	PCWP PAW PAO	8 to 12 mm Hg
Cardiac output	CO	4 to 8 L/min

[Modified from T. R. Des Jardins (1998). Cardiopulmonary anatomy and physiology—Essentials for respiratory care (3rd ed.). Albany, NY: Delmar Publishers, Inc. Used with permission.]

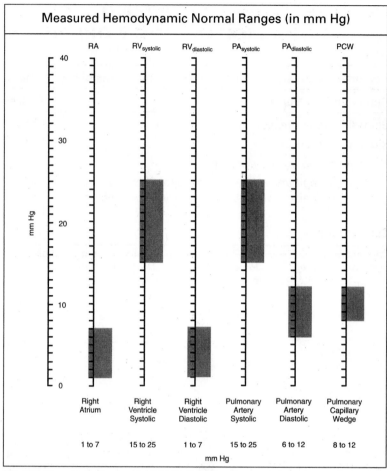

[Modified from T. R. Des Jardins (1998). Cardiopulmonary anatomy and physiology—Essentials for respiratory care (3rd ed.). Albany, NY: Delmar Publishers, Inc. Used with permission.]

Computed Hemodynamic Values

Hemodynamic Variable	Abbreviation	Normal Range
Stroke volume	SV	40 to 80 mL
Stroke volume index	SVI	33 to 47 L/beat/m2
Cardiac index	CI	2.5 to 3.5 L/min/m2
Right ventricular stroke work index	RVSWI	7 to 12 g·m/beat/m2
Left ventricular stroke work index	LVSWI	40 to 60 g·m/beat/m2
Pulmonary vascular resistance	PVR	50 to 150 dyne·sec/cm5
Systemic vascular resistance	SVR	800 to 1500 dyne·sec/cm5

[Modified from T. R. Des Jardins (1998). Cardiopulmonary anatomy and physiology—Essentials for respiratory care (3rd ed.). Albany, NY: Delmar Publishers, Inc. Used with permission.]

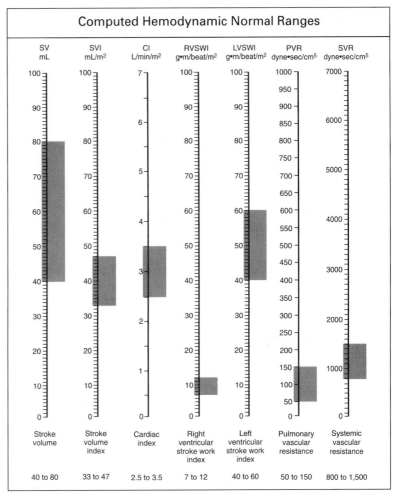

Computed Hemodynamic Normal Ranges

	SV mL	SVI mL/m²	CI L/min/m²	RVSWI g•m/beat/m²	LVSWI g•m/beat/m²	PVR dyne•sec/cm⁵	SVR dyne•sec/cm⁵
	Stroke volume	Stroke volume index	Cardiac index	Right ventricular stroke work index	Left ventricular stroke work index	Pulmonary vascular resistance	Systemic vascular resistance
	40 to 80	33 to 47	2.5 to 3.5	7 to 12	40 to 60	50 to 150	800 to 1,500

[*Modified from T. R. Des Jardins (1998).* Cardiopulmonary anatomy and physiology—Essentials for respiratory care *(3rd ed.). Albany, NY: Delmar Publishers, Inc. Used with permission.*]

INDEX